# Therapies for
# Viral Hepatitis

# Therapies for
# **Viral Hepatitis**

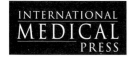
INTERNATIONAL
MEDICAL
PRESS

Edited by    **Raymond F Schinazi**
**Jean-Pierre Sommadossi**
**Howard C Thomas**

**International Medical Press**

125 High Holborn, London, WC1V 6QA, UK

2989 Piedmont Road, Atlanta, GA 30305, USA

International Medical Press • London • Atlanta
Manchester • Munich • Rome • Singapore • Sydney

**British Library Cataloguing in Publication Data**
A catalogue record for this book is available from the British Library

ISBN 1-901769-01-1

Printed and bound in the UK by The Bath Press

# CONTENTS

# SECTION VII: CLINICAL AND THERAPEUTIC STRATEGIES

## PART A: THE IMMUNOCOMPETENT INDIVIDUAL

## PART B: TRANSPLANT PATIENTS

## PART C: COINFECTIONS

## PART D: HEPATOCELLULAR CARCINOMA

# PREFACE

Viral hepatitis is one of the most common infectious diseases in the world and represents one of the decade's most significant public health challenges. It is estimated that more than 2 billion people worldwide have evidence of past or current hepatitis B virus (HBV) infection, and that 350 million are chronic carriers. This is put into perspective by a recent World Health Organization report, which indicates that HBV is the ninth leading cause of mortality in the world today, accounting for over 1.1 million deaths in 1996. Hepatitis C virus (HCV) is also widespread: approximately 3% of the world's population is infected with this virus and there may be more than 170 million chronic carriers. In addition, about one-third of individuals infected with human immunodeficiency virus (HIV) are coinfected with either HBV, HCV or both viruses.

Chronic infection with HBV and HCV has a major impact on health. Global statistics indicate that one-quarter of all chronic HBV carriers die from chronic active hepatitis, cirrhosis or primary liver cancer, and that this infection is responsible for 60–80% of the world's primary liver cancer. It is estimated that approximately 20% of chronically HCV-infected patients will develop cirrhosis, and that a further 1–5% will develop liver cancer over the next decade. Chronic infection with HBV or HCV is one of the major risk factors in the development of hepatocellular carcinoma (HCC); most patients who have HCC in the absence of HBV infection usually have evidence of HCV infection. The situation is confounded further in coinfected patients, as it is not yet clear if their response to therapy will be similar to that obtained in patients infected with either virus alone.

Current therapies for viral hepatitis remain unsatisfactory. Less than 25% of HCV-infected patients respond to FDA-approved therapies with long-term remission of liver disease. Why interferon α (IFN-α) and other antiviral agents induce viral clearance and improve liver disease in only a subpopulation of HBV-infected patients is not known. Their lack of utility in a high proportion of patients with HCV is also unexplained. Thus, the mechanism(s) by which infection with these viruses leads to liver injury and the factors determining the course and outcome of chronic infection, including therapy with antiviral agents, requires elucidation.

The challenges posed by viral hepatitis have prompted intense interdisciplinary research, particularly in the area of novel therapeutic agents and virally encoded targets, such as the HCV helicase, polymerase and serine protease. This book focuses on the latest advances in the search for new, more effective therapeutic options and also covers related topics. These include epidemiology and natural history; emerging viruses; viral diagnosis; the interaction between hepatitis B and C and the host immune system, and how this provides clues to disease pathogenesis; differences between the immunological responses associated with clearance of infection versus the chronic carrier state; drug discovery and clinical strategies; animal models, including an HBV transgenic mouse model and two new HCV mouse models; quasispecies; viral dynamics; extra-hepatic sites for viral replication; surrogate markers; drug resistance; transplantation; end-stage liver disease; hepatocellular carcinoma; and viral coinfections.

Therapeutic antiviral options aim to completely eliminate viral replication or to reduce viral burden to a level where the immune system can take over. The treatment options for HCV are widening, and include IFN, IFN in combination with ribavirin, aggressive IFN dosing regimens and novel antiviral drugs. For HBV, significant progress has been made with the development of lamivudine and famciclovir, although resistance can occur. HBV and HCV are characterized by high levels of replication and turnover, leading to a high incidence of resistant viruses and chronic progressive disease. The need to develop additional therapies and combined modalities that completely inhibit viral replication and the development of resistance is essential.

The breadth and scope of the data presented in this book provides insight into the most appropriate treatment approaches. Advances in our understanding of the molecular biology, immunology and pathogenesis of hepatitis viruses are increasing at a rapid pace. It is therefore particularly timely to attempt to bring together this burgeoning information in a book that deals with various aspects related to therapies for viral hepatitis and to provide an environment for an interdisciplinary dialogue. *Therapies for Viral Hepatitis* represents the synthesis of the latest research on this important group of viruses, which produce so much morbidity and mortality worldwide.

*Raymond F Schinazi*
*Jean-Pierre Sommadossi*
*and Howard C Thomas*

# ACKNOWLEDGEMENTS

We thank the authors of individual chapters for their contributions. We also express our thanks to Amy Juodawlkis and Janis Wright, and to the staff at International Medical Press, particularly Shaun Griffin, for assisting with the production of this book.

This book is dedicated to the memory of Felix S Schinazi, Piero Sommadossi, and to all those in the world who are suffering from, or who have suffered from, the physical, mental or social effects of viral diseases and associated cancers.

# BIOGRAPHIES

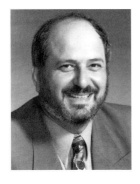 **Raymond F Schinazi** is Professor of Pediatrics and Chemistry and Director of the Laboratory of Biochemical Pharmacology at Emory University. He serves as the Senior Research Career Scientist and Scientific Director at the Georgia Research Center on AIDS and HIV Infections.

In 1976, Professor Schinazi received his PhD in chemistry from the University of Bath in England. He secured a postdoctoral position in pharmacology at Yale University with William Prusoff later that year. Between 1978 and 1980, Professor Schinazi was a postdoctoral fellow in infectious disease and immunology at Emory University. Professor Schinazi joined the Department of Pediatrics faculty at the Emory University School of Medicine in 1981. He has served on study sessions for the NIH and various other funding agencies, and is currently on the editorial board of five journals dealing with anti-infective agents – *Antimicrobial Agents and Chemotherapy, Antiviral Research, Antiviral Chemistry and Chemotherapy, Antiviral Therapy* and *International Antiviral News*. In 1996, Professor Schinazi was nominated and served on the Presidential Commission on AIDS. He has focused his research on the discovery of novel antiviral agents and the development of combined modalities to combat drug resistance.

Professor Schinazi has been involved in the discovery and development of many anti-HIV and anti-HBV compounds including lamivuudine, (–)-FTC, DXG, DAPD, FDOC, D-D4FC, stavudine, CS-87, CS-92, water-soluble buckyballs, porphyrins and polyoxometalates. His group continues to be interested in drug resistance associated with antiviral agents directed against HIV, HBV, herpesviruses and CMV. He is the founder and organizer of the Hawaii International Conference on Therapies for Viral Hepatitis.

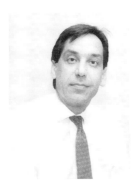 **Jean-Pierre Sommadossi** is Professor of Clinical Pharmacology and Associate Director, Liver Centre, University of Alabama at Birmingham.

He received his PhD in pharmacology in 1984 from the University of Marseilles in France. In 1985, after a postdoctoral fellowship at the Medical College of Virginia in Richmond, he was appointed Assistant Professor at the University of Alabama at Birmingham; he was made a full Professor in 1992.

Professor Sommadossi's research into the development of nucleoside analogues for the treatment of AIDS and hepatitis has led to a better understanding of the molecular pharmacology of these drugs and to the elucidation of their full mechanisms of action and toxicity, including the detailed molecular mechanism(s) involved in the lethal toxicity of FIAU observed in HBV-infected patients. Using *in vitro* and cell-based assays, his work has led to the discovery of novel inhibitors of HBV replication. Professor Sommadossi's work on antiviral drug development has attracted national and international attention, and he has given over 70 major presentations as an invited speaker during the past 5 years.

Professor Sommadossi is a former member of the AIDS Experimental Therapeutics Study Section, and serves on the editorial boards of *Antimicrobial Agents and Chemotherapy, Antiviral Research, Antiviral Chemistry and Chemotherapy* and *International Antiviral News;* he is also Section Editor for Hepatitis on *Antiviral Therapy.* Professor Sommadossi is co-founder of the Hawaii International Conference on Therapies for Viral Hepatitis. He has published more than 130 papers, most of which are related to the biochemistry, and molecular and clinical pharmacology of antiviral agents.

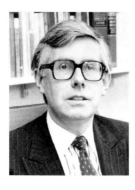 **Howard C Thomas** is Professor of Medicine at Imperial College School of Medicine and Head of the Department of Medicine A. He is a Consultant Hepatologist and General Physician at St Mary's Hospital in London, where he directs a research group studying the pathogenesis and therapy of chronic viral hepatitis.

Professor Thomas graduated in medicine in 1968 from Newcastle University and obtained his PhD from Glasgow University. As a lecturer in immunology, he described the induction of tolerance by the oral administration of protein antigens. In 1982 he started a programme of research on the pathogenesis and therapy of chronic hepatitis B at the Royal Free Hospital in London, and in 1986 was appointed to a Personal Chair of Medicine at London University. In 1987 he became Chair of Medicine at St Mary's School of Medicine.

His group subsequently described the HBe antigen-negative variant of HBV and the vaccine-escape variant. In 1995, working with Genelabs, his group contributed to the discovery of HGV. He was the first recipient of the Hans Popper Award for Hepatology and the Research Medal of the British Society of Gastroenterology. He is currently President of the British and European Societies for the Study of the Liver. Professor Thomas has over 350 publications and is the Editor of the *Journal of Viral Hepatitis.*

# CONTRIBUTORS

**Tsuyoshi Adachi**
Japan Tobacco, Osaka, Japan; and Center for Tsukuba Advanced Research Alliance, University of Tsukuba, Tsukuba, Japan

**Eugene V Agapov, MD, PhD**
Department of Molecular Microbiology, Box 8230, Washington University School of Medicine, 660 South Euclid Avenue, St Louis, MO 63110-1093, USA

**Alfredo Alberti, MD**
Department of Clinical and Experimental Medicine, University of Padova, Via Giustiniani, 2 35128 Padova, Italy

**Harvey Alter, MD**
Infectious Diseases Section and Department of Transfusion Medicine, National Institutes of Health, Bethesda, MD 20892, USA

**Miriam J Alter, PhD**
Hepatitis Branch, Centers for Disease Control and Prevention, 1600 Clifton Road, Atlanta, GA 30333, USA

**Cosme Alvarado-Esquivel, MD, PhD**
Instituto de Investigación Científica/Facultad de Medicina, Universidad Juarez del Estado de Durango, Avenida Universidad y Fanny Anitua, 34000 Durango, Dgo, México

**Antonio Ascione, MD**
Primario Fisiopatologia Epatica-Unitá Pancreas, Ospedale Cardarelli, via Caravaggio 89, 80126 Napoli, Italy

**Silvia Astretto, MD**
Ricertore Fisiopatologia Epatica-Unitá Pancreas, Ospedale Cardarelli, via Caravaggio 89, 80126 Napoli, Italy

**Mohammed A Attia, PhD**
Virology and Immunology Unit, National Cancer Institute, Cairo University, Fom El-Khalig, Kasr El-Aini Str., Cairo 11441, Egypt

**Betty H Baldwin, MS**
Department of Clinical Sciences, College of Veterinary Medicine, Cornell University, C2 005 Veterinary Medical Center, Ithaca, NY 14853, USA

**Angeline Bartholomeusz, PhD**
Victorian Infectious Diseases Reference Laboratory, 10 Wreckyn Street, North Melbourne, Victoria 3051, Australia

**Luisa Benvegnù, MD**
Department of Clinical and Experimental Medicine, University of Padova, Via Giustiniani, 2 35128 Padova, Italy

**Marina Berenguer, MD**
Veteran's Administration Medical Center, GI Section, 111B, 4150 Clement Street, San Francisco, CA 94121, USA

**Keril J Blight, PhD**
Department of Molecular Microbiology, Box 8230, Washington University School of Medicine, 660 South Euclid Avenue, St Louis, MO 63110-1093, USA

**Baruch S Blumberg**
Fox Chase Cancer Center, 7701 Burholme Avenue, Philadelphia, PA 19111, USA

**F Douglas Boudinot, PhD**
Center for Drug Discovery, Department of Pharmaceutical and Biomedical Sciences, The University of Georgia College of Pharmacy, Athens, GA 30602, USA

**Jens Bukh**
Hepatitis Viruses Section, Laboratory of Infectious Diseases, National Institutes of Allergy and Infectious Diseases, Building 7, Room 201, 7 Center Drive, MSC 0740, Bethesda, MD 20892-0740, USA

**Nigel J Burroughs, MA, PhD**
Mathematics Institute, University of Warwick, Coventry, CV4 7AL, UK

**Carmine Canestrini, MD**
Ricercatore, Fisiopatologia Epatica, Ospedale Cardarelli, via Caravaggio 89, 80126 Napoli, Italy

**Nicola Caporaso, MD**
Dipartimento di Scienze degli Alimenti, Università Federico II, Napoli, Italy

**Flair José Carrilho, MD, PhD**
Clinical Hepatology Branch, Department of Gastroenterology, University of São Paulo School of Medicine, Rua Silva Correia, 153, 41, 04537-040-São Paulo SP, Brazil

**Eduardo Carrillo-Maravilla, MD**
Centro Nacional de la Transfusión Sanguinea, Secretaria de Salud, Goya 35, 03920 Mexico, DF México

**John L Casey, PhD**
Division of Molecular Virology and Immunology, Georgetown University Medical Center, 5640 Fishers Lane, Rockville, MD 20852, USA

**Liliana Chemello, MA**
Department of Clinical and Experimental Medicine, University of Padova, Via Giustiniani, 2 35128 Padova, Italy

**Yung-Chi Cheng**
Yale University School of Medicine, New Haven, CT 016510, USA

**Yongseok Choi**
Center for Drug Discovery, Department of Pharmaceutical and Biomedical Sciences, The University of Georgia College of Pharmacy, Athens, GA 30602, USA

**Chung K Chu**
Center for Drug Discovery, Department of Pharmaceutical and Biomedical Sciences, The University of Georgia College of Pharmacy, Athens, GA 30602, USA

**Danni Colledge, B App Sci (Med Lab Sci)**
Victorian Infectious Diseases Reference Laboratory, 10 Wreckyn Street, North Melbourne, Victoria 3051, Sydney, Australia.

**Lynn D Condreay, PhD**
Glaxo Wellcome, Inc., Research Triangle Park, North Carolina, USA

**David A Cooper, MD, DSc**
National Centre in HIV Epidemiology and Clinical Research, University of New South Wales, Sydney, Australia

**Paul J Cote, PhD**
Division of Molecular Virology and Immunology, Georgetown University School of Medicine, 5640 Fishers Lane, Rockville, MD 20852, USA

**Erika Cretton-Scott, PhD**
Department of Clinical Pharmacology and The Liver Center, University of Alabama at Birmingham, Birmingham, AL 35294, USA

**Caemelo D'Asero, MD**
Primario Laboratorio di ricerca, Ospedale S. Pietro, Fatebenefratelli, Roma, Italy

**Shlomo Dagan, PhD**
XTL Biopharmaceuticals, Kiryat Weizmann, PO Box 370, Rehovot 76100, Israel

**Eleanor Dagostino**
Agouron Pharmaceuticals, 3565 General Atomics Court, San Diego, CA 92121, USA

**Beverly Dale, PhD**
Roche Molecular Systems, 1145 Atlantic Avenue, Alameda, CA 94501, USA

**Raffaele De Francesco, PhD**
Department of Biochemistry, Istituto di Ricerche di Biologia Molecolare 'P Angeletti', Via Pontina Km 30 2 600, I-00040 Pomezia, Rome, Italy

**Sija De Gendt**
Innogenetics NV, Industriepark Zwijnaarde 7, Box 4, B-9052 Gent, Belgium

**Massismo De Luca, MD**
Ricercatore Fisiopatologia Epatica, Ospedale Cardarelli, via Caravaggio 89, 80126 Napoli, Italy

**Xin-qing Deng**
Department of Epidemiology, School of Public Health, Shanghai Medical University, Shanghai, China

**Ding Ding**
Department of Epidemiology, School of Public Health, Shanghai Medical University, Shanghai, China

**Gerald Eder, MD, PhD**
Hans Popper Primate Center, Orth an der Donau, Austria

**Elwyn Elias, MD, FRCP**
Liver and Hepatobiliary Unit, Queen Elizabeth Hospital, Birmingham B15 2TH, UK

**Francesca Froio, MD**
Aiuto Laboratorio di Ricerca Ospedale S. Pietro Fatebenefratelli, Roma, Italy

**Kirk E Fry**
Genelabs Technologies, 505 Penobscot Drive, Redwood City, CA 94063, USA

**Phillip A Furman, PhD**
Triangle Pharmaceuticals, 4 University Place, 4611 University Drive, Durham, NC 27707, USA

**Alfonso Galeota Lanza, MD**
Ricercatore Fisiopatologia Epatica, Ospedale Cardarelli, via Caravaggio 89, 80126 Napoli, Italy

**J David Gangemi, PhD**
Greenville Hospital System/Clemson University, Clemson, South Carolina, USA

**John L Gerin, PhD**
Division of Molecular Virology and Immunology, Georgetown University School of Medicine, 5640 Fishers Lane, Rockville, MD 20852, USA

**Martina Gerotto, PhD**
Department of Clinical and Experimental Medicine, University of Padova, Via Giustiniani, 2 35128 Padova, Italy

**Gilles Gosselin, PhD**
Laboratoire de Chimie Bioorganiqu4e, UMR CNRS 5625, Case Courrier 008, Université Montpellier II, Sciences et Techniques du Languedoc, Place Eugène Bataillon, 34095 Montpellier, Cedex 5, France

**David R Gretch, MD, PhD**
Department of Laboratory Medicine, University of Washington Medical Center, Seattle, WA 98144, USA

**Karen Gutekunst, PhD**
Roche Molecular Systems, 4300 Hancienda Drive PO Box 9002, Pleasanton, CA 94566, USA

**Noriyuki Habuka**
Japan Tobacco, Osaka, Japan; and Center for Tsukuba Advanced Research Alliance, University of Tsukuba, Tsukuba, Japan

**Rodolfo Herrera-Luna**
Coordinación de Salud Comunitaria, Instituto Mexicano del Seguro Social, Insurgentes 253 Sur, 06700 Mexico, DF México

**Flor de Maria Herrera-Ortiz, MD**
Centro Nacional de la Transfusión Sanguinea, Secretaria de
Salud, Goya 35, 03920 Mexico, DF México

**Makoto Hijikata, PhD**
Institute for Virus Research, Kyoto University, Sakyo-ku,
Kyoto 606-8507, Japan

**Masami Hirota**
Institute for Virus Research, Kyoto University, Sakyo-ku,
Kyoto 606-8507, Japan

**Joon H Hong**
Center for Drug Discovery, Department of Pharmaceutical
and Biomedical Sciences, The University of Georgia College
of Pharmacy, Athens, GA 30602, USA

**William E Hornbuckle, DVM**
Department of Clinical Sciences, College of Veterinary
Medicine, Cornell University, C2 005 Veterinary Medical
Center, Ithaca, NY 14853, USA

**Zuzana Hostomska, PhD**
Agouron Pharmacuticals, 3565 General Atomics Court,
San Diego, CA 92121, USA

**Zdenek Hostomsky**
Agouron Pharmacuticals, 3565 General Atomics Court,
San Diego, CA 92121, USA

**Shiro Iino, MD**
Department of Medicine and Laboratory Medicine,
St Marianna University School of Medicine, Kawasaki,
216-8511 Japan

**Ehud Ilan, PhD**
XTL Biopharmaceuticals, Kiryat Weizmann,
PO Box 370, Rehovot 76100, Israel

**Jean-Louis Imbach, PhD**
Laboratoire de Chimie Bioorganique, UMR
CNRS 5625, Case Courrier 008, Université Montpellier II,
Sciences et Techniques du Languedoc, Place Eugène Bataillon,
34095 Montpellier, Cedex 5, France

**Michiharu Inudoh, MD**
Virology Division, National Cancer Center Research Institute,
Chuo-ku, Tokyo 104-0045, Japan

**Gilbert Jay, PhD, DSc**
Laboratory of Virology, The Jerome H Holland Laboratory,
15601 Crabbs Branch Way, Rockville, MD 20855, USA

**Naoya Kato, MD**
Second Department of Internal Medicine, Faculty
of Medicine, University of Tokyo, 7-3-1 Hongo, Bunkyo-ku,
Tokyo 113-8655, Japan

**Nobuyuki Kato, PhD**
Virology Division, National Cancer Center Research Institute,
Chuo-ku, Tokyo 104-0045, Japan

**Ronald C Kennedy, PhD**
Department of Microbiology and Immunology, University of
Oklahoma Health Sciences Center, Oklahoma City, OK 73190,
USA

**Jungsuh Kim, PhD**
Genelabs Technologies, 505 Penobscot Drive, Redwood City,
CA 94063, USA

**Alexander A Kolykhalov, PhD**
Department of Molecular Microbiology,
Box 8230, Washington University School of Medicine, 660
South Euclid Avenue, St Louis, MO 63110-1093, USA

**Brent E Korba, PhD**
Division of Molecular Virology and Immunology,
Georgetown University School of Medicine, 5640 Fishers
Lane, Rockville, MD 20852, USA

**Margaret James Koziel, MD**
Infectious Disease Laboratory, Harvard Institute of Medicine,
Beth Israel Deaconness Medical Center, 1 Deaconness Road,
Boston, MA 02215, USA

**Martin Krüger, MD**
Department of Gastroenterology and Hepatology,
Medizinische Hochschule Hannover, D-30623 Hannover,
Germany

**Keng-Hsin Lan, MD**
Second Department of Internal Medicine, Faculty of Medicine,
University of Tokyo, 7-3-1 Hongo, Bunkyo-ku, Tokyo 113-
8655, Japan

**Johnson YN Lau, MD**
Schering–Plough Research Institute, 2015 Galloping Hill
Road, Kenilworth, NJ 07033-0539, USA

**Jia-Yee Lee, PhD**
Victorian Infectious Diseases Reference Laboratory, 10
Wreckyn Street, North Melbourne, Victoria 3051, Australia

**Ximin Lin**
Department of Epidemiology, School of Public Health,
Shanghai Medical University, Shanghai, China

**Margaret Littlejohn, PhD**
Victorian Infectious Diseases Reference Laboratory, 10 Wreckyn
Street, North Melbourne, Victoria 3051, Australia

**Samuel Litwin, PhD**
Fox Chase Center, 7701 Burholme Avenue, Philadelphia, PA
19111, USA

**Stephen Locarnini, PhD, MBBS, MRC (Path)**
Victorian Infectious Diseases Reference Laboratory, 10 Wreckyn
Street, North Melbourne, Victoria 3051, Australia

**Gábor Lotz**
1st Institute of Pathology and Experimental Cancer Research,
Semmelweis Medical University, Budapest Üllöl út 26,
H-1085 Hungary

**Robert A Love, PhD**
Agouron Pharmacuticals, 3565 General Atomics Court, San Diego, CA 92121, USA

**Geert Maertens, PhD**
Department of Molecular Biology Innogenetics NV, Industriepark Zwijnaarde 7, Box 4, B-9052 Gent, Belgium

**Richard T Mahoney**
International Vaccine Institute, Seoul National University Campus, Shillim-Dong, Kwanak-Ku, Seoul, Korea 151-742

**Michael P Manns**
Department of Gastroenterology and Hepatology, Medizinische Hochschule Hannover, D-30623 Hannover, Germany

**Steve Margosiak**
Agouron Pharmacuticals, 3565 General Atomics Court, San Diego, CA 92121, USA

**William S Mason, PhD**
Fox Chase Cancer Center, 7701 Burholme Avenue, Philadelphia, PA 19111, USA

**Maria Cássia Jacintho Mendes Corrêa, MD**
Division of Infectious and Parasitic Diseases, Hospital das Clínicas, University of São Paulo - School of Medicine, Rua Caetés 855, 51, 05016-081 São Paulo SP, Brazil

**Ellen W Moomaw**
Agouron Pharmacuticals, 3565 General Atomics Court, San Diego, CA 92121, USA

**María del Carmen Morales-Macedo**
Centro Nacional de la Transfusión Sanguinea, Secretaria de Salud, Goya 35, 03920 Mexico, DF México

**Filomena Morisco, MD**
Dipartimento di Internistica Clinica e Sperimentale, Seconda Università Frederico II, Napoli, Italy

**John D Morrey, PhD**
Institute for Antiviral Research, Utah State University, Logan, UT 84322-5600, USA

**Joseph Moussali**
Service d'Hépato-Gastroentérologie Groupe Hospitalier Pitié-Salpêtrière, URA CNRS 1484, University Paris VI, Paris, France

**David Mutimer, MD, FRACP**
Liver and Hepatobiliary Unit, Queen Elizabeth Hospital, Birmingham B15 2TH, UK

**David R Nelson, MD**
Section of Hepatobiliary Diseases, Division of Gastroenterology, Hepatology and Nutrition, Department of Medicine, University of Florida, Gainesville, Florida, USA

**Fred Nunes, MD**
University of Pennsylvania, Philadelphia, PA 19104, USA

**Masao Omata, MD**
Second Department of Internal Medicine, Faculty of Medicine, University of Tokyo, 7-3-1 Hongo, Bunkyo-ku, Tokyo 113-8655, Japan

**Suzane Kioko Ono-Nita, MD**
Second Department of Internal Medicine, Faculty of Medicine, University of Tokyo, 7-3-1 Hongo, Bunkyo-ku, Tokyo 113-8655, Japan

**Pierre Opolon**
Service d'Hépato-Gastroentérologie Groupe Hospitalier Pitié-Salpêtrière, URA CNRS 1484, University Paris VI, Paris, France

**Hans E Parge**
Agouron Pharmaceuticals, 3565 General Atomics Court, San Diego, CA 92121, USA

**Jean-Michel Pawlotsky, MD, PhD**
Department of Bacteriology and Virology and INSERM U99, Hôpital Henri Mondor, Université Paris XII, 51 Avenue du Maréchal de Lattre de Tassigny, 94010 Creteil, France

**Simon F Peek, BVSc, DACVIM, MRCVS**
Department of Clinical Sciences, College of Veterinary Medicine, Cornell University, C2 005 Veterinary Medical Center, Ithaca, NY 14853, USA

**Christian Périgaud, PhD**
Laboratoire de Chimie Bioorganiqu4e, UMR CNRS 5625, Case Courrier 008, Université Montpellier II, Sciences et Techniques du Languedoc, Place Eugène Bataillon, 34095 Montpellier, Cedex 5, France

**Antonello Pessi, PhD**
Department of Biochemistry, Istituto di Ricerche di Biologia Molecolare 'P Angeletti', Via Pontina Km 30 2 600, I-00040 Pomezia, Rome, Italy

**Piero Piergrossi**
Laboratorio di ricerca, Ospedale S. Pietro Fatebenefratelli, Roma, Italy

**Deenan Pillay, PhD, MBBS, MRCPath**
PHLS Antiviral Susceptibility Reference Unit, Department of Infection, Birmingham University, Birmingham B15 2TH, UK

**Patrizia Pontisso, MD**
Department of Clinical and Experimental Medicine, University of Padova, Via Giustiniani, 2 35128 Padova, Italy

**Thierry Poynard**
Service d'Hépato-Gastroentérologie Groupe Hospitalier Pitié-Salpêtrière, 47–83 Boulevard de l'Hôpital, 75651 Paris Cedex 13, France

**Robert H Purcell**
Hepatitis Viruses Section, Laboratory of Infectious Diseases, National Institutes of Allergy and Infectious Diseases, Building 7, Room 201, 7 Center Drive, MSC 0740, Bethesda, MD 20892-0740, USA

David A Rand, PhD
Mathematics Institute, University of Warwick, Coventry
CV4 7AL, UK

Karen E Reed
Department of Molecular Microbiology, Box 8230,
Washington University School of Medicine, 660 South Euclid
Avenue, St Louis, MO 63110-1093, USA

Charles M Rice, PhD
Department of Molecular Microbiology, Box 8230,
Washington University School of Medicine, 660 South Euclid
Avenue, St Louis, MO 63110-1093, USA

Annelies Rombout
Innogenetics NV, Industriepark Zwijnaarde 7, Box 4, B-9052
Gent, Belgium

Rudi Rossau
Innogenetics NV, Industriepark Zwijnaarde 7, Box 4, B-9052
Gent, Belgium

Maurice Rosenstraus
Roche Molecular Systems, 1080 Route 202, Branchburg,
NJ 08876, USA

Rosario Ruiz-Astorga
Instituto de Investigación Científica/Facultad de Medicina,
Universidad Juarez del Estado de Durango, Avenida
Universidad y Fanny Anitua, 34000 Durango, Dgo, México

Lilia Ruiz-Maya
Coordinación de Salud Comunitaria, Instituto Mexicano del
Seguro Social, Insurgentes 253 Sur, 06700 Mexico, DF México

Shinya Satoh
Institute for Virus Research, Kyoto University, Sakyo-ku,
Kyoto 606-8507, Japan

Zsuzsa Schaff, MD, PhD
1st Institute of Pathology and Experimental Cancer Research,
Semmelweis Medical University, Budapest Üllöl út 26,
H-1085 Hungary

Raymond F Schinazi, PhD
Laboratory of Biochemical Pharmacology, Department of
Paediatrics, Emory University School of Medicine, Atlanta,
GA 30322, USA, and Veterans Affairs Medical Center,
Decatur, GA 30033, USA

Rolf Schulte-Hermann, MD, PhD
Institute of Cancer Research/Tumorbiology, University of
Vienna, 1090 Vienna, Austria.

Craig Shapiro, MD
Hepatitis Branch, Centers for Disease Control and Prevention,
1600 Clifton Road, Atlanta, GA 30333, USA

Michael H Shearer
Department of Microbiology and Immunology, University of
Oklahoma Health Sciences Center, Oklahoma City, OK
73190, USA

Kenneth E Sherman, MD, PhD
Hepatology and Liver Transplant Medicine, University of
Cincinnati School of Medicine, PO Box 670595, Cincinnati,
OH 45267, USA

Susan N Sherman, DPA
‰ Hepatology and Liver Transplant Medicine, University of
Cincinnati School of Medicine, PO Box 670595, Cincinnati,
OH 45267, USA

Kunitada Shimotohno, PhD
Institute for Virus Research, Kyoto University, Shogo-in,
Sakyo-ku, Kyoto 606-8507, Japan

Yasushi Shiratori, MD
Second Department of Internal Medicine, Faculty
of Medicine, University of Tokyo, 7-3-1 Hongo, Bunkyo-ku,
Tokyo 113-8655, Japan

Robert W Sidwell
Institute for Antiviral Research, Utah State University, Logan,
UT 84322-5600, USA

Jean-Pierre Sommadossi, PharmD, PhD
Department of Clinical Pharmacology and The Liver Center,
University of Alabama at Birmingham, Birmingham, AL
35294, USA

John R Stanley, MD
Department of Obstetrics and Gynecology, University of
Oklahoma Health Sciences Center, Oklahoma City, OK
73190, USA

Christian Steinkühler, PhD
Department of Biochemistry, Istituto di Ricerche di Biologia
Molecolare 'P Angeletti', Via Pontina Km 30 2 600, I-00040
Pomezia, Rome, Italy

Lieven Stuyver, PhD
Department of Nucleic Acid Chemistry, Innogenetics NV,
Industriepark Zwijnaarde 7, Box 4, B-9052 Gent, Belgium

Jesse Summers, PhD
University of New Mexico Cancer Center, University of New
Mexico, Albuquerque, NM 87131, USA

Bud C Tennant, DVM, MD
Department of Clinical Sciences, College of Veterinary Medicine,
Cornell University, T6023 VRT, Ithaca, NY 14853, USA

Thierry Thevenot
Service d'Hépato-Gastroentérologie Groupe Hospitalier Pitié-
Salpêtrière, URA CNRS 1484, University Paris VI, Paris, France

Howard C Thomas, PhD, FRCP, FRCPath
Hepatology Section, Department of Medicine A, Imperial
College School of Medicine, London, UK

Illia A Tochkov, MD, PhD
Department of Clinical Sciences, College of Veterinary
Medicine, Cornell University, C2 005 Veterinary Medical
Center, Ithaca, NY 14853, USA

Christian Trepo, MD
INSERM unit 271, 151 Cours Albert Thomas, 69003 Lyon,
France

Concetta Tuccillo, MD
Dipartimento di Internistica, Clinica e Sperimentale,
Università Frederico II, Napoli, Italy

D Lorne J Tyrrell, PhD, MD, FRCPC
Faculty of Medicine and Oral Health Sciences, 606 HMRC,
Univesity of Alberta, Edmonton, Alberta T6G 2S2 Canada

Hiroyuki Ueda, MD
Department of OB/GYN, Niigata University School of
Medicine, 1-757 Asahimachi-dori, Niigata, Japan

Caroline Van Geyt
Innogenetics NV, Industriepark Zwijnaarde 7,
Box 4, B-9052 Gent, Belgium

John Wages Jr
Genelabs Technologies, 505 Penobscot Drive, Redwood City,
CA 94063, USA

Allison M Watts
Department of Microbiology and Immunology, University of
Oklahoma Health Sciences Center, Oklahoma City, OK
73190, USA

Patricia Weber, PhD
Schering-Plough Research Institute, 2015 Galloping Hill Road,
K15-3-3855, Kenilworth, NJ 07033-0539, USA

John A Wickersham
Agouron Pharmacuticals, 3565 General Atomics Court,
San Diego, CA 92121, USA

Judith C Wilber, PhD
Nucleic Acid Diagnostics, Chiron Corporation,
4560 Horton Street, Emeryville, CA 94608, USA

Winnie WS Wong
Department of Medicine, 606 HMRC, Univesity of Alberta,
Edmonton, Alberta T6G 2B7, Canada

Teresa L Wright, MD
Veteran's Administration Medical Center, GI Section, 111B,
4150 Clement Street, San Francisco, CA 94121, USA

Ann Wyseur
Department of Nucleic Acid Chemistry, Innogenetics NV,
Industriepark Zwijnaarde 7, Box 4, B-9052 Gent, Belgium

Jie Xu
Department of Epidemiology, School of Public Health,
Shanghai Medical University, Shanghai, China

Zhi-Yi Xu
International Vaccine Institute, Seoul National University
Campus, Shillim-Dong, Kwanak-Ku, Seoul, Korea 151-742

Nanhua Yao, PhD
Schering-Plough Research Institute, 2015 Galloping Hill
Road, K15-3-3855, Kenilworth, NJ 07033-0539, USA

Hideo Yoshida, MD
Second Department of Internal Medicine, Faculty
of Medicine, University of Tokyo, 7-3-1 Hongo, Bunkyo-ku,
Tokyo 113-8655, Japan

Angel Zarate-Aguilar, MD
Coordinación de Salud Comunitaria, Instituto Mexicano del
Seguro Social, Insurgentes 253 Sur, 06700 Mexico, DF México

Shou-jun Zhao
Department of Epidemiology, School of Public Health,
Shanghai Medical University, Shanghai, China

Tianlun Zhou, MD
Fox Chase Cancer Center, 7701 Burholme Avenue,
Philadelphia, PA 19111, USA

Fabien Zoulim, MD, PhD
INSERM Unit 271, 151 Cours Albert Thomas, 69003 Lyon,
France

# Section I

---

## EPIDEMIOLOGY AND
## NATURAL HISTORY

# 1

# Epidemiology and prevention of chronic hepatitis B and C in North and South America

## Miriam J Alter and Craig N Shapiro*

## SUMMARY

Hepatitis B and C viruses are major causes of both acute and chronic liver disease. Prevention of hepatitis B is possible with the use of hepatitis B vaccine. Vaccination of infants is recommended for all countries. Additional programmes for the elimination of hepatitis B virus transmission include prenatal screening for hepatitis B virus infection, prophylaxis of infants born to infected women, vaccination of adolescents and vaccination of children and adults at high risk. The prevention of hepatitis C is problematic. Donor screening is effective in preventing transmission by transfusions or organ/tissue transplants, but most infections occur outside these settings, and no pre- or post-exposure prophylaxis is available. Identification of persons with unrecognized infection through screening programmes can provide benefits such as counselling to prevent transmission to others and evaluation for treatment with therapeutic agents.

## INTRODUCTION

Hepatitis B virus (HBV) and hepatitis C virus (HCV) are important causes of acute and chronic hepatitis, cirrhosis and hepatocellular carcinoma. Implementation of hepatitis B vaccination programmes has the potential to eliminate HBV transmission and the serious consequences of HBV infection. The availability of effective treatment for some people with HCV infection emphasizes the importance of identifying infected persons for medical evaluation and possible therapy. In this article, we review the disease burden and epidemiology of HBV and HCV infection in North and South America, and discuss prevention strategies for chronic HBV and HCV infection.

## EPIDEMIOLOGY OF HBV

### Extent of HBV infection

Numerous prevalence studies of HBV infection have been conducted that provide a fairly complete picture of the extent of infection in the Americas [1,2]. Geographic regions can be characterized by levels of endemicity. In regions of high endemicity, the rate of chronic infection (as determined by the presence of hepatitis B surface antigen) is high (>8% of the population) and the lifetime risk of HBV infection is >60%. In regions of intermediate endemicity, the rate of chronic infection is intermediate (2–7% of the population) and the lifetime risk of HBV infection is 20–60%. In regions with low endemicity, the rate of chronic infection is low (<2% of the population) and the lifetime risk of HBV infection is <20%. Areas of the Americas that correspond to regions with a high endemicity include the Amazon basin (parts of Venezuela, Colombia and Peru), Alaska, the Dominican Republic and Haiti. Areas with an intermediate rate of endemicity correspond to many countries surrounding the Amazon basin (Venezuela, Colombia, Ecuador, Peru, Bolivia, Brazil), and Honduras and Guatemala. Canada, the USA, Mexico, and southern South America (Chile, Argentina, Uruguay and Paraguay) have low rates of endemicity.

In the USA, there are an estimated 1–1.25 million chronically infected persons, and in the rest of Americas, there are an estimated 5.6 million infected persons (Table 1).

### Clinical features of HBV infection

HBV causes clinical illness in 30–50% of all individuals over the age of 5 years who are infected with the virus, but in less than 10% of those aged under 5 years. On average the incubation period for the disease is 60–90 days (range 45–180 days) and the acute case fatality rate is low at 0.5–1.0% [3,4]. There is a marked difference between the proportion of individuals aged under and over 5 years who become chronically infected after acute infection. Of infants and young children aged under 5 years, 30–90% become chronically infected, but of individuals over this age, 2–10% do so [5].

Table 1. Estimated number of persons in the Americas with chronic HBV infection

| Region | Estimated chronic infections (×1000) |
| --- | --- |
| USA | 1125 |
| Canada | 75 |
| Central America and Mexico | 1025 |
| Caribbean | 450 |
| South America | 4000 |
| Total | 6675 |

Adapted from [1].

Table 2. Type of exposure reported by people with acute hepatitis B in the USA, 1991–1996

| Exposure | Proportion of cases (%) |
| --- | --- |
| Heterosexual activity | 39 |
| Intravenous drug use | 14 |
| Homosexual activity | 13 |
| Household contact | 3 |
| Occupational exposure | 1 |
| Other high risk* | 24 |
| None identified | 5 |

Source: CDC.
*Route claimed to be unknown but many of these individuals have a high-risk behaviour or characteristic (for example, a history of other sexually transmitted diseases, imprisonment or illicit non-intravenous drug use).

Thus, adults account for most of the clinically apparent acute disease, but infants and children are disproportionately represented among those with chronic disease [6]. Among all age groups, an estimated 15–25% of those who become chronically infected with HBV die prematurely as a result of chronic liver disease.

## HBV transmission

HBV is extremely efficiently transmitted, primarily by percutaneous and mucous membrane exposure to infectious body fluids. Percutaneous exposures that have resulted in HBV transmission include transfusion of blood or blood products, sharing contaminated equipment during intravenous drug use, haemodialysis, acupuncture, and needlestick or other injuries from sharp instruments sustained by hospital personnel. Sexual (both heterosexual and homosexual) and perinatal transmission of HBV usually result from mucous membrane exposure to infectious blood or body fluids.

The various modes of transmission of HBV differ in their relative importance in different regions of the world [6]. In highly endemic regions, most transmission occurs perinatally or in early childhood. In intermediate endemic regions, infection commonly occurs in all age groups, although the high rate of chronic infection is primarily maintained by transmission occurring in infancy and early childhood. In low endemic regions, most infection occurs in adults, especially those who belong to known risk groups. In the USA, where the rate of chronic infection is low, the single largest risk factor group is that reporting heterosexual activity, which accounts for 39% of all transmission (Table 2).

## PREVENTION OF HBV TRANSMISSION

The mainstay for the prevention and control of chronic hepatitis B is primary prevention through the use of

the hepatitis B vaccine. The World Health Organization has recommended that all countries integrate hepatitis B vaccination into their routine infant immunization programme. Hepatitis B vaccination of infants is particularly important in countries of high and intermediate HBV endemicity, because of the high rates of infection in infants and children. This strategy is being implemented to various extents in the Americas. As of 1997, all countries in the Americas with regions of highly endemic HBV infection have initiated vaccination programmes in highly endemic regions (B Hersh, personal communication). Of the 40 countries in the Americas, 10 have initiated routine infant immunization countrywide. These include the USA, Canada, Cuba, French Guiana, Guadaloupe, Martinique, Puerto Rico, St Kitts and Nevis. Two countries (Brazil and Peru) are planning on initiating nationwide hepatitis B immunization programmes. The relatively high cost of the hepatitis B vaccine and competing health priorities, however, continue to be major impediments to the implementation of vaccination programmes in many countries.

Elements of a strategy for the elimination of HBV transmission in all age groups include routine infant vaccination, routine adolescent vaccination, HBV screening of pregnant women and administration of post-exposure prophylaxis to infants born to infected women, and vaccination of children and adults at increased risk for hepatitis B. The USA has adopted a multifaceted approach to eliminating HBV transmission, including screening all pregnant women for hepatitis B surface antigen and providing hepatitis B immunoglobulin (HBIG) and hepatitis B vaccine to infants born to infected women; routine hepatitis B vaccination of all infants; catch-up vaccination of high-risk children; vaccination of 11–12-year-old adolescents who have not previously been vaccinated; and vaccination of adults at high risk [7].

It has proved difficult to prevent the transmission of HBV between adults in the USA [8]. To date, the greatest success of the strategy for the immunization of adult high-risk groups has been among persons who are at risk of HBV infection through occupational exposure; however, even before the vaccine was introduced this group accounted for no more than 5% of cases. The majority of adults at risk of HBV infection are difficult to target because they do not belong to well-defined risk groups; identifying them and directing resources appropriately is a considerable challenge.

Even if HBV transmission is eliminated, a sizeable pool of persons with chronic HBV infection will remain for several generations and be at risk for the development of serious sequelae. Measures to control HBV infection among persons who have chronic HBV infection include screening to identify infected persons, screening (for example ultrasound and alphafetoprotein) among infected persons for the early detection of chronic sequelae, and treatment with antiviral agents. Impediments to implementation of these control measures include the problem that many populations in North and South America with highly endemic hepatitis B have poor access to healthcare and limited resources for screening and treatment. Furthermore, the most cost-effective strategies for screening and treatment remain to be determined.

# EPIDEMIOLOGY OF HCV

## Extent of HCV infection

Many studies examining the prevalence of HCV infection have measured antibody to HCV (anti-HCV) among blood donors [9,10]. Anti-HCV prevalence rates in blood donors among countries in the Americas have been relatively low (0.2–1.0%). This compares with high prevalence (5–20%) observed in Egypt, and intermediate prevalence (1.1–5.0%) found in countries such as the former Soviet Union and Japan.

Blood donors tend to be highly screened populations and therefore their anti-HCV prevalence rates might not reflect those in the general population [9]. For example, the third National Health and Nutrition Examination Survey (NHANES III) conducted in the USA from 1988 to 1994 provides data on the prevalence of HCV infection in a representative sample of the US civilian population [11]. In this study the overall prevalence of anti-HCV was 1.8%, corresponding to a reservoir of 3.9 million infected Americans; rates were higher in males than in females and higher in

blacks than in whites. The highest rates of HCV infection were found in adults aged 30–49 years.

The important contribution of HCV infection to chronic liver disease in the USA is evident from studies of the aetiology of chronic liver disease. In one such study conducted in Jefferson County, Alabama, HCV was associated with 40% of the cases of chronic liver disease identified by active surveillance during a 1 year period; 26% of the cases were associated with HCV alone and 14% were associated with both HCV and alcohol [Centers for Disease Control (CDC), Atlanta, Georgia, USA, unpublished results]. In contrast, HBV was associated with 11% of cases. A second study was conducted at Harlem Hospital in New York City, New York, USA. In Harlem, mortality from chronic liver disease is five times the national rate and chronic liver disease is the second most common cause of death [12]. HCV was associated with 58% of cases of chronic liver disease in this population; 12% of cases were associated with HCV alone and 46% with HCV in combination with alcohol (CDC, unpublished results). HBV in combination with alcohol was associated with 8% of cases. In both studies, patients whose chronic liver disease was associated with both HCV and alcohol had more severe disease than patients with either aetiology alone.

## Clinical features of infection

HCV causes clinical illness in 30–40% of individuals who become acutely infected with the virus. On average, the incubation period of the disease is 40–50 days (range 14–180 days) [13–15]. Infection with HCV persists in the vast majority of individuals (85–100%), even in the absence of biochemical evidence of liver disease, and an average of 70% of those infected develop chronic hepatitis [16,17]. To date, no effective neutralizing antibody response to HCV has been identified. In contrast to hepatitis B, there is no vaccine for hepatitis C and treatment is less effective.

## HCV transmission

The most efficient transmission of HCV is through direct percutaneous exposure to infectious blood, such as through transfusion of blood or blood products or transplantation of organs or tissues from infectious donors, and sharing of contaminated equipment among intravenous drug users [9]. Haemodialysis patients and healthcare workers who are exposed to needlestick injuries in an occupational setting are also at risk from exposure to infectious blood. Although HCV can be transmitted by sexual

**Table 3.** Types of exposure reported by people with acute hepatitis C in the USA, 1991–1996

| Exposure | Proportion of cases (%) |
|---|---|
| Intravenous drug user | 43 |
| Sexual/household | 17 |
| Transfusion | 3* |
| Occupational | 4 |
| Other high-risk† | 28 |
| None identified | 5 |

Source: CDC.
*None in 1995 or 1996.
†Route claimed to be unknown but many of these individuals have a high-risk behaviour or characteristic (for example, a history of other sexually transmitted diseases, imprisonment or illicit non-intravenous drug use).

or household exposure to an infected contact, exposure to multiple sexual partners or perinatal exposure, the efficiency of transmission in these settings appears to be low. There have been a small number of anecdotal reports of nosocomial transmission of HCV. The types of exposure reported by patients with acute hepatitis C in the USA between 1991 and 1996 are shown in Table 3.

HCV may be transmitted by sexual and household exposure to an infected contact, but the efficiency of transmission from these exposures appears to be low. Among male and female heterosexual and male homosexual patients attending clinics for sexually transmitted diseases who had no history of intravenous drug use, the prevalence of anti-HCV antibodies has been found to average 5% (range, 1–18%); factors associated with being anti-HCV-positive included greater numbers of sexual partners, a history of other sexually transmitted disease, and failure to use a condom. Among eight seroprevalence studies of long-term spouses of patients with chronic hepatitis C who had no other risk factors, the average anti-HCV prevalence was 5% [9]; however, five of these studies found none of the spouses to be anti-HCV positive, and three studies found that the prevalence of anti-HCV ranged from 2% to 15%. Among nine seroprevalence studies of non-sexual household contacts of patients with chronic hepatitis C, the average anti-HCV prevalence was also 4% [9]; two of these studies found none of the household contacts to be anti-HCV positive, and seven studies found that the prevalence of anti-HCV ranged from 1–11%. The presumed mechanism of transmission was inapparent percutaneous or permucosal exposure to infectious blood or body fluids containing blood. Although the infected contacts reported no other commonly recognized risk factors for hepatitis C, most of these studies were done in

countries where it has been suggested that transmission of HCV infection may be associated with common exposure in the community resulting from contaminated equipment used in traditional and non-traditional medical procedures in the past.

Perinatal transmission of HCV infection from anti-HCV-positive, anti-human immunodeficiency virus (HIV)-negative women has been documented in an average of 5% of their infants based on detection of anti-HCV, and in a similar proportion (6%) based on detection of HCV RNA [18]. Substantial and/or persistent elevations in alanine aminotransferase (ALT) levels as evidence of hepatitis developed in an average of 4% of all the infants followed and 67% of the HCV-infected infants. Among the studies of infants born to women co-infected with HCV and HIV, the average transmission rate was higher: 14% based on detection of anti-HCV and 17% based on detection of HCV RNA [18]. Hepatitis developed in 21% of all the infants followed and in 100% of the HCV-infected infants. In all of the studies that determined the HCV RNA status of the mother at the time of delivery, only mothers who were HCV RNA-positive transmitted HCV to their infants [18]. The apparent higher HCV transmission rate to infants from women co-infected with HIV may be the result of higher titres of HCV RNA compared with those in women infected only with HCV. In two studies of HCV-positive, HIV-negative women, the transmission of HCV to their infants was related to the titre of HCV RNA in the women at the time of delivery [19,20]. In one of these studies, transmission occurred only from women with titres >$10^6$ copies/ml [20]; in the other, transmission occurred only from one woman with a titre of $10^{10}$ copies/ml [19]. The data on the risk of HCV transmission from breast feeding are limited but suggest that breast feeding does not play a role in the transmission of the virus. In the five studies that have evaluated breast feeding among infants born to HCV-infected women, the average rate of infection was 4% in both breast-fed and bottle-fed infants [18].

## PREVENTION OF HCV TRANSMISSION

Preventative measures for HCV infection are limited. Although screening of blood, organ and tissue donors will virtually eliminate transmission of HCV by transfusions and transplants, the majority of HCV infections occur outside these settings. Initiatives to modify high-risk behaviour have the potential to reduce the transmission of HCV but require considerable resources. More effective therapies are needed for the vast majority of chronically infected people.

Prevention and control of HCV infection and HCV-related chronic disease should be the goals of public health efforts. Achieving these goals requires implementation of a comprehensive prevention strategy. This comprehensive strategy contains primary prevention activities that reduce the risk of contracting HCV infection and secondary prevention activities that reduce the risk of chronic disease in HCV-infected persons. Primary prevention activities include those that reduce or eliminate the risk of transmission from a number of sources, including: (i) blood, blood products or clotting factor concentrates; (ii) infected sexual, household or other contacts; (iii) high-risk behaviours, such as intravenous drug use and unprotected sex with multiple partners; and (iv) nosocomial (namely chronic haemodialysis) and occupational exposure to blood. Secondary prevention activities include those that reduce the risk of chronic disease by identifying HCV-infected persons through diagnostic testing and by providing appropriate medical management and antiviral therapy as described previously [21].

Because of the large number of people with chronic HCV infection, identification of these persons must be a major focus of a comprehensive prevention strategy. Identification of HCV-infected persons allows for counselling about prevention of further HCV transmission, evaluation for chronic liver disease, possible antiviral therapy and counselling concerning avoidance of potential hepatotoxins, such as alcohol, that may increase the severity of HCV-related liver disease. A number of traditional public health approaches must be used to effectively prevent and control HCV infection and its chronic disease outcomes. Health education, identification and testing of persons at risk of infection, counselling and surveillance are approaches that must be combined to achieve the primary and secondary prevention goals of the comprehensive strategy for HCV prevention and control. Immunization is not available as a primary prevention tool because development of a vaccine is not likely in the foreseeable future. Specific elements of a comprehensive HCV prevention and control strategy are: (i) identification, testing and counselling of at-risk persons; (ii) medical management of infected persons, including referral systems linking testing and medical evaluation sites; (iii) donor screening, education and infection control practices to reduce the risk of new infections; and (iv) surveillance and evaluation to monitor disease trends and measure the effectiveness of prevention programmes.

Because of its limited effectiveness, the extent to which currently available antiviral therapy will have an impact on the overall disease burden of hepatitis C is unclear. In addition, the impact of screening programmes for the early identification of persons eligible for antiviral therapy remains to be determined. Poor access to care, the high cost of treatment and limited resources among populations at increased risk for hepatitis C will also be barriers to the implementation of control programmes.

## REFERENCES

1. Fay OH and the Latin American Regional Study Group. Hepatitis B in Latin America: epidemiologic patterns and eradication strategy. *Vaccine* 1990; **8** (Supplement):S100–S106.
2. McQuillan GM, Towsend TR, Fields HA, Carroll M, Leahy M & Pok BF. Seroepidemiology of hepatitis B virus infection in the United States. *American Journal of Medicine* 1989; **87**:3S–10S.
3. Hoofnagle JH & Di Bisceglie AM. Serologic diagnosis of acute and chronic viral hepatitis. *Seminars in Liver Disease* 1992; **11**:73–83.
4. Centers for Disease Control, USA. *Hepatitis Surveillance Report* 1992; **54**.
5. McMahon BJ, Award WLM, Hall DB, Heyward WL, Bender TR & Francis DP. Acute hepatitis B virus infection: relation of age to the clinical expression of disease and subsequent development of the carrier state. *Journal of Infectious Diseases* 1985; **151**:599–603.
6. Margolis HS, Alter MJ & Hadler SC. Hepatitis B: evolving epidemiology and implications for control. *Seminars in Liver Disease* 1991; **11**:84–92.
7. Centers for Disease Control. Hepatitis B virus: a comprehensive strategy for eliminating transmission in the United States through universal childhood vaccination: recommendations of the Immunization Practices Advisory Committee (ACIP). *Mortality and Morbidity Weekly Report* 1991; **40**:1–25.
8. Alter MJ, Hadler SC, Margolis HS, Alexander WJ, Hu PY, Judson FN, Mares A, Miller JK & Moyer LA. The changing epidemiology of hepatitis B in the United States: need for alternative vaccination strategies. *Journal of the American Medical Association* 1990; **263**:1218–1222.
9. Alter MJ. Epidemiology of hepatitis C in the west. *Seminars in Liver Disease* 1995; **15**:5–14.
10. Mansell CJ & Locarnini SA. Epidemiology of hepatitis C in the east. *Seminars in Liver Disease* 1995; **15**:15–32.
11. McQuillan GM, Alter MJ, Moyer LA, Lambert SB & Margolis HS. A population based serologic study of hepatitis C virus infection in the United States. In *Viral Hepatitis and Liver Disease*, 1997; pp. 267–270. Edited by M Rizetto, RH Purcell, JL Gerin & G Verme. Turin: Edizioni Minerva Medica
12. McCord C & Freeman HP. Excess mortality in Harlem. *New England Journal of Medicine* 1990; **322**:173–177.
13. Koretz RL, Brezina M, Polito AJ, Quan S, Wilber J, Dinello R & Gitnick G. Non-A, non-B posttransfusion hepatitis. Comparing C and non-C hepatitis. *Hepatology* 1993; **17**:361–365.
14. Marranconi F, Mecenero V, Pellizzer GP, Bettini MC, Conforto M, Vaglia A, Stecca C, Cardone E & de Lalla F. HCV infection after accidental needlestick injury in health-care workers. *Infection* 1992; **20**:111.
15. Seeff LB. Hepatitis C from a needlestick injury. *Annals of Internal Medicine* 1991; **115**:411.

16. Alter MJ, Margolis HS, Krawczynski K, Judson FN, Mares A, Alexander WJ, Hu PY, Miller JK, Gerber MA, Sampliner RE, Meeks EL & Beach MJ. The natural history of community-acquired hepatitis C in the United States. *New England Journal of Medicine* 1992; **327**:1899–1905.

17. Shakil AO, Cory-Cantilena C, Alter HJ, Hayashi P, Kleiner DE, Tedeschi V, Krawczynski K, Conjeevaram HS, Sallie R, Di Bisceglie AM & The Hepatitis C Study Group. Volunteer blood donors with antibody to hepatitis C virus: clinical, biochemical, virologic, and histologic features. *Annals of Internal Medicine* 1995; **123**:330–337.

18. Mast EE & Alter MJ. Hepatitis C. *Seminars in Pediatric Infection and Disease* 1998; in press.

19. Lin HH, Kao JH, Hsu HY, Ni YH, Yeh SH, Hwang LH, Chang MH, Hwang SC, Chen PJ & Chen DS. Possible role of high-titer maternal viremia in perinatal transmission of hepatitis C virus. *Journal of Infectious Diseases* 1994; **169**:638–641.

20. Ohto H, Terazawa S, Sasaki N, Sasaki N, Hino K, Ishiwata C, Kako M, Ujiie N, Endo C, Matsui A, Okamoto H & Mishino S, the Vertical Transmission of Hepatitis C Collaborative Study Group. Transmission of hepatitis C virus from mothers to infants. *New England Journal of Medicine* 1994; **330**:744–750.

21. National Institutes of Health. National Institutes of Health Consensus Conference Panel Statement: Management of Hepatitis C. *Hepatology* 1997; **26**:2S–10S.

# 2 Epidemiology and control of hepatitis B and C in eastern Asia

Zhi-Yi Xu*, Shou-jun Zhao, Richard T Mahoney, Xin-qing Deng, Ximin Lin, Jie Xu and Ding Ding

## INTRODUCTION

Viral hepatitis A, B, C, D and E are important public health problems in eastern Asia. However, hepatitis B and C are the main concerns because of their severe and frequent sequelae, such as chronic hepatitis, cirrhosis and primary hepatocellular carcinoma. In eastern Asian countries, therefore, there are major programmes for the control of hepatitis B and C.

## HEPATITIS B

Epidemiological patterns and control programmes for hepatitis B virus (HBV) in eastern Asia are different from those in other areas in several ways. In eastern Asia there is high prevalence of infection, carrier rates, risk of maternal–infant transmission, ratio of chronic to acute disease and vaccination coverage of children.

### Prevalence of HBV infection

The prevalence of HBV markers [hepatitis B surface antigen (HBsAg), anti-HBs and anti-hepatitis B core protein (HBc)] is estimated at 50–70% in most countries of eastern Asia and increases with age (Fig. 1). The lifetime risk of HBV infection, as judged by the peak prevalence of HBV markers in elderly people, is approximately 80%. The annual incidence of HBV infection varies between 2–5% according to age [1,2]. Thus, Asians have high levels of exposure to HBV throughout life. Transmission was associated with the use of reusable syringes and needles for injection, toothbrush sharing, towel and cup sharing [2], and other personal contact including maternal–infant transmission and sexual activities. Lifestyles in eastern Asian countries, however, have been changing over the last 20 years as the economy has improved. The impact of these changes on HBV transmission should be taken into consideration in assessing hepatitis B control programmes.

## HBV carrier rate

The HBV carrier rate in most Asian countries is as high as 8–20%. The rapid increase in HBV carrier rate, however, was observed solely in children under 5 years of age (Fig. 1). In spite of the continuous increase of HBV infection with age, in both school children and adults, the carrier rate in these age groups remains at a stable level (Fig. 1). Only babies and young children are at a high risk of acquiring chronic HBV after an acute HBV infection. Throughout most of life, the annual rate of HBV clearance in chronic carriers is low, usually ranging from 1–2%. It is interesting to note that the annual clearance rate increases to 8% in carriers aged 50 years and above (Fig. 2), which explains the drop in carrier rates in this age group. There is no biological explanation for this increased rate of HBV clearance in older carriers.

Chronic HBV infection acquired in childhood can be reactivated in adulthood, usually between 20–40 years of age, and can result in clinical chronic liver disease. In a 10 year follow-up study, chronic liver disease was observed in 28% of chronic HBV carriers [3]. The mechanism of the reactivation of HBV chronic infection in adults remains unknown.

**Figure 1.** Prevalence rates of HBV infection and HBsAg by age (1985–1986)

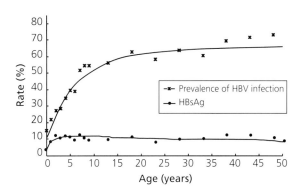

**Figure 2.** Annual rate of HBV clearance in chronic HBV carriers by age

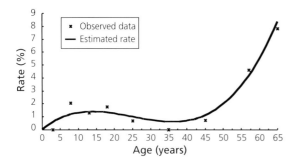

## Risk of maternal–infant transmission of HBV

A high prevalence of HBsAg (8–15%) and hepatitis B e antigen (HBeAg) (2.0–6.5%) has been observed in pregnant women in Asian populations. Infants born to HBV carrier mothers have a 20–40% chance of becoming chronic carriers, and this risk increases to 70–90% for those born to HBeAg-positive mothers. In a population-based cross-sectional study, 98 of 832 subjects (11.8%) tested HBsAg-positive. Among 85 people with HBV carrier mothers, 34 (40%) were HBsAg-seropositive; this rate, however, was 8.6% for those whose mothers were HBsAg-negative (Table 1). Thus, 34.7% (34/98) of the carriers in the community might have acquired HBV from their mothers.

Efficient maternal–infant transmission would play a role in perpetuating virus circulation from generation to generation. The maternal–infant transmission of HBV may occur in perinatal as well as in post-natal periods. The relative importance of the two transmission periods needs further study. It is interesting to note that an incidence rate of post-natally acquired HBsAg of 28% was reported in babies between 12–29 months of age born to carrier mothers [4].

## Chronic hepatitis B

From a nationwide survey conducted in China in 1978, the number of chronic hepatitis B patients was estimated to be 27 million (2.7%) [5]. Hence, chronic hepatitis B is a major disease burden for Asian countries. The annual incidence of acute hepatitis is usually about 1 per 1000 and 30% is caused by HBV [6]. Moreover, 54% of patients diagnosed with acute hepatitis B had the disease as a result of reactivation of the chronic carrier state acquired during childhood [2]. These patients tested IgG anti-HBc-positive (a marker of chronic hepatitis B) at the onset of the disease [2]. In a prospective study, patients who had shown IgG anti-HBc at the onset of the disease were persistent carriers, showed frequent relapse of hepatitis and were without seroconversion to anti-HBs (Table 2). On the other hand, during an 8–17 month follow-up, patients without IgG anti-HBc at the onset of the disease who were defined as suffering acute hepatitis B, cleared the virus,

**Table 1.** HBV carrier rate by maternal HBsAg seropositivity, Shanghai, 1984

| Age (years) | n | Maternal HBsAg | | | | |
| | | HBsAg-negative | % | n | HBsAg-positive | % |
|---|---|---|---|---|---|---|
| 0–9 | 186 | 10 | 5.3 | 24 | 5 | 20.5 |
| 10–19 | 89 | 3 | 3.4 | 25 | 9 | 36.0 |
| 20–29 | 323 | 36 | 11.1 | 30 | 15 | 50.0 |
| 30–39 | 135 | 13 | 9.6 | 6 | 5 | 83.3 |
| 40+ | 14 | 2 | 14.3 | 0 | 0 | 0 |
| Total | 747 | 64 | 8.6 | 85 | 34 | 40.0 |

**Table 2.** Clinical and serological findings from hepatitis B patients, by presence of IgG anti-HBc at onset of disease, during a 9–17 month follow-up

| IgG anti-HBc | Cases followed | Persistent HBsAg | | Seroconversion to anti-HBs | | Clinical relapse | |
| | | n | % | n | % | n | % |
|---|---|---|---|---|---|---|---|
| Negative | 24 | 0 | 0 | 19 | 79.2 | 0 | 0 |
| Positive | 24 | 24 | 100 | 0 | 0 | 8 | 33.3 |

recovered and had no relapse of hepatitis symptoms. In addition, 80% seroconverted to anti-HBs. Thus, the ratio of chronic to acute hepatitis B is about 200:1.

## Control of hepatitis B

For control of hepatitis B, most eastern Asian countries, such as China (mainland and Taiwan), Indonesia, Japan, Korea, Malaysia, Singapore, Thailand and others have integrated hepatitis B vaccination into their childhood immunization programmes. All babies, both born to HBV carrier and non-carrier mothers, receive the first dose of hepatitis B vaccine at birth and the second and third doses at 1–2 months and 6–12 months, respectively. In some areas, hepatitis B immunoglobulin (HBIg) is administered (for passive immunization) to babies of carrier mothers concurrently with the first dose of the vaccine. Universal infant hepatitis B immunization programmes were initiated in Asian countries between 1986 and 1990. In Shanghai, the first birth cohort received the vaccine in 1986 and were followed for 10 years; the carrier rate was 0.53% in 1995, compared to about 10% at the 1984 baseline (Table 3). The carrier rate in children born during 1986–1994, as shown in a cross-sectional study, was 0.41% (Table 3). Vaccine effectiveness was estimated at >95%. It is interesting to note that children aged 13–15 years in 1994 who could not have received the vaccine, also had a much lower HBsAg seropositivity in comparison with the baseline (Fig. 3). This was probably due to herd immunity and improved living conditions. The rates in individuals 15 years and older, however, were similar in the two cross-sectional studies conducted in 1984 (background) and 1994 (Fig. 3). Thus, the carrier rate and the rate of chronic hepatitis B in adults will remain unchanged for the next 30–50 years, until the vaccinated cohorts grow up.

In Taiwan, the rate of HBsAg positivity dropped from 10% to 0.9% after 10 years of universal infant immunization and catch-up immunization of preschool children [7]. In Thailand, a 4 year universal

**Figure 3.** HBsAg seropositivity pre- and post-hepatitis B immunization (Shanghai, 1995)

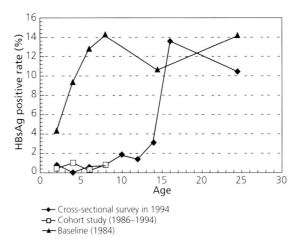

infant immunization programme was evaluated and it was found that HBsAg seropositivity decreased from 5.4% to 0.8% [8].

Failure of hepatitis B vaccine was observed in those babies whose mothers had a high serum HBV DNA concentration during pregnancy (Table 4). In both the vaccine group and the group with vaccine plus HBIg, vaccine failure was found only among those whose mothers had serum HBV DNA concentrations of 250 pg/ml or greater (Table 4). The rate of failure, however, was lower for the passive–active immunization group than for the group that was actively immunized.

Hence, the goal of eradicating HBV might be achievable in one generation if all babies are given hepatitis B vaccine and if the maternal virus load can be inhibited by chemotherapy.

## HEPATITIS C

The prevalence of hepatitis C virus (HCV) infection in the general population is low, ranging from 1–3%

**Table 3.** HBsAg seropositivity by year post-vaccination (cohort and cross-sectional studies, Shanghai, 1986–1995)

| Age (years) | Cohort study | | Cross-sectional study | | Background | |
|---|---|---|---|---|---|---|
| | HBsAg/$n$ | % | HBsAg/$n$ | % | HBsAg/$n$ | % |
| 1–2 | 2/432 | 0.46 | 1/128 | 0.78 | 2/81 | 2.47 |
| 3–4 | 7/716 | 0.98 | 0/431 | 0 | 6/96 | 9.37 |
| 5–6 | 3/924 | 0.32 | 2/361 | 0.55 | 5/39 | 12.82 |
| 7–8 | 5/653 | 0.77 | 2/295 | 0.68 | 8/56 | 14.28 |
| 9 | 0/468 | 0 | – | – | – | – |
| Total | 18/2915 | 0.53 | 5/1215 | 0.41 | 24/272 | 8.82 |

**Table 4.** HBV carrier rate in vaccinated infants by maternal HBV DNA level

| Vaccination regimen | Maternal HBV DNA (pg/ml) | | | |
|---|---|---|---|---|
| | 0–124 HBsAg/n % | 125–249 HBsAg/n % | 250–799 HBsAg/n % | 800+ HBsAg/n % |
| Vaccine alone | 0/46  0 | 0/4  0 | 17/45  37.7 | 3/6  50.0 |
| Vaccine plus HBIg | 0/24  0 | 0  0 | 4/28  14.3 | 1/1  100.0 |

[9,10]. In Japan, however, two community outbreaks were reported for which no specific source or route of transmission could be identified [11,12]. As in other areas of the world, the prevalence rate of HCV infection is very high in high-risk groups.

## Risk factors

The major risk factors for HCV infection are blood transfusion, intravenous drug use and plasma donation.

### Blood transfusion

Blood transfusion is the most important risk factor for HCV. The incidence rates of post-transfusion hepatitis C in several cities of China were in excess of 10% before 1997. The high risk associated with blood transfusion for surgical patients was a result of the lack of sensitive and reliable reagents for blood screening and the spread of HCV infection among blood donors.

### Intravenous drug use

Drug users sharing the same syringes and needles are at very high risk of HCV infection. The infection level was reported to be 60–97% in this group. Syringes and needles used by drug users are seriously contaminated. The use of reusable needles and syringes for medical injection in the general population, however, was not an important route for transmission of HCV. In a prospective study in a village where both hepatitis B and C were endemic and where only reusable and improperly sterilized syringes and needles were used, five new HBV infections (5.7%) were detected during a 1 year follow-up, but not a single HCV infection was found (Table 5). In both groups, repeated medical injections were reported in interviews. In this case, contamination of the syringes and needles might be serious enough for efficient transmission of HBV, but not for HCV. This observation provides an explanation for the low prevalence rate of HCV infection and high rate of HBV infection in the general population.

### Plasma donation

In several areas of China, plasma donation was performed with reusable and contaminated equipment before 1996. HCV infection was found in 10.8% of the professional donors who gave one donation, and 56.5% and 94.8% in those who gave 10–19 and 20–29 donations, respectively (Fig. 4), compared to 8.5% for those who donated blood alone.

## Control of hepatitis C

Efforts to control HCV include multiple blood screening with sensitive reagents, use of blood from volun-

**Table 5.** Incidence of HBV and HCV infection in susceptibles; a prospective study (China, 1994)

| | HBV Infection | HCV Infection |
|---|---|---|
| Susceptible (n) | 88 | 197 |
| Seroconversion | 5 | 0 |
| Annual incidence (%) | 5.7 | 0 |

The study was undertaken in a village with 775 subjects. The prevalence of HBV and HCV infections were 18.0% and 6.6%, respectively. Susceptible subjects were followed for 1 year.

**Figure 4.** Frequency of HCV infection and number of plasma donations among blood donors

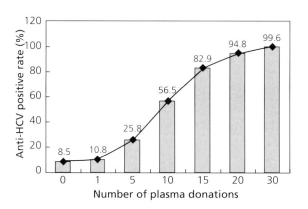

tary donors, education to stop sharing syringes and needles, use of disposable equipment for plasmaphoresis and treatment with interferon-α (IFN-α).

## Multiple blood screening with sensitive reagents

A prospective study has shown that the incidence of post-transfusion HCV infection was as high as 15.0% when the donated blood was prescreened by a single ELISA with locally produced, insensitive reagents. It was 2.5% when the blood was prescreened with ELISA kit reagents (Abbott Laboratories) and dropped to 1.6% when screened twice by locally produced and improved ELISA reagents, plus PCR for HCV RNA (Table 6). The strategy of multiple pre-screening of blood specimens collected at different time-points, for both anti-HCV and HCV RNA, allows the detection of the residual risk of post-transfusion hepatitis C from donors who are at the window phase of infection.

Use of disposable equipment for plasmaphoresis in China beginning in 1997 has almost eliminated the spread of HCV among the plasma donors.

## Interferon treatment

The lack of prophylactic vaccine, the high cost and unsatisfactory sensitivity of reagents for blood pre-screening and the low impact of education programmes on drug users and promiscuous individuals, have made preventive efforts extremely difficult. Thus, treatment is another choice for control. However, expensive interferon treatment provided a sustained efficacy in only 8–20% of chronic hepatitis C patients [13–15]. To analyse the economic aspects of the treatment, a cost-effectiveness study has been completed.

Sustained response to interferon treatment was assumed to be 15%. Medical expenses, including expenses for standard care or interferon-α, were obtained by special surveys in three cities of China. Annual rates of disease progression, from chronic

Figure 5. Comparison of cumulative medical expenses for 1000 chronic hepatitis C patients between IFN-α treatment and standard care over a period of 5–30 years

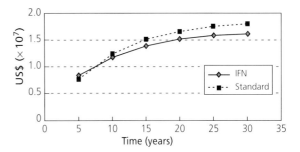

hepatitis C to compensated cirrhosis (4.4%), from compensated to decompensated cirrhosis (7.4%) and the death rate from decompensated cirrhosis (54.0%), were summarized from the literature [16–18]. The analysis has shown that of 1000 chronic hepatitis C patients treated with IFN-α, an additional 71 lives, 852 person-years and 1487 quality adjusted life-years would be saved, compared with the standard care group. The costs in the two groups, however, were similar. Actually, in the first 5–10 years of treatment, the cost of interferon exceeded those of standard care. After 10 years, however, the cumulative medical expenses were consistently higher for the standard care than for the interferon treatment (Fig. 5) because those cured in the interferon group no longer require treatment. Even when the interferon efficacy was set at the lower limit of 8%, the cost for a life saved was only US$21 197, and the costs for a life-year saved and for a quality-adjusted life-year saved were only US$1802 and US$1035, respectively. Therefore, interferon treatment is cost-effective for the treatment of chronic hepatitis C. A higher efficacy of IFN-α was reported when combined with ribavirin [19]. Thus, higher cost-effectiveness levels may be obtained with this combination.

Table 6. Post-transfusion HCV infection by reagent for screening of donors

| Reagent | Recipients | Anti-HCV+ | HCV RNA+ | ALT* elevation | Rate of infection (%) |
|---|---|---|---|---|---|
| ELISA | 133 | 20 | 7 | 13 | 15.4 |
| Two ELISAs plus PCR | 125 | 2 | 2 | 2 | 1.6 |
| Abbott ELISA | 122 | 3 | 1 | 2 | 2.5 |

*ALT, alanine aminotransferase.

# REFERENCES

1. Beasley RP & Hwang LY. Incidence of hepatitis B infection in preschool children in Taiwan. *Journal of Infectious Diseases* 1982; **46**:198–201.

2. Xu ZY. Epidemiology of hepatitis B. In *Viral Hepatitis in China, Virology Monograph Series 19*, 1992; pp. 99-110. Edited by YM Wen, ZY Xu & J Melnick. Basel: Karger.

3. Wu SM. Ten year follow up study of 52 chronic HBsAg carriers. *Chinese Journal of Infectious Diseases* 1984; **2**:36–39.

4. Postnatal infectivity of hepatitis B surface antigen-carrier mothers. *Journal of Infectious Diseases* 1983; **147**:185–190.

5. Li Y. Epidemiological study of viral hepatitis in China. *Chinese Journal of Microbiology and Immunology* 1986; **8** (Supplement):1–15.

6. Xu ZY & Fu TY. Study on sporadic acute hepatitis cases. *Chinese Journal of Infectious Diseases* 1983; **1**:192–195.

7. Chen HL, Chang MH & Hsu HY. Seroepidemiology of hepatitis B virus infection in children: ten years of mass vaccination in Taiwan. *Journal of the American Medical Association* 1996; **276**:906–908.

8. Chunsuttiwat S, Biggs B-A, Maynard J,Thampalo S, Laoboripat S & Bovoruson S. Integration of hepatitis B vaccination into the expanded programme on immunization in Chonberi and Chianmai provinces, Thailand. *Vaccine* 1997; **15**:769–774.

9. Christopher JM & Stephen AL. Epidemiology of hepatitis C in the East. *Seminars in Liver Diseases* 1995; **15**:15–20.

10. Lee SD, Chan CY & Wang YJ. Seroepidemiology of hepatitis C virus infection in Taiwan. *Hepatology* 1991; **13**:830–833.

11. Fukuda Y, Nagura H, Takayamam T, Imoto M, Shibatu M & Kudo T. Correlation between detection of antiviral antibody and histopathological disease activity in an epidemic of hepatitis C. *Archives of Virology* 1992; **126**:171–178.

12. Ishibashi M, Shinzawa H, Kuboki M, Tsuchida H & Takahashi T. Prevalence of Inhabitants with anti-hepatitis C virus antibody in an area following an acute hepatitis C epidemic: age- and area-related features. *Journal of Epidemiology* 1996; **6**:1–7.

13. Davis GL, Balart LA & Schiff ER. Treatment of chronic hepatitis C with recombinant interferon alfa. *New England Journal of Medicine* 1989; **321**: 1501–1506.

14. Di Bisceglie AM, Martin P & Kassianides C. Recombinant interferon alfa therapy for hepatitis C. *New England Journal of Medicine* 1989; **321**:1506–1510.

15. Chemello L, Bonneti P & Cavalleto L. Randomized trial comparing three regimens of alfa-2a-interferon in chronic hepatitis C. *Hepatology* 1995; **22**:700–706.

16. Muller R. Natural history of hepatitis C: clinical experience. *Journal of Hepatology* 1996; **24** (Supplement 2):52–54.

17. Fattovich G, Glustina G & Degos F. Morbidity and mortality in compensated cirrhosis type C; a retrospective follow up study of 384 patients. *Gastroenterology* 1997; **112**:463–472.

18. Seeff LB. Natural history of hepatitis C. *Hepatology* 1997; **26** (Supplement 1):21S–28S.

19. Reichard O, Norkrans G, Fryden A, Braconier J-H, Sonnerborg A & Weiland O. Randomized, double-blind, placebo-controlled trial of interferon alfa-2b with and without ribavirin for chronic hepatitis C. *Lancet.* 1998; **351**:83–87.

# 3 Prevalence of hepatitis B and C in Egypt and Africa

## Mohammed A Attia

## SUMMARY

Hepatitis B and C are, and will remain for some time, major health problems in Egypt and the entire continent of Africa. Both infections can lead to an acute or silent course of liver disease, progressing from liver impairment to cirrhosis and decompensated liver failure or hepatocellular carcinoma (HCC) in a 20–30 year period. In addition, hepatitis B and C infection rates differ in different settings, and prognosis may be worse in conjunction with schistosomiasis in Egypt, malaria in Sudan and human immunodeficiency virus (HIV) in other African populations. Unlike hepatitis B virus (HBV), for which the prospects for controlling the spread of infection by vaccination are promising, prospects for development of an effective vaccine against hepatitis C virus (HCV) are limited. As well as screening of blood for transfusion and using sterile needles for injection, preventive measures should be undertaken to reduce the risk of contact (often described as community-acquired infection). Until more is known about the unidentified routes of transmission in tropical and subtropical settings it will be difficult to be specific about the kind of measures which may be effective. Success may largely depend on changing habits within the population. Prevention should be the main goal of current efforts until low cost, effective therapies become available.

## PREVALENCE OF ACUTE HEPATITIS B AND C

Patients are considered to have acute B or C viral hepatitis if their aminotransferase levels are above normal and they have specific viral markers (HBsAg and anti-HBc antibodies for HBV, and anti-HCV antibodies for HCV). Subjects with obstructive jaundice, history of alcohol abuse or other non-infectious causes of liver injury are obviously not cases of viral hepatitis. Therefore, previous diagnoses of non-A non-B viral hepatitis included a wide range of causes, both infectious and non-infectious.

The variability of virus–host interaction generates different outcomes of infection. HCV causes chronic infection in more than 80% of individuals, with a wide spectrum of liver disease, ranging from an asymptomatic carrier state to severe forms of chronic hepatitis [1]. HBV infection, on the other hand, accounts for most clinically apparent acute hepatitis cases among adults, whereas children under 5 years of age usually (30–90%) become chronically infected [2].

In Egypt until the early 1980s it was difficult for epidemiologists, clinicians and pathologists to assign a patient with hepatitis to hepatitis A virus (HAV), HBV, or to other viral hepatitis infections, because of limited diagnostic tests and lack of specialized laboratories [3]. HCV was identified in 1989–90 as the cause of 80–90% of post-transfusion hepatitis [4]. Acute viral hepatitis and progression of a high proportion of cases over time into serious chronic liver damage and HCC are recognized public health problems, the prevalence of which has not been accurately measured in Egypt or elsewhere in Africa. A rate of acute viral hepatitis of 53.7% was calculated in 1974–75 for HBV in a population of 2032000 in Alexandria, Egypt [3]. An attack rate of 9.4 for total hepatitis and 5 for HBV per 10000 of the population was calculated. The male to female ratio was 2:1, with a mean duration of hospitalization of 14.1 days. Hospital bed occupancy rate was 71.3%. The calculated fatality rate was 1.6%, being higher for patients aged 45 years or more. In one other large study, out of about 18000 samples collected by the Egyptian Organization for Biological Products and Vaccines [5] from different geographical settings in Egypt in the period 1975–1979, 2894 were from patients admitted to Abbasia Fever Hospital in Cairo, and HBV infection accounted for 46.4% of the acute hepatitis cases (Table 1). In another prospective study carried out on children with acute hepatitis in Qalyubia, HBV was found in 17% of the cases, whereas no anti-HCV antibodies could be detected [6]. In contrast, out of 1023 subjects with chronic liver disease, HCV antibodies were detected in 74%. In 89 biopsied patients (in the same study) with histological evidence of chronic active or chronic persistent

Table 1. Prevalence of HBV-specific markers in the Egyptian population, 1975–1979

| Population group | (n) | HBsAg-positive (%) | Anti-HBs-positive (%) |
|---|---|---|---|
| Children | | | |
| Below 1 year old | 98 | 1 | – |
| 1–2 years old | 66 | 15.2 | – |
| 12–19 years old | 2956 | 4.1 | 18.4 |
| Blood donors | | | |
| Professional | 1107 | 3.2 | 56.4 |
| Volunteer | 882 | 5.0 | 35.6 |
| Recruits | 3030 | 5.2 | 42.6 |
| Acute hepatitis | 2894 | 46.4 | 40.4 |
| Geographical areas | | | |
| Sinai | 132 | 3.8 | 31.8 |
| New valley | 632 | 7.3 | 42.2 |
| Aswan | 425 | 8.7 | 22.3 |
| Rural | 5187 | 4 | 54 |

Based on [5].

hepatitis, cirrhosis or cancer, HCV was the only marker present in 63% [7].

Among black Africans, HBV was detected in 10% of Sudanese children with acute hepatitis [8], and in 62–90% of Nigerian patients with histologically characterized chronic liver disease, whereas anti-HCV antibodies were detected in only 4% [9]. In southern Sudan, 20% of 666 patients attending six public clinics in the city of Juba were HBsAg-positive, whereas only two (3%) were seropositive for HCV [10].

## PREVALENCE OF INFECTION

For unknown reasons, Egyptians have the highest worldwide prevalence of HCV infection. The first evidence was provided by a study on Egyptian blood donors living in Saudi Arabia, which indicated an anti-HCV antibody prevalence of 19.2% [11], compared to 0.5% from Bedouins and 4.2% in non-Bedouins [12] born in Saudi Arabia. Subsequent studies conducted in Egypt confirmed the high anti-HCV antibody prevalence, of 6–38% in blood donors enrolled from the general population in Cairo and adjacent areas in the Nile delta [13–17]. In a more recent study by Arthur et al. [18] from US Naval Medical Research Unit 3 (NAMRU-3) in Cairo, serum samples were collected from 2644 blood donors in 24 of Egypt's 26 governorates. The study indicated that the prevalence of anti-HCV antibodies was high not only in Cairo and adjacent areas but also in many other regions of the country. It ranged from 0% in the

North Sinai governorate to 38.2% in the Beni Suef governorate adjacent to the Nile (Table 2; Fig. 1). The HCV antibody prevalence was greater than 20% in more than half of the 26 governorates, and greater than 30% in six. Another study from the same research unit [7] was conducted on 740 tourism workers whose residences were distributed throughout Egypt. After adjusting for age (ranging from 25–40 years with an average of about 25–27 years in each region), the seroprevalence was highest, at approximately 20%, in the Nile delta north of Cairo. The governorates in the Nile valley south of Cairo had an intermediate prevalence of 13%, and the lowest prevalences of 7% and 9% were observed in the Cairo and Sinai areas, respectively (Table 3).

In an attempt to determine the route and chronology of HCV spread in the Egyptian population, 120 stored serum samples collected in 1977 from HBsAg-positive patients presenting to the largest fever hospital in Cairo were screened in the same research unit for HCV infection [19]: 18% were HCV-positive in a recombinant immunoblot assay compared to 7% of a comparable group of 95 patients presenting to the same hospital in 1993–94. HCV infections were therefore well established in the Egyptian population in 1977. Wide dissemination of the infection at that time was attributed to a number of factors, among which is the reuse of inadequately sterilized needles and syringes in the mass treatment of schistosomiasis with tartar emetic. This began in the 1950s and continued up until 1982 when oral praziquantel

Table 2. Overall prevalence of HBV and HCV antibodies in blood donors in 24 of the 26 governorates in Egypt

| Governorate/DR* | Number of samples | Number (%) containing specific IgG antibodies | |
| | | Anti-HBV | Anti-HCV |
| --- | --- | --- | --- |
| 1 Alexandria/1 | 136 | 33 (24) | 15 (11) |
| 2 Assiut/3 | 139 | 59 (42) | 34 (24) |
| 3 Aswan/3 | 58 | 15 (26) | 2 (3) |
| 4 Beheira/4 | 193 | 69 (36) | 43 (22) |
| 5 Beni Suef/3 | 89 | 40 (45) | 34 (38) |
| 6 Cairo/1 | 349 | 97 (28) | 68 (19) |
| 7 Damietta/4 | 45 | 10 (22) | 17 (38) |
| 8 Daqahliya/4 | 181 | 58 (32) | 51 (28) |
| 9 Fayoum/– | 0 | – (–) | – (–) |
| 10 Gharbiya/4 | 169 | 74 (44) | 56 (33) |
| 11 Giza/1 | 99 | 48 (48) | 24 (24) |
| 12 Ismailia/2 | 56 | 23 (41) | 9 (16) |
| 13 Kafr El-Sheikh/4 | 134 | 47 (35) | 36 (27) |
| 14 Matrouh/2 | 28 | 5 (18) | 5 (18) |
| 15 Menoufiya/4 | 136 | 62 (46) | 32 (24) |
| 16 Minya/3 | 154 | 67 (44) | 57 (37) |
| 17 North Sinai/2 | 30 | 7 (23) | 0 (0) |
| 18 Port Said/2 | 29 | 13 (45) | 6 (21) |
| 19 Qalyubiya/4 | 136 | 68 (50) | 43 (32) |
| 20 Qena/3 | 135 | 81 (60) | 44 (33) |
| 21 Red Sea/2 | 30 | 13 (43) | 5 (17) |
| 22 Sharqiya/4 | 130 | 60 (46) | 38 (29) |
| 23 Sohag/3 | 129 | 66 (51) | 25 (19) |
| 24 South Sinai/2 | 29 | 15 (52) | 5 (17) |
| 25 Suez/2 | 30 | 12 (40) | 7 (23) |
| 26 Wadi El-Gedid/– | 0 | – (–) | – (–) |
| Total | 2644 | 1042 (39.4) | 656 (24.8) |

Based on [18].
*DR, degree of relative risk according to locality; 1 and 2, low risk; 3, intermediate risk; 4, high risk.

became available. This may explain the strikingly higher prevalence of anti-HCV antibodies in elderly people in areas of the Nile delta. Possible exposure in the general population may also have occurred during nationwide immunization programmes, such as the smallpox vaccination campaigns in the 1940s. Once the virus became established, transmission almost certainly occurred from blood transfusion administered before routine HCV screening of blood and blood products began in 1993–1994.

In community-based fragmentary studies from tropical and subtropical Africa, the seroprevalence of immunoblot-confirmed anti-HCV antibodies was 0.75% of 3077 black African volunteer blood donors in Natal and South African areas. A prevalence of 3% was reported from Djibouti and of 3.2% in a cohort

of refugees from Mozambique in south-eastern Africa, mostly in older individuals. In HCV-endemic areas of equatorial Africa however, the prevalence is considerably higher; anti-HCV antibody was confirmed by an immunoblot assay in 6.5% of 1172 subjects over 5 years of age in eastern Gabon and in 6.7% of 1421 subjects in Guinea Conakry in west central Africa. The overall prevalence of HCV infection among black Africans throughout the continent is much lower than figures reported from anywhere in Egypt (Fig. 2). With one exception, where anti-HCV was 24% in a rural population in Gabon, one may conclude that HCV infection is moderately endemic in black Africa, in contrast to the unique hyperendemic figures of HCV infection in the Egyptian population.

In contrast, HBV infection is widespread throughout continental Africa (Fig. 2). Recently, it has been estimated that there are 50 million chronic carriers of HBV in Africa, with a 25% mortality risk [20]. In Egypt, 1042/2644 (39.4%) of subjects had evidence of HBV infection, ranging from 18 to 60% in different governorates [18]. Similar intermediate to high rates of HBV infection have been reported from several regions in Africa. The overall prevalence of HBV infection was 56% in a cohort of refugees from Mozambique in south-eastern Africa and the HBsAg carrier rate was 13.2% [21]. In sub-Saharan Africa the overall HBsAg carrier rate in the general population is 5 to 20%, which is among the highest in the world [22]. In rural Sudan, the overall prevalence of HBV antibodies was 63.9%; the prevalence of HBsAg was 18.7% [23]. The HBsAg prevalence was highest in children less than 5 years of age (32.3%) and the infection rate increased from 48.4% in this age group to 88.5% in individuals of 50 years or more. These infection and carrier rates are comparable to rates in other areas of black Africa, and indicate a relatively higher degree of exposure to HBV in rural Africa.

## GENOTYPE PREVALENCE

The distribution of different types and subtypes of HCV is mostly geographically restricted, with Africa showing an enormous variety of different subtypes [24]. Genotype 4 is the most widely distributed in many African regions. This genotype has been detected in 80% of chronic carriers in Egypt but genotype 1 is also present [25,26]. Genotype 4 is also dominant in Burundi and Gabon together with genotype 5 (which is most prevalent in South Africa). Genotype 4 is found with genotypes 1 and 3 in Tanzania, and with 2 in Guinea Conakry. The co-existence of different HCV types and subtypes raises

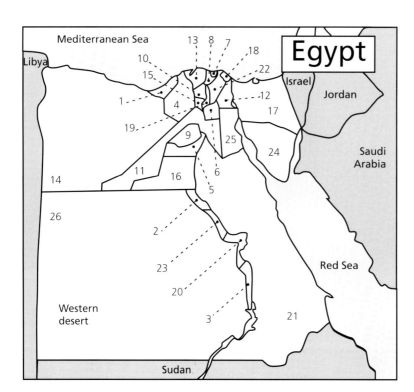

**Figure 1.** Map of Egypt showing the 26 governorates listed in Table 2.

Modified from RR Arthur *et al. Transactions of the Royal Society of Tropical Medicine and Hygiene* 1997; **91**:271–274, with permission.

questions about mechanisms of transmission and clinical importance in relation to such a wide spectrum of variants.

Recently HBV has been classified into six different genotypes, A to F. These also show a restricted geographical distribution, with genotype A (64%) prevalent in central Africa and genotype E (86%) in Guinea (west Africa) [24]. Further studies will allow the clinical relevance of particular HBV types and subtypes to be determined and hopefully allow optimization of therapeutic outcome.

## RISK FACTORS FOR INFECTION

In Egypt it is estimated that 400 000 units of donated blood are transfused annually [14]. Taking into account the motivation of selling blood as a risk factor

**Table 3.** Distribution of HCV infection among tourism workers adjusted for age (25–40 years) throughout Egypt

| Region | Anti-HCV positive (%) |
| --- | --- |
| Cairo, Giza | 7.3 |
| Sinai areas | 8.9 |
| Nile valley south of Cairo | 12.6 |
| Nile delta north of Cairo | 20.5 |

Based on [7].

[16,18], paid blood donors who repeatedly donate blood have a higher HCV infection rate than unpaid volunteer donors [16,27]. To minimize the risk of post-transfusion HCV infection, mandatory screening of all blood donors for anti-HCV antibodies was instituted by the Egyptian Ministry of Health in June 1993 and professional blood donors were replaced with volunteer unpaid blood donors. Routine screening for anti-HCV antibodies in blood banks began in 1993–1994. The number of post-transfusion hepatitis infections has since been substantially reduced. Screening for HBV serological markers started in the 1980s. The delay in screening for anti-HCV antibodies and early exclusion of HBV-infected blood donors probably caused an increase in the HCV infectious pool among Egyptians during that lag period. However, this cannot explain the higher prevalence of HBV infection (39.4%) over that of HCV (24.8%) in the general population [18]. One explanation is that HBV infection occurs at a younger age than HCV infection. HBV becomes detectable in 8% of Egyptian children at 1–3 years old, whereas HCV does not reach a similar level until the age of 9 [13]. The seroprevalence of HBV therefore begins earlier and progresses to higher peaks.

Childhood as a risk factor and as a reservoir of HBV infection has been supported by a number of studies in Africa. Evidence from rural Gabon [28],

Figure 2. Distribution of HBV and HCV antibodies and HCV genotypes in the general population of Africa

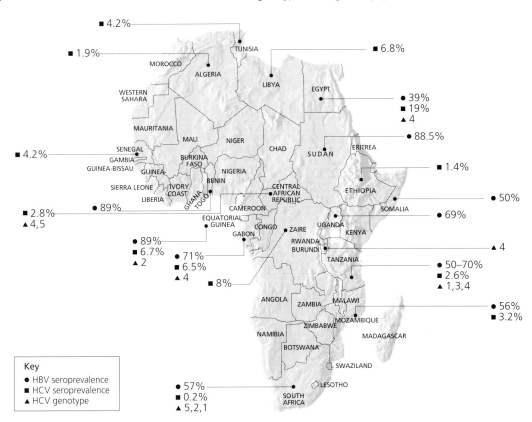

Sudan [23] and sub-Saharan Africa [22] shows that most HBV infections are acquired between 6 months and the pre-school age of 5–6 years. It is disturbing that when HBsAg carriers were tested for HBV DNA in rural Gabon, all HBV DNA carriers were children less than 11 years of age. In the 2–9 years old group, 71% of the HBsAg-positive children tested were HBV DNA carriers [28]. These results strongly suggest that HBV transmission occurs predominantly in childhood by the horizontal rather than the perinatal route.

Association between hepatitis B and C forms another risk in Egypt and elsewhere in Africa. HCV prevalence was higher among individuals who had HBV infection. Out of 1042 subjects who were anti-HBc positive, 36% had HCV infection, whereas only 18% of HBV-negative subjects were HCV-seropositive [18]. Similar studies in Tunisia, Senegal, Burundi and Madagascar also showed higher prevalence of anti-HCV antibodies in HBsAg-positive patients than in HBsAg-negative patients. Combined infection may cause more liver damage over time than single infection. The livers of patients that are seropositive for both HBsAg and anti-HCV were mostly decompensated (57%), whereas 14.3% presented with no

evidence of active liver disease [29].

The association with schistosomiasis is another important risk factor for HCV infection in Egypt. The risk remains significant after adjustment for age, gender, marital status and residence [30]. Mechanisms by which schistosomiasis leads to a high prevalence of HCV infection can be speculated upon. People living in the Nile delta who are over 40 or 50 years of age were mostly exposed to mass treatment with tartar emetic, given as a series of 15 injections, for their schistosomiasis. They could have become infected through reuse of contaminated needles and syringes before the shift to oral praziquantel in 1982 [31]. Previous parenteral antischistosomal therapy was also associated with HBsAg positivity [32]. Another possibility is that schistosomiasis-induced immune suppression [33] and the inhibition of a protective intrahepatic cytotoxic T lymphocyte response to HCV [34] can result in delayed virus clearance and provoke viral replication and liver damage. Similarly, in the Gezira region of Sudan, parenteral therapy of malaria proved to be an independent risk factor for HBV infection [23], which may also apply to other African regions (infections with related species of Plasmodia are established in west Africa and throughout the malaria belt). In developing countries, reuse of unsterile syringes and needles is still an important risk factor.

HIV is another risk marker for hepatitis in tropical and subtropical Africa, where HIV infection is widespread. In central Africa, HBV infection is significantly more correlated to HIV, shown by the very high HBsAg carrier rate (40.1%) in HIV-infected adults compared to controls (11%) [35]. In the Ivory Coast in west Africa, co-infection by HBV and hepatitis D virus (HDV) is a common occurrence, but found to be significantly more frequent in HIV-1-infected adults than in a control group with acute viral hepatitis [36]. In this African setting co-infection leads to accelerated disease and more efficient sexual and perinatal transmission [37].

Intravenous drug abuse is a risk factor in western countries, where 75% to 80% of users may become carriers of the virus [38]. Parenteral drug abuse is not known to be common in Egypt, neither it is thought to be important in tropical Africa. However, other population groups could be infected from the numerous blood donations provided by a relatively small number of users of illicit drugs [16].

Exposure to infective serous exudates, vaginal secretions, menstrual fluid, semen as well as blood may explain transmission during sexual intercourse, especially between long-term heterosexual or homosexual partners. This may also explain increased transmission rates in association with other venereal diseases. However, conflicting results do exist in studies from South Africa and other western communities such as Sweden [38]. Transmission from carriers to close non-sexual family contacts directly, or indirectly through fomites, saliva and blood may also occur. There have been two small cohort studies that looked at such risks. One of the two studies, from South Africa on HBV, gave positive results [39], whereas the other, from Egypt on HCV, gave negative results [30]. The impact of close living and the risk of intrafamilial transmission will not be fully determined until detailed epidemiological studies have been carried out in different tropical settings on both viruses.

Many individuals in Egypt and in other regions of Africa could get infected by other risk modes, including percutaneous infections through tribal scarification, tattooing, and ear and nose piercing. In one report, a history of scarification was not significantly associated with HCV infection but it was with HBV infection [10]. Other possible vehicles that are suspected, though not verified, include insect bites.

Flaviviruses such as yellow fever and dengue have an insect vector, and HCV is a member of the same family.

## WHO IS MOST AT RISK IN EGYPT AND AFRICA?

Egyptian and African populations at highest risk of HBV and HCV infections are those who are most exposed to risk factors (Table 4). Transfusion recipients are still at risk of transfusion-associated hepatitis B or C, despite mandatory screening of blood donors for HBsAg and anti-HCV antibodies. Anti-HCV antibodies may not be detected even with the latest commercially available tests until 10–12 weeks after initial infection, whereas HCV RNA can be detected within a few days to 1 week after infection, during the seronegative window. Adding to the same problem of post-transfusion hepatitis is the circulation of possible HBV mutants [40] which escape detection when screening blood donors for HBsAg by standard methods. People at high-risk are therefore multi-transfused haemophiliacs, thalassaemics, leukaemics and patients with maintained haemodialysis. Seropositivity is significantly associated in these groups with duration of illness and number of blood transfusions.

Rural populations both in Egypt and other African areas have a higher incidence of viral hepatitis. On top of the low hygiene in these rural areas, habitual and tribal traditions of scarification and tattooing (al-washm in Egypt) are still ongoing practices, providing routes by which many individuals may become infected.

Populations with other endemic infections are more prone to co-infection with hepatitis viruses and have a worse prognosis. People with a history of schistosomiasis in Egypt [13] or living in the African malaria belt [23,41] and AIDS patients in central and southern Africa are associated with an increased risk of HBV and HCV infection. Many AIDS patients have markers of HBV replication [42]. Household contacts have a higher prevalence of HBV and HCV infections when a member of the family is infected. In a study from South Africa, evidence of HBV infection among children was present in 73.7% of 186 household contacts of index-carrier (HBsAg-positive) cases, 48.7% of 150 contacts of index-past infection (anti-HBs-positive) and 38.2% of 207 contacts of index-negative cases. This potential risk indicates that intrafamilial horizontal person-to-person transmission is important in black South Africans [39] and elsewhere among other poor and rural populations in Africa.

Table 4. Risk groups of Egyptian/African populations

| Risk factor/group | Infection rate (%) | | | |
| | HBV | | HCV | |
| | Egyptian | African | Egyptian | African |
| --- | --- | --- | --- | --- |
| Rural | 60 | 98 | 33 | 0.8 |
| Urban | 24 | 56 | 11 | 1.7 |
| Professional blood donor | – | – | 27 | – |
| Volunteer blood donor | 53 | – | 17 | 3.2 |
| Haemodialysis | 80 | – | 67 | 21 |
| Chronic liver disease | 51 | 17 | 50 | 33 |
| HCC | 47.6 | 55.5 | 72.1 | 38 |
| HBc antibody positive | – | – | 36 | 4 |
| HBc antibody negative | – | – | 18 | 2 |
| Anaesthetists | 25.7 | – | 8.6 | – |
| Internal medicine | 11.1 | – | – | – |

Healthcare personnel including surgeons, anaesthetists, dentists and other physicians, nurses and laboratory technicians have a higher incidence of HBV and HCV infections, which increases with exposure to patients or blood products. Infection from patients to health workers has been documented following percutaneous exposure to blood. In one report, from Assiut University Hospital in upper Egypt approximately 25% of anaesthetists, with a higher risk of exposure, were anti-HBc-positive compared to 11% of medical staff practising internal medicine [43]. Possible transmission of HBV and HCV infections by HCV RNA-positive saliva has been of concern to dentists. In New York city, 9% of dental surgeons and 1% of other dentists were anti-HCV positive [44]. In South Africa a study showed that both dental students and staff are exposed to a significantly higher risk of contracting hepatitis B.

## TRANSMISSION

Despite the lack of explanation for the extraordinarily high HCV infection rates in Egypt, parenteral exposure remains the most efficient route of transmission. Blood transfusion-associated HCV infection has been responsible for only a minority of reported cases, the risk of which declined as a result of donor testing. In addition to blood transfusion, individuals most at risk in western countries were those with a past history of intravenous drug abuse, which is not an important source of infection among high-risk population groups in Egypt. Though inefficient compared to parenteral transmission, sexual and intrafamilial non-parenteral routes should be considered in highly endemic areas. There exists, however, little evidence of sexually transmitted HCV in Egypt [30]. Although it may be inferred from other studies that sexual partners are at an increased risk, it does not necessarily follow that sexual intercourse is the source of that risk. Studies looking for HCV infection in sexual partners of haemophiliacs revealed no increased prevalence of HCV [45]. If it exists in western countries, the risk of sexual transmission is small and certainly not sufficient to account for the very high prevalence in Egypt. The possible increased risk of HCV infection by sexual transmission may be demonstrated in association with a history of other sexually transmitted diseases. In a report from Sweden, HCV carriers were most likely to have antibodies to herpes simplex virus type 2. However, a study from South Africa showed no evidence of increased HCV prevalence in those with sexually transmitted disease [46].

Contact-associated transmission cannot be excluded in households in the highly endemic populations of Egypt and Africa. These include inadvertent exposure through shared razors and toothbrushes, and exposure to skin lesion exudates and contaminated fomites. Traditional scarification and tattooing practices are widely performed in rural populations of upper and lower Egypt, and reuse of contaminated instruments is certainly a possible means by which many individuals can become infected. A positive association was demonstrated between hepatitis C and tattooing in Taiwan [47]. Future studies should therefore take into account the prevalence of hepatitis C in Egyptian villages and in African regions where tattooing and scarification are presently performed. Other inadvertent percutaneous routes of transmission which have not been studied include insect bites and blood shedding or tropical ulcers, where large volumes of serosanguinous exudate may result in a high level of environmental virus and therefore increase the possibility of contamination of cuts and bites on the skin [38].

Perinatal transmission of HCV from infected women to their babies is still controversial. In one study, seropositivity was detected in 4.3% of 1536 pregnant women attending an antenatal clinic in Alexandria, Egypt [48]. In another study, 12 out of 44 mothers (18–34 years old) were anti-HCV-positive, and 11 of their newborns were seropositive. This was confirmed in six out of the 11 reactive cord blood samples by a line immunoblot assay. HCV RNA, however, was detected in three mothers and only one cord blood sample by double nested PCR [49]. In another study, 131 out of 1000 (13%) pregnant women were anti-HCV antibody-positive; 10 of the seropositives were examined for HCV by RT–PCR in a follow-up after 3, 6 and 9 months. HCV RNA was detected in five infants born to seven HCV RNA-positive mothers (71%). However, the detection of HCV RNA in these infants showed different presentations, in which the virus persisted continuously in one infant with elevated transaminases in two. The mothers of the anti-HCV seropositive infants were either diabetic, bilharzial or HBsAg-positive, suggesting that perinatal infection is more efficient in these settings [50]. However, evaluation of the risk of perinatal transmission from such small studies is difficult because of the sample size and the duration of follow-up, and methods of serological testing are highly variable [51]. The data available fails to show whether the virus is highly infectious by this perinatal route in the Egyptian series. Yet, it has been estimated that in HBV hyperendemic populations most transmission occurs perinatally and early childhood infection is common [52].

## NATURAL HISTORY AND PROGNOSIS

A number of factors, both viral and environmental, interact to influence the course of infection. Patients seeking medical treatment are only those with advanced liver disease. It is difficult at this stage to relate HCV genotypes or viral load to differences in the severity of the disease [38]. Viral titres are low in the serum of most HCV carriers, but patients co-infected with HBV may have high levels of viraemia and accelerated liver disease. HBV is therefore considered a risk marker for co-infection and for severe liver damage in the Egyptian population, where HCV infection is hyperendemic. Patients who are co-infected with HBV may have a worse prognosis and develop fulminant hepatitis. HCV is only rarely the sole cause of fulminant hepatitis, and it has not been reported in Egypt. Other factors like schistosomiasis, which is also hyperendemic in Egypt, and malaria and HIV in other parts of Africa are settings which promote HBV and HCV replication, viral persistence and enhanced progression to severe liver damage.

Adverse prognoses have been reported to be associated elsewhere with HCV genotype 1. In Egypt and most of Africa, genotype 4 is the dominant genotype [25,53]. All genotypes are likely to elicit different immune responses and therefore have different progression to long-term liver disease.

Co-infection by HDV suppresses the replication of HBV, and is a common occurrence within the African continent. However, co-infection with both HBV and HDV, but not with HBV alone, is significantly more frequent in asymptomatic HIV-infected black adults in west Africa [36]. Contamination of foodstuffs with aflatoxin increases the risk of progression to HCC in individuals infected with HBV. The risk is more serious in most African regions, where the HBsAg carrier rate is among the highest in the world. For unknown reasons, HBeAg positivity rates are much lower in black Africans of childbearing age than in women in the Far East, thus accounting for a much lower rate of perinatal infection [20]. Several factors, acting alone or in combination, appear to be linked to regional and/or socioeconomic factors and play a major role in the clinical outcome of HBV infection.

## TREATMENT, CONTROL AND PREVENTION

Vaccination is one of the strategies for enviromental intervention, to decrease the heavy toll of disease associated with HBV and other hepatitis viruses. This includes screening of all pregnant women for HBsAg and providing anti-HBV immunoglobulin and vaccine to infants born to infected mothers. In view of the high HBV carrier rates in the general population of Africa, universal immunization of all infants was recommended through the Expanded Programme on Immunization (EPI). In 1986, introduction of the hepatitis B vaccine was initiated in The Gambia in west Africa. The rate of HBV infection dropped to less than 5% in children who received all four doses of HBV vaccine [54].

In countries integrating HBV vaccination in their routine childhood immunization programme, more than 90% of children are covered. However, 110 countries (55%), representing 33% of HBV carriers worldwide, have no vaccination programmes [51]. Vaccination strategy should include adolescents and adults at high risk, especially those who are likely to acquire HBV infection through occupational exposure.

Prospects of an effective vaccine against HCV are poor, as there is little evidence of a neutralizing antibody response to infection [55]. Passive protection with a specific immunoglobulin is probably not feasible for the same reason. In addition, the extreme heterogeneity of the virus, with many genotypes, subtypes and variants, will restrict the efficiency of vaccines derived from only one virus strain. Loss of HCV viraemia following treatment with α-interferon (α-IFN) may be achieved in up to 50% of the patients, with serum transaminases returning to normal levels. The other half of these patients may relapse during or after treatment. This kind of poor response rate is unlikely to have any impact in a hyperendemic area like Egypt, as patients usually present with advanced disease. This is especially true in view of the very high cost of α-IFN therapy [38].

In Egypt and other tropical countries in Africa, prevention of HBV and HCV transmission depends on avoiding the risk of contact. With HCV, this necessitates knowing about the mechanisms and routes of infection in a hyperendemic setting in tropical or subtropical populations. So far, HCV transmission can be reduced only by screening of blood donors but will depend largely on educational measures and/or changing habits.

## REFERENCES

1. Alter MJ, Margolis HS, Krawczynski K, Judson FN, Mares A, Alexander WJ, Hu PY, Miller JK, Gerber MA, Sampliner RE, Meeks EL & Beach MJ. The natural history of community acquired hepatitis C in the United States. *New England Journal of Medicine* 1992; **327**:1899–1905.
2. McMahon BJ, Alward WLM, Hall DB, Heyward WI, Bender TR & Francis DP. Acute hepatitis B virus infection: relation of age to the clinical expression of disease and subsequent development of the carrier state. *Journal of Infectious Diseases* 1985; **151**:599–603.
3. Sallam SA & Wahdan MH. Viral hepatitis in Alexandria. *Journal of the Egyptian Public Health Association* 1981; **56**:324–344.
4. Choo QL, Weiner AJ, Overby LR, Houghton M & Bradley DW. Hepatitis C virus: the major causative agent of viral non-A non-B hepatitis. *British Medical Bulletin* 1990; **46**:423–441.
5. Egyptian Organization for Biological Products and Vaccines, Ministry of Public Health. Activities of viral hepatitis B in Egypt. *Annual Report* 1979; 49–70.
6. El-Dafrawi MS & El-Dakhakhni MY. Viral profile (HAV, HBV, HCV and Delta-agent) in children with acute hepatitis. *Egyptian Medical Journal* 1992; **9**:23–29.
7. Arthur RR. Epidemiology of HCV infections in Egypt. *Medicine and the Community* 1996; **6–7**:4–7.
8. Hyams KC, Hussain MA, Al-Arabi MA, Al-Huda-

Atallah N, El-Tigani A & McCarthy MC. Acute sporadic hepatitis in Sudanese children. *Journal of Medical Virology* 1991; **33**:73–76.
9. Ojo OS, Thursz M, Thomas HC, Ndububa DA, Adeodu OO, Rotimi O, Lawai AA, Durosinmi MA, Akonai AK, Fatusi AO & Goldin RD. Hepatitis B virus markers, hepatitis D virus antigen and hepatitis C antibodies in Nigerian patients with chronic liver disease. *East African Medical Journal* 1995; **72**:719–721.
10. McCarthy MC, El-Tigani A, Khalid IO & Hyams KC. Hepatitis B and C in Juba southern Sudan: results of a serosurvey. *Transactions of the Royal Society of Tropical Medicine and Hygiene* 1994; **88**:534–536.
11. Saeed AA, Al-Admawi AM, Al-Rasheed A, Fairclough D, Bacchus R, Ring C & Garson J. Hepatitis C virus infection in Egyptian volunteer blood donors in Riyadh. *Lancet* 1991; **338**:459–460.
12. Abdelaal M, Rowbottom D, Zawawi T, Scott T & Gilpin C. Epidemiology of hepatitis C virus: a study of male blood donors in Saudi Arabia. *Transfusion* 1994; **34**:135–137.
13. Darwish MA, Faris R, Clemens JD, Rao MR & Edelman R. High seroprevalece of hepatitis A, B, C and E viruses in residents in an Egyptian village in the Nile Delta: a pilot study. *American Journal of Tropical Medicine and Hygiene* 1996; **54**:554–558.
14. Kamel MA, Ghaffar YA, Wasef MA, Wright M, Clark LC & Miller FD. High HCV prevalence in Egyptian blood donors. *Lancet* 1992; **340**:427.
15. Wegdan AA, Berry ME, Ismail MA & El-Kholy A. Prevalence of antibodies to hepatitis C virus in Egyptian blood donors. *Egyptian Journal of Medical Microbiology* 1994; **3**:381–384.
16. Bassily S, Hyams KC, Fouad RA, Samaam MD & Hibbs RG. A high risk of hepatitis C infection among Egyptian blood donors: the role of parenteral drug abuse. *American Journal of Tropical Medicine and Hygiene* 1995; **52**:503–505.
17. Hegazi LA & Hasab-Allah MA. Prevalence of antibodies of HCV in Egypt: a survey of 5221 apparently healthy individuals. *Medical Journal of Cairo University* 1996; **64**:167–176.
18. Arthur RR, Hassan NF, Abdallah MY, El-Sharkawy MS, Saad MD, Hackbart BG & Imam IZ. Hepatitis C antibody prevalence in blood donors in different governorates in Egypt. *Transactions of the Royal Society of Tropical Medicine and Hygiene* 1997; **91**:271–274.
19. Arthur RR, Iman ZI, Magdi DS, Hackbart BG & Mossad SB. HCV in Egypt in 1977. *Lancet* 1995; **346**:1239–1240.
20. Kiire CF. The epidemiology and prophylaxis of hepatitis B in sub-Saharan Africa: a view from tropical and subtropical Africa. *Gut* 1996; **38** (Supplement 2):95–112.
21. Bos P, Steale AD, Peenze I & Aspinall S. Seroprevalence of hepatitis B and C virus infection in refugees from Mozambique in southern Africa. *East African Medical Journal* 1995; **72**:113–115.
22. Kiire CF. Hepatitis B infection in sub-Saharan Africa. *Vaccine* 1990; **8** (Supplement 1):S107–S112.
23. Hyams KC, Al-Arabi MA, El-Tigani AA, Messiter JF, Al-Gaali AA & George JF. Epidemiology of hepatitis B in the Gezira region of Sudan. *American Journal of Tropical Medicine and Hygiene* 1989; **40**:200–206.
24. Stuyver L, Rossau R & Maertens G. Line probe assays for the detection of hepatitis B and C virus genotypes. *Antiviral Therapy* 1996; **1** (Supplement 3):53–57.

25. Attia MA, Abdel-Hadi S, Alam El-Din HM & Abdel-Rahman H. Seroprevalence of hepatitis C amongst Egyptian pediatric acute leukemics and their siblings of NCI, Egypt: genotyping and risk of intrafamilial transmission. *Proceedings of the American Society of Clinical Oncology* 1996; **15**:370.

26. Rapicetta M. Molecular structure of HCV and diagnostic assays. *Medicine and the Community* 1996; **6-7**:14–16.

27. Attia MAM, Zekri AN, Goudsmit J, Boom R, Khaled HM, Mansour MT, De Wolf F, Alam-El-Din HM & Sol CJA. Diverse patterns of recognition of hepatitis C virus core and nonstructural antigens by antibodies present in Egyptian cancer patients and blood donors. *Journal of Clinical Microbiology* 1996; **34**:2665–2669.

28. Richard-Lenoble D, Traore O, Kombila M, Roingeard P, Dubois F & Goudeau A. Hepatitis B, C, D, and E markers in rural equatorial African villages (Gabon). *American Journal of Tropical Medicine and Hygiene* 1995; **53**:338–341.

29. Rafla H & Abdel-Masih MA. Study of HBV and HCV infection in chronic liver disease. *Medical Journal of Cairo University* 1993; **61** (Supplement 1):203–210.

30. Darwish MA, Raouf TA, Rushdy P, Constantine NT, Rao MR & Edelman R. Risk factors associated with a high seroprevalence of hepatitis C virus infection in Egyptian blood donors. *American Journal of Tropical Medicine and Hygiene* 1993; **49**:440–447.

31. McNeeley DF, Habib MA, Morgan SH, Azziz FA & Cline BL. Changes in antischistosomal drug usage patterns in rural Qalyubia, Egypt. *American Journal of Tropical Medicine and Hygiene* 1990; **42**:157–159.

32. Hyams KC, Mansour MM, Massoud A & Dunn MA. Parenteral antischistosomal therapy: a potential risk factor for hepatitis B infection. *Journal of Medical Virology* 1987; **23**:109–114.

33. Actor IK, Shirai M, Kullberg MC, Buller RML, Sher A & Benzofsky JA. Helminth infection results in decreased virus-specific CD8 and cytotoxic T-cell and TH$_1$ cytokine responses as well as delayed virus clearance. *Proceedings of the National Academy of Sciences, USA* 1993; **90**:948–952.

34. Koziel MJ, Dudley D, Wong JT, Dienstag J, Houghton M, Ralston R & Walker BD. Intrahepatic cytotoxic T lymphocytes specific for hepatitis C virus in persons with chronic hepatitis. *Journal of Immunology* 1992; **149**:3339–3344.

35. Tswana SA & Moyo SR. The interrelationship between HBV-markers and HIV antibodies in patients with hepatocellular carcinoma. *Journal of Medical Virology* 1992; **37**:161–164.

36. Soubeyrand J, Niamikey EK, Quattara SA, Diallo D, Leleu JP & Beda BY. HIV 1 seropositivity and hepatitis B and D viruses in West Africa. *Pathologie et Biologie* 1990; **38**:899–902.

37. Manzini P, Saracco G, Cerchier A, Riva C, Musso A, Ricotti E, Palomba E, Scolfaro C, Verme G, Bonino F & Tovo PA. Human immunodeficiency virus infection as risk factor for mother-to-child hepatitis C virus transmission, persistence of anti-hepatitis C virus in children is associated with the mother's anti-hepatitis C virus immunoblotting pattern. *Hepatology* 1995; **21**:328–332.

38. Tibbs CJ. Tropical aspects of viral hepatitis: hepatitis C. *Transactions of the Royal Society of Tropical Medicine and Hygiene* 1997; **91**:121–124.

39. Abdool-Karim SS, Theipal R & Coovadia HM. Household clustering and intra-household transmission patterns of hepatitis B virus infection in south Africa. *International Journal of Epidemiology* 1991; **20**:495–503.

40. Gaobep M, Aspinall S & Bos P. Hepatitis B viral markers in bushmen at Schidtsdrift, South Africa: baseline studies for immunization. *East African Medical Journal* 1995; **72**:421–423.

41. Adebajo AD, Smith DJ, Hazlemen BL & Wreghitt TG. Seroepidemiological associations between tuberculosis, malaria, hepatitis B and AIDS in West Africa. *Journal of Medical Virology* 1994; **42**:366–368.

42. Kashala O, Mubikay I, Kayembi K, Mukeba P & Essex M. Hepatitis B virus activation among central Africans infected with human immunodeficiency virus (HIV) type 1: pre-S2 antigen is predominantly expressed in HIV infection. *Journal of Infectious Diseases* 1994; **169**:628–632.

43. El-Qadhi SA & El-Kabsh M. Study of the prevalence of hepatitis C and B virus infection among anesthetists in Assiut University Hospital. *Assiut Medical Journal* 1994; **18**:213–216.

44. Klein RS, Freeman K, Taylor PE & Stevens CE. Occupational risk for hepatitis C virus infection among New York City dentists. *Lancet* 1991; **338**:1539–1542.

45. Brettler DB, Maunucci PM, Gringeri A, Rasko JE, Forsberg AD, Rumi MG, Garsia RJ, Rickard KA & Colombo M. The low risk of hepatitis C virus transmission among sexual partners of hepatitis C-infected hemophilic males: an international multicentre study. *Blood* 1992; **80**:540–543.

46. Schoub BD, Johson S, McAnerey JM & Blackburn NK. The role of sexual transmission in the epidemiology of hepatitis C virus in black South Africans. *Transactions of the Royal Society of Tropical Medicine and Hygiene* 1992; **86**:431–433.

47. Ko YC, Ho MS, Chiang TA, Chang SJ & Chang PY. Tattooing as a risk of hepatitis C virus infection. *Journal of Medical Virology* 1992; **38**:288–291.

48. Hassan NF. Prevalence of hepatitis C antibodies in patient groups in Egypt. *Transactions of the Royal Society of Tropical Medicine and Hygiene* 1993; **78**:638.

49. Mansour TM, Abdel-Wahab AA, El-Shinawy NM, Gazar NM, Attia MAM & El-Zayadi A. Is vertical transmission of HCV a reality? *Medical Journal of Cairo University* 1994; **62**:883–889.

50. El-Ghoneimy S & Hadhoud A. Materno-fetal transmission of hepatitis C virus. *Egyptian Journal of Medical Microbiology* 1995; **4**:361–365.

51. Alter M. Epidemiology and disease burden of hepatitis B and C. *Antiviral Therapy* 1996; **1** (Supplement 3):9–14.

52. Margolis HS, Alter MT & Hadler SC. Hepatitis B: evolving epidemiology and implications for control. *Seminars in Liver Disease* 1991; **11**:84–92.

53. Dusheiko G, Schmilovir-Weiss H, Brousi D, McOmish F, Yap PL, Sherlock S, McIntyre N & Simmonds P. Hepatitis C virus genotypes: an investigation of type-specific differences in geographic origin and disease. *Hepatology* 1994; **19**:13–18.

54. Ryder RW, Whittle HC, Sanneh AB, Ajdukiewicz AB, Tulloch S & Younnet B. Persistent hepatitis B virus infection and hepatoma in Gambia, West Africa. A case-control study of 140 adults and their 603 family contacts. *American Journal of Epidemiology* 1992; **136**:1122–1131.

55. Iwarson S, Norkrans G & Wejstal R. Hepatitis C: natural history of a unique infection. *Clinical Infectious Diseases* 1995; **20**:1361–1370.

# 4 Magnitude of hepatitis B and C in Latin America

Flair José Carrilho* and
Maria Cássia Jacintho Mendes Corrêa

## SUMMARY

Infections with hepatitis B and C viruses are common in Latin America. They may lead to end-stage liver disease, cirrhosis and hepatocellular carcinoma, and are therefore an important and emerging public health problem. The objective of this chapter is to discuss some epidemiological aspects of these important viral infections in Latin America.

## HEPATITIS B

The prevalence of different hepatitis B virus (HBV) serum markers varies in different Latin American countries (Table 1). The prevalence of HBV surface antigen (HBsAg) in blood donors varies from 0.2% in Puerto Rico to 2.8% in Venezuela [1]. This variation probably depends on the different assays used to detect the markers and on the geographical region being studied. The prevalence of HBV serum markers in countries of the Amazon basin (Brazil, Venezuela, Colombia, Peru and Bolivia) is higher than that observed in other areas of Latin America [2].

In Brazil, the prevalence of HBV serum markers also varies depending on the geographical region being analysed (Table 2). Prevalence is higher in states in the north and northeast of the country when compared to states in the south and southeast [3]. The seroprevalence may reach 2.8% to 10.3% of the entire population in these areas. In Espirito Santo and Parana, southeastern states, the prevalence of HBV serum markers has been reported to vary between 3.2% and 8.3%, respectively.

The prevalence of acute HBV infection varies throughout Latin America (Table 3) depending on the geographical area and on the population group being studied.

There is little information available on the prevalence of acute viral hepatitis in Brazil, although the prevalence of acute hepatitis B seems to be significantly higher among healthcare workers [4].

## MODES OF TRANSMISSION AND RISK GROUPS

### Blood and its derivatives

In areas where the prevalence of HBV infection is low, blood and its derivatives are responsible for most cases of transmission. The probable routes of infection are blood transfusions, accidental inoculation of small amounts of blood (surgical and dental interventions), injections, tattoos, acupuncture and laboratory accidents. In areas of intermediate and high prevalence of HBV infection, other modes of transmission may also be important, such as perinatal transmission, transmission through haematophagous insects and transmission through exudative cutaneous lesions [5–7].

HBsAg has been detected in *Triathomineos* [6,7] but replication of HBV has not been demonstrated in these or other insects [8]. HBsAg has also been found in exudative cutaneous ulcers [9]. This fact could

Table 1. Prevalence of HBV serum markers in 7487 samples from blood donors of 13 Latin American countries [54]

| Country | HBsAg (%) | Anti-HBs (%) | Anti-HBc (%) |
|---|---|---|---|
| Argentina | 0.8 | 14.7 | 9.4 |
| Barbados | 1.4 | 9.0 | 11.9 |
| Brazil | 2.1 | 26.7 | 27.6 |
| Chile | 0.4 | 3.8 | 5.3 |
| Colombia | 1.0 | 25.1 | 18.1 |
| Costa Rica | 0.6 | 17.3 | 16.7 |
| Ecuador | 2.0 | 29.4 | 21.9 |
| Mexico | 1.6 | 11.6 | 9.0 |
| Puerto Rico | 0.2 | 9.2 | 10.1 |
| Dominican Republic | 4.1 | 55.3 | 81.1 |
| Dutch Guyana | 2.3 | 28.1 | 37.9 |
| Peru | 2.2 | 20.2 | 20.4 |
| Venezuela | 2.8 | 11.6 | 15.5 |

Table 2. Prevalence of HBV serum markers in blood donors and in normal adults in Brazil [1,2,54–58]

| Region | Cases | HBsAg (%) | Anti-HBs (%) | Tests* |
|---|---|---|---|---|
| South | | | | |
| Rio Grande do Sul | 31244 | 0.9–1.2 | 8.0 | RIA/EIA |
| Paraná | 70548 | 0.3–1.7 | 25.4 | HPR/RIA |
| Francisco Beltrão | 6061 | 8.3 | – | EIA |
| Southeast | | | | |
| São Paulo | 62402 | 0.3–1.3 | 25.9 | HPR/RIA |
| Rio de Janeiro | 41654 | 0.6–3.1 | 26.7 | RIA/EIA |
| Espirito Santo | 5200 | 3.2 | – | HPR |
| Minas Gerais | 22470 | 1.6 | – | RIA |
| Central | | | | |
| Goiás | ? | 0.9 | – | RIA |
| Mato Grosso | 222 | 1.2–4.5 | 39.6 | EIA |
| Northeast | | | | |
| Bahia | 871 | 4.2 | – | RIA |
| Sergipe | 930 | 2.0 | – | HPR |
| North | | | | |
| Amazonas | 1354 | 2.8–10.3 | 89.7 | RIA/EIA |
| Pará | 734 | 5.6 | 36.2 | EIA |
| Amapá | 748 | 0.9 | 16.6 | EIA |

*HPR, reverse passive haemagglutination; RIA, radio immunoassay; EIA, enzyme immunoassay.

explain the transmission of HBV infection among Indian children in the Amazon, where the practice of fighting, as sport or fun, is common.

## Perinatal transmission

In Bahia (northeast Brazil) transmission of HBsAg during pregnancy has been shown to be 27.3% [10]. This mechanism of transmission, according to some authors, is unusual [11].

## Sexual transmission

HBV can be transmitted through saliva, semen, vaginal secretions and menstrual blood. Such routes of transmission probably explain the high infection rates observed among the sexual or household contacts of HBV-infected patients.

It seems that prostitutes may represent an important reservoir of infection in some areas. In Chile, the prevalence of HBV infection among prostitutes was 3.0% and in the control group it was 0.3% [12]. A similar study in Brazil showed the prevalence of HBV infection to be 3.6% in a group of prostitutes and 3.0% in the control group [13].

Table 3. Prevalence of acute hepatitis B in Latin America

| Countries | Children (≤14 years) | Adults | All ages | Reference |
|---|---|---|---|---|
| Argentina | 4.0 | 35.5 | – | 59–61 |
| Brazil | | | | |
| Southeast | 5.0 | 30.1 | 21.0 | 62–66 |
| Northeast | 16.0 | 54.0 | – | 67 |
| North | – | – | 25.0 | 68 |
| Chile | 2.0 | 7.0 | – | 69–70 |
| Colombia | 0.0 | 25.0 | – | 71 |
| Costa Rica | – | – | 10.0 | 72 |
| Honduras | – | 67.0 | – | 73 |
| Mexico | 13.0 | – | – | 74 |
| Peru | – | 42.0 | – | 75 |

## HIGH RISK GROUPS

Because of the frequency of contact with HBV, poor hygiene conditions, promiscuity or immunodeficiency, certain population groups are at a higher risk of acquiring HBV infection; these include healthcare workers, haemodialysis patients, haemophiliacs, patients with hepatosplenic schistosomiasis, patients with leprosy, male homosexuals, prostitutes, drug addicts and household contacts of HBV carriers. Table 4 shows the seroprevalence of HBV markers in such population groups in Brazil.

## FAMILIAL CLUSTERING

Studies in Brazil have shown that relatives of index hepatitis B cases of Oriental and Western ethnic origin have a high family aggregation rate for HBV serum markers, varying between 74.2% and 90.5% [14–17].

As shown in Table 5, the presence of serum HBsAg was significantly higher in the group of Oriental origin than in the group of Western origin (44.6% and 12.3%, respectively; $P<0.0001$).These studies have also shown that mothers transmit HBV to their children more frequently than fathers, independent of ethnic origin. It has also been shown that HBV-infected mothers of Oriental origin transmit HBV infection more frequently to their children than do HBV-infected mothers of Western origin. In relatives of Oriental origin, the occurrence of HBsAg was more prevalent in consanguineous relatives than in those who were non-consanguineous. Anti-HBs antibody was more prevalent in the non-consanguineous relatives of Oriental origin. In relatives of Western origin anti-HBs was more prevalent in the non-consanguineous group. There was no difference for HBsAg in relatives of Western origin.

## HEPATITIS C

Hepatitis C virus (HCV) infection occurs throughout Latin America and until the recent introduction of serological tests for HCV, the prevalence of this infection was not known. Among the risk factors for HCV infection are previous blood transfusion, surgery,

Table 4. Prevalence of HBsAg and anti-HBs in high risk groups in Brazil

| Group | HBsAg (%) | Anti-HBs (%) | Reference |
|---|---|---|---|
| Haemodialysis | 7.8–19.2 | 8.9–36.0 | 76–78 |
| Leprosy | 2.3 | 57.6 | 13 |
| Schistosomiasis | 1.5–23.3 | 28.5 | 79,80 |
| Haemophialics | 8.7 | 87.3 | 81 |
| IVDU | 4.5 | 63.6 | 82 |
| Alcoholics | 13.0 | 33.5 | 83 |
| Male homosexuals | 6.7–23.0 | 57.0–73.0 | 13, 84 |
| Prostitutes | 7.6 | – | 85 |
| Healthcare workers | 3.0–11.1 | 26.3 | 54,78,86, |
| Household contacts | 4.0–7.1 | 68.0–85.6 | 87,88 |

intravenous drug use (IVDU), sexual promiscuity, tattooing practices, exposure to blood and haemodialysis. Other risk factors have been identified.

In Brazil, previous blood transfusion, IVDU and sexual contact have been identified as the most frequent risk factors involved in transmission of HCV [18]. The route of transmission could not be determined in 9.0% to 57.6% of the HCV infection cases studied in Brazil, according to different reports [19–21].

Population studies on the prevalence of HCV infection are not common in Brazil. Three different studies have shown prevalence to vary between 0% and 3% [22–24].

The use of screening assays for HCV in blood banks has uncovered a large population of asymptomatic carriers. Table 6 shows the prevalence of antibody to HCV in blood donors in different Latin American countries. According to the data in the table, the seroprevalence varies from 0.2% in El Salvador to 3.4% in the northeast of Brazil. The introduction of more sensitive tests (EIE-II/III and immunoblot-II/III) has decreased the seroprevalence throughout Latin America (unpublished data).

Table 5. Prevalence of HBsAg and anti-HBs in relatives of HBV-infected patients from oriental (Group I) and western (Group II) ethnic origin [14,88]

| | HBsAg | | | Anti-HBs | | |
|---|---|---|---|---|---|---|
| Relationship | Group I n (%) | Group II n (%) | P | Group I n (%) | Group II n (%) | P |
| Parents | 21 (52.4) | 29 (20.7) | <0.05 | 16 (56.3) | 29 (41.4) | NS |
| Mother | 12 (83.3) | 16 (25.0) | <0.01 | 8 ( 25.0) | 16 (43.7) | <0.05 |
| Father | 9 (11.1) | 13 (15.4) | NS | 8 (87.5) | 13 (38.5) | NS |
| Siblings | 68 (73.5) | 51 (13.7) | <0.001 | 62 (20.9) | 51 (25.5) | NS |
| Children | 30 (33.3) | /1 (/.0) | <0.01 | 30 (3.3) | 71 (8.5) | NS |
| Spouses | 14 (7.1) | 25 (4.0) | NS | 14 (85.7) | 25 (68.0) | NS |
| Others | 134 (35.1) | 36 (19.4) | NS | 122 (41.8) | 33 (24.2) | NS |
| Total | 267 (44.6) | 212 (12.3) | <0.001 | 244 (35.2) | 209 (26.8) | NS |

# MODES OF TRANSMISSION AND RISK GROUPS

## Haemophiliacs

HCV infection is the most important cause of hepatitis in this group of patients. In Brazil, Chile and Peru, the prevalence of anti-HCV antibodies has been shown to vary between 51.0% and 87.2% [25–27].

## Intravenous drug use

Use of intravenous drugs represents a major mode of transmission of HCV infection worldwide. HIV infection seems to increase the risk of acquiring HCV infection.

Studies in Brazil have shown IVDU to be an important risk factor in both HIV-positive patients and HIV-negative patients [18,28]. A study in Buenos Aires, Argentina showed that 57.3% of HIV-positive male intravenous drug users and 20% of HIV-positive female intravenous drug users also carried anti-HCV antibodies. A study from Lima, Peru shows that 2.0% of a population of IV drug users, who were negative for HIV infection, were anti-HCV antibody-positive [27].

## Sexual transmission

Conflicting data have emerged from studies investigating sexual transmission of HCV infection. Data from different studies suggest that sexual transmission may occur, although transmission between spouses via other routes cannot be ruled out at present.

In Brazil, different studies have revealed that 2.4% to 21% of the sexual partners of HCV-infected patients were also infected with HCV [18,29,30]. A study among the spouses of HIV/HCV-infected patients in Buenos Aires, Argentina showed that 10.3% of them were also infected with HCV [31].

The seroprevalence of HCV among prostitutes in Argentina has been shown to be 2.9% [32]. In Santiago, Chile, no cases of HCV infection were detected among 25 prostitutes submitted to a third-generation ELISA assay for HCV [26]. In homosexuals, the seroprevalence of anti-HCV antibodies has been found to be above that found in low-risk volunteer blood donors. In Brazil, it varies between 4.5% to 7.9% [33,34]. In Chile, 9.0% of a homosexual population studied was shown to be infected with HCV [26].

**Table 6.** Frequency of serum anti-HCV in blood donors and normal adults in Latin America*

| Country | Anti-HCV (%) | Year | Test | Reference |
| --- | --- | --- | --- | --- |
| Argentina | 0.5–2.8 | 1987–96 | EIA-II | 89,90 |
| Brazil | | | | |
| South | 1.1–2.1 | 1991–97 | EIA-II | 91 |
| Southeast | 0.8–2.8 | 1991–97 | EIA-II | 92,93 |
| Central | 1.0–1.4 | 1988–95 | EIA-II | 94,95 |
| Northeast | 1.7–3.4 | 1991–95 | EIA-I/II | 96,97 |
| North | 0.9–2.4 | 1989–97 | EIA-II | 98,99 |
| Chile | 0.2–0.5 | 1991–93 | EIA-I | 100–102 |
| Cuba | 0.6–1.5 | 1991 | EIA-I | 103–105 |
| Dutch Guyana | 0.4 | 1991 | EIA-I | 106 |
| El Salvador | 0.2–1.2 | 1993 | – | 100,101 |
| French Guyana | 1.5 | 1997 | EIA-II | 106 |
| Guatemala | 0.6–0.9 | 1993 | – | 100,101 |
| Honduras | 0.4–0.8 | 1990–93 | – | 100,101,107,108 |
| Jamaica | 0.3 | 1995 | – | 109 |
| Mexico | 0.1–1.47 | 1991–94 | – | 100,101,110 |
| Nicaragua | 0.4–1.7 | 1993 | – | 100,101 |
| Panama | 0.3 | 1993 | – | 101 |
| Peru | 0.7–1.6 | 1990–94 | EIA-I/II | 111,112 |
| Uruguay | 0.4–0.5 | 1993 | – | 100,101 |
| Venezuela | 0.6–1.2 | 1990 | EIA-I | 113 |

*Normal adults are members of the general population who do not donate blood.

Table 7. HCV genotypes in Latin America

| Country | n | 1a | 1b | 1 | 2 | 2a | 2b | 3a | 3 | 4 | 4+5 | Mixed | Unclassified | Method | Reference |
|---|---|---|---|---|---|---|---|---|---|---|---|---|---|---|---|
| Argentina | | | | | | | | | | | | | | | |
| Buenos Aires | 434 | 30.3% | 68.5% | 58.5% | 25.6% | – | – | – | 8.3% | 0.9% | – | 6.7% | – | LIPA | 114 |
| Rosario | 212 | 19.3% | 29.7% | 4.7% | 1.4% | 31.6% | 0.5 | 8.9 | – | 0.9% | – | 1.8% | 0.9% | LIPA | 115 |
| Brazil | | | | | | | | | | | | | | | |
| North/northeast | 66 | 31.0% | 50.0% | – | – | – | – | – | 18.2% | – | – | – | – | PCR | 116 |
| Southeast | 548 | 26.7% | 42.2% | – | 2.5% | – | – | – | 27.9% | – | 0.7% | – | – | PCR | 116 |
| South | 85 | 27.0% | 24.7% | – | 3.5% | – | – | – | 44.7% | – | – | – | – | PCR | 116 |
| São Paulo | 423 | 24.6% | 39.7% | – | 3.1% | – | – | – | 32.6% | – | 0.9% | – | – | PCR | 116 |
| Brazil | 705 | 27.2% | 40.8% | – | 2.4% | – | – | – | 29.0% | – | 0.6% | – | – | PCR | 116 |
| Chile | | | | | | | | | | | | | | | |
| Santiago | 164 | 3.0% | 73.8% | – | 1.2% | – | – | 20.7% | – | – | 1.2% | – | – | RFLP | 117 |
| Puerto Rico | 35 | 11.4% | 65.7% | – | 2.8% | – | – | 20.0% | – | – | – | – | – | RFLP | 118 |
| Venezuela | 122 | – | – | 66.0% | 20.0% | – | – | – | 2.5% | 0.8% | – | 10.0% | – | RFLP | 119 |
| Dominican Rep. | 33 | 59.5% | 3.6% | – | – | 7.1% | 2.4% | – | – | – | – | 19.0% | 5.9% | ? | 120 |

## HIV-positive patients

The detected prevalence of anti-HCV antibodies in HIV-infected patients varies according to the risk factors involved for HCV and HIV infection and according to the serological assay used. In Brazil this co-infection varies between 8.02% and 53.8% in three different groups of patients, according to different reports [34–37]. Another Brazilian study showed that 68.8% of HIV/HCV-co-infected patients were intravenous drug users, 15.5% were homosexual males, 13.3% were the sexual partners of HIV/HCV-infected patients without a history of IVDU or transfusion and 2.2% had received transfused blood [28].

In Buenos Aires, Argentina, the prevalence of serum anti-HCV in this group of patients was 72.4% [31]. Another report from Argentina has shown that 72.0% of HIV/HCV patients were IV drug users, 34% were homosexual and 66% had promiscuous sexual habits [38].

## Patients with chronic renal disease

Patients with chronic renal disease on haemodialysis programmes or after renal transplantation also constitute a group at high risk for HCV infection. The seroprevalence of anti-HCV antibodies in this group of patients has been shown to vary between 7.0% and 48.1% in different reports from Brazil [2,39]. In Chile the seroprevalence is 29.8% [40]. In Lima, Peru, it is 61.0% [27] and in Cuba it is 34.8% [41].

## Alcoholism

Alcoholism is common among HCV-infected patients. In Brazil this association has been reported to be vary between 12.2% to 25.7% and 27.7%, according to different reports [42–44]. In others countries of Latin America this association has been reported to be 16.0% in Tucuman, Argentina [45], and 17.0% in Santiago, Chile [26].

## Schistosomiasis

Data from Brazil shows a high prevalence of HCV infection in patients with schistosomiasis. This association may be caused by previous blood transfusion or surgery [46–48].

## Pregnancy

The prevalence of anti-HCV antibodies in pregnancy varies all over the world and the same seems to happen in Latin America. Data from Manaus, Brazil shows the prevalence of anti-HCV antibodies to be 0.6% in this group of patients [49]. In Buenos Aires, Argentina, the prevalence of anti-HCV antibodies has been reported to be 2.6% [50]. In Santiago, Chile, the prevalence has been reported to be 1.9% [26].

## Hepatocellular carcinoma and HCV

HCV infection may lead to chronic liver disease,

cirrhosis and hepatocellular carcinoma. In Brazil, HCV infection has been demonstrated in 26.9% of patients with hepatocellular carcinoma [51]. This association varies in different geographic areas of Brazil. If this association is analysed according to these areas, we can observe that it may vary between 12.5% in Rio Grande do Sul (south Brazil), to 45% in Bahia (northeast Brazil). In Chile this association has been reported to be 49% [26].

## HCV genotypes

The prevalence of different HCV genotypes in some countries in Latin America is shown in Table 7. The most frequently identified genotype is type 1b in Argentina, Brazil, Chile and Puerto Rico, followed by genotypes 1a and 3. Genotype 2 was identified in 25% of cases in Argentina and Venezuela, and genotype 3 has been identified in 44.7% of cases in some areas in Brazil. Data from Argentina shows that genotype 3a was the most frequent in IVDU, either infected or not infected with HIV [52–53], confirming previous results from western countries.

## REFERENCES

1. Mazzur S, Nath N & Fang C. Distribución de marcadores de virus da hepatite B (VHB) en la sangre de donantes de 13 paises del hemisférico occidental: actas del taller latinoamericano de la Cruz Roja sobre hepatitis. *Boletim da Oficina Sanitária Panamericana* 1980; 89:239–248.
2. Carrilho FJ & Silva LC. Epidemiologia. In *Hepatites Agudas e Crônicas*, 1995; pp. 73–95. Edited by LC Silva. São Paulo: Sarvier.
3. Carrilho FJ, Baldy JLS & Takata PK. Prevalence and study of asymptomatic carriers of hepatitis B surface antigen in blood donors in Londrina, South of Brazil. *Gastroenterologia Endoscopia Digestiva, S Paulo* 1984; 3:13–20.
4. Focaccia R. Etio-epidemiologia das hepatitis virais tipo A e B. Contribuiçao ao estudo da prevalência e risco de contágio em funcionários hospitalares. Tese de Mestrado, 1982. Faculdade de Medicina da Universidade de Sao Paulo, Brasil.
5. Brotman B, Prince AM & Godfrey HR. Role of arthropods in transmission of hepatitis B virus in the tropics. *Lancet* 1973; 1:1305–1308.
6. Granato C, Amato Neto V & Moreira AAB. Importância de triatomídeos na transmissao do vírus da hepatite tipo B. *Revista da Sociedade Brasileira de Medicina Tropical* 1986; 19:121.
7. Rosa H, Lemos ZP & Porto JD. Role of triatoma (cone-nose bugs) in transmission of hepatitis-B antigen. *Revista do Instituto de Medicina Tropical de Sao Paulo* 1977; 19:310–312.
8. Lopes MH, Shiroma M, Carrieri GCB, Ciarávolo RMC, Oba IT, Granato C, Siqueira ML & Amato Neto V. Prevalência da infecção pelo vírus da hepatite B em escolares de zona rural do Vale do Ribeira do Estado de São Paulo. *Revista da Sociedade Brasileira de Medicina Tropical* 1991; 24 (Supplement 2):156.
9. Snydman DR, Hindman SH & Wineland MD. Nosocomial viral hepatitis B. A cluster among staff with subsequent transmission to patients. *Annals of Internal Medicine* 1976; 85:573–577.
10. Silva LC, Motta E, Mano MJ & Lyra LG. Transmissao vertical do AgHBs e passiva do anti-HBs em Salvador - Bahia. *Anais da IX Jornada Latino Americana de Hepatologia*. São Paulo, Brasil, 1986.
11. Organizacion Mundial de la Salud. Progress en el estudio de la hepatitis vírica. *Série de Informes Técnicos*, 1977, Genebra no. 602:3–69.
12. Velasco M. New information, new problems in viral hepatitis. A rapid literature review. *Hepatology* 1978; 6:1–3.
13. Mendes TF, Cruz PRS & Pitella AMM. Transmissao sexual do vírus da hepatite B. *Moderna Hepatologia* 1982; 7:1–6.
14. Carrilho FJ. Estudo comparativo da prevalência de marcadores do vírus da hepatite B (AgHBs e anti-HBs) em familiares de hepatopatas crônicos AgHBs-positivos de ascendência oriental (japonesa) e ocidental. Dissertação de Mestrado. 1987. Faculdade de Medicina da Universidade de São Paulo, Brasil.
15. Carrilho FJ, Gayotto LCC, Silva LC, Fonseca LEP, Cançado ELR. Sexual transmission of HBV within Brazilian spouses of oriental and occidental origin. *Acta Hepatologica* 1991; 1:25.
16. Ono-Nita SK. Comportamento da infecção pelo vírus da hepatite B em grupos familiares de origem oriental e ocidental. Dissertação de Mestrado. 1995. Faculdade de Medicina da Universidade de São Paulo, Brasil.
17. Barone AA. Prevalência do estado de portador e de formas graves de hepatite por vírus B em três famílias de pacientes de origem oriental. Tese de Doutoramento. 1986. Faculdade de Medicina da Universidade São Paulo, Brasil.
18. Tengan FM. Fatores de risco associados à infecção pelo vírus da hepatitite C. Tese de Doutoramento. 1997. Faculdade de Medicina da Universidade de São Paulo, Brasil.
19. Mendes LCA, Carrilho FJ, Silva LC, Fonseca LEP, Cançado ELR, Alves VAF, Deguti MM, Laudanna AA & Gayotto LCC. Hepatite crônica C. Dados epidemiológicos de uma casuística de 404 pacientes. *Gastroenterologia Endoscopia Digestiva, S Paulo* 1995; 14:137. Abstract TL-1.
20. Cheinquer H, Coelho-Borges S, Fonseca ASK, Lunge VR, Ikuta N & Cheinquer N. Hepatite crônica C em Porto Alegre, RS: Aspectos epidemiológicos, laboratoriais e histológicos. *Gastroenterologia Endoscopia Digestiva, S Paulo* 1995; 16:197. Abstract PO-74.
21. Pacheco M, Bigatão AM, Figueiredo VM, Blum VF, Ferraz ML & Silva AE. Estudo comparativo entre antecedentes epidemiológicos de pacientes com hepatite crônica C e doadores de sangue anti-HCV positivos. *Gastroenterologia Endoscopia Digestiva, S Paulo* 1995; 16:197. Abstract PO-76.
22. Silva L, Paran R, Mota E, Cotrim HP, Boennec-McCurtey ML, Vitvitinky L, Padua A, Trepo C & Lyra L. Prevalence of hepatitis C virus in urban and rural population of Northeast Brazil: pilot study. *Arquivos de Gastroenterologia* 1995; 32:168–171.
23. Martins RMB, Porto SOB, Vanderborght BOM, Rouzere CD, Cardoso DDP & Yoshida CFT. Short report: Prevalence of hepatitis C viral antibody among Brazilian children, adolescents, and street youths. *American Journal of Tropical Medicine and Hygiene*

1995; **53**:654–655.

24. Focaccia R. Prevalência das hepatites virais A, B, C e E. Estimativa de prevalência na população geral da cidade de São Paulo, medida por marcadores séricos, em amostragem populacional estratificada com sorteio aleatório e coleta domiciliar. 1998. Tese de Livre Docência. Faculdade de Medicina da Universidade de São Paulo, Brasil.

25. Mattos AA, Silvério AO, Araújo FSB & Bailon CR. Estudo da prevalência de marcadores virais em hemofílicos. *Gastroenterologia Endoscopia Digestiva, S Paulo* 1997; **16**:187. Abstract PO 36.

26. Velasco M, Muñoz G, Hurtado C, Gil LC, Alegria S & Larrondo-Lillo M. Rol preponderante del virus hepatitis C en Chile como factor etiológico de daño hepático crónico. *Archivos Argentinos Enfermedades Aparato Digestivo*, 1996; **10**:89, Abstract p.161.

27. Figueroa BR, Watts DM, Sanchez JL, Sjogren MH, Chauca G, Gallahan J, Hinostrosa S, Ramos Garcia S, Carrillo L, Cárdenas R, Cabezas C, Rodriguez G & Estacio RC. Prevalencia de hepatitis C en el Peru. *Archivos Argentinos Enfermedades Aparato Digestivo*, 1996; **10**:89, Abstract p.118.

28. Mendes Corrêa MCJ, Duarte MIS, Guastini C, Barone AA. Hepatitis C in patients with the immunodeficiency virus. *5th Conference on Retrovirus and Opportunistic Infections*. Chicago, USA, 1–5 February 1998; Abstract 494.

29. Figueiredo VM, Cruz CN, Oliveira PM, Lopes EP, Silva AE & Ferraz ML. Evidência da transmissão sexual do vírus da hepatite C: estudo sorológico em cônjuges. *Gastroenterologia Endoscopia Digestiva, S Paulo* 1995; **14**:150. Abstract PO 54.

30. Brasil L, Botelho R, Castilho M, Braga W, Borborema C, Ferreira L & Fonseca JC. Estudo familiar da infecção pelo vírus da hepatite C de pacientes com doença hepática crônica tipo C. *Archivos Argentinos Enfermedades Aparato Digestivo* 1996; **10**:89. Abstract P 162.

31. Gonzalez J, Castro R, Alonso A, Cañizal R, Vasquez A, Deluchi & Benetucci J. Transmision heterosexual de HCV y HIV en parejas en riesgo de infeccion. *Archivos Argentinos Enfermedades Aparato Digestivo* 1996; **10**:59. Abstract P 101.

32. Bertolachini S, Daruich JR, Rey JÁ, Maurizi D, Barberio P, Kohan A & Findor JÁ. Seroprevalence of anti-HCV in female sexual workers. *Archivos Argentinos Enfermedades Aparato Digestivo* 1996; **10**:7. Abstract TL 3.

33. Carvalho AP, Edelenyi MP, Nogueira C, Coelho HSM & Schechter M. Prevalência do anti-VHC em população de baixo e alto risco para doenças sexualmente transmissíveis. *Anais XXXII Congresso Brasileiro de Gastroenterologia*. Natal, Brazil, 25–29 October 1992; p. 88.

34. Rocha MDC, Elias JA, Grimm L, Penteado SM, Haber IR, Tanibata PR & Lima, MPJS. Soroprevalência de HIV, hepatite B, hepatite C e sífilis em população com comprometimento de risco HIV. *Revista da Sociedade Brasileira de Medicina Tropical* 1994; **27**(Suppl. I):353.

35. Edelenyi-Pinto M, Carvalho AP, Nogueira C, Ferreira JO & Schechter M. Prevalence of antibodies to hepatitis C virus in populations at low and righ risk for sexually transmitted diseases in Rio de Janeiro. *Memorias do Instituto Oswaldo Cruz* 1993; **88**:305–307.

36. Ferraz ML, Diaz R, Yoshida C, Castelo A & Silva AE. Prevalence of hepatitis B, hepatitis Delta and Hepatitis C seromarkers in HIV seropositive patients in São Paulo, Brazil. *Scientific Meeting of International Association for Study of the Liver Diseases*. Brighton, United Kingdom, 1992; p. 175.

37. Gonçalves Jr EL, Pavan MHP, Aoki FH, Lazarini MSK & Gonçalves NSL. Marcadores sorológicos para hepatite B e C em pacientes infectados pelo HIV. *Anais do IX Congresso da Sociedade Brasileira de Infectologia*. Recife, Brazil, 1996; Abstract 328.

38. Arpa A, Lischitz A, Blancat R, Romano G & Gil S. Experience in patients with human immunodeficiency virus positive serology in the medical clinic unit to Valez Sarsfield Hospital. *Revista da Associação Medica Argentina* 1995; **108**:9–16.

39. Flores AL, Mattos AA, Goldani JC, Garcia V, Garcia E, Becker M & Asquidamini S. Marcadores virais da hepatite em uma unidade de hemodiálise. *Gastroenterologia Endoscopia Digestiva, S Paulo* 1997; **16**:187. Abstract PO 46.

40. Rodriguez MI, Estay R, Soto JR, Wolff C, Plubins L, Child R & Armas R. Prevalence of hepatitis C virus antibodies in a hemodialysis unit. *Revista Medica Chilena* 1993; **121**:152–155.

41. Garcia W, Escobar MP, Rodriguez V, Falcon D & Martinez E. Prevalencia de anti-VHC en pacientes con insuficiencia renal cronica. *XXV Congreso Panamericano de Gastroenterologia*. Santo Domingo, Republica Dominicana, 17–21 Noviembre 1997; Abstract p. 40.

42. Both CT & Mattos AA. Prevalência e repercussão do vírus da hepatite C em alcoolistas. *Gastroenterologia Endoscopia Digestiva, S Paulo* 1995; **14**:149. Abstract PO 49.

43. Corrêa EBD, Meirelles CZ, Ramos Jr MT & Borini O. Prevalência dos marcadores dos vírus das hepatites B e C em etilistas hepatopatas crônicos. *Gastroenterologia Endoscopia Digestiva, S Paulo* 1995; **14**:149. Abstract PO 111.

44. Amaral ISA, Moia LJMP, Barbosa MSB, Conde SRS, Miranda ECBM, Moraes MLF, Soares MCP, Araujo M & Pinheiro MC. Análise de 141 casos de doença hepática crônica alcoólica isolada ou associada a infecção viral. *Gastroenterologia Endoscopia Digestiva, S Paulo* 1997; **16**:206. Abstract PO 112.

45. Palazzo FH, Capelli ME, Sarmiento M, Weller C, Boscarino G & Rodriguez C. Incidencia de marcadores para virus B y C en alcoholistas cronicos en una poblacion hospitalaria. *Archivos Argentinos Enfermedades Aparato Digestivo* 1996; **10**:95. Abstract P 173.

46. França AVC, Carrilho FJ, Lins ALGP, Silva LC, Santos VA, Bassit L, Carvalho AS, Alquezar AS & Laudanna AA. Marcadores séricos do vírus da hepatite C em pacientes com esquistossomose forma hepatointestinal e hepatesplênica. *Revista do Instituto de Medicina Tropical de São Paulo* 1993; **35** (Supplement 10):S39.

47. Lima RA, Domingues ALC, Magalhães V, Lucena TAL, Moura IMF, Lira EC & Guimarães RX. Ocorrência de hepatite C em pacientes com esquistossomose mansoni. Resultados preliminares. *Revista da Sociedade Brasileira de Medicina Tropical* 1992; **25** (Supplement): 17.

48. Pereira LMMB. Hepatotropic viruses and autoimmunity in schistosomiasis in Brazil. PhD Thesis. Open University of Great Britain, London, 1993.

49. Perdiz RHO, Perdiz RO, Ferreira CA, Castilho MC, Botelho R & Fonseca JC. Estudo da prevalência de infecção pelos vírus das hepatites B, C e D em gestantes. *Gastroenterologia Endoscopia Digestiva, S Paulo* 1995; **14**:148. Abstract PO 46.

50. Rey J, Daruich JR, Bruch IE, Santarelli MT, Bianchi G,

Kohan AI & Findor JÁ. HCV infection in pregnancy in the metropolitan area of Buenos Aires. *Archivos Argentinos Enfermedades Aparato Digestivo* 1996; **10**:23. Abstract P 35.

51. Gonçalves CS, Pereira FEK, Gayotto LCC & Brazilian Society of Hepatology. Hepatocellular carcinoma in Brazil: report of a national survey (Florianópolis, SC, 1995). *Revista Instituto Medicina Tropical, S Paulo* 1997; **39**:165–170.

52. Padró I, Jones D, Pagani D, Farroni A, Taborda M, Fay O, Bortolozzi R & Lupo S. Incidencia de hepatitis virales B y C en pacientes HIV positivos. *Archivos Argentinos Enfermedades Aparato Digestivo* 1996; **10**:50. Abstract P 83.

53. Campodonico M, Taborda M, Banchio C, Gramajo H, Lupo S, Bortolozzi R, Fay O & Fay F. Infección por virus C de la hepatitis en pacientes drogadictos endovenosos (IVDU): determinación de la presencia de HCV-RNA y genotipo del HCV presente en ellos. Relación com la infección por virus de la inmunodeficiencia humana (HIV). *Archivos Argentinos Enfermedades Aparato Digestivo* 1996; **10**:24. Abstract TL 38.

54. Campos EP, Colauto EMR & Curi PR. Hepatitis B investigaçao em faumacêuticos, barbeiros-manicures e dentistas da cidade de Botucatu - São Paulo. *A Folha Médica, S Paulo* 1985; **90**:93–96.

55. Moreira SDR, Pianovski MAD, Aldenucci M, Silva AC & Voss SZ. Alta prevalência de HBsAg e anti-HBcT em doadores de sangue da região sudoeste do Paraná. *Gastroenterologia Endoscopia Digestiva* 1995; **14**:173.

56. Alves JG, Tyll J, Brum A, Ezetelna H, Mello MAS, Moneró F & Hatum BM. Incidência de HBsAg em 90. 632 doadores de sangue. *Gastroenterologia Endoscopia Digestiva, S Paulo* 1998;**17**:559, Abstract PO98.

57. Azevedo RA, Silva AE, Ferraz ML, Marcopito LF & Baruzzi RG. Prevalência dos marcadores sorológicos do HBV e HDV em crianças do Parque Indígena do Xingu. *Gastroenterologia Endoscopia Digestiva* 1995; **14**:141.

58. Bensabath G & Boshell J. Presença do antígeno 'Austrália' em populaçoes do interior do Estado do Amazonas, Brasil. *Revista do Instituto de Medicina Tropicalde Sao Paulo* 1973; **15**:284–288.

59. Findor KA, Igartua EB & Domecq P. Epidemiologia de la hepatitis viral em Buenos Aires. *VIII Jornadas Latino Americanas de Hepatologia.* Lima, Perú, 1983. Abstract 25.

60. Findor KA, Igartua EB & Domecq P. Epidemiologia de la hepatitis viral en Buenos Aires. *Boletim da Sociedade Latino Americana de Hepatologia*, 1984; p.5, Abstract.

61. Organizaçao Pan-Americana da Saude. 1985. *Hepatitis in the Americas.* PAHO collaborating group.

62. Koff RS, Pannuti CS & Pereira MLG. Hepatitis A and non-A, non-B viral hepatitis in Sao Paulo, Brazil: epidemiological, clinical, and laboratory comparisons in hospitalized patients. *Hepatology* 1982; **2**:445–448.

63. Pannuti CS, Mendonça JS & Pereira MLG. Sporadic acute viral hepatitis A, B and non-A, non-B. A prospective study of 150 consecutive cases in Sao Paulo, Brazil. *Tropical and Geographical Medicine* 1985; **37**:136–138.

64. Pannutti CS, Pereira M, Hansson B, Feinstone SM, Dienstag JL & Koff RS. Epidemiological-clinical studies of hepatitis A and non-A, non-B viral hepatitis in Sao Paulo, Brazil. *Gastroenterology* 1980; **78**:1315, Abstract.

65. Silva LC, Carrilho FJ & Chavez BA. Frequency of A, B and non-A, non-B hepatitis in Sao Paulo liver unit. *Gastroenterology* 1983; **84**:1369.

66. Silva LC, Carrilho FJ & Di Pietro A. Epidemiological aspects of acute viral hepatitis in Sao Paulo, Brasil. *Revista do Instituto de Medicina Tropical de São Paulo* 1986; **28**:400–405.

67. Lyra LG, Rebouças G & Fontes F. Australia antigen in acute hepatitis and leptospirose in Salvador, Bahia. *Revista do Instituto de Medicina Tropical de São Paulo* 1975; **17**:361–367.

68. Fonseca JCF, Simonetti, SR & Tavares AM. Aspectos epidemiológicos da infecçao pelo vírus da hepatite delta (HDV) e portadores assintomáticos do vírus da hepatite B (HBV) no Estado do Amazonas, Brasil. *Revista da Sociedade Brasileira de Medicina Tropical* 1986; **19**:120.

69. Velasco M, Puelma E & Katz R. Marcadores virales de la hepatitis aguda: estudio de 291 niños y adultos en Chile. *Revista Medicina do Chile* 1982; **110**:542–546.

70. Zacarias J, Rakela J & Velasco M. Prevalencia de los virus de hepatitis en las hepatitis agudas en niños. *Revista Chilena Pediatria* 1983; **54**:316.

71. Ljungren K, Patarroyo ME & Engle R. Viral hepatitis and delta agent in Colombia. *International Symposium on Viral Hepatitis*, California, USA, 1984; Abstract 616.

72. Villarejos VM, Visona KA & Eduarte CA. Evidence for viral hepatitis other than type A or type B among persons in Costa Rica. *New England Journal of Medicine* 1975; **293**:1350–1352.

73. Figueiroa MS & Rivas JÁ. Antigeno Australiano en pacientes con hepatitis en Honduras. *Boletim da Oficina Sanitária Panamericana* 1974; **76**:155–160.

74. Calderon E, Ridaura G. & Iegorreta J. Hepatitis infecciosa. Presencia del antígeno HBs. *Boletin Medico del Hospital Infantil de Mexico* 1975; **32**:1145.

75. Figueiroa R, Soriano C & Padron. Antigeno de superfície HB en población hospitalaria del Seguro Social del Perú - 1980. *Boletim da Sociedade LatinoAmericana de Hepatologia* 1983, p.4. Abstract.

76. Ianhez LE, Cuelar MKS & Romao JE Jr. Hepatopatia em pacientes transplantados que adquiriram o vírus B da hepatite pós-transplante. *Revista do Hospital das Clínicas da Faculdade de Medicina de São Paulo* 1985; **40**:58–61.

77. Romao JE Jr. Hepatite B em hemodiálise. *Jornal Brasileiro de Nefrologia* 1984; **6**:2–3.

78. Kopstein J, Ugalde CB & Fiori AMC. Hemodiálise e hepatite a vírus B. *Jornal Brasileiro de Nefrologia* 1984; **6**:9–11.

79. Guimarães RX. Frequência do antígeno Australia em indivíduos normais, índios do Parque Nacional do Xingu e portadores de esquistossomose mansônica. Tese de Doutoramento. 1973. Escola Paulista de Medicina - São Paulo, Brasil.

80. Lyra LG. Esquistossomose e vírus B (do início ao estágio atual). *Moderna Hepatologia* 1983; **8**:1–7.

81. Brandão-Mello CE, Gonzaga AL & Pitella AM. Hepatitis A and B virus serum markers in haemophiliacs. *Boletim da Sociedade Brasileira de Hematologia e Hemoterapia* 1985; **7**:114.

82. Mendes TF, Kutz H & Mexas PPF. Infection by the hepatitis B virus in patients of a general hospital. *Arquivos de Gastroenterologia de São Paulo* 1979; **16**:73–80.

83. Mincis M, Guimarães RX & Farinazzo Neto J. Marcadores imunológicos do vírus B da hepatite em alcoólatras e indivíduos normais. *Revista Paulista de Medicina* 1984; **102**:205–213.

84. Ferraz MLG, Vilela MP & Silva AE. Marcadores

sorológicos do VHB e anticorpo delta em homossexuais masculinos brasileiros. *Revista Paulista de Medicina* 1985; **103**:228–230.

85. Varela H, Motta E & Contrin H. Importância do comprometimento sexual na disseminaçao da infecçao pelo vírus da hepatite B e sua associaçao com doenças sexualmente transmissíveis. *Anais da IX Jornadas Latino Americanas de Hepatologia*, Sao Paulo, Brasil, 1986; Abstract 119.

86. Carrilho FJ & Baldy JLS. Prevalência do AgHbs em pessoal da área de Odontologia. *Anais do Congresso Médico da Associação Médica de Londrina,* Brazil 1979; p.15, Abstract.

87. Alvaryz FG, Ribeiro JFS, Gurfinkel S & Nogueira CM. Hepatite pós-transfusional NANB/C: positividade do anti-HCV em 47 casos. *Anais XXXII Congresso Brasileiro de Gastroenterologia*. Natal, Brazil, 25–29 October, 1992; Abstract 87.

88. Carrilho FJ, Porta G, Antonelli R, Deperon S, Carvalho J, Alquezar AS & Silva LC. Estudo dos marcadores do vírus da hepatite B em familiares de pacientes com hepatite crônica B. *Anais do Il Simposium Internacional Hispanoparlante de Hepatologia*. Cocoyoc, México, 1985; p.71. Abstract.

89. Daruich JR, Rey JA, Pinchuk L, Bruch Igartua E, Zeilicoff R, Michelini J, Manero E, Palermo C, Sordá J, Ameijeiras B, Nakatsuno M & Findor JA. Prevalencia de marcadores sericos del HCV en poblacion general en Buenos Aires, Argentina. *Archivos Argentinos Enfermedades Aparato Digestivo* 1996; **10**:73. Abstract TL 09.

90. Perez-Bianco R & Santarelli MT. Analysis of a aational serological survey for diseases transmitted by blood transfusion. *Medicina, B Aires* 1993; **53**:491–496.

91. Brandão ABM, Torres R, Oliveira BR, Coral GP, Magalhães RB & Bredemeir M. Prevalência do anti-VHC (Elisa-II) em doadores de sangue e sua correlação com os níveis de ALT e com o anti-HBc. Porto Alegre, Rs. *Gastroenterologia Endoscopia Digestiva, S Paulo* 1995; **14**:147. Abstract PO-41.

92. Lopes MH, Cavalheiro NP, Suematsu S & Barone AA. Infecção pelo vírus da hepatite C em marcadores de área do vale do Ribeira, São Paulo. *Revista da Sociedade Brasileira de Medicina Tropical* 1994; **27**(Supplement I): 384.

93. Pereira JL, Lousada NA, Tarnapolsky A & Frederick CJ. Anti-HCV por método ELISA II em doadores de sangue na cidade do Rio de Janeiro. *Anais XXXII Congresso Brasileiro de Gastroenterologia*. Natal, Brazil, 25–29 October 1992; Abstract 88.

94. Martins RBM, Vanderborght BOM, Rouzere CD, Santana CL, Santos CO, Mori DN, Ferreira RG & Yoshida CFT. Anti-HCV related to HCV PCR and risk factors analysis in a blood donor population of Central Brazil. *Revista do Instituto de Medicina Tropical de São Paulo* 1994; **36**:501–506.

95. Silva MC, Gomes MC, Rodrigues GM & Leite MLCB. Positive serology in blood donors in the Federal District (Brazil). *Revista de Saude do Distrito Federal* 1996; **7**:13–25.

96. Garbes Netto PG & Yoshida CT. Considerações sobre a prevalência da infecção pelo vírus da hepatite C. *Revista da Sociedade Brasileira de Medicina Tropical* 1994; **27** (Supplement I): 380.

97. Stabnov IM, Stabnov LMD, Esberard EBC & Peçanha AJ. Vírus da hepatite C. *Jornal Brasileiro de Medicina* 1996; **71**:62–76.

98. Fonseca JCF. Prevalência dos marcadores do VHB nos

índios Ticuna (Alto Solimoes). Amazonas 1986. Personal communication.

99. Gayotto LCC. Soro epidemiologia da hepatite pelo vírus B: experiência brasileira. *Revista Paulista de Medicina* 1985; **103**:219–221.

100. Fay O, Schatzmayer H, Visona C, Brahn J, Garrassini, N, Russi C, Rey J & Chiera A. Prevalence of HCV antibodies in Latin America. *Hepatology* 1994; **19**:601

101. Saez-Alquezar A. Hepatite C. Aspectos epidemiológicos e metodologias. *Anais do I Simpósio Nacional de Hepatite C*. São Paulo, Brazil, 24–25 May, 1996: pp. 12–21.

102. Silva HC, Giaconi XP & Vargas CM. Hepatitis C virus. *Boletin do Hospital San Juan de Dios* 1991; **38**:148–154.

103. Galban EG, Padron G, Arus ES, Gonzalez O, Rodrigues Z, Mora S & Brito M. Antibodies against the hepatitis C virus. Study in blood donors. Cuba, 1991. *Gastroenterologia y Nutrición, Caracas* 1992; **46**:10–14.

104. Fano RV, Gonzalez OM, Longres AM & Perez MH. Prevalence of hepatitis C virus antibodies in a blood bank. *Revista de Cuba Med Mil* 1995; **24**:94–96.

105. Galvan EG, Collado FM & Mora S. Seroprevalence of hepatitis C virus in different population groups and associated risk factors, Cuba 1991. *Revista Cubana de Medicina General Integral* 1993; **9**:52–62.

106. Talarmin A, Kasanji M, Cardoso T, Pouliquen JF, Sankale-Suzanon J & Sarthou JL. Prevalence of antibodies to hepatitis A, C and E viruses in different ethnic groups in French Guiana. *Journal of Medical Virology* 1997; **52**:430–435.

107. Grispan SK & Grave de Peralta L. Seroprevalence of hepatitis B and C in blood donors. *Revista de Medicina de Honduras* 1993; **61**:42–44.

108. Vinelli E, Visona K & Nuila L. Prevalence of hepatitis C virus and other viral markers in volunteer blood donors of the Cruz Roja Hondurena. *Revista de Medicina de Honduras* 1990; **58**:166–169.

109. King SD, Dodd RY & Haynes AG, Grace A, Wynter HH, Sullivan MT, Searjeant GR, Choo KE & Michael E. Prevalence of antibodies to hepatitis C virus and others markers in Jamaica. *West Indian Medical Journal* 1995; **44**:545–557.

110. Guerrero JFR, Castaneda A & Rodriguez MM. Prevalence and risk factors associated to hepatitis C in blood donors in Durango, Mexico. *Salud Publica Mexicana* 1996; **38**:94–100.

111. Hyams KC, Phillips IA, Tejada A, Wignal FS, Roberts CR & Escamilla J. Three year incidence study of retroviral and viral hepatitis transmission in a Peruvian prostitute population. *Journal of Acquired Immune Deficiency Syndromes* 1993; **6**:1353–1357.

112. Barham WB, Figueiroa R, Phillips IA & Hyams KC. Chronic liver disease in Peru: role of viral hepatitis. *Journal of Medical Virology* 1994; **42**:1994.

113. Muller G, Zabaleta M, Caldera LH, Bianco N & Machado IV. Hepatitis C in Venezuela. Preliminary report. *Gastroenterologia y Nutrición , Caracas* 1990; **44**:336–342.

114. Del Pino N, Fernandez JL, Silva M, Diaz Lestrem M, Tanno H, Valtuille R, Cavalli N, Marangunich L, Rendo P, Viola L & Bio Sidus. Genotipos del virus de la hepatitis C en pacientes de la Argentina. *Archivos Argentinos Enfermedades Aparato Digestivo* 1996; **10**: 22. Abstract TL 33.

115. Vanderborgth B, Campodonico M, Banchio L, Benetti S, Gramajo H, Tanno H & Fay O. Prevalencia de genotipos del virus C de la hepatitis en distintas pobla-

ciones infectadas por dicho virus. *Archivos Argentinos Enfermedades Aparato Digestivo* 1996; **10**:11. Abstract TL 12.

116. Campiotto S, Pinho JRR, Da Silva LC, Coelho HSM, Carrilho FJ, Sumita LM, Guz B, Silva AO & Bernardini P. Distribuição dos genótipos do vírus da hepatite C nas diferentes regiões do Brasil. Dados preliminares. *Gastroenterologia Endoscopia Digestiva, S Paulo* 1998; **17**:550. Abstract 64.

117. Muñoz G, Venegas M, Velasco M, Thiers V, Guglielmetti A, Lamas E, Larrondo-Lillo M, Brahm J, Hurtado C & Brechot C. Análisis de genotipos del virus hepatitis C en enfermedad hepática crónica y portadores asintomáticos en Chile. *Gastroenterologia Endoscopia Digestiva, S Paulo* 1998; **17**:562. Abstract 108.

118. Martin JR, Castro F, Rodriguez Medina JR, Perez W, Gallagher J & Torres EA. Prevalencia de genotipos de hepatitis C y respuesta a interferon alfa 2b en una poblacion puertorriqueña. *XXV Congreso Panamericano de Gastroenterologia*. Santo Domingo, Republica Dominicana, 17–21 Noviembre 1997; Abstract p. 45.

119. Pujol FH, Loureiro CL, Devesa M, Blitz L, Parra K, Beker S & Liprandi F. Determination of genotypes of hepatitis C virus in Venezuela by restriction fragment length polymorphism. *Journal of Clinical Microbiology* 1997; **35**:1870–1872.

120. Terao H, Shuto R, Nishisono A, Shichijo A, Aono H, Mifune K, Jonchong B, Montás B, Pimentel D, Castro Bella M & Solano Fernández F. *XXV Congreso Panamericano de Gastroenterologia*. Santo Domingo, Republica Dominicana, 17–21 Noviembre 1997; Abstract p. 43.

# 5

# Hepatitis B and C virus infections in Mexico: genotypes and geographical distribution in blood donors and patients with liver disease

Cosme Alvarado-Esquivel*, Ann Wyseur,
Flor de Maria Herrera-Ortiz, Lilia Ruiz-Maya,
Rosario Ruiz-Astorga, Angel Zarate-Aguilar,
Eduardo Carrillo-Maravilla, Rodolfo Herrera-Luna,
Maria del Carmen Morales-Macedo, Geert Maertens
and Lieven Stuyver

## SUMMARY

To determine hepatitis B virus (HBV) and hepatitis C virus (HCV) genotypes and the prevalence of HBV precore mutants in Mexican blood donors and patients with liver disease, we studied 516 blood donors and 235 patients with liver disease. Of the 516 donors, 386 were tested using HCV genotyping; these included 297 donors positive for anti-HCV by confirmation assay, 73 donors with indeterminate anti-HCV confirmation assay, and 16 donors with elevated alanine aminotransferase (ALT) but seronegative for HBV and HCV. The remaining 130 donors were hepatitis B surface antigen (HBsAg)-positive and were tested for HBV genotypes. Of the 235 patients with liver disease, 191 were tested for HCV genotypes. All suffered from chronic disease, and included 109 patients positive for anti-HCV antibodies by confirmation assay, 14 patients with an indeterminate anti-HCV confirmation assay, and 68 patients seronegative for HBV and HCV. A total of 106 out of the 235 patients were tested for HBV genotypes, of whom 67 had chronic and 39 acute hepatitis. Sixty-two chronic patients were seronegative for HBV and HCV, and the remaining 44 were positive for HBV markers including five chronic and 39 acute patients. We used PCR, a line probe assay (LiPA HBV; research version) and INNO-LiPA HCV II (Innogenetics, Gent, Belgium) for HBV and HCV genotyping, respectively; the LiPA HBV also allows determination of the presence or absence of precore mutants. HCV RNA was detected in 162 (43.8%) out of 370 donors having a positive or indeterminate anti-HCV confirmation assay. HCV genotypes 1, 1a, 1b, 2a/2c, 2b and 3a were found in 3 (1.9%), 28 (17.3%), 76 (46.9%), 20 (12.3%), 24 (14.8%) and 9 (5.6%) donors, respectively. Two sera could not be classified (1.2%). None of the 16 donors with elevated ALT but seronegative for HBV and HCV were HCV RNA-positive. HBV DNA was detected in 30 (23.1%) out of 130 HBsAg-positive donors. HBV genotypes A,D and F were found in two (6.7%), 13 (43.3%) and 15 (50%) donors, respectively. A mutation in the precore region (codon 28; TTG→TAG) was observed in one (3.3%) case. HCV RNA was present in 49 (26.7%) out of the 191 chronic patients studied. HCV subtypes 1a, 1b, 2a/2c, 2b and 3a were found in 5 (10.2%), 30 (61.2%), 5 (10.2%), 6 (12.3%) and two (4.1%) patients, respectively. One serum (2%) could not be classified. HBV DNA was detected in 15 (22.4%) of 67 chronic patients. HBV genotypes D and F were found in 14 (93.3%) and 1 (6.7%) patient, respectively. Only one precore mutation was observed (6.7%). HBV DNA was positive in 24 (62%) of 39 acute patients.

---

HBV genotypes A, D and F were found in three (12%), 16 (67%) and five (21%) patients, respectively. We conclude that: in Mexico most HCV infections result from genotypes 1a, 1b, 2b, 2a/2c and 3a, with 1b causing more than half of infections; HBV infections in Mexico result from genotypes D, F and A; and that HBV precore mutants are rare in Mexican blood donors and in chronically infected patients.

## INTRODUCTION

Of the seven known hepatotropic viruses (A, B, C, D, E, G and GB), HCV and HBV are responsible for most cases of chronic hepatitis, liver cirrhosis and hepatocellular carcinoma (HCC) worldwide [1–3]. HCV is a positive-strand RNA virus [4] that belongs to a third genus of the family *Flaviviridae* [5] and is made up of at least 11 types and 70 subtypes, which are not evenly spread throughout the world [6,7]. Most of the HCV infections in the Americas, Western Europe and Australia are caused by HCV types 1, 2 and 3 [4,8–14]. HCV type 3 variants are a major cause of HCV infection in India [15], while HCV type 4 predominantly circulates in African countries and the Middle East [3,13,16,17]. In Asian countries, HCV types 1 and 2 infections predominate [18–21]. HCV type 1 infection is more frequently associated with severe hepatitis than other genotypes, and most of the HCV subtype 1b infections are more resistant to interferon-α therapy than infections with other genotypes [3,14,22]. In addition, patients with HCC are frequently infected by HCV type 1 [3].

For its part, HBV is a circular, partially double-stranded DNA virus that belongs to the family *Hepadnaviridae* [23,24]. HBV was initially classified according to several antigenic determinants (a, d, y, w and r) into some 10 subtypes [23,25]. Recently, a new classification of HBV into genotypes was proposed, based on the assignment of genetic variants into six different genotypic groups, termed A, B, C, D, E and F [26]. The distribution of HBV genotypes around the world is geographically restricted. HBV types A and D are common in Europe, HBV types A and E are dominant in Africa, whereas HBV types B, C and F are prevalent in Asia and South America [7].

Little knowledge is available concerning the HBV and HCV genotypes circulating in Mexico. In addition, the frequency of HBV mutants in Mexico is unknown. This study was designed to determine the profile of HCV and HBV genotypes, and the frequency of HBV precore mutants in Mexican patients and blood donors.

## METHODS

### Blood donors

A total of 516 blood donors were studied for HBV and HCV genotyping. Serum samples were collected from 1992 to 1996 in two referral blood banks. The blood donors originated from the majority of Mexican States including five northern, 10 central and six southern States.

After serological testing, the blood donors could be grouped as follows: 297 donors positive for both anti-HCV enzyme immunoassay (EIA) and anti-HCV confirmation assay; 73 with positive anti-HCV EIA but indeterminate anti-HCV confirmation assay; 130 HBsAg-positive blood donors; and 16 with elevated ALT but seronegative for HBV and HCV.

### Patients

A total of 235 patients with liver disease were studied for HBV and HCV genotyping. Samples were collected from 1991 to 1996. The patients originated from the States of Mexico, Jalisco, Michoacan and Oaxaca. The patients were grouped as follows: 109 patients positive for both anti-HCV EIA and anti-HCV confirmation assay; 14 with positive anti-HCV EIA but indeterminate anti-HCV confirmation assay; 68 seronegative for HBV and HCV; and 44 positive for HBV markers. Of the latter, 39 patients suffered from acute hepatitis; they originated from seven indigenous villages of Oaxaca State. The remaining five HBV patients suffered from chronic liver disease (Table 1).

### Serological tests

Serum samples were analysed by a second generation HCV EIA (Abbott Diagnostics) for HCV antibodies. HCV EIA-positive samples were further analysed by INNO-LIA HCV III (Innogenetics) or RIBA-2 (Chiron Corporation, Emeryville, California, USA) for confirmation of anti-HCV antibodies. Serum HBV markers were detected by commercially available EIA kits for HBsAg, anti-HBs antibodies (HBsAb), HBeAb, immunoglobulin M (IgM) HBcAb, IgG HBcAb and HBeAg (Abbott Diagnostics).

### HCV RNA detection and genotyping

HCV RNA in serum was detected by reverse transcription–nested PCR (RT–PCR) as reported elsewhere [10]. Briefly, RNA was extracted from 50 μl of serum by a modification of a previously described method [27]

Table 1. Diagnosis and serological profiles of the patients with liver disease studied

| Serology | Diagnosis | | | | Total |
| --- | --- | --- | --- | --- | --- |
| | Acute hepatitis | Chronic hepatitis | Cirrhosis | HCC* | |
| Positive anti-HCV confirmation assay | 0 | 77 | 28 | 4 | 109 |
| Indeterminate anti-HCV confirmation assay | 0 | 13 | 1 | 0 | 14 |
| Seronegative for HCV and HBV | 0 | 52 | 16 | 0 | 68 |
| Positive for HBV markers | 39 | 3 | 2 | 0 | 44 |
| Total | 39 | 145 | 47 | 4 | 235 |

*HCC, hepatocellular carcinoma.

using TRIzol LS reagent (Gibco BRL). The primers used were complementary to the 5′-untranslated region (UTR) of the different HCV types. RNA was transcribed to cDNA and then amplified by RT–PCR under the following conditions: 40 cycles at 95°C for 1 min, 50°C for 1 min and 72°C for 1 min. PCR products were separated on 2.5% agarose gels, stained with ethidium bromide and visualized by UV illumination.

HCV genotyping was carried out by INNO-LiPA HCV II (Innogenetics) as reported earlier [6]. This method allows the genotyping of seven major HCV types and at least 22 subtypes. All positive serum samples for HCV types 1 and 2 were further analysed by 5′UTR/core LiPA (Innogenetics) as described previously [28]. These methods allow correct genotyping of HCV type 1 and HCV type 2 into subtypes 1a, 1b, 1c, 1d, 6a, 7a and 9a, and subtypes 2a, 2b and 2c, respectively [28]. The RT–PCR conditions used were: 40 cycles at 94°C for 1 min, 45°C for 1 min and 72°C for 1 min.

### HBV DNA detection and genotyping

HBV DNA was extracted from 10 µl of serum. An equal volume of 0.2 M NaOH was added, and the solution was incubated at 37°C for 60 min at room temperature. Thereafter, 20 ml of 0.1 M HCl was added and the solution was centrifuged at $14000\times g$ for 15 min. HBV DNA in the supernatants was subsequently amplified with pre-S and core primers [7] by nested PCR under the following conditions: 40 cycles at 95°C for 1 min, 45°C for 1 min and 72°C for 1 min.

HBV genotyping was performed by a research version of LiPA HBV (Innogenetics). This method permits the genotyping of the six HBV genotypes, and allows detection of HBV precore mutants at codon 28 (TGG→TAG), codon 29 (GGC→GAC) and codon 28 plus 29 (TGGGGC→TAGGAC).

### Statistical analysis

The significance of the differences between the groups was determined by the $\chi^2$ test and by the Mann-Whitney U test. $P<0.05$ was considered significant.

## RESULTS

### Blood donors: HCV and HBV genotypes

Out of the 297 blood donors positive for both anti-HCV EIA and anti-HCV confirmation assay, 156 (52.5%) were HCV RNA-positive. Six (8.2%) out of the 73 blood donors with indeterminate anti-HCV had detectable HCV RNA. None of the 16 blood donors with elevated ALT, but seronegative for HBV and HCV, were HCV RNA-positive. Overall, HCV RNA was detected in 162 (43.8%) out of the 370 blood donors showing HCV antibody markers. Sera of all 162 blood donors were genotyped. Thirty out of the 130 HBsAg-positive blood donors were HBV DNA-positive.

HBV type F and HBV type D were predominant, followed by HBV type A. One blood donor (3.3%) with HBV type F infection showed a precore stop codon mutation at codon 28 (Table 2).

### Patients: HCV and HBV genotypes

Forty-five (41.3%) out of the 109 anti-HCV-positive patients were HCV RNA-positive. Two (14.3%) out of the 14 patients with indeterminate anti-HCV had detectable HCV RNA. Two (2.9%) out of the 68 patients seronegative for HBV and HCV were HCV RNA-positive. Overall, 49 (25.7%) out of the 191 patients studied were HCV RNA-positive.

Two out of the five HBV seropositive patients with chronic liver disease were positive for HBV DNA. One patient was infected by HBV type D and one patient

**Table 2.** Geographical distribution of HCV and HBV genotypes in Mexican blood donors

| Origin Region/State | Number tested* | HCV RNA+ | HCV genotypes | | | | | | | Number tested‡ | HBV DNA+ | HBV genotypes | | | Precore mutations |
|---|---|---|---|---|---|---|---|---|---|---|---|---|---|---|---|
| | | | 1 | 1a | 1b | 2a/2c | 2b | 3a | NC† | | | A | D | F | |
| **North** | | | | | | | | | | | | | | | |
| Baja California Sur | 4 | 2 | | | 1 | | 1 | | | 6 | 0 | | | | |
| Coahuila | 4 | 2 | 1 | | 1 | | | | | 1 | 1 | 1 | | | |
| Durango | 3 | 3 | | 1 | 1 | | 1 | | | 1 | 1 | 1 | | | |
| Sinaloa | 4 | 3 | | 1 | 1 | 1 | | | | 3 | 1 | | | 1 | |
| Zacatecas | 3 | 1 | | 1 | | | | | | 0 | 0 | | | | |
| **Central** | | | | | | | | | | | | | | | |
| Colima | 4 | 2 | | 1 | | | | 1 | | 4 | 0 | | | | |
| Distrito Federal | 109 | 50 | 1 | 7 | 27 | 5 | 9 | 1 | | 13 | 1 | | 1 | | |
| Guerrero | 11 | 3 | | | | 3 | | | | 5 | 2 | | | 2 | |
| Hidalgo | 9 | 2 | | | 2 | | | | | 3 | 0 | | | | |
| Jalisco | 48 | 13 | | 2 | 5 | 4 | 1 | 1 | | 6 | 1 | | 1 | | |
| Mexico | 97 | 48 | | 5 | 27 | 5 | 7 | 3 | 1 | 41 | 10 | | 4 | 6 | |
| Michoacan | 20 | 9 | | 2 | 5 | | 1 | | 1 | 2 | 1 | | | 1 | |
| Puebla | 5 | 2 | | 1 | | | | 1 | | 0 | 0 | | | | |
| San Luis Potosi | 2 | 1 | | | 1 | | | | | 1 | 0 | | | | |
| Tlaxcala | 6 | 3 | | 2 | 1 | | | | | 0 | 0 | | | | |
| **South** | | | | | | | | | | | | | | | |
| Campeche | 4 | 2 | 1 | | | | | 1 | | 3 | 1 | | | 1 | |
| Chiapas | 9 | 3 | | | | 1 | 1 | 1 | | 8 | 1 | | | 1 | |
| Oaxaca | 9 | 4 | | 1 | | 1 | 1 | 1 | | 6 | 0 | | | | |
| Quintana Roo | 6 | 2 | | 1 | 1 | | | | | 1 | 0 | | | | |
| Tabasco | 12 | 6 | | 3 | 2 | | 1 | | | 26 | 10 | | 7 | 3 | 1¶ |
| Veracruz | 1 | 1 | | | 1 | | | | | 0 | 0 | | | | |
| **Total** | 370 | 162 | 3 | 28 | 76 | 20 | 24 | 9 | 2 | 130 | 30 | 2 | 13 | 15 | 1 |
| (%) | | (43.8) | (1.9) | (17.3) | (46.9) | (12.3) | (14.8) | (5.6) | (1.2) | | (23.1) | (6.7) | (43.3) | (50.0) | (3.3) |

*Blood donors with positive and indeterminate anti-HCV confirmation assay.
†NC, Not classified.
‡HBsAg-positive blood donors.
¶One mutation was observed in an HBV type F isolate.

was infected by HBV type F. We were able to perform HBV PCR in 62 chronic patients seronegative for HBV and HCV. Thirteen (21%) out of the 62 patients were HBV DNA-positive. All 13 chronic patients were infected by HBV type D. A precore stop codon mutation was observed in one patient (7.7%) from this group with chronic hepatitis.

Twenty-four (61.5%) out of the 39 acute hepatitis B patients were HBV DNA-positive. Three (12.5%) patients were infected with HBV type A, 16 (66.7%) with HBV type D and 5 (20.8%) with HBV type F. No mutations were observed (Tables 3 and 4).

## DISCUSSION

Genotyping is important for epidemiological studies, for tracing infectious sources, and for the development of reliable diagnostic tests and vaccines. In this study, we investigated 516 blood donors and 235 patients with liver disease from Mexico. We observed that most of the

HCV infections in both blood donors and patients with liver disease were associated with genotypes 1b, 1a, 2b, 2a/2c and 3a, and all Mexican HBV infections were due in decreasing prevalence, to genotypes F, D and A. We did not observe regional differences in HCV genotype distribution. The distribution of HCV genotypes in Mexico is therefore more or less identical to the ones determined in the USA and South America [9,10,12], except for a markedly higher prevalence of subtype 1b infections in blood donors. With respect to the regional distribution of HBV genotypes, HBV type A was found only in two northern States of Mexico ($P<0.01$), HBV type D was found in central and southern Mexico, and HBV type F was evenly distributed throughout Mexico.

Using INNO-LiPA HCV II, we were able to determine the HCV genotypes in the vast majority of the samples tested; only three (1.4%) out of 211 samples need to be further studied by analysis of the core or NS5B regions.

These three unclassified HCV isolates were from

**Table 3.** HCV and HBV genotype distribution in patients with liver disease

| | | | | HCV RNA PCR and LiPA | | | | | | |
|---|---|---|---|---|---|---|---|---|---|---|
| | | | | HCV genotypes | | | | | | |
| Serology | Diagnosis | Number tested | HCV RNA+ | 1 | 1a | 1b | 2a/2c | 2b | 3a | NC* |
| Patients with positive anti-HCV confirmation assay | Chronic hepatitis | 77 | 33 | | 4 | 18 | 5 | 5 | 1 | |
| | Cirrhosis | 28 | 10 | | | 9 | | | | 1 |
| | HCC | 4 | 2 | | | 2 | | | | |
| | Total | 109 | 45 | 0 | 4 | 29 | 5 | 5 | 1 | 1 |
| | (%) | | (41.3) | | (8.9) | (64.5) | (11.1) | (11.1) | (2.2) | (2.2) |
| Patients with indeterminate anti-HCV confirmation assay | Chronic hepatitis | 13 | 2 | | 1 | 1 | | | | |
| | Cirrhosis | 1 | 0 | | | | | | | |
| | Total | 14 | 2 | 0 | 1 | 1 | 0 | 0 | 0 | 0 |
| | (%) | | (14.3) | | (50) | (50) | | | | |
| Patients seronegative for HBV and HCV | Chronic hepatitis | 52 | 2 | | | | | 1 | 1 | |
| | Cirrhosis | 16 | 0 | | | | | | | |
| | Total | 68 | 2 | 0 | 0 | 0 | 0 | 1 | 1 | 0 |
| | (%) | | (2.9) | | | | | (50) | (50) | |
| All patients | Total | 191 | 49 | 0 | 5 | 30 | 5 | 6 | 2 | 1 |
| | (%) | | (25.7) | | (10.2) | (61.2) | (10.2) | (12.3) | (4.1) | (2.0) |

| | | | HBV DNA PCR and LiPA | | | | |
|---|---|---|---|---|---|---|---|
| | | | | HBV genotypes | | | |
| Serology | Diagnosis | Number tested | HBV DNA+ | A | D | F | Precore Mutations |
| Patients seropositive for HBV | Acute hepatitis | 39 | 24 | 3 | 16 | 5 | |
| | Chronic hepatitis | 3 | 2 | | 1 | 1 | |
| | Cirrhosis | 2 | 0 | | | | |
| | Total | 44 | 26 | 3 | 17 | 6 | 0 |
| | (%) | | (59.1) | (11.5) | (65.4) | (23.1) | |
| Patients seronegative for HBV and HCV | Chronic hepatitis | 47 | 11 | | 11 | | 1 |
| | Cirrhosis | 15 | 2 | | 2 | | |
| | Total | 62 | 13 | 0 | 13 | 0 | 1 |
| | (%) | | (21) | | (100) | | (7.7) |
| All patients | Total | 106 | 39 | 3 | 30 | 6 | 1 |
| | (%) | | (36.8) | (7.7) | (76.9) | (15.4) | (2.6) |

*NC, not classified.

three States of central Mexico: two of them were found in blood donors from Mexico and Michoacan States, and one isolate was found in a patient from Jalisco State.

HCV subtype 1b infection was more frequent in chronic hepatitis patients (51.4%), cirrhosis patients (90%; $P<0.01$), and patients with hepatocellular carcinoma (100%) than among blood donors (46.9%). We observed a low prevalence of HCV subtype 3a infection in Mexico. As HCV subtype 3a infection is common in intravenous drug users [29], the low prevalence maybe explained by the paucity of intravenous drug users in the present study.

In this study, only 52.5% of blood donors with confirmed antibodies against HCV, and 41.3% of patients with confirmed antibodies against HCV, were HCV RNA-positive. Although such a figure was expected in blood donors, the number of HCV RNA-positive patients is certainly lower than expected [17,30]. Although the low percentage of RT–PCR-positive samples might be real, it is most likely due to a suboptimum preservation of the samples during the transportation from the different Mexican States to Mexico City.

Similarly, we observed a low number of HBV DNA-positive subjects (23.1%) in the group of HBsAg-positive blood donors.

Table 4. Overall distribution of HCV genotypes in Mexico

| Diagnosis | HCV RNA$^+$ | HCV genotypes | | | | | | |
|---|---|---|---|---|---|---|---|---|
| | | 1 | 1a | 1b | 2a/2c | 2b | 3a | NC* |
| Blood donors | 162 | 3 | 28 | 76 | 20 | 24 | 9 | 2 |
| | (%) | (1.9) | (17.3) | (46.9) | (12.3) | (14.8) | (5.6) | (1.2) |
| Chronic hepatitis | 37 | | 5 | 19 | 5 | 6 | 2 | |
| | (%) | | (13.5) | (51.4) | (13.5) | (16.2) | (5.4) | |
| Cirrhosis | 10 | | | 9 | | | | 1 |
| | (%) | | | (90) | | | | (10) |
| HCC | 2 | | | 2 | | | | |
| | (%) | | | (100) | | | | |
| All | 211 | 3 | 33 | 106 | 25 | 30 | 11 | 3 |
| | (%) | (1.4) | (15.7) | (50.2) | (11.9) | (14.2) | (5.2) | (1.4) |

*NC, not classified.

Using LiPA HBV, we were able to determine the HBV genotype in all of the samples studied. HBV type D infection was more common in acute hepatitis (66.7%), chronic hepatitis (92.3%) and in cirrhosis (100%), compared with blood donors (43.3%). (Blood donors versus chronic hepatitis patients: $P<0.01$; blood donors versus chronic and cirrhotic patients together: $P<0.01$). The frequency of HBV type F infection was higher in blood donors (50%) than that observed in acute hepatitis patients (20.8%; $P<0.05$), chronic hepatitis patients (7.7%; $P<0.01$) and cirrhosis patients (0%). (Blood donors versus chronic hepatitis and cirrhosis patients together: $P<0.01$).

We were able to obtain HBV DNA-positive results in six out of seven indigenous villages of Oaxaca. HBV type D alone was responsible for the hepatitis B infections in two villages. In three villages we found two or three HBV genotypes (D, F and/or A), and in one village the only subject tested had HBV type F infection. Overall, HBV type D infection was responsible for the majority (66.7%) of the acute hepatitis cases followed by HBV type F (20.8%) and A (12.5%). Since HBV type D was found as a single isolate in two villages (Petlapa and Tagui) and the same genotype infected the majority of subjects of the neighbouring villages, it is highly probable that the source of the HBV type D infections was located at the villages of Petlapa and Tagui.

High frequencies of HBV type D infection have been found in Belgium, France and Saudi Arabia, while a high frequency of HBV type F is predominant in Venezuela [7]. Our patients with liver disease and negative HBV and HCV serum markers were more frequently infected by HBV (21%) than by HCV (2.9%) ($P<0.01$). It is not clear why these patients had negative HBV and HCV serum markers. However, this study shows the importance of PCR testing in clarifying the cause of liver disease.

Only 38 (7.4%) out of the 516 blood donors and 85 (36.2%) out of the 235 patients studied had risk factors, suggesting that the majority of HCV and HBV infections in Mexico are community-acquired. However, in Mexico, blood donors with risk factors are excluded before donation. Therefore, the frequency of risk factors in blood donors could be underestimated.

There was no correlation between HCV or HBV genotypes and age, gender, ALT level or risk factors of the subjects studied.

In conclusion, at least three HCV types composed of at least five different subtypes and three HBV genotypes circulate in Mexico. Infection by HCV subtype 1b and HBV type D occurred more frequently in patients with liver disease than in blood donors. In contrast, HBV type F infection seemed to be associated with milder forms of hepatitis.

## ACKNOWLEDGEMENTS

This study was supported by Innogenetics, Gent, Belgium, and 1WT940072 and Eureka EU680 grants. CAE was supported by a grant of the Secretaría de Educación Pública of the Mexican Government, Mexico City, Mexico. Fred Shapiro edited the manuscript.

## REFERENCES

1. Tzonou A, Trichopoulos D, Kaklamani E, Zavitsanos X, Koumantaki Y & Hsieh CC. Epidemiological assessment of interactions of hepatitis-C virus with

seromarkers of hepatitis-B and -D viruses, cirrhosis and tobacco smoking in hepatocellular carcinoma. *International Journal of Cancer* 1991; **49**:377–380.

2. Merican I, Sherlock S, McIntyre N & Dusheiko GM. Clinical, biochemical and histological features in 102 patients with chronic hepatitis C virus infection. *Quarterly Journal of Medicine* 1993; **86**:119–125.

3. Dusheiko G, Schmilovitz-Weiss H, Brown D, McOmish F, Yap PL, Sherlock S, McIntyre N &, Simmonds P. Hepatitis C virus genotypes: an investigation of type-specific differences in geographic origin and disease. *Hepatology* 1994; **19**:13–18.

4. Choo QL, Kuo G, Weiner AJ, Overby LR, Bradley DW & Houghton M. Isolation of a cDNA clone derived from a blood-borne non-A, non-B viral hepatitis genome. *Science* 1989; **244**:359–362.

5. Francki RIB, Fauquet CM, Knudson DL & Brown F. Classification and nomenclature of viruses. Fifth report of the International Committee on Taxonomy of Viruses. *Archives of Virology* 1995; (Supplement 2):223.

6. Stuyver L, Wyseur A, Van Arnhem W, Hernandez F & Maertens G. Second-generation line probe assay for hepatitis C virus genotyping. *Journal of Clinical Microbiology* 1996; **34**:2259–2266.

7. Stuyver L, Rossau R & Maertens G. Line probe assays for the detection of hepatitis B and C virus genotypes. *Antiviral Therapy* 1996; **1** (Supplement 3):52–57.

8. Inchauspe G, Zebedee S, Lee DH, Sugutani M, Nasoff M & Prince AM. Genomic structure of the human prototype strain H of hepatitis C virus: comparison with American and Japanese isolates. *Proceedings of the National Academy of Sciences, USA* 1991; **88**:10292–10296.

9. Cha TA, Beall E, Irvine B, Kolberg J, Chien D, Kuo G & Urdea MS. At least five related, but distinct, hepatitis C viral genotypes exist. *Proceedings of the National Academy of Sciences, USA* 1992; **89**:7144–7148.

10. Stuyver L, Rossau R, Wyseur A, Duhamel M, Vanderborght B, Van Heuverswyn H & Maertens G. Typing of hepatitis C virus isolates and characterization of new subtypes using a line probe assay. *Journal of General Virology* 1993; **74**:1093–1102.

11. Kleter GE, Van Doorn LJ, Brouwer JT, Schalm SW, Heijtink RA & Quint WG. Sequence analysis of the 5′ untranslated region in isolates of at least four genotypes of hepatitis C virus in the Netherlands. *Journal of Clinical Microbiology* 1994; **32**: 306–310.

12. Mahaney K, Tedeschi V, Maertens G, Di Bisceglie AM, Vergalla J, Hoofnagle JH & Sallie R. Genotypic analysis of hepatitis C virus in American patients. *Hepatology* 1994; **20**:1405–1411.

13. McOmish F, Yap PL, Dow BC, Follett EA, Seed C, Keller AJ, Cobain TJ, Krusius T, Kolho E, Naukkarinen R et al. Geographical distribution of hepatitis C virus genotypes in blood donors: an international collaborative survey. *Journal of Clinical Microbiology* 1994; **32**:884–892.

14. Tisminetzky SG, Gerotto M, Pontisso P, Chemello L, Ruvolletto MG, Baralle F & Alberti A. Genotypes of hepatitis C virus in Italian patients with chronic hepatitis C. *International Hepatology Communications* 1994; **2**:105–112.

15. Panigrahi AK, Roca J, Acharya SK, Jameel S & Panda SK. Genotype determination of hepatitis C virus from

Northern India: identification of a new subtype. *Journal of Medical Virology* 1996; **48**:191–198.

16. Oni A & Harrison TJ. Genotypes of hepatitis C virus in Nigeria. *Journal of Medical Virology* 1996; **49**:178–186.

17. Stuyver L, Fretz C, Esquivel C, Boudifa A, Jaulmes D, Azar N, Lunel F, Leroux-Roels G, Maertens G & Fournel JJ. Hepatitis C virus (HCV) genotype analysis in apparently healthy anti-HCV-positive Parisian blood donors. *Transfusion* 1996; **36**:552–558.

18. Takada N, Takase S, Enomoto N, Takada A & Date T. Clinical backgrounds of the patients having different types of hepatitis C virus genomes. *Journal of Hepatology* 1992; **14**:35–40.

19. Wang Y, Okamoto H, Tsuda F, Nagayama R, Tao QM & Mishiro S. Prevalence, genotypes, and an isolate (HC-C2) of hepatitis C virus in Chinese patients with liver disease. *Journal of Medical Virology* 1993; **40**:254–260.

20. Ng WC, Guan R, Tan MF, Seet BL, Lim CA, Ngiam CM, Sjaifoellah Noer HM & Lesmana L. Hepatitis C virus genotypes in Singapore and Indonesia. *Journal of Viral Hepatitis* 1995; **2**:203–209.

21. Lee DS, Sung YC & Whang YS. Distribution of HCV genotypes among blood donors, patients with chronic liver disease, hepatocellular carcinoma, and patients on maintenance hemodialysis in Korea. *Journal of Medical Virology* 1996; **49**:55–60.

22. Pozzato G, Kaneko S, Moretti M, Croce LS, Franzin F, Unoura M, Bercich L, Tiribelli C, Crovatto M, Santini G et al. Different genotypes of hepatitis C virus are associated with different severity of chronic liver disease. *Journal of Medical Virology* 1994; **43**: 291–296.

23. Tiollais P, Purcel C & Dejean A. The hepatitis B virus. *Nature* 1985; **317**:489–495.

24. Pugh JC & Bassendine MF. Molecular biology of hepadnavirus replication. *British Medical Bulletin* 1990; **46**:329–353.

25. Thomas HC & Scully LJ. Antiviral therapy in hepatitis B infection. *British Medical Bulletin* 1985; **41**: 374–380.

26. Okamoto H, Tsuda F, Sakugawa H, Sastrosoewignjo RI, Imai M, Miyakawa Y & Mayumi M. Typing hepatitis B virus by homology in nucleotide sequence: comparison of surface antigen subtypes. *Journal of General Virology* 1988; **69**:2575–2583.

27. Chomczynski P & Sacchi N. Single step method of RNA isolation by acid guanidinium thiocyanate–phenol–chloroform extraction. *Analytical Biochemistry* 1987; **162**:156–159.

28. Stuyver L, Wyseur A, van Arnhem W, Lunel F, Laurent-Puig P, Pawlotsky JM, Kleter B, Bassit L, Nkengasong J, van Doorn LJ et al. Hepatitis C virus genotyping by means of 5′-UR/core line probe assays and molecular analysis of untypeable samples. *Virus Research* 1995; **38**:137–157.

29. Pawlotsky JM, Tsakiris L, Roudot-Thoraval F, Pellet C, Stuyver L, Duval J & Dhumeaux D. Relationship between hepatitis C virus genotypes and sources of infection in patients with chronic hepatitis C. *Journal of Infectious Diseases* 1995; **171**:1607–1610.

30. Van der Poel CL, Cuypers HT & Reesink HW. Hepatitis C virus six years on. *Lancet* 1994; **344**:1475–1479.

# 6  Natural history and clinical aspects of hepatitis C virus infection

## Harvey Alter

## SUMMARY

Hepatitis C virus (HCV) persists in the majority of those it infects. Although acute infection usually provokes a strong antibody response, neither humoral nor cell-mediated immune responses appear sufficient to clear the virus in the majority of cases. This can be explained, in part, by the selection of quasispecies that are not neutralized by antibodies raised against the original infectious strain of the virus. Despite viral persistence, disease manifestations are minimal in the majority of infected subjects. The paradox of HCV infection is that the disease seems clinically benign in the majority of carriers and yet serious and sometimes fatal outcomes are repeatedly documented. The factors that place HCV-infected individuals at most risk of progressing to severe liver disease are not yet clear, but might include age at time of infection, genetic susceptibility, cofactors such as alcohol, or viral factors such as the infecting dose, the array of quasispecies or the viral genotype. The most clearly documented contributor to severe outcome is alcoholic liver injury superimposed on viral injury; the net deleterious effect might be more than additive. Long-term prospective studies indicate that, within the first two to three decades of HCV infection, only a minority of individuals (<20%) will have serious outcomes (clinical cirrhosis, hepatocellular carcinoma (HCC) or end-stage liver disease). Although the proportion with severe liver disease will increase with time, it is probable that the lifespan of the majority of HCV-infected adults will be unaffected by this generally indolent and slowly progressive infection.

## PERSISTENCE OF INFECTION

HCV commonly causes a persistent infection and chronic hepatitis. The estimated risk of progression to chronic hepatitis in HCV-infected individuals varies between studies, but most indicate that 60–80% of people infected develop chronic hepatitis and that a still higher proportion have persistent viraemia. In prospective studies at the National Institutes of Health

(NIH), Maryland, USA [1], 85% of patients were found to be chronically infected and 15% appeared to resolve their infection, as indicated by long-term loss of HCV RNA and normalization of alanine aminotransferase (ALT) levels. There is now some early evidence that a small proportion of patients who are chronically HCV infected might spontaneously resolve the infection.

The resolution of HCV infection was also examined in an NIH study of asymptomatic individuals found to be anti-HCV positive at the time of blood donation [2]. This study included 248 anti-HCV-positive, recombinant immunoblot assay (RIBA) confirmed donors, who were followed for at least 9 months. Approximately 15% of donors had specific anti-HCV antibody, but no detectable viraemia and no evidence of liver disease, suggesting recovery from a previous HCV infection. Hence, studies both in prospectively followed transfusion recipients and in blood donors lead to the same proportion of people who recover (15%) or become chronically infected (85%). In those people followed prospectively from the time of exposure, the incubation period, degree of elevation of the ALT level and extent of viraemia were not predictive of whether the infection would resolve or become chronic.

The reason for HCV persistence in the majority of infected individuals is not fully understood. However, it is clear that the lack of immunological control of the infection is not a consequence of failure to raise antibodies. Indeed, a variety of HCV-specific antibodies usually develop. These antibodies are directed against multiple antigens derived from coding regions along the entire HCV genome. Although these antibodies provide useful targets for diagnostic tests, they do not contain the virus sufficiently to prevent persistent infection.

Since readily detectable antibodies against HCV do not seem to be protective, considerable effort has been expended to measure neutralizing antibody responses. These studies have used chimpanzees and short-term culture systems as models of infectivity. The most extensive work has involved the mixture of infectious inocula of known HCV strain (early acute-phase H strain) with serum from the same patient taken at various time points during the course of chronic HCV infection [3]. The mixture was then inoculated into chimpanzees and infectivity assessed in this model. Initially, it was shown that serum derived 9 years after the acute infection could not neutralize the HCV strain that was present at the time of acute infection. Furthermore, it was shown by cloning and sequencing that an animal that had been infected with one strain of HCV and had then recovered could be re-infected not only with a different HCV strain, but even with the same strain [3]. These experiments suggested that protective antibodies did not develop during the course of HCV infection. However, subsequent studies in the chimpanzee showed that neutralizing antibodies did form, but that they were highly strain-specific and could not block the emergence of alternative strains that resulted in persistent infection. Similar conclusions were derived from *in vitro* studies that measured the binding and entry of HCV into immortalized lymphocyte or other cell lines [4]. These studies showed that HCV-infected patients could develop antibodies that blocked the adherence and uptake of HCV into tissue culture cells. Again, these responses were transient and highly strain-specific. Studies of cell-mediated immunity have been still more difficult, but a similar conclusion has been reached. Lymphocytes derived from HCV-infected liver have been shown to react with HCV in a similar strain-specific manner [5].

The current concept is that specific neutralizing and cell-mediated responses to HCV do occur, but they generally cannot eradicate the infection. Instead, the immune pressure selects for another strain of the HCV quasispecies, which then emerges as the predominant strain. In this manner, the virus continues to elude the immune response and maintains a persistent infection despite demonstrable neutralizing and cytotoxic immune responses. In the final analysis, the ability of the virus to mutate rapidly and to exist simultaneously as multiple closely related, but immunologically distinct, variants (a quasispecies) allows it to evade immune surveillance and to establish persistent viraemia in the majority of infected individuals.

## NATURAL HISTORY OF INFECTION

Given that HCV often persists in association with chronic hepatitis, it is appropriate to consider the natural history of the infection. The potential course of HCV infection is well illustrated by a Japanese patient who underwent serial liver biopsies during the course of progressive hepatitis C [6]. This individual received a blood transfusion and 2 months later experienced acute hepatitis, which was confirmed by liver biopsy. Over the course of the next 18 years, liver biopsies documented the progression from acute hepatitis to HCC with intervening sequential stages of chronic persistent hepatitis, chronic active hepatitis, active hepatitis with bridging fibrosis, and cirrhosis. This case depicts what is now considered to be the classical sequence of clinical and histological events that occur during the natural history of HCV infection: slowly progressive hepatocellular inflammation that evolves in stages to the culminating events of cirrhosis and HCC.

Although this classical sequence provides a useful basic reference, it does not indicate the proportion of infected people who follow this course, nor the characteristics of the infected individual or of the virus that might alter this natural history and result in more benign outcomes. Several studies have therefore been designed to characterize the natural history of HCV infection in more detail and to identify prognostic parameters that might predict disease outcome.

Several studies have demonstrated both the marked variability and the potential severity of disease outcome. At the NIH, we conducted a study in which 39 individuals with histologically confirmed transfusion-associated hepatitis C were followed for up to 20 years. At the initial biopsy, 69% had mild-to-moderate chronic active hepatitis, 8% had chronic persistent hepatitis, 10% had cirrhosis and 13% had severe chronic active hepatitis. Follow-up biopsies were obtained 1–5 years later in 20 of these individuals, at which time 30% had improved histology, 45% had stable histology and 25% had progressive liver disease. Combining the initial and follow-up biopsies, eight patients (20%) developed cirrhosis. Of the eight patients with cirrhosis, three died of HCV-induced liver failure, three developed severe liver disease, but died of their underlying heart disease before the onset of liver failure, one died of unrelated causes 10 years after biopsy documentation of cirrhosis and had no clinical evidence of liver disease at the time of death, and one has survived for 20 years after the histological documentation of cirrhosis without clinical evidence of liver disease. The dichotomy between severe and seemingly benign outcomes in those with documented cirrhosis is currently unexplained, but might relate to cofactors, such as alcohol, or to host factors that are poorly defined and difficult to study.

A study in Spain [7] compared the clinical status of 211 individuals with community-acquired (sporadic) hepatitis C with that of 77 individuals with post-trans-

Table 1. Comparison of outcomes of sporadic and post-transfusional forms of chronic hepatitis C in a study in Spain

| Disease stage | Sporadic (n = 211) | Post-transfusion (n = 77) | P |
|---|---|---|---|
| Apparent remission | 13 (6%) | 8 (10%) | NS |
| Cirrhosis | 83 (39%) | 23 (30%) | NS |
| Decompensated cirrhosis | 31 (15%) | 10 (13%) | NS |
| Hepatocellular carcinoma | 15 (7%) | 2 (2%) | NS |
| Death | 20 (9%) | 3 (4%) | NS |
| Follow-up (months) | 112±51 | 120± 57 | NS |

NS, not significant.
Data from [7].

fusion hepatitis C. After a mean follow-up period of >10 years, there were no significant differences between the two groups in the severity of the clinical or histological outcomes (Table 1). This study demonstrated that the source of infection did not appear to influence clinical outcome. The trends observed were similar to the NIH study, but overall, a more severe outcome was observed over a shorter interval.

A still more severe outcome was observed among patients referred for therapy to a tertiary care centre in California, USA [8]. Among 131 patients with chronic HCV infection, 46% developed cirrhosis and 11% HCC. These high rates reflected a selection bias in that only the more severe cases were referred to this tertiary care treatment centre and might also have reflected a high proportion of Asian patients who had a disproportionately high rate of HCC. Although Asians constituted only 17% of the study group, they accounted for 36% of the cases of HCC (Table 2).

These severe outcomes need to measured against the more benign outcome of HCV infection measured in a carefully controlled, multicentre, long-term

Table 2. Types of liver disease according to race in post-transfusional hepatitis C patients referred to a tertiary care centre in California, USA

| Ethnicity | Patients | Chronic hepatitis | Chronic active hepatitis | Cirrhosis | HCC |
|---|---|---|---|---|---|
| White (77%) | 101 | 25% | 21% | 46% | 9% |
| Asian (17%) | 22 | 5% | 18% | 54% | 23% |
| African–American (8%) | 8 | 12% | 50% | 38% | 0% |
| Total | 131 | 20% | 23% | 46% | 11% |

Data from [8].

prospective study [9]. This prospective study assessed overall mortality and liver-related mortality among patients who had developed post-transfusion hepatitis in the 1970s, compared with two groups of matched controls who had been similarly transfused during open-heart surgery, but who had not developed hepatitis. After 20 years of follow-up, the overall mortality was identical among hepatitis cases and controls. There was a slight, but significant, increase in liver-related mortality in those with a history of hepatitis, but the vast majority of patients with documented HCV infection either lacked clinical, biochemical or histological evidence of severe liver disease or had died of other causes. The overall pattern suggested that although HCV infection could lead to severe liver disease, it rarely did so in the first two decades after infection. The study projected that less than 15% of HCV-infected individuals would develop cirrhosis over that 20 year interval.

The low frequency of cirrhosis during the first two decades of HCV infection has been confirmed in a large cohort study of Irish women who were inadvertently exposed to HCV from a contaminated lot of Rh immunoglobulin [10,11]. Subsequently, an investigative team headed by Kenny-Walsh (manuscript in preparation) performed liver biopsies on 376 of the immunoglobulin recipients who were HCV RNA positive 17 years after their initial exposure. While 98% had some degree of histologic inflammation, this was predominantly either minimal (41%) or mild (52%). Similarly, although some degree of fibrotic change was seen in 51%, only 2% had developed cirrhosis over this 17 year interval. Thus, the follow-up of this large cohort who were inadvertently infected with a single strain of HCV (genotype 1b) shows an even more benign outcome of HCV infection than did the multicentre transfusion study of Seeff et al. [9] Both studies indicate that the probability of cirrhosis in the first two decades is less than 15% and is considerably lower in a young population of women infected during child-bearing years compared to a population that was predominantly male and generally older than 50 when they were transfused at the time of open-heart surgery.

## PREDICTORS AND PROGRESSION OF LIVER FIBROSIS

Were it not for the potential to progress to severe hepatic fibrosis and cirrhosis, chronic HCV infection would be almost devoid of clinical symptoms and signs. It is only after significant fibrosis occurs that important clinical manifestations, including liver failure and HCC, appear. The corollary to this is that the natural or therapeutic prevention of cirrhosis would, for the most part, abrogate the clinical relevance of chronic HCV infection. Thus it is important to know the factors that predispose to and predict the development of fibrosis, the rate at which fibrosis progresses and the overall likelihood that an HCV-infected individual will develop cirrhosis within a given time span or over a lifetime. Many studies have now tried to address these issues.

Poynard [12] headed a multicentre collaborative study in France that investigated 2235 patients with biopsy proven chronic hepatitis C, none of whom had been treated with interferon prior to the time of biopsy. The study assessed the effect of nine factors on fibrosis progression. Three independent factors were associated with an increased rate of fibrosis progression: age at the time of infection that exceeded 40 years; daily alcohol consumption of 50 g or more; and male gender. There was no association between fibrosis progression and HCV genotype, the estimated duration of infection, level of viraemia, cause of infection or the histological activity grade. Using a formula that calculated fibrosis units (ratio of the fibrosis stage to the estimated duration of infection), they calculated that the median rate of fibrosis progression per year was 0.133 fibrosis units, where one unit was equivalent to one fibrosis stage. This translated to a 7.5 year interval from one fibrosis stage to the next, where stage zero was no fibrosis and stage 4 was cirrhosis. Hence, the median estimated duration of infection to cirrhosis was 30 years. The study also estimated that in the absence of treatment, 33% of patients would progress to cirrhosis in less than 20 years and 31% would never progress to cirrhosis or would not do so in less than 50 years. These conclusions are drawn from a massive database employing a standardized method of biopsy interpretation. This is a very important study in our understanding of the natural history of HCV infection.

Fattovich and associates [13] studied 384 patients in Italy with compensated cirrhosis. These patients were then followed for a mean period of 5 years. The 5 year risk for developing HCC was 7%, was 18% for decompensated liver disease and 9% for death from liver disease. Conversely, the survival probability was 91% at 5 years and 79% at 10 years. Hence, not only is the progression to cirrhosis measured in multiple decades, but even after the development of cirrhosis, further progression to fatal outcomes may take an additional decade or more. This relatively indolent natural course of cirrhosis raised the issue of whether antiviral therapy started after the development of cir-

rhosis could delay or abrogate further progression to end-stage liver disease or HCC. In the Fattovich study, 53% were treated with interferon during the period of follow-up. The estimated 5 year survival probability was 96% and 95% for treated and untreated subjects, respectively. While this study did not support the efficacy of interferon in patients with established cirrhosis, other studies examining interferon alone or in combination with ribavirin are in progress.

Serfaty [14] also looked at the rate of progression among patients with compensated cirrhosis at the time of enrolment and found more rapidly developing severe outcomes. During a median follow-up of 40 months in 103 patients, HCC developed in 11%, decompensation in 18% and liver-related mortality in 16%. The annual incidence of HCC was 3.3%. Survival probability was 96% at 2 years and 84% at 4 years. There was a significant association between severe outcomes and the serum albumin level at entry, suggesting that the more severe outcomes in this study as compared to that of Fattovich et al [13]. may have reflected more advanced cirrhosis at the time of enrolment.

Also in contrast to the Fattovich study, the probability of survival at 4 years in the Serfaty cohort was significantly better ($P < 0.0001$) in interferon-treated patients (92%) compared to patients who were not treated (63%).

## DURATION OF INFECTION AND AGE AS DETERMINANTS OF DISEASE OUTCOME

There is a need to reconcile the severe outcomes observed in some studies and the very mild clinical course demonstrated in the, large, carefully controlled prospective study of Seeff et al. [9]. Indeed, this gives rise to one of the key questions in clinical hepatology: what distinguishes those who develop clinically severe liver disease in response to HCV infection from those who do not? The answer to this is unknown, but one hypothesis is that the varying outcomes might merely reflect the indolent nature of HCV infection and the long time necessary for the evolution to cirrhosis and HCC. The long interval to disease presentation was well characterized in a study conducted in Japan [6]. Among 106 individuals with transfusion-associated non-A, non-B hepatitis, the vast majority of whom subsequently proved to have hepatitis C, the mean interval from initial infection to the clinical diagnosis of chronic hepatitis was 13.6 years, that to the diagnosis of clinical cirrhosis was 17.8 years and that to

Table 3. Interval from date of blood transfusion to clinical diagnosis of hepatitis C-related chronic liver disease in a study in Japan

| Disease status | Patients | Time after transfusion (years) (mean±SD) |
|---|---|---|
| Chronic hepatitis | 82 | 13.6 ± 8.2 |
| Cirrhosis | 17 | 17.8 ± 10.6 |
| Hepatocellular carcinoma | 7 | 23.4 ± 7.5 |

Data from [6].

Table 4. Interval from date of blood transfusion to clinical diagnosis of hepatitis C-related chronic liver disease in a study in the USA

| Time after transfusion Disease status | Patients | Years (mean ± SD) |
|---|---|---|
| Chronic hepatitis | 27 | 13.7 ± 10.9 |
| Chronic active hepatitis | 30 | 18.4 ± 11.2 |
| Cirrhosis | 60 | 20.6 ± 10.1 |
| Hepatocellular carcinoma | 14 | 28.3 ± 11.5 |

Data from [8].

the presentation of HCC was 23.4 years (Table 3). In the US based study of 131 individuals with post-transfusion hepatitis discussed previously [8], the mean intervals from the onset of infection to the diagnosis of chronic hepatitis, chronic active hepatitis, cirrhosis and HCC were 13.7, 18.4, 20.1 and 28.3 years, respectively (Table 4).

In some cases, HCV infection can remain indolent for even longer than the results of these studies suggest. This phenomenon is illustrated by an individual studied at the NIH, who was presumably infected at age 10 years, when transfused following a car accident. The patient recovered and was then asymptomatic and disease-free until age 56 years when he was found to have elevated ALT levels during a routine medical examination. A liver biopsy taken at that time showed chronic active hepatitis with bridging fibrosis, but he remained asymptomatic. At age 62 years, he volunteered to donate blood, but was excluded because he had an elevated ALT level and had antibodies to HCV. Apart from the transfusions when he was 10 years old, there had been no intervening parenteral exposures; he specifically denied additional transfusions, tattoos, acupuncture, injection drug use or work in a healthcare setting. When admitted to our study at age 62, he had splenomegaly and abnormal coagulation indices, suggesting cirrhosis with portal hypertension. After 1 year of follow-up, a sonogram revealed an intrahepatic mass that was confirmed by computer-aided tomography scanning and accompanied by a rise in α-fetoprotein, and he was found to have inoperable HCC. Hence, in this case, the presumed elapsed time from HCV infection to severe clinical outcome was 53 years.

The long interval from infection to clinical disease in this case and in the studies discussed previously raises the possibility that all HCV-infected patients might have a severe outcome if they did not succumb to intercurrent illnesses and if they were followed for a long enough period. No study has followed a large cohort of patients for a sufficient length of time to

confirm or exclude this possibility. However, many patients still have no apparent liver disease or very mild disease after 10–20 years, while others show diminishing evidence of inflammation over time, suggesting that HCV infection is not uniformly progressive and that many patients might have stable hepatitis for many decades and perhaps for their entire natural life. A small proportion could spontaneously clear HCV infection and others will clear the infection with interferon therapy or other therapeutic interventions. One important implication of the generally slow progression of HCV-related disease and the long time that elapses before severe outcomes occur is that the emphasis for treatment should perhaps be switched from adults, whose natural lifespan might not exceed the natural duration of chronic hepatitis C, to infants, children and young adults whose long anticipated lifespan might allow sufficient time for the more serious consequences of HCV infection to evolve.

In addition to the duration of infection, age at the time of infection might be an important determinant of disease outcome. There is a general impression that patients older than 50 at the time of infection have more severe chronic sequelae than persons infected at younger ages. In the Poynard study [12], age above 40 was found to be an important discriminating factor predictive of more rapid and frequent progression to fibrosis. Kage et al. [15] found that the evolution from chronic hepatitis C to cirrhosis occurred more frequently in patients aged over 50 years and that the interval to cirrhosis was 1.8 times shorter than in patients who were less than 50 years old.

An analysis of mortality from liver disease and liver cancer among 4865 haemophiliacs in the United Kingdom revealed that for patients with severe haemophilia who were not infected with HIV, the cumulative risk of death from chronic or unspecified liver disease in the 25 years from first exposure was 1.4% for all ages, 0.1% for those first exposed before age 25, 2.2% for those exposed at ages 25–44 and

44% for those first exposed after age 45. Hence, not only was the duration of infection important, but also the age at which infection was acquired, the risk increasing with increasing age.

The more rapid progression to cirrhosis in older patients sets up an interesting treatment paradox. If the rate of disease progression was the same at all ages, then one might not be inclined to treat patients over age 60–70 because of the low likelihood that they would have a deleterious hepatitis outcome before succumbing to natural causes or other underlying diseases. However, if such patients have a rapid progression to cirrhosis, then they might be strong candidates for therapeutic intervention. This dilemma will lessen as the efficacy of antiviral therapy increases and the toxicity profile decreases.

It appears that persons who were infected as young adults have a very slow progression of HCV infection. This was shown in the cohort of Irish women who were infected with a contaminated lot of anti-D immunoglobulin [10,11]. After 17 years only 2% had cirrhosis. Similarly, preliminary data from a study of air force recruits who were infected with HCV in World War II shows no excess mortality as compared to controls at least 50 years after the onset of infection (Leonard Seeff, personal communication); these patients are now being recalled for liver biopsy to determine long-term morbidity. Not much is known at present regarding the rate of hepatitis progression in non-immunosuppressed infants and children. Preliminary data suggest the rate of progression is slow, but, as noted above, this is counterbalanced by the long natural life-span that could allow sufficient time for cirrhosis to occur even if the evolution were very slow. There is critical need to do long-term follow-up studies in HCV-infected children.

## ALCOHOL AS A COFACTOR

Another possible determinant of disease outcome is the presence of a cofactor that might speed disease progression. One candidate cofactor is alcoholism. Accumulating evidence from many studies indicates that alcohol consumption considerably worsens the

prognosis of individuals who are infected with HCV. Perhaps the most graphic example of this is the Dionysos study [16]. This study involved 6917 people comprising 69% of the populations of two villages in northern Italy. This large population was first screened by ALT testing to determine the proportion of people who had evidence of hepatocellular inflammation. Those with evidence of chronic hepatitis were then evaluated for probable cause. While the most common cause of ALT elevation was excess consumption of alcohol, a relatively low proportion (3%) of alcoholic patients had cirrhosis or HCC in the absence of an associated hepatitis virus infection. The most common cause of severe liver disease was the combination of excess alcohol consumption and infection with either hepatitis B virus or HCV (Table 5). The risk of developing cirrhosis was ninefold higher and the risk of HCC 31-fold higher in those with combined alcoholic and viral liver disease, compared with those with alcoholic liver disease alone.

Corrao and Arico [17] performed a case control study of 285 cirrhotic patients who were admitted for the first time for liver decompensation. The odds ratio for developing cirrhosis (as compared to anti-HCV negative teetotallers) was 9 for anti-HCV positive, non-drinkers; 15 for anti-HCV-negative, heavy drinkers; and 147 for anti-HCV-positive, heavy drinkers. Thus alcohol and HCV interacted to make the risk markedly greater than either factor alone.

## RISK OF A FATAL OUTCOME

Based on studies conducted in my laboratory and in the published literature, it is possible to speculate about the outcome of HCV infection over the first two decades of infection. Considering an initial population of 100 HCV-infected individuals, it would appear that 85 (85%) will develop chronic infection and that 15 (15%) will spontaneously resolve their infection. Of the 85 with chronic infection, 17 (20%) will develop cirrhosis and 68 (80%) will either have stable chronic liver disease or die from unrelated causes. Of those with cirrhosis, a maximum of 75% (13 patients) will die as a result of their liver disease and the others will either

**Table 5.** Dionysos study: increased risk of serious outcome associated with excess alcohol consumption and viral hepatitis in two Italian villages

| Risk factor | Patients | Cirrhosis | HCC |
|---|---|---|---|
| Excessive alcohol intake | 707 | 20 (2.8%) | 1 (0.2%) |
| Alcohol + HBV or HCV infection | 32 | 8 (25%) | 2 (6.2%) |

Data from [16].

**Figure 1.** Estimated risk of fatal outcome within first two decades among people infected with hepatitis C

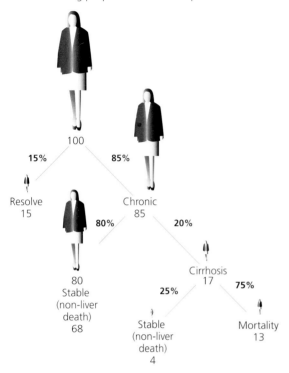

remain stable or die from unrelated causes (Fig.1). Hence, the frequency of liver-related mortality in the first 20 years of infection is only in the range of 13% in this model. In the third and subsequent decades, some patients with stable disease will presumably progress to more severe outcomes. The exact proportion cannot be accurately estimated, but if the mortality curve maintained the same slope over time, then HCV-related mortality would be less than 30% in 40 years.

In conclusion, there is no doubt that hepatitis C is a serious illness that can lead to cirrhosis, end-stage liver disease and HCC. At present, it is the leading indication for liver transplantation. Nonetheless, and paradoxically, HCV infection is also frequently asymptomatic and very benign and non-progressive over many decades. It is probable that the majority of infected individuals will succumb to other diseases or natural causes before they ever manifest any clinical evidence of their HCV infection. Except for incidental discovery, most HCV-infected individuals would never become aware of their infection and would have no clinical sequelae from that infection. It is important to hold HCV infection in this more balanced perspective so as to not unduly alarm those who have this infection as an incidental finding and to render treatment decisions more rational until highly effective therapy is developed and we can readily treat the asymptomatic carrier state as well as the disease.

## REFERENCES

1. Alter HJ. To C or not to C: these are the questions. *Blood* 1995; **85**:1681–1695.
2. Conry-Cantilena C, VanRaden M, Gibble J, Melpolder J, Shakil AO, Viladomiu L, Cheung L, DiBisceglie A, Hoofnagle J, Shih JW, Kaslow R, Ness P & Alter HJ. *New England Journal of Medicine* 1998; in press.
3. Farci P, Alter HJ, Govindarajan S, Wong DC, Engle R, Lesniewski RR, Mushawar IK, Desai SM, Miller RH, Ogata N & Purcell RH. Lack of protective immunity against reinfection with hepatitis C virus. *Science* 1992; **258**:135–140.
4. Shimizu YK, Yoshikura H, Hijikata M, Iwamoto A, Alter HJ & Purcell RH. Neutralizing antibodies against hepatitis C virus and the emergence of neutralization escape mutant viruses. *Journal of Virology* 1994; **68**:1494–1500.
5. Koziel MJ, Dudley D, Wong JT, Dienstag J, Houghton M, Ralston R & Walker BD. Intrahepatic cytotoxic T lymphocytes specific for hepatitis C virus in persons with chronic hepatitis. *Journal of Immunology* 1992; **149**:3339–3344.
6. Kiyosawa K, Akahane Y, Nagata A, Koike Y & Furuta S. Significance of blood transfusion in non-A, non-B chronic liver disease in Japan. *Vox Sanguinis* 1982; **43**:45–52.
7. Sanchez-Tapias JM, Barrera J, Costa J, Ercilla MG, Pares A, Comalrrena L, Soley F, Bruix J, Calvet X, Gil MP, Mas A, Bruguera M, Castillo R & Rodes J. Hepatitis C virus infection in patients with non-alcoholic chronic liver disease. *Annals of Internal Medicine* 1990; **112**:921–924.
8. Tong MJ, El-Farra S, Reikes R & Co RL. Clinical outcomes after transfusion-associated hepatitis C. *New England Journal of Medicine* 1995; **332**: 1463–1466.
9. Seeff LB, Buskell-Bales Z, Wright EC, Durako SJ, Alter HJ, Iber FL, Hollinger FB, Gitnick G, Knodell RG, Perillo RP, Stevens CE & Hollingsworth CG. Long-term mortality after transfusion-associated non-A, non-B hepatitis. *New England Journal of Medicine* 1992; **327**:1906–1911.
10. Power JP, Lawlor E, Davidson F, Holmes EC, Yap PL & Simmonds P. Molecular epidemiology of an outbreak of infection with hepatitis c virus in recipients of anti-D immunoglobulin. *Lancet* 1995; **345**:1211–1213.
11. Power JP, Lawlor E, Davidson F, Yap PL, Kenny-Walsh E, Whelton MJ & Walsh TJ. Hepatitis C viraemia in recipients of Irish intravenous anti-D immunoglobulin. *Lancet* 1994; **344**:1166–1167.
12. Poynard T, Bedossa P & Opolon P. Natural history of liver fibrosis progression in patients with chronic hepatitis C. *Lancet* 1997; **349**:825–832.
13. Fattovich G, Giustina G, Degos F, Tremolada F, Diodati G, Almasio P, Nevens F, Sohno A, Mura D, Brouwer JT, Thomas H, Njapoum C, Casarin C, Bonetti P, Fuschi P, Basho J, Tocca A, Bhalla A, Galossini R, Noventa F, Schalm SW & Realdi G. Morbidity and mortality in compensated cirrhosis type C: a retrospective follow-up study of 384 patients. *Gastroenterology* 1997; **112**:463–472.
14. Serfaty L, Aumaitre H, Chazouilleres O, Bonnand AM, Rosmorduc O, Poupon RE & Poupon R Determinants of outcome of compensated hepatitis C virus-related cirrhosis. *Hepatology* 1998; **27**:1443–1444
15. Kage M, Shimamatu K, Nakashima E Kojiro M, Inoue O & Yano M. Long-term evolution of fibrosis from

chronic hepatitis to cirrhosis in patients with hepatitis C: morphometric analysis of repeated biopsies. *Hepatology* 1997; **25**:1028–1031.

16. Bellentani S, Tribelli C, Saccoccio G, Soddle M, Fratti N, DeMartin C, Christianni G & The Dionysos Study Group. Prevalence of chronic liver diseases in the general population of northern Italy: the Dionysos Study. *Hepatology* 1994; **20**:1442–1450.

17. Corrao G & Arico S. Independent and combined action of hepatitis C virus infection and alcohol consumption on the risk of symptomatic liver cirrhosis. *Hepatology* 1998; **27**:914–919.

# Section II

## IMMUNOLOGY, PATHOGENESIS AND EMERGING VIRUSES

# 7

# The immunopathogenesis of hepatitis B virus infection

## Margaret James Koziel

## INTRODUCTION

Hepatitis B virus (HBV) is a major health problem in many countries, leading to disease in up to 5% of the world's population. The spectrum of HBV disease ranges from acute, self-limited hepatitis to chronic liver disease. Although the incidence of acute HBV infection is dropping in many countries due to universal vaccination programs, approximately 350 million people are already chronically infected with hepatitis B, and 1 million of these die yearly as a result of HBV-induced liver cirrhosis or cancer. HBV infection causes at least 60% of the primary liver cancer worldwide, which in many nations is one of the leading causes of cancer-related deaths.

Manifestations of disease in HBV infection are a result of a balance between host and viral factors. Immune responses, especially the cellular immune response, are important in both resolution of HBV infection and protection from disease, but also to tissue injury. For example, immunodeficient individuals who develop HBV infection appear to have both a higher rate of carriage than normal individuals and higher viral titres [1]. Similarly, prednisone and other immunosuppressive agents may result in some transient improvement in transaminitis in chronic HBV carriers, yet the subsequent level of viraemia is higher [2]. Following the withdrawal of immunosuppressive medications, there is often a flare of hepatitis, accompanied by a rebound viraemia [3,4]. However, it is also clear from animal models and human studies that the cellular immune response may play an important role in disease pathogenesis [5].

This chapter will review our current understanding of host immunity to HBV, with the goal of illuminating potential targets for manipulation of the immune response. Our current understanding of the precise role of immune responses is limited by the lack of tissue culture systems and suitable animal models in which to study disease pathogenesis. For example, although HBV will replicate in primary human hepatocytes, such cells are difficult to obtain and grow for long periods of time in culture. Thus, it is still unclear whether HBV is cytopathic, whether variants of HBV display different replication kinetics unrelated to their interaction with host factors [6], and whether the immune system can readily kill HBV-infected hepatocytes. The lack of a small-animal model in which to study HBV pathogenesis has also limited our understanding of disease pathogenesis. Although the chimpanzee can develop acute and chronic HBV infection, these studies are limited by the expense and difficulty of performing such studies outside of selected centres; the relatively mild disease that chimpanzees develop; and the limited ability to manipulate the chimpanzee immune system *in vivo* and *in vitro*. Similarly, although the duck, ground squirrel, and woodchuck models of HBV infection have provided insight into the molecular virology of HBV and are valuable test systems for candidate antiviral agents, their role in facilitating understanding of immunity against HBV is limited, because for the most part the immune system in these animals is undefined. Transgenic mice expressing HBV antigens have provided insight into mechanisms of liver cell injury [5], but because these animals express HBV antigens during the period of neonatal development, they are not suitable models for the questions of what constitutes immunity during acute infection, and what host factors permit the establishment of chronic infection.

## IMMUNE RESPONSES AGAINST VIRAL INFECTIONS

Viruses are obligate intracellular pathogens which utilize many host macromolecules during the course of the viral replication cycle. Following infection of the cell, which in the case of HBV is usually the hepatocyte but may also include other cells, a variety of cellular and humoral responses occur which are aimed at elimination of the virus (Fig. 1). Many of the earliest responses are non-specific and will not be discussed in great detail in this review. These non-specific effector

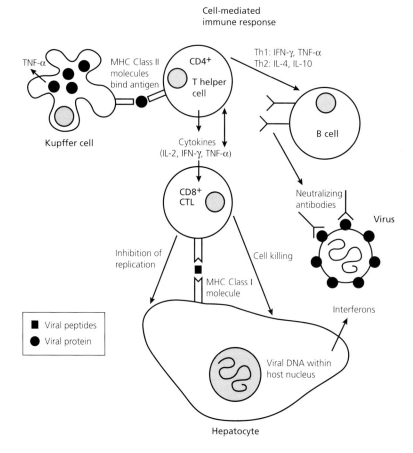

**Cell-mediated immune response**

TNF-α

Kupffer cell

MHC Class II molecules bind antigen

CD4⁺ T helper cell

Th1: IFN-γ, TNF-α
Th2: IL-4, IL-10

B cell

Cytokines (IL-2, IFN-γ, TNF-α)

CD8⁺ CTL

Neutralizing antibodies

Virus

Inhibition of replication

Cell killing

MHC Class I molecule

Interferons

■ Viral peptides
● Viral protein

Viral DNA within host nucleus

Hepatocyte

**Figure 1.** The immune response against viruses in the liver

Viral infection of an MHC class I-expressing cell, such as a hepatocyte, leads to activation of at least three arms of the acquired immune system. Release of free viral antigens leads to production of specific antibody, at least some of which is neutralizing. Viral antigens are also endocytosed by Kupffer cells, which likely serve as antigen presenting cells (APCs), which in turn present these antigens as peptides bound to the major histocompatibility complex (MHC) class II molecules. CD4⁺ cells recognise these peptide fragments and release cytokines that direct B and CD8⁺ cells. CD8⁺ and cytolytic T cells (CTLs) also recognize viral proteins as small peptide fragments bound to the MHC class I molecule on the cell surface. These CTLs can control viral replication through killing of the infected cell, as well as non-cytolytic inhibition of viral replication.

mechanisms include the interferon system, which is a family of related proteins that act against many phases of the viral replication cycle; complement, which can serve to disrupt the viral envelope and lead to enhanced opsonization of viruses by phagocytic cells; and natural killer (NK) cells, which are very primitive cells that non-specifically lead to lysis of infected cells. Few studies to date have specifically examined the role of innate immunity in determining the outcome of acute HBV infection. It is known that the type I interferons (IFN)-α and -β can effectively inhibit HBV replication [7]. Although adequate NK cell activity is likely critical in most acute viral infections, the role of these cells is not understood in HBV infection, with variable reports of either increased or decreased NK cell function in acute HBV infection [8,9]. Interestingly, there was a recent report of mutation in the mannose binding protein (MBP) of Caucasians with persistent HBV infection [10]. MBP is a lectin that is critical to innate immunity against a variety of microorganisms, including viruses, through activation of the complement cascades and phagocytosis. The large HBV surface antigen (large HBs) encoded by the

pre-S1 open reading frame contains numerous mannose oligosaccharides, and thus might be susceptible to MBP binding; a mutation in MBP might alter the relative kinetics of viral replication and the immune response. This report awaits further confirmation and examination in animal studies. Finally, non-specific activation of Kupffer cells, which are the resident macrophages within the liver, may result in the production of cytokines, such as tumour necrosis factor alpha (TNF-α), which have important effects upon viral replication and transcription.

## ACQUIRED IMMUNITY: ANTIBODY AND CELLULAR IMMUNE RESPONSES

Following these non-specific responses, immune responses which are directed specifically against viral proteins become important. In most human infections, the simultaneous function of several arms of the immune system is important in limiting viral replication. The two major arms of the immune system are the humoral arm, which consists of B lymphocytes that produce antibody; and the cellular arm, which is composed of a variety of cell types including macrophages and lymphocytes. Antibody responses are often directed against several viral proteins, although usually it is antibody responses against viral envelope proteins which serve as neutralizing antibodies. Such antibodies are particularly important in the prevention of viral infection, since they may prevent viral attachment and entry into the cells by adsorption of the viral particles. Antibodies may also enhance opsonization of viral particles by phagocytic cells, such as macrophages and neutrophils. Epitopes recognized by B cells are generally conformational and dependent on post-translational modifications such as glycosylation. Thus, neutralizing antibodies are often specific for a particular serological type of the virus, an issue which is particularly relevant in discussion of vaccine escape mutants of HBV and long-term use of anti-hepatitis B immunoglobulin (HBIg) in prophylaxis of recurrent liver disease after orthotopic liver transplantation [6]. Induction of neutralizing antibodies alone during prophylactic vaccination is often sufficient to completely prevent against many viral infections, including HBV, irrespective of whether this is the only mechanism operative in the defence against the viral infection during the course of natural infection. Some investigators believe that neutralizing antibodies are the only component of the immune system that is important in protection against viral infection, and that the cellular immune response is detrimental to the host. This is controversial, however, and evidence for the protective role of cellular immune responses will be discussed.

## CELLULAR IMMUNE RESPONSES

Once a virus has achieved entry into the cell, it is protected against antibody neutralization and opsonization, and the cellular immune system is the dominant means of limitation of viral spread. Both CD8+ and CD4+ T cells function as a result of the specific interaction of T cell receptor (TCR) with a complex consisting of processed viral protein and a major histocompatibility complex (MHC) class I or class II molecule. Thus, CD8+ T cells are restricted by the MHC class I molecule, since they only function as a result of this specific interaction, and CD4+ T cells are restricted by MHC class II. CD4+ cells play a central role in control of immune responses, by stimulating the activity of antibody-producing B cells, as well as induction of cytotoxic T lymphocytes (CTLs). CD4+, MHC class II-restricted T cells generally recognize protein fragments which are the result of endocytosis of soluble antigens and subsequent proteolysis within

acidified cellular compartments of the antigen presenting cell (APC) (reviewed in ref. [11]). Since hepatocytes do not express MHC class II molecules on their surface, during viral hepatitis the resident APC is probably the Kupffer cell, although circulating B cells may also function as APCs [12]. Recognition of viral peptides by MHC class II-restricted CD4+ cells results in the production of cytokines, which in turn regulate the activity of B and CD8+ T cells. CD4+ cells may also have cytolytic function [13], although the role of these cells in human HBV infection is not well established.

## CTLs ARE CRITICAL IN THE HOST IMMUNE RESPONSE TO VIRAL INFECTION

In animal models of viral infection, MHC class I-restricted CTLs have been shown to be an important host defence [14]. The CTL response is in fact uniquely suited to the potential clearance of viruses. As intracellular pathogens, the replicative cycle of viruses includes a phase of potential complete vulnerability to CTLs. Enveloped viruses become uncoated upon viral entry, at which point the viral genome serves as a template for synthesis of new viral proteins to be packaged into progeny virions. At the same time that new viral proteins are being produced, a process of cytoplasmic proteolysis is occurring, in which viral proteins are degraded by the proteosome complex and transported to the endoplasmic reticulum (ER) [15]. In the ER, peptides (typically 8–10 amino acids in length) associate with nascent MHC class I molecules, and are transported ultimately to the cell surface as a trimolecular complex consisting of β2 microglobulin, MHC class I and peptide. This trimolecular complex serves as a target for recognition by CTLs. Following recognition of the infected cell by the CTL, activation of the lymphocyte leads to production of perforin/granzyme complex, which results in apoptosis and death of the infected cell. Activated CTLs also express Fas ligand (FasL) on the cell surface, which interacts with Fas, a cell surface molecule. Binding of FasL to the Fas molecule, which is present in abundant amounts on hepatocytes, results in activation of another series of apoptotic molecules [16]. Upon activation, CTLs also produce a number of other soluble factors, such as cytokines, which effect viral replication and the recruitment of other cell types to the area of infection.

The most compelling evidence for a protective role of virus-specific CTLs, particularly MHC class I-restricted CTLs, comes from adoptive transfer experiments [17]. For example, in lymphocytic choriomeningitis virus (LCMV) infection, immunocompetent animals generate a brisk virus-specific CTL response which results in clearance of the virus. Mice which do not mount a CTL response (for example, those animals infected *in utero* or in the neonatal period) develop productive infection following virus challenge, and the virus persists throughout the life of the animal [18]. However, adoptive transfer of MHC class I restricted, LCMV-specific CTLs results in reconstitution of effective immunity and in the clearance of virus from these animals. The ability of CTLs to terminate an established viral infection has also been shown in a murine model of respiratory syncytial virus infection [19]. In humans, the presence of virus-specific CTLs has been associated with recovery from viral infection in both influenza and cytomegalovirus (CMV) [20,21]. In adoptive transfer experiments in humans, transfer of CMV-specific CTLs have been associated with the lack of development of CMV pneumonia [22], although the numbers of subjects are still limited. Together, these data indicate a clear antiviral effect of CTLs, and have prompted numerous laboratories to investigate the role of HBV-specific CTLs in recovery from acute infection.

## ACUTE HBV INFECTION: MECHANISMS OF VIRAL CLEARANCE

During acute HBV infection, multiple arms of the immune system are activated and probably must act in concert in order to achieve viral clearance. Coincident with the development of transaminitis during acute HBV infection, antibodies specific for HBV proteins develop [23]. The earliest antibody to appear is IgM directed against core antigen (HBcAg). This is produced by virtually all infected patients, and both IgM and IgG anti-HBc may persist for years after infection. Antibody to e antigen (anti-HBe) is not universally produced, but at least in some patients may be associated with termination of viral replication. The development of anti-HBs marks the resolution of the acute phase of the illness. This antibody is neutralizing, and presence of it alone is sufficient to protect from viral infection [24].

During acute, self-limited HBV infection there is also a vigorous CD4+ response directed against multiple epitopes within HBcAg, HBeAg and HBsAg. The precise onset of specific cellular immune responses is not known but is probably within weeks of the infection. Although both HBsAg and HBcAg are targets of the CD4+ response, HBcAg is the dominant antigen in most cases of acute self-limited HBV infection [25]. In particular, a CD4+ response against the HBcAg 50–69 epitope is present in almost all cases of acute, self-limited

HBV infection, whereas it is absent in all cases of chronic infection. The development of a vigorous CD4+, MHC class II-restricted response against core is temporally associated with the clearance of HBV from the serum, and is likely essential for efficient control of viraemia through several mechanisms. HBc-specific CD4+ cells contribute to the induction of HBV-specific CTLs, the kinetics of which parallels the CD4+ response [26–28]. In addition to activation of HBV-specific CTLs, these HBc-specific CD4+ cells may provide help to HBs-specific B cells through 'intermolecular help'. HBV env-specific B cells can bind HBV virions via the receptors for the HBs and then process the viral antigens, including HBcAg, for presentation to CD4+ cells. HBc-specific CD4+ T cells in turn can provide help via cytokine release for the env-specific B cells [29]. Production of anti-HBsAb is T-cell dependent [30], so a weak T-cell response results in a lower antibody titre. Although HBc is the dominant epitope, epitopes within HBs are also recognized by CD4+ cells from individuals with acute HBV infection but not chronic. These CD4+ response may persist for many years after the resolution of acute HBV infection, in part because of persistence of low levels amounts of antigen [31].

The mechanism whereby these CD4+ responses produce an effect is through production of cytokines. T helper (Th) cells have been broadly categorized into two subsets, which produce distinct cytokines and may influence the outcome of infection. The different subsets are defined by cytokine production: Th1 (or type 1) produce interleukin (IL)-2, interferon gamma (IFN-γ) and TNF-α and enhance cellular immunity; whereas Th2 (or type 2) produce IL-4, IL-5, IL-6, IL-10 and help B cells produce antibodies and control allergic and immunological reactions (reviewed in ref. [32]). The influence of the dominant Th response on outcome from infection is best characterized in murine models of the protozoan infection *Leishmania major* [33], although it has also been seen in bacterial, fungal and helminthic infections [34–38]. The role of polarized Th cell responses in outcome from viral infections has been studied only recently. The vigorous cellular immune response seen in acute self-limited HBV infection is accompanied by a predominant type 1 response [39], whereas T-cell clones from persons with chronic HBV infection predominantly produce a type 2 response [40]. Moreover, among chronic carriers, those with a response to IFN therapy had substantial increases in IL-12 and Th1 cytokines compared to IFN non-responders [41]. However, it is not clear why this occurs. To some extent, this is probably secondary to the host genetic background, as certain murine haplotypes preferentially express a type 1 or 2 response when immunized with HBcAg [42]. Alternatively, different HBV antigens drive different immune responses. In mice, HBcAg preferentially elicits Th1-like cells and HBeAg preferentially elicits Th0 or Th2-like cells [43].

## CTL RESPONSES IN ACUTE HBV INFECTION

CTL responses play a major role in elimination of infected hepatocytes through destruction of infected hepatocytes and non-cytolytic control of viral replication. Although CTLs are technically more difficult to characterize in the laboratory, the use of strategies to predict putative CTL epitopes in short synthetic peptides enhanced our understanding of CTL responses in HBV infection. The hallmark of persons who have acute self-limited HBV infection is the presence of a strong, polyclonal and multispecific CTL response to HBV [44,45]. During acute self-limited HBV infection, CTL responses are directed against multiple epitopes present with the core, envelope and polymerase gene products. Because of the technical method used to identify these CTLs, most of the epitopes thus far identified are recognized in the context of the MHC molecule, human leucocyte antigen (HLA)-A2.1 [28,46], although epitopes restricted by HLA-A31 and HLA-Aw68 have also been identified. In contrast to the CD4+ response, the envelope and polymerase proteins are major targets of the CTL response [28]. In part this may be accounted for by the unique antigen presentation of HBsAg, which can enter the MHC class I antigen processing pathway through two distinct routes [47]. Multiple epitopes are recognized in a majority of HLA-A2.1-positive individuals, notably core 18–27, envelope 183–191, envelope 250–258, envelope 335–343, and polymerase 455–463 [28,48]. This CTL response persists after clinical recovery from HBV infection [49], and is also detectable during spontaneous flares of disease in persons with chronic HBV infection that are followed by a resolution of persistent infection [50]. Of interest, it was recently shown that even in those persons who appear to recover completely from acute HBV infection, there may be low-level persistence of virus, which may help maintain this vigorous memory response [49].

## NON-CYTOLYTIC CONTROL OF HBV REPLICATION

CTLs mediate apoptosis of infected cells through the release of lytic granules and Fas/FasL binding, but this recognition of antigen and subsequent activation of

the T cell also triggers CTLs to produce a number of cytokines. Depending on the relative kinetics of viral replication versus cell death, soluble mediators may be more important than actual cell killing in control of viral replication [51]. Moreover, in infections of solid organs such as the liver, it is likely that cytokines play a crucial role in controlling viral replication, since even in an initially vigorous immune response, CTLs would be unlikely to achieve contact with all infected cells in the liver [52]. In a series of elegant studies, Guidotti and colleagues have shown that production of IFN-$\gamma$ and TNF-$\alpha$ by virus-specific CTLs may amplify the ability of the CTLs to clear viral infection in a transgenic mouse model of fulminant HBV infection [53]. Following adoptive transfer of cloned HBV-specific CTLs into transgenic mice expressing a full-length replicative form of HBV, the CTLs produced both IFN-$\gamma$ and TNF-$\alpha$, which led to down-regulation of HBV gene expression. Blockade of the cascade of events occurs when animals are pretreated with antibodies to TNF-$\alpha$ prior to adoptive transfer of HBV-specific CTLs [53]. This inhibition of viral replication occurs even when CTLs from perforin-knockout mice are used [54], suggesting that apoptotic cell death and production of cytokines are separate events in controlling viral replication. Activation of other virus-specific lymphocytes, such as occurred during infection with an unrelated virus, also led to cytokine production and down-regulation of HBV gene expression in this animal model [55].

## PERSISTENT HBV INFECTION

Five per cent of adults and 95% of neonates infected with HBV develop persistent infection. The viral or host factors which permit this development have not been defined. It is well known that age at acquisition determines the likelihood of chronic infection, with neonatal infection representing the highest risk period [56], but whether this is due to a relative immune hyporesponsiveness in neonates or high levels of HBeAg leading to tolerance [57] is unknown. In adults, the CD4+ response found in the peripheral blood mononuclear cells (PBMCs) in persons with chronic HBV infection is quantitatively much less vigorous than that observed in acute self-limited HBV infection [26,58]. HBV-specific CD4+ cells can still be found in the liver, albeit at a lower frequency than is seen in the PBMCs of persons with acute self-limited HBV infection [59]. Several groups have reported an association between a particular MHC class II allele, DRB*1302, and a resistance to chronic HBV infection in Gambian and Caucasian persons [60,61]. However, the reason for this resistance to chronic infection has not been linked to either a particular T-cell response or pattern of cytokine response in humans, although it is tempting to speculate that this underlies this genetic pattern. Similar to what is seen in the CD4+ response, HBV-specific CTL responses are present at much lower frequency in chronic HBV infection, where such responses cannot be identified among PBMCs [45]. Although a low-level CTL response can be found among liver-infiltrating lymphocytes in chronic HBV infection [62], such a response is ineffective at viral clearance and may instead contribute to liver damage [44]. In addition to a quantitative deficit of HBV-specific CD4+ and CD8+ cells in persons who develop chronic infection, these individuals may also be prone to produce type 2 cytokines [40].

In addition to quantitative defects in cellular responses to HBV, the virus may have specific mechanisms to evade host immune defences. Some of these defences have been demonstrated in other viral infections but not in HBV infection: for example, adenoviruses use a specific set of gene products to interfere with the proper maturation and assembly of MHC class I molecules on the cell surface [63]. Numerous investigators have attempted to define whether HBV infection results in changes in MHC class I expression in infected liver, with variable and contradictory results. Recently, it was reported that the HBx protein interacts with a subunit of the catalytic proteosome, which is a key component in the processing of viral antigens for recognition by CTLs [64]; this suggests that the pleiotropic HBx protein might alter antigen processing such that persistent infection is favoured. Other strategies are undoubtedly used by HBV but remain undefined.

One mechanism which has been well defined in animal models of chronic viral infection is immune escape by viral variation within antigenic epitopes. For example, in a group of vaccinated infants of chronically infected mothers, a few infants developed infection despite the presence of apparently protective titres of HBsAb [6]. Sequencing of the virus in these infected infants revealed a point mutation in HBsAg, specifically in the highly antigenic 'a' determinant. Similar findings have been noted in recipients of HBIg for prophylaxis of HBV infection after orthotopic liver transplantation [65]. These mutations apparently result in a loss of the ability of antibodies to neutralize the viral isolates. Such immune escape is also important for CTL epitopes, since only a single amino acid change within a CTLs epitope may abrogate recognition by CTLs [66]. For example, mice transgenic for a specific T-cell receptor (TCR) that only mount a CTL response against a single epitope within LCMV were challenged with a well characterized

isolate of LCMV [67]. Viral persistence in these animals is associated with a single amino acid change within a CTL epitope, resulting in a failure of the CTL response in these animals. In human infections, escape mutations within CTL epitopes associated with a persistent viral infection have been demonstrated in Epstein–Barr virus (EBV) and human immunodeficiency virus (HIV) infection [68,69]. In two HLA-A2-positive individuals chronically infected with HBV, mutations within the epitope recognized by HLA-A2-restricted CTLs were found [70]. These variant sequences were not recognized by CTLs that recognized the wild-type strain, and also acted as antagonists which appeared to interfere with binding of the wild-type epitope to the TCR. However, sequencing of multiple isolates from chronically infected persons has revealed little evidence of mutations within CTL epitopes, suggesting that immune escape from CTLs is a rare event [71]. A better understanding of the host and viral factors that permit the development of chronic infection is needed.

## THE ROLE OF CELLULAR IMMUNE RESPONSES IN DISEASE PATHOGENESIS

Despite the evidence that CTLs are an important component of recovery from viral infection, in some animal models of infection these same virus-specific cellular immune responses are the mediators of tissue injury. Although HBV-specific immune responses in the periphery appear to be less vigorous, the immune reaction within the liver appears to continue [62,72]. The role of these persistent, ineffective immune responses in liver damage is suggested by several lines of evidence. Histologically, hepatitis is marked by hepatocyte swelling and necrosis with a mononuclear cell infiltrate, enriched for CD8+ cells, seen in portal tracts and variably within the hepatic lobule [73]. In a transgenic mouse model of HBV infection, adoptive transfer of murine CD8+, HBV-specific CTLs can mediate liver cell necrosis [5,74]. This model demonstrates that tissue damage by CTLs is a multistep process (Fig. 2). The initial event is antigen recognition by the HBV-specific CTLs [74], which triggers apoptosis in the infected hepatocyte [75]; apoptotic hepatocytes are seen in biopsy specimens as the acidophilic Councilman bodies. *In vivo*, CTLs probably use several overlapping pathways to induce apoptosis in cells, including both perforin/granzyme and Fas/FasL [16,76]. Interaction of Fas/FasL is critical in this animal model, as anti-Fas antibodies can block the development of hepatitis [77].

The CTLs induce death directly in a minority of infected cells, however, the number of infected hepatocytes far outnumbers that of CTLs and the tissue architecture of the liver inhibits free access of CTLs to all tis-

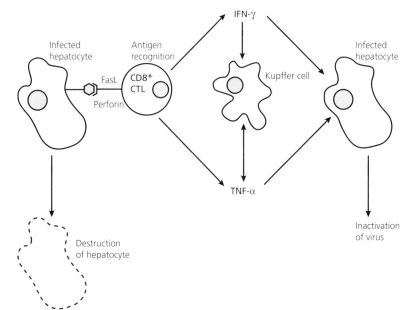

**Figure 2.** A model for HBV pathogenesis

CTLs specific for HBV are present within the hepatic parenchyma, but kill a minority of infected cells. Cytokines such as IFN-γ and TNF-α produced by the CTL recruit and activate other inflammatory cells, leading both to tissue destruction and control of viral replication. The balance between liver cell destruction and non-cytolytic control of the virus determines the clinical outcome.

sues. Therefore, cytokines also play an important role in tissue injury. Following antigen recognition, the CTLs also produce cytokines that lead to the recruitment of antigen non-specific inflammatory cells, such as macrophages and NK cells [75]. This step can be prevented by antibodies against IFN-γ and by the macrophage inhibitor carrageenan. In another transgenic mouse model, liver-specific expression of IFN-γ produced a transaminitis and histological appearance similar to that of human chronic active hepatitis [78]. In most HBV transgenic mice, this process is relatively mild; however, in mice that overexpress HBsAg, which renders the hepatocytes sensitive to lysis by IFN-γ [79] the disease progresses to fulminant hepatic failure. There is a marked mononuclear cell infiltrate with Kupffer cell hyperplasia, resembling the fulminant hepatitis seen in humans. TNF-α produced by activated Kupffer cells may induce apoptosis in hepatocytes [16], and may cause hepatocyte necrosis independent of macrophage activation [80]. In summary, many of the manifestations of liver damage in chronic HBV infection appear to be initiated by antigen-recognition by CTLs; however, there is an important role of cytokines and antigen non-specific cells in the pathogenesis of disease.

## PROSPECTS FOR MANIPULATION OF THE IMMUNE RESPONSE IN CHRONIC HBV INFECTION

Given the central role of cellular immunity in disease pathogenesis, strategies have been proposed to manipulate this cellular immune response in favour of protec-

tion from disease rather than pathogenesis. Given the central role of cellular immunity in tissue injury, one strategy involved blockade of immune responses. Trials of prednisone in chronic HBV infection, however, resulted in a worsening of disease, as well as the significant side effects caused by the immunosuppressants [2]. In those instances of acute fulminant HBV infection, where the problem may lie in an exuberant immune reaction, the use of small molecules to block components of the apoptotic cascade have been tested. Recently, use of a tripeptide inhibitor of a key protease in the cascade was shown to prevent the fulminant hepatitis caused by anti-Fas antibodies [81], raising the possibility that this or similar molecules might also be useful in fulminant HBV infection. If it was possible to separate the recruitment of antigen non-specific cells from the process of antigen recognition, this might also decrease the inflammation, thus reducing morbidity from chronic active hepatitis and mortality from hepatocellular carcinoma, which nearly always occurs on the background of longstanding liver inflammation. However, the same cytokines that appear to mediate the recruitment of antigen non-specific cells also appear to inhibit viral replication; until additional cytokines are identified, this is unlikely to be a realistic target for intervention.

Another strategy uses the rationale that the magnitude of the immune response is lower in persons with chronic HBV infection than persons with acute self-limited HBV infection, and so therapics should be designed to augment immunity. Immunization of adult carriers with recombinant HBs subunit vaccine was ineffective in reducing HBV DNA [82], which is not surprising since antibody alone cannot eliminate intracellular organisms. Since CTLs are capable of eliminating persistent infections, the more promising approach is induction of cellular immune responses. In one interesting case report, persistent HBV infection was eliminated in the recipient of an allogeneic bone marrow graft from an HBV-immune donor [83], suggesting that the cellular immunity transferred in the graft eliminated chronic HBV infection. Obviously this approach is impractical, but the emerging knowledge that vigorous, polyclonal immune responses are likely to be critical in the control of HBV infection, as well as greater understanding of the principles of vaccination, has led to strategies to boost cellular immune responses through 'therapeutic' vaccination. Vaccines containing single or multiple CTL epitopes have been shown to induce protective immunity and cure persistent infection in animal models [84,85], although the peptide must be delivered with an adjuvant or as part of a live viral vector [86].

The first requirement for such vaccines is a knowledge of the epitopes recognized. Although initial mapping of CTL epitopes was performed using cloned cells and overlapping peptides that spanned the protein of interest, these studies are technically laborious and expensive to perform. In the past several years, numerous groups have delineated the requirements for binding of peptides to MHC class I molecules, and have found that motifs exist which predict which peptide sequences bind to a given MHC class I molecule. Some investigators have used the predicted motifs to scan viral sequences for sets of peptides [87], then tested these peptides for affinity binding to purified MHC class I molecules in an effort to avoid the large amount of labour necessary to define viral epitopes through screening of CTL clones. In general, the strength of binding of a particular peptide to purified MHC molecules has correlated with the immunogenicity [88], although whether this translates into more efficient control of viral replication is controversial [89]. In HBV infection, the identification of HLA-A2.1 has expedited the identification of HLA-A2-restricted epitopes in acute and chronically infected individuals [44], as well as transgenic animals expressing HLA-A2.1 [88].

Based on the observation that the CD8+ CTL response is strong in acutely infected individuals and weak or undetectable in chronically infected individuals, a 'therapeutic' vaccine for HBV was developed [90]. The goal of this vaccine is the induction of CTL responses against an epitope in HBcAg, core 18–27, that is recognized by the majority of HLA-A2-positive individuals with acute self-limited HBV infection. In Phase I studies, the vaccine was able to induce a CTL response even in HBV-naive individuals. However, in persons with chronic HBV infection, the vaccine resulted in only modest decrease in HBV DNA levels (Frank Chisari, personal communication), suggesting the need for additional epitopes in chronically infected individuals. Recently, common motifs that predict binding to multiple MHC class I alleles (superfamilies) have been described [91–93]; for example, members of the A3 superfamily, which includes A3, A11, A31, and A*6801 recognize A, I, L, M, V, S or T at position two and R or K at the C terminus. This has facilitated identification of additional epitopes recognized in acute self-limited HBV infection [94]. Inclusion of other epitopes into a vaccine might result in the vigorous, polyclonal immune response that is the hallmark of acute self-limited HBV infection, but this remains to be proven.

Genetic immunization (or a 'DNA vaccine') has also been shown to be highly effective in eliciting both antibody-mediated and cellular immune responses, especially the CTL response [95,96]. This technique, which involves the intramuscular or intradermal injection of plasmid DNA encoding the proteins of interest, has been used in a wide variety of animal models to induce protective immunity against a variety of pathogens [97]. Some of the advantages of the technology include the relative ease of preparation compared to live virus vectors and stability at room temperature. Several groups have reported induction of immune responses against HBV in both mice and chimpanzees [98,99], including a mouse strain previously considered to be a nonresponder at the CTL level [100]. Moreover, these vaccines can overcome tolerance in HBV transgenic mice, suggesting that this strategy may be useful in chronically infected persons [99]. However, these have not been tested in human trials of persistent viral infection and perhaps should be approached with caution; in an animal model of persistent LCMV infection, DNA vaccination was capable of curing the animal, but at a cost of enhanced pathology [101].

## SUMMARY AND CONCLUSIONS

In summary, although our understanding of HBV pathogenesis is limited by our current experimental systems, we can still conclude the following. In acute self-limited HBV infection, there is a vigorous, polyclonal CD4+ and CD8+ immune response. The CD4+ response is directed toward production of adequate amounts of antibody as well as priming of a vigorous CTL response. The CD8+ CTL response is directed at multiple epitopes, and can probably eliminate viral replication in the majority of infected cells. Control of HBV replication occurs not only through death of infected cells, but also through the production of cytokines that inhibit viral replication. In contrast, individuals with chronic HBV infection never mount a vigorous CD4$^+$ or CD8$^+$ response. There is a low level cellular immune response in the liver, but this appears to result in liver cell injury. Given our knowledge of the immune responses against HBV and the mechanisms of liver damage, it may be possible to design rational strategies to manipulate the immune system to the benefit of the infected person.

# REFERENCES

1. Horvath J & Raffanti SP. Clinical aspects of the interactions between human immunodeficiency virus and the hepatotropic viruses. *Clinical Infectious Diseases* 1994; **18**:339–347.
2. Perillo R, Schiff E, Davis G, Bodenheimer H, Lindsay K, Payne J, Dienstage J, O'Brien C, Tamburro C, Jacobsen I, *et al.* A randomized, controlled trial of interferon alfa-2b alone and after prednisone withdrawal for the treatment of chronic hepatitis B. *New England Journal of Medicine* 1990; **323**:295–301.
3. Bird GL, Smith H, Portmann B, Alexander GJ & Williams R. Acute liver decompensation on withdrawal of cytotoxic chemotherapy and immunosuppressive therapy in hepatitis B carriers. *Quarterly Journal of Medicine* 1989; **73**:895–902.
4. Thung SN, Gerber MA, Klion F & Gilbert H. Massive hepatic necrosis after chemotherapy withdrawal in a hepatitis B virus carrier. *Archives of Internal Medicine* 1985; **145**:1313–1314.
5. Chisari FV. Hepatitis B virus transgenic mice: insights into the virus and the disease. *Hepatology* 1995; **22**:1316–1325.
6. Carman W. Molecular variants of hepatitis B virus. *Clinics in Laboratory Medicine* 1996; **16**:407–428.
7. Caselmann WH, Meyer M, Scholz S, Hofschneider PH & Koshy R. Type I interferons inhibit hepatitis B virus replication and induce hepatocellular gene expression in cultured liver cells. *Journal of Infectious Diseases* 1992; **166**:966–971.
8. Colucci G, Colombo M, Del Ninno E & Paronetto F. In situ characterization by monoclonal antibodies of the mononuclear cell infiltrate in chronic active hepatitis. *Gastroenterology* 1983; **85**:1138–1145.
9. Scully LJ, Brown D, Lloyd C, Shein R & Thomas HC. Immunological studies before and during interferon therapy in chronic HBV infection: identification of factors predicting response. *Hepatology* 1990; **12**:1111–1117.
10. Thomas HC, Foster GR, Sumiya M, McIntosh D, Jack DL, Turner MW & Summerfield JA. Mutation of gene of mannose-binding protein associated with chronic hepatitis B viral infection. *Lancet* 1996; **348**:1417–1419.
11. Pieters J. MHC class II restricted antigen presentation. *Current Opinion in Immunology* 1997; **9**:89–96.
12. Lanzavecchia A. Mechanisms of antigen uptake for presentation. *Current Opinion in Immunology* 1996; **8**:348–354.
13. Franco A, Guidotti LG, Hobbs MV, Pasquetto V & Chisari FV. Pathogenetic effector function of CD4-positive T helper 1 cells in hepatitis B virus transgenic mice. *Journal of Immunology* 1997; **159**:2001–2008.
14. Gotch F, Gallimore A & McMichael A. Cytotoxic T cells—protection from disease progression—protection from infection. *Immunology Letters* 1996; **51**:125–128.
15. Lehner PJ & Cresswell P. Processing and delivery of peptides presented by MHC class I molecules. *Current Opinion in Immunology* 1996; **8**:59–67.
16. Berke G. Killing mechanisms of cytotoxic lymphocytes. *Current Opinion in Hematology* 1997; **4**:32–40.
17. Riddell SR & Greenberg PD. Principles for adoptive T cell therapy of human viral diseases. *Annual Review of Immunology* 1995; **13**:545–586.
18. Tishon A, Borrow P, Evans C & Oldstone MB. Virus-induced immunosuppression. 1. Age at infection relates to a selective or generalized defect. *Virology* 1993; **195**:397–405.
19. Munoz JL, McCarthy CA, Clark ME & Hall CB. Respiratory syncytial virus infection in C57BL/6 mice: clearance of virus from the lungs with virus-specific cytotoxic T cells. *Journal of Virology* 1991; **65**:4494–4497.
20. Qiunnan G, Kirmani N, Rook A, Manischewitz J, Jackson L, Moreschi G, Santos G, Saral R & Burns W. Cytotoxic T cells in cytomegalovirus infection: HLA-restricted T lymphocytes and non-T lymphocyte responses correlate with recovery from cytomegalovirus infection in bone-marrow-transplant recipients. *New England Journal of Medicine* 1982; **307**:6–13.
21. McMichael AJ, Gotch FM, Noble GR & Beare PA. Cytotoxic T-cell immunity to influenza. *New England Journal of Medicine* 1983; **309**:13–17.
22. Riddell SR, Reusser P & Greenberg PD. Cytotoxic T cells specific for cytomegalovirus: a potential therapy for immunocompromised patients. *Reviews of Infectious Diseases* 1992; **11**.
23. Milich DR, Sallberg M & Maruyama T. The humoral immune response in acute and chronic hepatitis B virus infection. *Springer Seminars in Immunopathology* 1995; **17**:149–166.
24. Howard CR & Allison LM. Hepatitis B surface antigen variation and protective immunity. *Intervirology* 1995; **38**:35–40.
25. Ferrari C, Bertoletti A, Penna A, Cavalli A, Valli A, Missale G, Pilli M, Fowler P, Giuberti T, Chisari FV, *et al.* Identification of immunodominant T cell epitopes of the hepatitis B virus nucleocapsid antigen. *Journal of Clinical Investigation* 1991; **88**:214–222.
26. Ferrari C, Penna A, Bertoletti A, Valli A, Antoni AD, Giuberti T, Cavalli A, Petit MA & Fiaccadori F. Cellular immune response to hepatitis B virus-encoded antigens in acute and chronic hepatitis B virus infection. *Journal of Immunology* 1990; **145**:3442–3449.
27. Penna A, Chisari FV, Bertoletti A, Missale G, Fowler P, Giuberti T, Fiaccadori F & Ferrari C. Cytotoxic T lymphocytes recognize an HLA-A2-restricted epitope within the hepatitis B virus nucleocapsid antigen. *Journal of Experimental Medicine* 1991; **174**:1565–1570.
28. Nayersina R, Fowler P, Guilhot S, Missale G, Cerny A, Schlicht HJ, Vitiello A, Chesnut R, Person JL, Redeker AG, *et al.* HLA A2 restricted cytotoxic T lymphocyte responses to multiple hepatitis B surface antigen epitopes during hepatitis B virus infection. *Journal of Immunology* 1993; **150**:4659–4671.
29. Milich DR, McLachlan A, Thornton GB & Hughes JL. Antibody production to the nucleocapsid and envelope of the hepatitis B virus primed by a single synthetic T cell site. *Nature* 1987; **329**:547–549.
30. Milich DR. T- and B-cell recognition of hepatitis B viral antigens. *Immunology Today* 1988; **9**:380–386.
31. Penna A, Artini M, Cavalli A, Levrero M, Bertoletti A, Pilli M, Chisari FV, Rehermann B, Del Prete G, Fiaccadori F & Ferrari C. Long-lasting memory T cell responses following self-limited acute hepatitis B.

*Journal of Clinical Investigation* 1996; **98**:1185–1194.

32. O'Garra A & Murphy K. Role of cytokines in determining T-lymphocyte function. *Current Opinion in Immunology* 1994; **6**:458–466.

33. Sher A, Gazzinelli RT, Oswald IP, Clerici M, Kullberg M, Pearce EJ, Berzofsky JA, Mosmann TR, James SL & Morse HC 3rd. Role of T-cell derived cytokines in the downregulation of immune responses in parasitic and retroviral infection. *Immunological Reviews* 1992; **127**: 183–294.

34. Daugelat S & Kaufmann SH. Role of Th1 and Th2 cells in bacterial infections. *Chem Immunology* 1996; **63**:66–97.

35. Urban JF Jr, Katona IM, Paul WE & Finkelman FD. Interleukin 4 is important in protective immunity to a gastrointestinal nematode infection in mice. *Proceedings of the National Academy of Sciences, USA* 1991; **88**:5513–5517.

36. Cenci E, Mencacci A, Del Sero G, Bistoni F & Romani L. Induction of protective Th1 responses to *Candida albicans* by antifungal therapy alone or in combination with an interleukin-4 antagonist. *Journal of Infectious Diseases* 1997; **176**:217–226.

37. Spaccapelo R, Del Sero G, Mosci P, Bistoni F & Romani L. Early T cell unresponsiveness in mice with candidiasis and reversal by IL-2: effect on T helper cell development. *Journal of Immunology* 1997; **158**:2294–2302.

38. Matyniak JE & Reiner SL. T helper phenotype and genetic susceptibility in experimental Lyme disease. *Journal of Experimental Medicine* 1995; **181**:1251–1254.

39. Penna A, Del Prete G, Cavalli A, Bertoletti A, D'Elios MM, Sorrentino R, D'Amato M, Boni C, Pilli M, Fiaccadori F & Ferrari C. Predominant T-helper 1 cytokine profile of hepatitis B virus nucleocapsid-specific T cells in acute self-limited hepatitis B. *Hepatology* 1997; **25**:1022–1027.

40. Bertoletti A, D'Elios MM, Boni C, De Carli M, Zignego AL, Durazzo M, Missale G, Penna A, Fiaccadori F, Del Prete G & Ferrari C. Different cytokine profiles of intrahepatic T cells in chronic hepatitis B and hepatitis C virus infections. *Gastroenterology* 1997; **112**:193–199.

41. Rossol S, Marinos G, Carucci P, Singer MV, Williams R & Naoumov NV. Interleukin-12 induction of Th1 cytokines is important for viral clearance in chronic hepatitis B. *Journal of Clinical Investigation* 1997; **99**:3025–3033.

42. Milich DR, Peterson DL, Schodel F, Jones JE & Hughes JL. Preferential recognition of hepatitis B nucleocapsid antigens by Th1 or Th2 cells is epitope and major histocompatibility complex dependent. *Journal of Virology* 1995; **69**:2776–2785.

43. Milich DR, Schodel F, Hughes JL, Jones JE & Peterson DL. The hepatitis B virus core and e antigens elicit different Th cell subsets: antigen structure can affect Th cell phenotype. *Journal of Virology* 1997; **71**:2192–2201.

44. Chisari FV & Ferrari C. Hepatitis B virus immunopathogenesis. *Annual Review of Immunology* 1995; **13**:29–60.

45. Rehermann B, Fowler P, Sidney J, Person J, Redeker A, Brown M, Moss B, Sette A & Chisari FV. The cytotoxic T lymphocyte response to multiple hepatitis B virus polymerase epitopes during and after acute viral hepatitis. *Journal of Experimental Medicine* 1995; **181**:1047–1058.

46. Bertoletti A, Chisari F, Penna A, Guilhot S, Galati L, Missale G, Fowler P, Schlicht H-J, Antonella V, Chesnut R, *et al*. Definition of a minimal optimal cytotoxic T-cell epitope within the hepatitis B virus nucleocapsid protein. *Journal of Virology* 1993; **67**:2376–2380.

47. Schirmbeck R, Melber K & Reimann J. Hepatitis B virus small surface antigen particles are processed in a novel endosomal pathway for major histocompatibility complex class I-restricted epitope presentation. *European Journal of Immunology* 1995; **25**:1063–1070.

48. Penna A, Fowler P, Bertoletti A, Guilhot S, Moss B, Margolskee RF, Cavalli A, Valli A, Fiaccadori F, Chisari FV, *et al*. Hepatitis B virus (HBV)-specific cytotoxic T-cell (CTL) response in humans: characterization of HLA class II-restricted CTLs that recognize endogenously synthesized HBV envelope antigens. *Journal of Virology* 1992; **66**:1193–1198.

49. Rehermann B, Ferrari C, Pasquinelli C & Chisari FV. The hepatitis B virus persists for decades after patients' recovery from acute viral hepatitis despite active maintenance of a cytotoxic T lymphocyte response. *Nature Medicine* 1996; **2**:1104–1108.

50. Rehermann B, Lau D, Hoofnagle JH & Chisari FV. Cytotoxic T lymphocyte responsiveness after resolution of chronic hepatitis B virus infection. *Journal of Clinical Investigation* 1996; **97**:1655–1665.

51. Kagi D & Hengartner H. Different roles for cytotoxic T cells in the control of infections with cytopathic versus noncytopathic viruses. *Current Opinion in Immunology* 1996; **8**:472–477.

52. Guidotti LG & Chisari FV. To kill or to cure: options in host defense against viral infection. *Current Opinion in Immunology* 1996; **8**:478–483.

53. Guidotti LG, Ando K, Hobbs MV, Ishikawa T, Runkel L, Schreiber RD & Chisari FV. Cytotoxic T lymphocytes inhibit hepatitis B virus gene expression by a noncytolytic mechanism in transgenic mice. *Proceedings of the National Academy of Sciences, USA* 1994; **91**:3764–3768.

54. Guidotti LG, Ishikawa T, Hobbs MV, Matzke B, Schreiber R & Chisari FV. Intracellular inactivation of the hepatitis B virus by cytotoxic T lymphocytes. *Immunity* 1996; **4**:25–36.

55. Guidotti LG, Borrow P, Hobbs MV, Matzke B, Gresser I, Oldstone MB & Chisari FV. Viral cross talk: Intracellular inactivation of the hepatitis B virus during an unrelated viral infection of the liver. *Proceedings of the National Academy of Sciences, USA* 1996; **93**:4589–4594.

56. Hyams KC. Risks of chronicity following acute hepatitis B virus infection: a review. *Clinical Infectious Diseases* 1995; **20**:992–1000.

57. Milich DR, Jones JE, Hughes JL, Maruyama T, Price J, Melhado I & Jirik F. Extrathymic expression of the intracellular hepatitis B core antigen results in T cell tolerance in transgenic mice. *Journal of Immunology* 1994; **152**:455–466.

58. Jung MC, Diepolder HM & Pape GR. T cell recognition of hepatitis B and C viral antigens. *European Journal of Clinical Investigation* 1994; **24**:641–650.

59. Ferrari C, Penna A, Giuberti T, Tong MJ, Ribera E, Fiaccadori F & Chisari FV. Intrahepatic, nucleocapsid antigen-specific T cells in chronic active hepatitis B. *Journal of Immunology* 1987; **139**:2050–2058.

60. Höhler T, Gerken G, Notghi A, Lubjuhn R, Taheri H, Protzer U, Löhr H, Schneider P, Zum Büschenfelde K & Rittner C. HLA DRB*1301 and *1302 protect against chronic hepatitis B. *Journal of Hepatology* 1997; **26**:503–507.

61. Thursz MR, Kwiatkowski D, Allsopp CE, Greenwood BM, Thomas HC & Hill AV. Association between an MHC class II allele and clearance of hepatitis B virus in the Gambia. *New England Journal of Medcine* 1995; **332**:1065–1069.

62. Barnaba V, Franco A, Alberti A, Balsano C, Benvenuto R & Balsano F. Recognition of hepatitis B virus envelope proteins by liver-infiltrating lymphocytes in chronic HBV infection. *Journal of Immunology* 1989; **143**:2650–2655.

63. Fruh K, Ahn K & Peterson PA. Inhibition of MHC class I antigen presentation by viral proteins. *Journal of Molecular Medicine* 1997; **75**:18–27.

64. Huang J, Kwong J, Sun EC & Liang TJ. Proteasome complex as a potential cellular target of hepatitis B virus X protein. *Journal of Virology* 1996; **70**:5582–5591.

65. Carman WF, Trautwein C, van Deursen FJ, Colman K, Dornan E, McIntyre G, Waters J, Kliem V, Muller R, Thomas HC & Manns MP. Hepatitis B virus envelope variation after transplantation with and without hepatitis B immune globulin prophylaxis. *Hepatology* 1996; **24**:489–493.

66. Mescher MF. Molecular interactions in the activation of effector and precursor cytotoxic T lymphocytes. *Immunological Reviews* 1995; **146**:177–210.

67. Aebischer T, Moskophidis D, Rohrer U, Zinkernagel R & Hengartner H. *In vitro* selection of lymphocytic choriomeningitis escape mutants by cytotoxic T lymphocytes. *Proceedings of the National Academy of Sciences, USA* 1991; **88**:11047–11051.

68. de Campos-Lima P-O, Gavioli R, Zhang Q-J, Wallace L, Dolcetti R, Rowe M, Rickinson AB & Masucci MG. HLA-A11 epitope loss isolates of Epstein–Barr virus from a highly A11+ population. *Science* 1993; **260**:98–100.

69. McMichael AJ & Phillips RE. Escape of human immunodeficiency virus from immune control. *Annual Review of Immunology* 1997; **15**:271–296.

70. Bertoletti A, Sette A, Chisari FV, Penna A, Levrero M, De Carli M, Fiaccadori F & Ferrari C. Natural variants of cytotoxic epitopes are T-cell receptor antagonists for antiviral cytotoxic T cells. *Nature* 1994; **369**:407–410.

71. Rehermann B, Pasquinelli C, Mosier SM & Chisari FV. Hepatitis B virus (HBV) sequence variation of cytotoxic T lymphocyte epitopes is not common in patients with chronic HBV infection. *Journal of Clinical Investigation* 1995; **96**:1527–1534.

72. Lohr HF, Gerken G, Schlicht HJ, Meryer zum Buschenfelde KH & Fleischer B. Low frequency of cytotoxic liver-infiltrating T lymphocytes specific for endogenous processed surface and core proteins in chronic hepatitis B. *Journal of Infectious Diseases* 1993; **168**:1133–1139.

73. Dienes H, Hutteroth T, Hess G & Meuer S. Immunoelectron microscopic observations on the inflammatory infiltrates and HLA antigens in hepatitis B and non-A, non-B. *Hepatology* 1987; **7**:1317–1325.

74. Moriyama T, Guilhot S, Klopchin K, Moss B, Pinkert CA, Palmiter RD, Brinster RL, Kanagawa O & Chisari FV. Immunobiology and pathogenesis of hepatocellular injury in hepatitis B virus transgenic mice. *Science* 1990; **248**:361–364.

75. Ando K, Moriyama T, Guidotti L, Wirth S, Schreiber R, Hans-Jurgen S, Huang S-N & Chisari F. Mechanisms of class I restricted immunopathology. A transgenic mouse model of fulminant hepatitis. *Journal of Experimental Medicine* 1993; **178**:1541–1554.

76. Nakamoto Y, Guidotti LG, Pasquetto V, Schreiber RD & Chisari FV. Differential target cell sensitivity to CTL-activated death pathways in hepatitis B virus transgenic mice. *Journal of Immunology* 1997; **158**:5692–5697.

77. Kondo T, Suda T, Fukuyama H, Adachi M & Nagata S. Essential roles of the Fas ligand in the development of hepatitis. *Nature Medicine* 1997; **3**:409–413.

78. Toyonaga T, Hino O, Sugai S, Wakasugi S, Abe K, Shichiri M & Yamamura K-I. Chronic active hepatitis in transgenic mice expressing interferon-γ in the liver. *Proceedings of the National Academy of Sciences, USA* 1994; **91**:614–618.

79. Gilles PN, Guerrette DL, Ulevitch RJ, Schreiber RD & Chisari FV. HBsAg retention sensitizes the hepatocyte to injury by physiological concentrations of interferon-gamma. *Hepatology* 1992; **16**:655–663.

80. Orange J, Salazar-Mather T, Opal S & Biron C. Mechanisms for virus-induced liver disease: Tumor necrosis factor-mediated pathology independent of natural killer and T cells during murine cytomegalovirus infection. *Journal of Virology* 1997; **71**:9248–9258.

81. Rodriguez I, Matsuura K, Ody C, Nagata S & Vassalli P. Systemic injection of a tripeptide inhibits the intracellular activation of CPP32-like proteases in vivo and fully protects mice against Fas-mediated fulminant liver destruction and death. *Journal of Experimental Medicine* 1996; **184**:2067–2072.

82. Dienstag JL, Stevens CE, Bhan AK & Szmuness W. Hepatitis B vaccine administered to chronic carriers of hepatitis B surface antigen. *Annals of Internal Medicine* 1982; **96**:575–579.

83. Ilan Y, Nagler A, Adler R, Tur-Kaspa R, Slavin S & Shouval D. Ablation of persistent hepatitis B by bone marrow transplantation from a hepatitis B-immune donor. *Gastroenterology* 1993; **104**:1818–1821.

84. Klavinskis LS, Tishon A & Oldstone MB. Molecularly engineered vaccinia which expresses an immunodominant T-cell epitope induces cytotoxic T lymphocytes that confer protection from lethal virus infection. *Journal of Virology* 1989; **63**:4311–4316.

85. Randall RE & Young DF. Peptide-induced antiviral protection by cytotoxic T cells. *Proceedings of the National Academy of Sciences, USA* 1991; **88**:991–993.

86. Schulz M, Zinkernagel R & Hengartner H. Peptide-induced antiviral protection by cytotoxic T cells. *Proceedings of the National Academy of Sciences, USA* 1991; **88**:991–993.

87. Falk K & Ramensee H-G. Consensus motifs and peptide ligands of MHC class I molecules. *Seminars in Immunology* 1993; **5**:81–94.

88. Sette A, Vitiello A, Reherman B, Fowler P, Nayersina R, Kast WM, Melief CJ, Oseroff C, Yuan L, Ruppert J, et al. The relationship between class I binding affinity and immunogenicity of potential cytotoxic T cell epitopes. *Journal of Immunology* 1994; **153**:5586–5592.

89. Alexander-Miller MA, Leggatt GR & Berzofsky JA. Selective expansion of high- or low-avidity cytotoxic T lymphocytes and efficacy for adoptive immunotherapy. *Proceedings of the National Academy of Sciences, USA* 1996; **93**:4102–4107.

90. Vitiello A, Ishioka G, Grey HM, Rose R, Farness P, LaFond R, Yuan L, Chisari FV, Furze J, Bartholomeuz R, et al. Development of a lipopeptide-based therapeutic vaccine to treat chronic HBV infection. I. Induction of a primary cytotoxic T lymphocyte response in humans. *Journal of Clinical Investigation* 1995; **95**:341–349.

91. Sidney J, Southwood S, del Guercio MF, Grey HM, Chesnut RW, Kubo RT & Sette A. Specificity and degeneracy in peptide binding to HLA-B7-like class I molecules. *Journal of Immunology* 1996; **157**:3480–3490.

92. del Guercio MF, Sidney J, Hermanson G, Perez C, Grey HM, Kubo RT & Sette A. Binding of a peptide antigen to multiple HLA alleles allows definition of an A2-like supertype. *Journal of Immunology* 1995; **154**:685–693.

93. Sidney J, del Guercio MF, Southwood S, Engelhard VH, Appella E, Rammensee HG, Falk K, Rötzschke O, Takiguchi M, Kubo RT, *et al.* Several HLA alleles share overlapping peptide specificities. *Journal of Immunology* 1995; **154**:247–259.

94. Bertoni R, Sidney J, Fowler P, Chesnut RW, Chisari FV & Sette A. Human histocompatibility leukocyte antigen-binding supermotifs predict broadly cross-reactive cytotoxic T lymphocyte responses in patients with acute hepatitis. *Journal of Clinical Investigation* 1997; **100**:503–513.

95. Tang D-C, DeVit M & Johnston SA. Genetic immunization is a simple method for eliciting an immune response. *Nature* 1992; **356**:152–154.

96. Ulmer JB, Donnelly JJ, Parker SE, Rhodes GH, Felgner PL, Swarki VJ, Gromkowski SH, Deck RR, DeWitt CM & Friedman A. Heterologous protection against influenza by injection of DNA encoding a viral protein. *Science* 1993; **259**:1745–1749.

97. Donnelly JJ, Ulmer JB, Shiver JW & Liu MA. DNA vaccines. *Annual Review of Immunology* 1997; **15**:617–648.

98. Geissler M, Tokushige K, Chante CC, Zurawski VR Jr & Wands JR. Cellular and humoral immune response to hepatitis B virus structural proteins in mice after DNA-based immunization. *Gastroenterology* 1997; **112**:1307–1320.

99. Davis HL, Brazolot Millan CL, Mancini M, McCluskie MJ, Hadchouel M, Comanita L, Tiollais P, Whalen RG & Michel ML. DNA-based immunization against hepatitis B surface antigen (HBsAg) in normal and HBsAg-transgenic mice. *Vaccine* 1997; **15**:849–852.

100. Schirmbeck R, Bohm W, Ando K, Chisari FV & Reimann J. Nucleic acid vaccination primes hepatitis B virus surface antigen-specific cytotoxic T lymphocytes in nonresponder mice. *Journal of Virology* 1995; **69**:5929–5934.

101. Martins LP, Lau LL, Asano MS & Ahmed R. DNA vaccination against persistent viral infection. *Journal of Virology* 1995; **69**:2574–2582.

# 8

# Pathogenesis of chronic hepatitis C virus infection

## David R Nelson* and Johnson YN Lau

## INTRODUCTION

The importance of hepatitis C virus (HCV) infection lies in its ability to cause insidious and progressive liver damage in the majority of those infected. Acute infection is typically mild and often subclinical, yet there is a high rate of chronicity after HCV infection. At least 70% of the individuals who contract HCV will develop chronic infection and hepatitis, 20–50% of these will eventually progress to cirrhosis, and 1% to 2% will develop liver cell cancer after a 10–20 year period [1]. In addition to the personal costs of morbidity and mortality to individual patients and their families, the clinical impact of HCV infection is immense. At present, HCV-related cirrhosis is one of the leading indications for liver transplantation worldwide. However, despite advances in our knowledge of the epidemiology and molecular virology of HCV, the mechanisms of hepatocellular injury in HCV infection are not completely understood.

Studies of the immunopathogenesis of HCV in patients with chronic hepatitis C have been difficult. After infection with HCV is established, multiple factors influence the host–virus interaction, resulting in an unique, individual disease pattern (Table 1). Viral factors include direct cytopathic effects, replication efficiency, nucleotide substitution rates and mutations (diversity) that have specific biological consequences. Host factors may include the competence of the immune system, local and systemic cytokine production, and the humoral and cellular immune responses. Other environmental factors, especially alcohol abuse, may alter the progression of liver disease. Indirect evidence suggests that HCV may be cytopathic at high levels and this may lead to a unique pattern of rapidly progressive fibrosing cholestatic liver disease in a small proportion of immunosuppressed patients. However, in most patients with chronic HCV infection, there is a growing body of evidence that the host immune response plays the major role in controlling HCV infection and causing

**Table 1.** Factors involved in the pathogenesis of chronic HCV infection

Virus
- Direct cytopathic effects
- Replication efficiency
- Nucleotide substitution rate & diversity (quasispecies)
- Genotype (?)

Immune Response
- Immune competence/genetic predisposition (?)
- Humoral
- Cellular
- Cytokine (local/systemic)

Environmental
- Alcohol
- Drugs (immunosuppression)
- Viral coinfection

hepatocellular damage. This review will focus on recent advances in the understanding of the interaction between HCV and the host immune system and its potential implications on disease pathogenesis.

## IMMUNE-MEDIATED MECHANISMS

The host immune response to HCV infection is made up of a non-specific immune response, including interferon production and natural killer cell activity, and a HCV-specific immune response, including humoral and cellular components, which accompany all viral infections (Fig. 1). Antibodies to structural and non-structural HCV proteins are produced during infection, and form the basis for detecting host exposure to the virus. The cellular immune response is also activated in these patients, resulting in the production of CD4+ and CD8+ cells that recognize and respond to various processed HCV antigens. However, neither the humoral nor the cellular immune response appears sufficient to eradicate infection in most patients. Although a small proportion of subjects who contract HCV may clear the virus (<15%), the

*Corresponding author

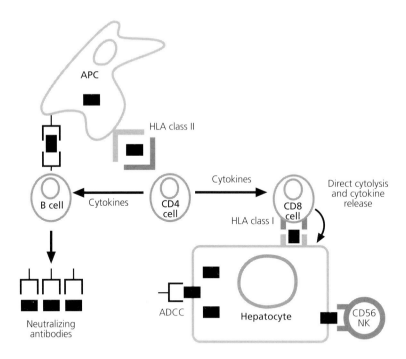

**Figure 1.** The host immune response to HCV infection

Viruses are endocytosed by local presenting cells (APCs), which present antigen to CD4⁺ cells in the form of peptides bound to the class II molecules. Upon antigen recognition, CD4⁺ cells release cytokines that regulate the activity of B cells and CD8⁺ cells. B cells produce antibodies that can neutralize circulating virus and may also participate in antibody-dependent cellular cytotoxicity (ADCC). The infected hepatocyte processes and presents HCV antigens on its cell surface. CD8⁺ cytolytic cells (CTLs) can recognize HCV peptides in the context of an HLA class I molecule and help control viral replication through killing of infected hepatocytes, as well as non-cytolytic, cytokine-mediated inhibition of viral replication.

infection more commonly persists (80%) and is characterized by progressive liver disease in a significant proportion of patients.

## HUMORAL IMMUNE RESPONSE TO HCV

Following exposure to HCV, viraemia develops within one week. In the immunocompetent host, this is followed in several weeks by elevated levels of transaminases and then a delayed antibody seroconversion. In most patients infected with HCV, a wide variety of antibodies are generated to both structural and non-structural regions of the virus. In fact, HCV was originally identified using the humoral response to HCV as a probe for the screening of molecular clones [2]. Antibodies against conserved epitopes of the putative envelope proteins (E1 and E2) are also found in more than 90% of patients with chronic HCV infection [3]. Despite its current diagnostic utility, the clinical significance of antibodies to HCV polypeptides with respect to control of infection and the pathogenesis of liver disease is still largely unknown.

The clinical significance of the humoral immune response is poorly defined. Some have reported a rapid progression of HCV-related liver disease in patients with impaired B-cell immunity (hypogammaglobulinaemia) [4], suggesting that B-cell immunity may play a role in controlling disease progression. It

has also been shown that certain anti-HCV antibodies, such as anti-NS4, may decline or even disappear in patients who recover from acute hepatitis or respond to interferon (IFN) therapy [5]. Core-specific IgM has also been reported to decline with successful IFN therapy and the antibody titre may correlate with disease activity [6]. However, other studies have failed to show an association [7]. Thus, although statistical correlations between anti-HCV levels and clinical features may exist, they are not sufficiently uniform to suggest a common pathogenic mechanism.

The persistence of infection in the majority of the HCV-infected individuals, despite the presence of HCV-directed antibodies, suggests that such antibodies fail to induce viral clearance. Antibodies against envelope proteins often have neutralizing ability and may prevent viral entry into cells or target the virus for elimination by scavenger cells. A series of experiments by Farci *et al.* provides insight into this issue [8,9]. They have shown that chimpanzees that cleared an initial infection, as judged by normal alanine aminotransferase (ALT) levels and the absence of HCV RNA, could be reinfected by either heterologous or autologous challenge, despite the development of a competent humoral response [8]. In a second study, the authors performed *in vitro* neutralization followed by chimpanzee challenge to show that a serum obtained 11 years after infection had no neutralizing effect, whereas a serum obtained two years after infection was able to neutralize the infecting strain [9]. Sequential analysis of viral isolates revealed significant genetic divergence between the acute-phase strain and the predominant strain at two years, although the latter strain was present during the acute phase of infection [9]. This data supports the quasispecies nature of the virus and the selection of strains that lack the corresponding epitopes by immune pressure. Overall, this evidence suggests those neutralizing responses are highly strain-specific and that the quasispecies nature of the virus allows other strains to emerge when the predominant strain is under immune pressure. This represents a major obstacle in the development of an effective vaccine, since vaccine development is dependent upon induction of neutralizing antibodies to conserved epitopes of the envelope proteins.

Most studies have focused on the protective role of antibodies in HCV infection and there has been limited information on antibody-mediated hepato cellular cytotoxicity. Antibodies may contribute to hepatocellular damage through direct cytotoxicity, complement activation, or antibody-dependent cellular cytotoxicity (ADCC). Intrahepatic lymphoid aggregates containing a germinal centre of activated B cells are commonly observed in patients with chronic HCV infection and may represent a host B-cell response to HCV infection [10]. Furthermore, serum interleukin 4, a cytokine known to activate B cells, is also shown to be elevated in a small proportion of patients with chronic HCV infection [11]. However, for the antibodies produced by these activated B cells to contribute to hepatocellular damage, they must recognize antigen on the hepatocyte cell membrane. To date, HCV antigens (core, E1, E2, NS3 and NS4) have only been detected in the cytoplasm of infected hepatocytes; membranous distribution has not been observed *in vivo* or *in vitro* [12]. These data support the belief that antibody-mediated pathways are unlikely to play an important role in mediating hepatocellular damage.

The humoral immune response to HCV may also contribute to extrahepatic and autoimmune immunopathology. More than half of the patients with chronic HCV infection show marked expansion of CD5+ B lymphocytes in their peripheral blood [13]. Activation of this subset of cells has been associated with autoimmune diseases such as rheumatoid arthritis [14], and their expansion may be linked to the development of autoimmunity, and possibly B-cell lymphomas in patients with HCV infection. Moreover, chronic HCV infection has been linked to the development of autoantibodies, including liver/kidney

microsomal autoantibodies (anti-LKM antibodies), the antibody sometimes associated with type 2 autoimmune hepatitis. The exact relationship between HCV infection and this type of autoimmunity is unknown but the majority of such patients also have circulating antibodies to a human-derived epitope known as GOR [15]. Recent data suggests that these antibodies may result from molecular mimicry between the HCV core sequence and GOR [16]. Regardless, these autoantibodies have no clinical implications and it appears that a role in disease pathogenesis, if it exists, is minor [17,18].

## CELLULAR IMMUNE RESPONSE

The cellular immune defence against viral infection involves both non-specific and antigen-specific phases. Eradication of viral infection is probably dependent upon classical CD4+ and CD8+ cytotoxic T-lymphocyte (CTL) responses. Intracellular and extracellular viral proteins present quite different challenges to the immune system, both in terms of recognition and of appropriate response. Unlike antigen recognition by B-cell immunoglobulin receptors, the two general classes of T cells do not recognize native antigen, but rather recognize short antigenic peptides that have been 'processed' and presented on the cell surface. For an appropriate response, it is necessary for the T cell receptor to recognize a ligand composed of a processed viral immunogenic peptide bound to a major histocompatibility complex (MHC) molecule on the surface of an antigen presenting cell (APC) or target cell. Processed peptides are generally presented to CD8+ T cells by MHC class I molecules, which are expressed on virtually all cells, or to CD4+ T cells by the MHC class II molecules which are found on specialized APCs. The mechanisms by which CD4+ and CD8+ effector cells resolve viral infection and contribute to hepatocellular damage in HCV remain to be elucidated.

### CD4+ T cell response

The CD4+ T cell response to viral proteins is usually critical for host protection, since it augments antibody production by B cells and stimulates CD8+ T cells, including those that are specific for virus-infected cells [19,20]. Without CD4+ cells, induction of new immune responses is impaired and CTL memory cannot be maintained *in vivo*. Numerous studies have described human leukocyte antigen (HLA) class II-restricted CD4+ T cell responses in HCV-infected individuals, usually by measuring proliferative T cell responses or the production of IFN-γ when cells are exposed to recombinant viral proteins. Boterelli *et al.* found HLA class II-restricted CD4+ T cell mediated proliferative responses to several recombinant proteins derived from different regions of HCV, with NS4 being the most immunogenic HCV antigen [21]. Of particular interest, HCV RNA-positive individuals without clinical or histological evidence of liver disease had a significantly higher CD4+ proliferative response to the HCV core protein (73%) than patients with chronic hepatitis (10%). Lechmann *et al.* have recently provided evidence for an association between the elimination of HCV infection and strong T helper proliferative responses to the core, NS4A and NS5B regions [22]. This association of a more benign course of infection with a T-helper response to core protein has been reported by other investigators [23]. This suggests that CD4+ cells may control or protect against, rather than mediate, hepatocellular damage.

Most of the CD4+ proliferative data has been generated by analysing peripheral blood responses as opposed to intrahepatic ones. One drawback to the study of T cell responses in the peripheral blood is that it may not necessarily reflect the pattern of T cell responses in the liver. Study of the hepatic CD4+ cell population has the advantage of analysing cells that function at the site of HCV infection. Minutello *et al.* found that the NS4 protein was able to stimulate CD4+ cells isolated from liver biopsies in 3 of 19 patients [24]. There was no response to any of the other recombinant HCV-derived proteins. It is of interest that the NS4-specific clones derived from the peripheral blood had T cell receptors that were different to those on the intrahepatic clones, suggesting compartmentalization of the T-lymphocyte response to the liver. Lohr *et al.* identified liver-derived T cell clones that had a proliferative response to conserved regions of core, E1 and NS4 [25]. Of note, proliferative responses to HCV core peptides were significantly greater in patients with active liver disease than in HCV carriers with normal liver tests, suggesting a possible correlation between the CD4+ response to the core protein and disease activity. Interestingly, Bertoletti and colleagues have studied the intrahepatic CD4+ cell response and failed to detect HCV antigen-specific T cell clones [26]. These findings suggest that virus non-specific T cells are the dominant population in the inflammatory infiltrates within the liver.

It is clear that CD4+ T cells are present in patients with chronic HCV infection and respond to both structural (core) and non-structural (NS4) proteins. CD4+ cells are important for providing help for B cells and local cytokine production in the liver, but may also augment HCV-specific CTL activity. Quantitatively, individuals who have a more vigorous proliferative response to HCV antigens are more likely to clear HCV after acute infection and clear viraemia after interferon therapy [23]. When infection persists, CD4+ cells contribute to the inflammatory infiltrate within the liver and may help mediate ongoing hepatocellular injury. Future functional studies of specific CD4+ T cells, as well as studies of their response during IFN therapy and virus elimination, will enhance our understanding of the pathogenetic role of this effector arm.

## Cytokine response

Cytokines are regulatory molecules that play an important role in orchestrating several physiological and pathological processes. CD4+ T cells, which are central to the induction of antiviral responses, are separated into Th1 (T-helper 1) and Th2 subtypes, and an inactive Th0 type, based on the profile of their cyokine production. Th1 cells secrete interleukin 2 (IL-2) and interferon γ, which are required for host antiviral immune responses including CTL generation and natural killer (NK) cell activation. Th2 cells produce IL-4 and IL-10, which help augment antibody production, play a prominent role in allergic and anti-helminthic responses, and exert a negative regulatory effect on the Th1 response [27,28]. It is now recognized that these cytokines can be produced by cells other than CD4+ T cells. It has therefore been suggested that these cytokine responses should be referred to as Th1-like and Th2-like responses [29].

It has been postulated that an imbalance in Th1 and Th2 cytokine production is implicated in disease progression or inability to clear infections. In acute self-limiting HCV infection, circulating helper T cell clones have been shown to predominantly produce interferon-γ, suggesting a Th0/Th1-like pattern [30]. Tsai *et al.* have recently found that patients who are able to clear an acute hepatitis C infection and who do not progress to chronic disease have a strong Th1, but no Th2 cytokine response [31]. In contrast, those who developed a chronic infection had a milder Th1 response and all of them had a Th2 response. It has therefore been speculated that this Th2 type of response may have an inhibitory impact on the patients' immune function. In a study by Reiser *et al.*, a proportion of patients with chronic hepatitis C, but not controls, had increased serum levels of IL-4 and IL-10, suggesting that this Th2-like response is activated, at least in a proportion of patients [11].

Whether this Th2 response is secondary to an increased Th1 response and whether the increased Th2 response has a role in viral persistence and disease pathogenesis remains to be established.

Once persistent infection occurs, cytokines may also play a role in mediating hepatocellular injury. Bertoletti et al. studied the intrahepatic CD4$^+$ response and demonstrated that the majority of liver-infiltrating T cells were Th1 cells able to secrete IFN-$\gamma$ but unable to secrete IL-4 or IL-5, cytokines that are commonly secreted by Th2 cells [26]. Others have shown that circulating T cells release IFN-$\gamma$ and TNF-$\alpha$ upon peptide stimulation, also suggesting a Th1 cytokine profile [32]. Plasma levels of TNF-$\alpha$ have been found to correlate with biochemical markers of hepatocellular damage in HCV patients [33]. Napoli et al. looked at the role of cytokines in the mechanism of liver injury in chronic HCV patients. They found that patients with severe chronic hepatitis C or cirrhosis had an enhanced expression of both IFN-$\gamma$ and IL-2 compared with controls and those with mild disease [34]. In contrast, controls and patients with milder inflammation had higher expression of IL-10 compared with patients with overt liver disease. In addition, the mRNA levels of IFN-$\gamma$ and IL-2 correlated with fibrosis and portal inflammation, suggesting that Th1 cytokines might play a role in mediating hepatocellular damage. Interestingly, Cacciarelli and colleagues showed that the levels of Th2 cytokines were markedly greater than those of Th1 cytokines during chronic HCV infection [35]. IFN-$\alpha$ treatment diminished the Th2 cytokine response in parallel to the decrease in viral load. Reiser et al. confirmed that a proportion of patients with chronic HCV infection had elevated serum IL-4 and IL-10 levels, and found Th2 cell markers in inflammatory infiltrates within the liver, although Th2 cells represented a minority of the infiltrating mononuclear cells [11]. Given the ability of IL-4 and IL-10 to inhibit immune cell function, Th2 cells may provide an autoregulatory mechanism whereby the host immune response is able to partially offset the potentially detrimental effects of the Th1 response.

From the existing data, it appears that the Th1 response is activated in the liver in response to HCV infection. Local production of these cytokines by virus-specific and non-specific T cells may represent an attempt by the immune system to maximize the efficiency of controlling the infection and target cell killing via an increase in the target cell molecules necessary for recognition or inhibition of viral replication. This attempt to control viral replication is apparently ineffective in eliminating the infection in the case of chronic HCV infection, with a resultant increase in liver cell damage once persistent infection is established. The Th2 cascade probably represents an autoregulatory response which originates mainly outside of the liver and attempts to confine the Th1 response to the liver in order to prevent systemic effects. One cannot rule out that this Th2 response may play a role in viral persistence but definite evidence supporting this is lacking.

## CD8$^+$ CTL response

The CD8$^+$ CTL arm of the cellular immune system may be important in the control of HCV infection and the pathogenesis of liver injury. CTLs have been found to offer protection against a number of viral infections in vivo. In their attempt to control the viral infection by eliminating viral infected cells, tissue damage occurs. In patients with chronic HCV infection, an insufficient HCV-specific CTL response may be responsible for viral persistence. An ongoing HCV-specific CTL response without viral elimination might thereby contribute to chronic hepatocellular damage.

The importance of the CTL response during acute infection has recently been studied. Using a chimpanzee model, Cooper et al. prospectively analysed the humoral and intrahepatic CTL responses during the acute phase of HCV infection [36]. Four individuals that progressed to chronic infection either failed to display HCV-specific CTLs or developed a CTL response that remained narrowly focused during the early course of infection. In contrast, in both individuals that resolved, termination of viraemia correlated precisely with an early, class I-restricted, polyspecific CTL response against multiple HCV proteins, some of which were conserved. Termination of viraemia did not correlate however, with the presence of anti-HCV antibodies, which persistently remained undetectable in one of the two patients that resolved. Of interest, one and a half years later, HCV-specific CTLs were still detectable, attesting to the durability of the CTL response.

HCV-specific cytotoxic, CD8$^+$ T lymphocytes have been isolated from the liver or peripheral blood mononuclear cells (PBMCs) in a significant proportion of patients with chronic HCV infection. Immunophenotyping studies have demonstrated that activated CD8$^+$ T lymphocytes make up a significant proportion of the intrahepatic-activated cell population in patients with chronic hepatitis C [37]. There is also up-regulated expression of adhesion molecules in the inflamed portal tracts, which may reflect a pathway for the recruitment and priming of hepatic T cells [38].

Intrahepatic CD8+, HCV-specific CTLs have been isolated from the liver of chronic HCV infection using a non-specific stimulation strategy. Koziel *et al.* demonstrated that HCV-specific CTLs are present in the livers of patients with chronic HCV infection [39,40]. They also showed that the HCV-specific CTLs are restricted by MHC class I molecules, suggesting that MHC subtypes might present different processed viral peptides to their CTLs and affect the severity of cell injury.

The presence of HCV-specific CTLs in chronic HCV infection has been confirmed by a number of groups, and target epitopes from within both structural and non-structural regions have been identified [41–44]. To define the role of HCV-specific CTLs in pathogenesis and host–virus interaction, our laboratory has isolated hepatic lymphocytes from 35 patients with chronic HCV infection. Using recombinant vaccinia viruses that expressed the prototypic 1a strain to screen for HCV-specific CTLs, hepatic HCV-specific CTLs were detected from bulk-expanded CD8+ cells in half of the patients. Three of these individuals were infected with strains that were not type 1a, suggesting that the CTL response in these individuals had cross-genotype CTL responses. The immunodominant CTL epitopes were most commonly located within the HCV structural antigens (core, E1 and E2). CTL responses to non-structural regions occured in a smaller subset of patients. HCV-specific CTLs could not be detected in peripheral blood without HCV-specific stimulation, suggesting a tissue-dependent prevalence of HCV-specific CTL activity [45]. This is not surprising since the liver is the primary site of HCV replication and is the logical recruiter of HCV-specific CTLs. In an elegant set of experiments, Cerny *et al.* estimated the frequency of HCV-specific CTLs in PBMCs from patients with chronic hepatitis C to be only 1 per 30,000 to 1 per 300,000. We have recently determined CTL precursor (pCTL) frequencies for peripheral and intrahepatic CTLs using linear regression analysis [46]. The frequency of intrahepatic pCTLs specific for the structural region of HCV ranged from 240–1000/total CD8+ cells, while peripheral frequencies ranged from $2.5 \times 10^3$ to $30 \times 10^3$/total CD8+ cells. There was an approximately 10–100 fold difference in the frequencies of intrahepatic and peripheral pCTLs specific for HCV structural epitopes. Thus, the frequent detection of HCV-specific CTL activity in hepatic CD8+ cells suggests a preferential compartmentalization of the anti-HCV CTL response in the liver. As described earlier, a similar tissue-specific localization has also been reported for CD4+cells [24].

Our laboratory has also provided indirect evidence supporting a role for HCV-specific CTLs in the control of viral replication and production of hepatocellular damage in chronic HCV infection. Patients with HCV-specific CTL activity from bulk-expanded liver CD8+ T cells were found to have higher serum ALT levels and more active histological disease compared with patients who had levels of CTL activity that were not detectable using our assay. Of interest, both portal and periportal inflammatory activity on liver biopsy correlated with the presence of CTL activity. These findings complement the immuno-histochemical studies of intrahepatic inflammatory infiltrates that have demonstrated an increase in CD8+ cells in the periportal areas, especially in areas of piecemeal necrosis [47]. In the same set of experiments we were also able to show that patients with HCV-specific CTL activity had HCV RNA levels that were reduced by 0.5–1 log, suggesting that HCV-specific CTL activity is important in regulating HCV infection. Rehermann *et al.*, using a multiwell stimulation technique, found a correlation between the overall CTL response and the likelihood of having no detectable virus by a branched-chain DNA assay [48]. Hiroishi and colleagues found that, among a group of individuals with the HLA-B44 allele, the presence of a CTL response against an epitope in HCV core was associated with a lower viral titre [49]. A similar role for CTLs in other viral infections has been demonstrated. For example, in lymphocytic choriomeningitis virus infection, introduction of virus-specific CTL activity reduces viral titres by 4–5 logs [50]. The CD8+ CTL response may lead to viral clearance either through direct lysis of infected cells or through cytokine-mediated inhibition of the virus. It is likely that the balance between viral clearance and hepatocellular damage is determined by the relative activities of, and interactions between, HCV-specific CD8+ and CD4+ cells within the liver.

## Mechanism of action of CTLs

The mechanisms by which CTLs destroy virus-infected hepatocytes are just beginning to be clarified. Apoptosis is an important mechanism of immune-mediated cell death [51]. By secreting molecules, such as the pore-forming protein perforin and a series of granule serine proteinases (granzymes), CTLs can directly induce the death of target cells by forming holes in their membranes [52]. CTL-mediated cytotoxicity can also result from the interaction between the Fas/Apo1 receptor and its ligand expressed on the surface of the activated CD8+ cells [53]. This mechanism is supported by the observation that hepatic expression of c-Fas is increased in patients with chronic HCV infection, particularly among hepatocytes adjacent to infiltrating lymphocytes. The binding of Fas to its ligand, FasL, would be expected to render the hepatocytes susceptible to death [54,55]. Finally, CTLs can disrupt viral replication by producing lymphokines such as IFN-γ and TNF-α, which are known to directly inhibit viral replication in infected cells [56]. Koziel and colleagues were able to demonstrate that liver-derived HCV-specific CTLs produce TNF-α and IFN-γ when they recognize HCV-infected target cells. Other cytokines, such as granulocyte–macrophage colony-stimulating factor (GM–CSF) and IL-8, which can act as a neutrophil chemotactic factor, are also produced by HCV-specific CTLs. In addition, IFNs can upregulate expression of MHC class I molecules on the surface of infected cells, which may enhance their ability to be recognized by CTLs [57].

## Influence of HLA

The human leukocyte antigen is a crucial genetic factor that initiates or regulates immune response by presenting foreign antigens to T lymphocytes. The association between HLA polymorphism and disease susceptibility is currently under investigation. An association between some HLA alleles and the asymptomatic state of HCV infection has been reported. In Italian and Japanese subjects, the DR5 and DR13 alleles, respectively, are more frequently found in symptom-free HCV carriers than in patients with progressive liver disease [58,59]. This data suggests that the particular class II molecules protect against HCV-induced liver injury. Kuzushita and colleagues have reported that extended haplotypes, which include the class I B54 allele, are closely associated with the progression of liver injury, whereas certain extended class II haplotypes are associated with low hepatitis activity in chronic HCV infection [60]. The same group has also recently reported a primary association of hepatitis activity with the transporter molecule that is associated with antigen processing for HLA class I molecules [61]. These results suggest that the particular HLA alleles or the extended haplotypes spanning the class I to class II loci may be associated with susceptibility or resistance to HCV, and may influence the clinical course of HCV infection.

## DIRECT VIRAL CYTOPATHICITY

A virus can induce direct cytopathic injury either through a direct toxic effect on cell viability or by interference with normal cellular function by viral gene products. Thus, viruses may interfere with the synthesis of cellular macromolecules, increase lysosomal permeability, or alter cellular membranes. There is some evidence to suggest that HCV can, in certain circumstances, induce tissue damage directly. First, HCV is a member of the family *Flaviviridae*, and other members of this family, such as yellow fever virus, often cause direct cytopathic injury to infected cells [62]. Second, histological examination of HCV-infected livers occasionally reveals a hepatocyte that exhibits cytopathic changes in the absence of adjacent inflammation. Direct cytopathicity is usually recognized by morphological alterations of cellular architecture such as cell shrinkage, cell rounding and nuclear pycnosis. This finding suggests that HCV may exert a direct cytopathic effect in some infected cells [63,64]. Recent clinical observations have also suggested a role for HCV in direct cytopathicity. In an immunocompromised heart transplant recipient who acquired HCV infection from the donor organ, very high-level hepatic RNA expression has been reported. This patient subsequently developed subfulminant hepatic failure, characterized by coagulopathy and marked cholestasis [65]. Since this initial report, various liver transplant centres have described a similar disease pattern in a small number of liver transplant patients with recurrent HCV infection. These patients also developed rapidly progressive graft dysfunction, and had liver biopsy findings that resembled the fibrosing cholestatic hepatitis seen in liver transplant recipients with severe hepatitis B recurrence, in which clinical and biochemical liver failure was associated with minimal liver inflammation. This suggests that the high-level expression of HBV was directly cyopathic in this clinical setting [66,67]. The severe liver dysfunction in these patients is usually associated with an atypical histological picture of pericellular fibrosis, marked intracellular cholestasis and only mild inflammation. This pathology (fibrosing cholestatic hepatitis) is reminiscent of the cytopathic changes seen in hepatitis B virus-infected immunosuppressed patients and therefore suggests that HCV might be directly cytopathic at high levels of intracellular virus [68]. The relative paucity of intrahepatic lymphocytes in these individuals with markedly depressed cell-mediated immunity, and the marked increase in the expression of HCV, suggests that it is the presence of HCV itself that is the cause of the liver damage. Thus, while direct evidence is lacking, these clinical data provide supportive evidence that HCV, when expressed at very high levels, may cause direct cytopathicity in the liver.

If intracellular viral accumulation is essential for direct cytopathicity, one would expect a correlation between viral load and hepatocellular damage. Indeed, a correlation between serum HCV RNA, as measured by branched DNA (bDNA) signal amplification, has been noted and suggests that cytopathicity may contribute to hepatocellular damage in cells expressing high levels of HCV [69]. Higher hepatic HCV RNA levels were also reported in patients with chronic active hepatitis compared with those with chronic persistent hepatitis [70]. However, *in situ* detection of HCV (*in situ* PCR and immunohistochemistry) has failed to demonstrate a correlation between hepatic expression of HCV antigen or RNA and biochemical or histological markers of disease activity [71,72]. One may interpret this lack of a convincing correlation between hepatic HCV expression and hepatocellular damage as critical evidence against a direct cytopathic effect of HCV. However, direct liver damage may occur only when intracellular HCV antigen accumulation exceeds a critical threshold, and this level may not be reached in most infected hepatocytes in patients with chronic HCV infection.

If HCV is cytopathic at high levels, one would expect that high-level expression of HCV proteins must alter hepatocellular structure or function. HCV structural proteins, which contain a hydrophobic sequence that guides the structural proteins to the endoplasmic reticulum for processing and glycosylation, may play a role in viral cytopathicity. Evidence for this hypothesis was recently provided in cell lines expressing HCV structural proteins. In cells that persistently express these proteins, there was mitochondrial and endoplasmic reticulum proliferation, distention of the endoplasmic reticulum, and hepatocellular ballooning, as seen in liver transplant recipients with early severe HCV recurrence [73]. It is possible that overexpression of HCV structural proteins may interfere with the regular cellular protein processing, thereby leading to ballooning (from dilation of endoplasmic reticulum) and loss of cellular function (cholestasis and reduced production of proteins like coagulation factors). However, recent transgenic mouse models with high-level expression of HCV structural proteins did not show similar findings. In fact, the transgenic livers remained histologically normal [74]. Taken together, these observations suggest that direct cytopathic injury due to expression of HCV structural proteins might be possible, but probably depends on either the level of viral expression, or factors other than protein expression. It is possible that

high-level expression of some HCV gene products may enhance cellular susceptibility to cytokines or other mediators of liver cell injury. *In vitro*, it was reported that high level expression of HCV core leads to an enhanced sensitivity to the effects of TNF-α [75]. The core protein has also recently been shown to interact with the TNF receptor [76].

Evidence arguing against direct cytopathicity can also be found in the clinical setting. First, a small number of patients have recently been identified as healthy carriers, in other words they have persistently normal serum ALT levels despite the presence of detectable HCV RNA in the blood [77,78]. Since HCV is known to replicate in the liver, this would suggest that HCV is not directly cytopathic to hepatocytes. As discussed earlier, the level of HCV expression may not reach the threshold level that induces cytopathic changes. Second, in the majority of patients with chronic HCV infection, the typical histological picture of HCV is notable for lymphoid infiltration of the liver, and not cytopathic changes in the infected cells.

In summary, it appears that under normal host–virus interactions, there is little evidence to suggest that direct cytopathicity plays a significant role in liver cell injury. But, when host conditions are altered to allow for unusually high levels of viral replication and viral protein expression (for example, during immune suppression), HCV may induce direct hepatocellular damage. The development of cell culture systems and animal models will allow further clarification of this issue.

## ENVIRONMENTAL FACTORS

Other factors such as viral coinfection, alcohol abuse and drugs may interact with the host–virus relationship to alter the pathogenesis of HCV infection. Studies have suggested that chronic hepatitis C is worsened by the superimposition of HBV infection, and that this combination increases the risk of carcinogenesis [79,80]. The relationship between HCV infection and alcoholic liver disease is well documented. Chronic alcoholism may allow a higher level of HCV replication [81] and is a major factor in promoting progression of liver disease in persons with chronic HCV infection [82]. It is unclear whether HCV infection and chronic alcoholism are independent risk factors for chronic liver disease or whether they are additive or synergistic in their effects. Regardless, cessation of alcohol intake remains one of the most important interventions to limit further progression of liver disease in patients with chronic HCV infection.

# CONCLUSIONS

HCV-infected patients with chronic liver disease have evidence of circulating HCV-specific antibodies and a polyclonal, multispecific T cell response. CD4[+] proliferative responses and HCV-specific CTLs directed against one or more viral antigens are readily detected in those individuals who develop chronic HCV infection and appear to compartmentalize within the liver. Cytokines, which are produced locally within the liver and systemically, may play an important role in controlling viral replication and contributing to hepatocellular damage. However, neither the humoral nor cellular immune response, nor the cytokine response appears sufficient to eradicate infection in most patients. In its attempt to clear the virus from the liver, the immune system contributes to the hepatocellular injury seen in the majority of chronically infected patients. A better understanding of the host's immune response may provide further insight on the pathogenetic mechanisms involved in development of chronic hepatitis and aid the development of more effective therapeutic strategies.

# ACKNOWLEDGEMENTS

This work was carried out at the Department of Medicine at the University of Florida. David R. Nelson is supported by a GlaxoWellcome Institute of Digestive Health Clinical Investigator Award and the Digestive Health Foundation Hepatology Research Award. Johnson Y.N. Lau was supported by the American Liver Foundation Hans Popper Liver Scholar Award and a NIH R01AI41219.

# REFERENCES

1. Kiyosawa K, Sodeyama T, Tanaka E, Gibo Y, Yoshizawa K, Nakano Y Furuta S, et al. Interrelationship of blood transfusion, non-A, non-B hepatitis and hepatocellular carcinoma: analysis by detection of antibody to hepatitis C virus. Hepatology 1990; 67:671–675.
2. Choo QL, Kuo G, Weiner AJ, Overby LR, Bradley DW & Houghton Ml. Isolation of a cDNA clone derived from a blood borne non-A, non-B hepatitis genome. Science 1989; 244:359–362.
3. Ray R, Khanna A, Lagging LM, Meyer K, Choo QL, Ralston R, Houghton M & Becherer PR. Peptide immunogen mimicry of putative E1 glycoprotein-specific epitopes in hepatitis C virus. Journal of Virology 1994; 68:4420–4226.
4. Bjorkander J, Cunningham-Rudles C, Lundin P, Olsson R, Soderstrom R & Hanson LA. Intravenous immunoglobulin prophylaxis causing liver damage in 16 of 77 patients with hypogammaglobulinaemia or IgG subclass deficiency. American Journal of Medicine 1988; 84:107–111.
5. Diodati G, Bonetti P, Noventa F, Casarin C, Rugge M, Scaccabarozzi S, Tagger A, et al. Treatment of chronic hepatitis C with recombinant human interferon-2a: results of a randomized controlled clinical trial. Hepatology 1994; 19:1–5.
6. Nagayoma R, Miyake K, Tsuda F, Okamoto H. IgM antibody to a hepatitis C virus core peptide (CP14) for monitoring activity of liver disease in patients with acute or chronic hepatitis C. Journal of Medical Virology 1994; 42:311–317.
7. Lau GKK, Lesniewski R, Johnson RG, Davis GL, Lau JY. Immunoglobulin M and A in chronic hepatitis C virus infection. Journal of Medical Virology 1994; 44:1–4.
8. Farci P, Alter HJ, Govindarajan S, Wong DC, Engle R, Lesniewski RR, Mushahwar IK, et al. Lack of protective immunity against reinfection with hepatitis C virus. Science 1992; 258:135–140.
9. Farci P, Alter HJ, Wong DC, Miller RH, Govindarajan S, Engle R, Shapiro M & Purcell RH. Prevention of hepatitis C virus infection in chimpanzees after antibody-mediated in vitro neutralization. Proceedings of the National Acadamy of Sciences, USA 1994; 91:7792–7796.
10. Desmet VJ, Gerber M, Hoofnagle JH, Manns M & Scheuer PJ. Classification of chronic hepatitis: diagnosis, grading and staging. Hepatology 1994; 19:1513–1520.
11. Reiser M, Marousis CG, Nelson DR, Lauer G, Gonzalez-Peralta RP, Davis GL & Lau JYN. Serum interleukin 4 and interleukin 10 levels in patients with chronic hepatitis C virus infection. Journal of Hepatology 1997; 26:471–478.
12. Selby MJ, Choo QL, Berger K, Kuo G, Glazer E, Eckart M, Lee C, Chien D, Kuo C & Houghton M. Expression, identification and subcellular localization of the proteins encoded by the hepatitis C viral genome. Journal of General Virology 1993; 74:1103–1113.
13. Pozzato G, Moretti M, Crovatto M, Modolo ML, Gennari D & Santini G. Lymphocyte subsets in HCV-positive chronic liver disease. Immunology Today 1994; 15:137–138.
14. Jarvis JN, Kaplan J & Fine N. Increase in CD5+ B-cells in juvenile rheumatoid arthritis. Relationship to IgM rheumatoid factor expression and disease activity. Arthritis and Rheumatology 1992; 35:204.
15. Lenzi M, Cassani F, Ballardini G, Bianchi FB, Mishiro S; Unoura M, Kaneko S & Kobayashi K. Anti-HCV, anti-GOR, and autoimmunity. Lancet 1992; 339: 871–872.
16. Lau JYN, Mizokami M, Davis G, Kolberg JA, Urdea M, Orito E, Polito A, DiNello R & Quan S. Relationship between the presence of circulating anti-GOR and hepatitis C viremia/genotype. Journal of Hepatology 1995; 22:707.
17. Lau JYN, Davis GL, Orito E, Qian KP, Mizokami M. Significance of antibody to the host cellular gene derived epitope GOR in chronic hepatitis C virus infection. Journal of Hepatology 1994; 17:253–257.
18. Liani G, Lecce R, Badolato MC, et al. Anti-GOR antibodies in anti-hepatitis C virus positive subjects with and without virus replication and liver disease. Journal of Hepatology 1994; 20:845.
19. Sprent J & Webb SR. Function and specificity of T cell subsets in the mouse. Advances in Immunology 1987; 41:39–133.
20. Kita H, Moriyama T, Kaneko T, Hiroishi K, Harase I, Miura H, Nakamura I, Inamori H, et al. A helper T cell antigen enhances generation of hepatitis C virus-

specific cytotoxic T lymphocytes in vitro. *Journal of Medical Virology* 1995; **45**:386–391.

21. Botarelli P, Brunetto MR, Minutello MA, Calvo P, Unutmaz D, Weiner AJ, Choo QL, *et al*. T-lymphocyte response to hepatitis C virus in different clinical courses of infection. *Gastroenterology* 1993; **194**: 580–587.

22. Lechmann M, Ihlenfeldt HG, Braunschweiger I, Giers G, Jung G, Matz B, Kaiser R, Sauerbruch T & Spengler U. T and B cell responses to different hepatitis C virus antigens in patients with chronic hepatitis C infection and in healthy anti-hepatitis C virus-positive blood donors without viremia. *Hepatology* 1996; **24**:790–795.

23. Hoffman RM, Diepolder HM, Zachoval R, Zweibel FM, Jung MC, Scholz S, Nitscho H, Riethmuller G & Pape GR. Mapping of immunodominant CD4+ T lymphocyte epitopes of hepatitis C virus antigens and their relevance during the course of chronic infection. *Hepatology* 1995; **21**:632–638.

24. Minutello MA, Pleri P, Unutmaz D, Censini S, Kuo G, Houghton M, Brunetto MR, Bonino F & Abrignani S. Compartmentalization of T lymphocytes to the site of disease: intrahepatic CD4+ T cell-specific for the protein NS4 of hepatitis C virus in patients with chronic hepatitis C. *Journal of Experimental Medicine* 1993; **178**:17–25.

25. Lohr HF, Schlaak JF, Kollmannsperger S, dienes HP, Meyer zum Buschenfelde KH & Gerken D. The role of cellular immune response in chronic HCV infection. *Hepatology* 1994; **20**:A533.

26. Bertoletti A, D'Elios MM, Boni C, De Carli M, Zignego AL, Durazzo M, Missale G, *et al*. Different cytokine profiles of intrahepatic T cells in chronic hepatitis B and hepatitis C virus infections. *Gastroenterology* 1997; **112**: 193–199.

27. Mosmann TR & Coffman RL. Th1 and Th2 cells: Different patterns of lymphokine secretion lead to different functional properties. *Annual Review of Immunology* 1989; **7**:145–173.

28. Fiorentino DF, Zlotnik A, Viera P, Mosmann TR, Howard M, Moore KW & O'Garra A. IL-10 acts on the antigen presenting cell to inhibit cytokine production by Th1 cells. *Journal of Immunology* 1991; **146**:3444–3451.

29. Clerici M & Shearer GM. The Th1-Th2 hypothesis of HIV infection: new insights. *Immunology Today* 1994; **15**:575–581.

30. Diepolder HM, Zachoval R, Hoffmann RM, Wierenga EA; Santantonio T, Jung MC; Eichenlaub D & Pape GR. Possible mechanism involving T-lymphocyte response to non-structural protein 3 in viral clearance in acute hepatitis C infection. *Lancet* 1995; **346**:1006–1007.

31. Tsai SL, Liaw YF, Chen MH, Huang CY & Kuo GC. Detection of type 2-like T-helper cells in hepatitis C virus infection: implications for hepatitis C virus chronicity. *Hepatology* 1997; **25**:449–458.

32. Diepolder HM, Zachoval R, Wierenga E, Jung MC, Korherr C, Zweibel FM, Riethmuller G Paumgartner G & Pape GR. Nonstructural protein 3 of hepatitis C virus is the most immunogenic HCV antigen for CD4+ T lymphocytes in acute hepatitis C. *Hepatology* 1994; **20**:229A.

33. Nelson DR, Lim HL, Fang JWS, *et al*. The tumor necrosis-a system in chronic hepatitis C. *Digestive Disease and Science* 1998; in press.

34. Napoli J, Bishop A, McGuinness P, Painter DM & McCaughan GW. Progressive liver injury in chronic hepatitis C infection correlates with increased intra-hepatic expression of Th1-associated cytokines.

*Hepatology* 1996; **24**:759–765.

35. Cacciarelli TV, Martinez OM, Gish RG, Villanueva JC & Krams SM. Immunoregulatory cytokines in hepatitis C virus infection: pre- and post-treatment with interferon alfa. *Hepatology* 1996; **24**:6–9.

36. Cooper S, Erickson A, Chein D, Weiner A, Houghton M, Parham P, Walker C. CD8+ CTL directed against multiple hepatitis C viral proteins early in the course of infection correlate with immunity and endure following viral clearance. *US–Japan Hepatitis Joint Panel Meeting*, Pacific Grove, California, USA, 1998.

37. Onji M, Kikuchi T, Kumon I Masumoto T, Ndano S, Kajino K, Horikee N & Ohta Y. Intrahepatic lymphocyte subpopulations and HLA class I antigen expression by hepatocytes in chronic hepatitis C. *Hepatogastroenterology* 1992; **39**:340–343.

38. Garcia-Monzon C, Sanchez-Madrid F, Garcia-Buey L, Garcia-Arroyo A, Garcia-Sanchez A & Moreno-Otero R. Vascular adhesion molecule expression in viral chronic hepatitis: evidence of neoangiogenesis in portal tracts. *Gastroenterology* 1995; **108**:231–241.

39. Koziel MJ, Dudley D, Wong JT, Dienstag J, Houghton M, Ralston R & Walker BD. Intrahepatic cytotoxic T lymphocytes specific for hepatitis C virus in persons with chronic hepatitis. *Journal of Immunology* 1992; **149**:3339–3344.

40. Koziel MJ, Dudley D, Afdhal N, Choo QL, Houghton M, Ralston R & Walker BD. Hepatitis C virus-specific cytotoxic T lymphocytes recognize epitopes in the core and envelope proteins of HCV. *Journal of Virology* 1993; **67**:7522–7532.

41. Kita H, Moriyama T, Kaneko T, Harase I, Nomura M, Miura H, Nakamura I, Yazaki Y & Imawari M. HLA B44-restricted cytotoxic T lymphocytes recognizing an epitope on hepatitis C virus nucleocapsid protein. *Hepatology* 1993; **18**:1039-1044.

42. Erickson AL, Houghton M, Choo QL, Weiner AJ, Ralston R, Muchmore E & Walker CM. Hepatitis C virus-specific CTL responses in the liver of the chimpanzees with acute and chronic hepatitis C. *Journal of Immunology* 1993; **151**:4189–4199.

43. Cerny A, McHutchinson JG, Pasquinelli C, Brown ME, Brothers MA, Grabscheid B, Fowler P, Houghton Mn & Chisari FV. Cytotoxic T lymphocyte response to hepatitis C virus-derived peptides containing the HLA A2.1 binding motif. *Journal of Clinical Investigation* 1995; **95**:521–530.

44. Tsai SL, Chen PJ, Hwang LH, Kao JH, Huang JH, Chang TH & Chen DS. Immune response to a hepatitis C nonstructural protein in chronic hepatitis C virus infection. *Journal of Hepatology* 1994; **21**:403–411.

45. Nelson DR, Marousis CG, Davis GL, Rice CM, Wong J, Houghton M & Lau JYN. The role of hepatitis C virus-specific cytotoxic T lymphocytes in chronic hepatitis C. *Journal of Immunology* 1997; **158**: 1473–1481.

46. Nelson DR, Bhardwaj B & Lau JYN. HCV-specific CTL: evidence for intrahepatic compartmentalization and participation in disease pathogenesis. *Hepatology* 1997; **26**:361A.

47. Onji M, Kikuchi Y, Kumon, Masumoto T, Ndano S, Kajino K, Horikee N & Ohta Y. Intrahepatic lymphocyte subpopulations and HLA class I expression by hepatocytes in chronic hepatitis C. *Hepatogastroenterology* 1992; **39**:340–343.

48. Rehermann B, Chang K, Mchutchinson J, Kokka R, Houghton M, Rice C & Chisari FV. Differential cytotoxic T-lymphocyte responsiveness to the hepatitis

B and C viruses in chronically infected patients. *Journal of Virology* 1996; **70**:7092–7102.

49. Hiroishi K, Kita H, Kojima M, Okamoto H, Moriyama T, Kaneko T, Ishikawa T, Ohnishi S, Aikawa T, Tanaka N, Yazaki Y, Mitamura K & Imawari M. Cytotoxic T lymphocyte response and viral load in hepatitis C virus infection. *Hepatology* 1997; **25**:705–712.

50. Byrne JA & Oldstone MBA. Biology of cloned cytotoxic T lymphocytes specific for lymphocytic choriomeningitis virus: clearance of virus *in vivo*. *Journal of Virology* 1984; **51**:682–686.

51. Patel T, Gores GJ. Apoptosis and hepatobiliary disease. *Hepatology* 1995; **21**:1725–1741.

52. Kagi D, Vignaux F, Ledermann B, *et al*. Fas and perforin pathways as major mechanisms of T cell mediated cytotoxicity. *Science* 1994; **265**:528–530.

53. Shi L, Kraut RP, Aebersold R & Greenberg AH. A natural killer cell granule protein that induces DNA fragmentation and apoptosis. *Journal of Experimental Medicine* 1992; **175**:553–566.

54. Fang JWS, Gonzalez-Peralta RP, Gottschall JA, *et al*. Hepatic expression of c-Fas and apoptosis in chronic hepatitis C virus infection. *Hepatology* 1994; **20**:250A.

55. Hiramatsu N, Hayashi N, Katayama K, Mochizuki K, Kawanishi Y, Kasahara A; Fusamoto H, Kamada T. Immunohistochemical detection of Fas antigen in liver tissue of patients with chronic hepatitis C. *Hepatology* 1994; **19**:1354–1359.

56. Chisari FV. Hepatitis B virus transgenic mice: models of viral immunobiology and pathogenesis. *Current Topics Microbiology and Immunology* 1996; **206**:149.

57. Pestka S, Langer JA, Zoon KC & Samuel CE. Interferons and their actions. *Annual Review of Biochemistry* 1987; **56**:727–777.

58. Kuzushita N, Hayashi N, Katayama K, Hiramatsu N; Yasumaru M; Murata H; Shimizu Y, Yamazaki T, Fushimi H, Kotoh K, Kasahara A, Fusamoto H & Kamada T. Increased frequency of HLA DR13 in hepatitis C virus carriers with persistently normal ALT levels. *Journal of Medical Virology* 1996; **48**:1–7.

59. Peano G, Menardi G, Ponzetto A & Fenoglio LM. HLA-DR5 antigen. A genetic factor influencing the outcome of hepatitis C virus infection? *Archives of Internal Medicine* 1994; **154**:2733–2736.

60. Kuzushita N, Hayashi N, Moribe T, Katayama K, Kanto T, Nakatani S, Kaneshige T, Tatsumi T, Ito A, Mochizuki K, Sasaki Y, Kasahara A & Hori M. Influence of HLA haplotypes on the clinical courses of individuals infected with hepatitis C virus. *Hepatology* 1998; **27**:240–244.

61. Hayashi N, Kuzushita N. Association of HLA and TAP2 gene polymorphisms on the clinical outcome of HCV infection. *US–Japan Hepatitis Joint Panel Meeting*, Special NIH Conference, Pacific Grove, California, 1998.

62. Feinstone SM. The virology of hepatitis C. *Journal of Gastroenterology and Hepatology* 1991; **1**:26–28.

63. Bamber M, Murray AK, Weller IVD, *et al*. Clinical and histological features of a group of patients with sporadic non-A, non-B hepatitis. *Journal of Clinical Pathology* 1981; **34**:1175.

64. Dienes HP, Popper H, Arnold W & Lobeck H. Histologic observations in human non-A, non-B hepatitis. *Hepatology* 1982; **2**:562–571.

65. Lim HL, Lau GKK, Davis GL, Dolson DJ & Lau JY. Cholestatic hepatitis leading to hepatic failure in a patient with organ-transmitted hepatitis C virus infection. *Gastroenterology* 1994; **106**:248–251.

66. Dickson RC, Caldwell SH, Ishitani MB, Lau JY, Driscoll CJ, Stevenson WC, McCullough CS & Pruett TL. Clinical and histologic patterns of early graft failure due to recurrent hepatitis C in four patients after liver transplantation. *Transplantation* 1996; **61**:701–705.

67. Schluger LK, Sheiner PA, Thung SN, Lau JY, Min A, Wolf DC, Fiel I, Zhang D, Gerber MA, Miller CM & Bodenheimer HC Jr. Severe recurrent cholestatic hepatitis C following orthotopic liver transplantation. *Hepatology* 1996; **23**:971–976.

68. Lau JY, Bain VG, Davies SE, O'Grady JG, Alberti A, Alexander GJ & Williams R. High level expression of hepatitis B viral antigen in fibrosing cholestatic hepatitis. *Gastroenterology* 1992; **102**:956–962.

69. Lau JY, Davis GL, Kniffen J, Qian KP, Urdea MS, Chan CS, Mizokami M, Neuwald PD, Wilber JC. Significance of serum hepatitis C RNA levels in chronic HCV. *Lancet* 1993; **341**:1501–1504.

70. Jeffers LJ, Dailey PJ, Coelho-Little E, *et al*. Correlation of HCV RNA quantitation in sera and liver tissue of patients with chronic hepatitis C. *Gastroenterology* 1993; **106**:A866.

71. Gonzalez-Peralta RP, Fang JWS, Davis GL, Gish RG, Kohara M, Mondelli MU, Urdea MS, Mizokami M & Lau JY. Significance of hepatic expression of hepatitis C viral antigens in chronic hepatitis C. *Digestive Disease and Science* 1995; **40**:2595–2601.

72. Lau JY, Davis GL, Wu SP, Gish RG, Balart LA, Lau JY. Hepatic expression of hepatitis C virus RNA in chronic hepatitis C: Study by in situ reverse-transcription polymerase chain reaction. *Hepatology* 1996; **23**:1318–1323.

73. Wu PC, Fang JWS, Dong C, Choo QL, Houghton M Lau JYN. Ultrastructural changes in cells expressing HCV structural proteins - implications on pathogenesis. *Hepatology* 1996; **24**:263A.

74. Kawamura T, Furusaka A, Koziel M, Chung RT, Wang TC, Schmidt EV & Liang JT. Transgenic expression of hepatitis C virus structural proteins in the mouse. *Hepatology* 1997; **25**:1014–1021.

75. Ruggieri A, Harada T, Matsuura Y & Miyamura T. Sensitization to Fas-mediated apoptosis by hepatitis C virus core protein. *Virology* 1997; **229**:68–76.

76. Zhu N, Khoshnan A, Schneider R, Matsumoto M, Dennert G, Ware C & Lai MM. Hepatitis C virus core protein binds to the cytoplasmic domain of tumor necrosis factor (TNF) receptor 1 and enhances TNF-induced apoptosis. *Journal of Virology* 1998; **72**: 3691–3697.

77. Kodama T, Tamaki T, Katabami S, Katamuma A, Yamashita K, Azuma N, Kamijo K, Kinoshita H, Yachi A. Histological findings in asymptomatic hepatitis C virus carriers. *Journal of Gastroenterology and Hepatology* 1993; **8**:403–405.

78. Shindo M, Arai K, Sokawa Y & Okuno T. The virological and histological states of anti-hepatitis C virus-positive subjects with normal liver biochemical values. *Hepatology* 1995; **22**:418–425.

79. Fong TL, Di Bisceglie AM, Waggoner JG, Banks SM & Hoofnagle JH. The significance of antibody to hepatitis C in patients with chronic hepatitis B. *Hepatology* 1991; **14**:64–67.

80. Benvegnu L, Fattovich G, Noventa F, Tremolada F, Chemello L, Cecchetto A & Alberti A. Concurrent hepatitis B and C virus infection and risk of hepatocellular carconima in cirrhosis: a prospective study. *Cancer* 1994; **27**:2442–2448.

81. Oshita M, Hayashi N, Kasahara A, Hagiwara H, Mita E, Naito M, Katayama K, Fusamoto H & Kamada T.

Increased serum hepatitis C virus RNA levels among alcoholic patients with chronic hepatitis C. *Hepatology* 1994; **20:**1115–1120.

82. Rosman AS, Paronetto F, Galvin K, Williams RJ & Lieber CS. Hepatitis C virus antibody in alcoholic patients: Association with the presence of portal and/or lobular hepatitis. *Archives of Internal Medicine* 1993; **153:**965–969.

# 9 Pathomorphology and apoptosis in viral hepatitis

## Zsuzsa Schaff*, Gábor Lotz, Gerald Eder and Rolf Schulte-Hermann

## PATHOMORPHOLOGICAL CHARACTERISTICS OF VIRAL HEPATITIS

Viral hepatitis is a diffuse inflammatory reaction of the liver caused by hepatotropic viruses. Acute hepatitis is characterized by a combination of hepatocellular degeneration, necrosis and regeneration, as well as portal and lobular inflammatory infiltration. The proportion of these components varies according to the particular virus, the host response and the passage of time [1]. Several histological classifications of acute hepatitis exist, based on the different patterns of necrosis: spotty (focal necrosis), confluent, bridging or piecemeal [2].

Piecemeal necrosis is the key feature of chronic active hepatitis, as described by Popper *et al.* [3]. It is defined as a gradual destruction of single or small numbers of hepatocytes at the border or interface of the mesenchymal–parenchymal margin and is associated with an inflammatory reaction; Scheuer *et al.* refer to this process as interface hepatitis [2]. Very close contact between the cell membranes of hepatocytes and lymphocytes has been detected in chronic hepatitis [4]. Lymphocytes destroy the periportal parenchyma, the limiting plate of the lobule is broken and lymphocytes replace the hepatocytes.

It is generally accepted that, based on histological examination alone, it is difficult to differentiate reliably between the forms of hepatitis caused by different hepatotropic viruses [1,2]. However, there are certain characteristic histopathological features caused by different viruses – for example, the bile duct damage, microvesicular fat and lymphoid follicles observed in hepatitis C virus (HCV) infection (Fig. 1a,b) [1,5]. Recent results suggest that the relationship between the expression of HCV core protein and cellular lipid metabolism might be responsible for the accumulation of fat in the hepatocytes [6].

There have been many discussions on the nomen-clature and classification of chronic hepatitis (CH) after the definition in 1968 [7], which recommended a simple division of CH into chronic persistent (CPH), chronic active (CAH) and chronic lobular (CLH) forms. These terms can still be meaningful but only if used in association with an aetiological desig-

**Figure 1.** Chronic hepatitis C

**(a)**

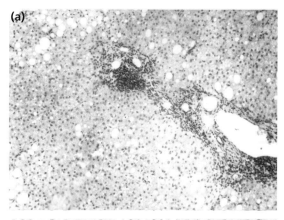

**(b)**

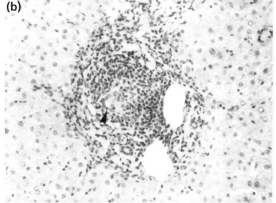

(a) Liver section stained with haematoxylin and eosin, showing portal lymphoid aggregates and fatty degeneration. (b) Bile canalicular alteration (arrow) surrounded by lymphoid aggregate.

---

*Corresponding author

nation [8]. Based on aetiology, the following forms of CH have been distinguished: CH-B (caused by hepatitis B virus; HBV), CH-C (caused by HCV), CH-D (caused by hepatitis D virus; HDV), autoimmune CH, drug-induced CH and cryptogenic CH [8].

The activity of the necro-inflammatory reaction can be assessed using a histological grading system. The first numerical scoring system for CH was proposed by Knodell and colleagues in 1981 [9]. In this system, the portal, periportal, intralobular necrosis and inflammation and fibrosis are scored independently and combined to give the histology activity index [9]. Recent editorials and reviews [8,10–13] consider CH to be a spectrum of disease caused by a common inflammatory reaction, the histological presentation of which oscillates in grade, can be modified by structural alterations such as fibrosis or cirrhosis, and can have different prognostic and therapeutic implications, according to its aetiology.

More recently, the original histology activity index [9] has been further divided into the grade and stage of the disease – terms borrowed from the field of oncology. Grade describes the intensity of the necro-inflammatory activity in CH, whereas the stage measures the fibrosis and architectural distortion of the liver [8]. Numerical scores are used to quantify both grading (total scores of 18) and staging (total scores of 4 or 6), providing a semi-quantitative evaluation of the observed histological features. The METAVIR group in France examined liver biopsy specimens from patients with CH-C; 27 histological features were scored and a relatively simple algorithm was constructed [14]. The international group that has formulated a recent semi-quantitative scoring system emphasizes that "...each pathologist is, however, free to use whatever system he or she wishes" [10]. Intra- and inter-observer variations in the histopathological assessment may also be important [15]. The greatest advantage of the scoring of liver biopsy specimens arises in therapeutic trials. The individual elements of grading should, however, be evaluated separately when the effect of a particular antiviral therapy is studied [13,15]. Semi-quantitative scoring seems to be important in clinical trials but the numerical scoring might be less relevant in routine reporting of liver biopsy specimens [10–13].

Several studies have analysed the relationship between histology and genotypes in CH-C [16–22]. More active necro-inflammatory reaction ('grade') was found to be associated with HCV genotype 1, raised serum aminotransferase (ALT) levels and HCV RNA titre [16,17]. In other studies, however, more active liver disease was more frequently related to HCV

serotype 2 than to serotype 1 [18]. In another study, HCV genotypes were not found to have a significant effect on the severity and outcome of liver disease [21].

## MECHANISM OF CELL DEATH

It is now generally appreciated that apoptosis and necrosis can co-exist in human diseases [23] and may both contribute to liver cell death [24]. Necrosis is defined by loss of the permeability barrier of the plasma membrane, resulting in cytolysis [24]. Apoptosis is defined as nuclear DNA and cell fragmentation with the preservation of plasma membrane and organelle integrity [24]. Typical apoptotic cells can be observed in acute and chronic hepatitis as large Councilman bodies (Fig. 2a,b), or smaller, membrane-bound cell fragments, many of which have already been phagocytosed by neighbouring cells and macrophages. It has been suggested that the elimina-

**Figure 2.** Councilman (apoptotic) body in viral hepatitis

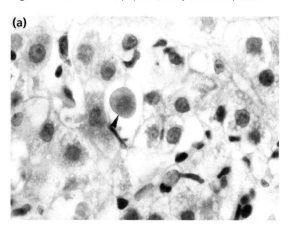

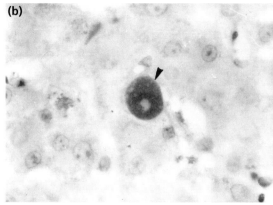

Arrowheads indicate Councilman bodies
(a) Liver section stained with haematoxylin and eosin.
(b) DNA fragmentation resulting from apoptosis detected by terminal deoxynucleotidyl transferase-mediated dUTP–digoxigenin nick-end labelling (TUNEL) reaction.

**Figure 3.** Possible mechanisms of hepatocyte death

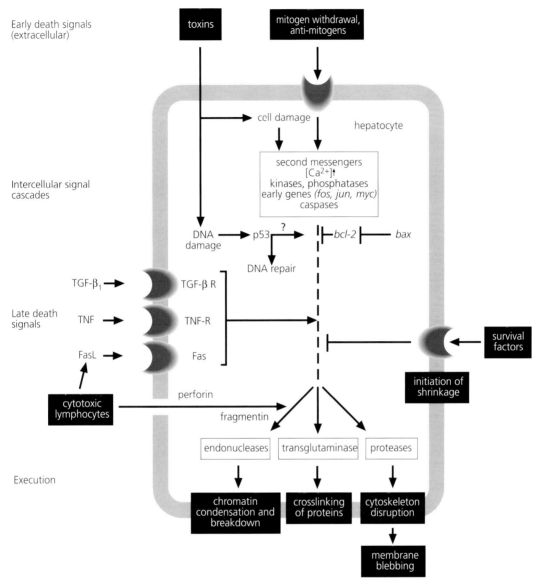

See text for details.

tion of virus-infected cells by apoptosis, rather than necrosis, might significantly benefit the host. Apoptotic bodies will be phagocytosed while their membranes are still intact, which should prevent the release of virions and other intracellular constituents, thereby preventing tissue inflammation [25]. In contrast, (lytic) necrosis of cells might lead to viral dissemination.

The biochemical and molecular events occurring during cell death have been studied extensively and the genes and proteins involved in the active self-destruction of cells have been the focus of intensive research efforts (Fig. 3) [25]. Cellular ATP levels and mitochondrial functions are currently recognized as key factors determining whether an active or passive mode of cell death will occur in a given cell [23]. In the liver, active cell death may occur after intoxication with chemicals such as ethanol, in viral hepatitis, in immune diseases, during or after ischaemia, and in carcinoma.

Active cell death begins with a preparatory phase, during which events favouring or inhibiting active cell death will lead to a point of no return [25]. Proteases are probably very important in the preparatory phase in viral hepatitis. Cytotoxic T lymphocytes (CTLs) and natural killer cells are known to inject a pore-forming protein (perforin), which is integrated into the membrane and a group of proteases (known as fragmentins) into the target cells [26] (Fig. 3). Serine proteases are responsible for the appearance of apoptotic changes in the nucleus of the target cell [26]. Recently a family of cysteine proteases named caspases have been identified as key players in the intracellular signal transduction pathway; they may also serve in the final stage of execution, providing a kind of 'death command' that leads to an almost simultaneous incapacitation of a variety of different cell organelles and cell functions [27–29].

Apoptosis is a very important mechanism of counterbalancing cell proliferation [24,25]. The *bcl-2* gene family is a critical regulator of apoptosis [30–32], and its products have been shown to localize to mitochondria, nuclear membranes and the endoplasmic reticulum [31,32]. Bcl-2 can block or delay the apoptotic death of a virus-infected cell, and viral *bcl-2* homologues can contribute to viral latency or result in a persistent viral infection in the absence of cell lysis [33]. Other genes, such as *p53*, *myc*, *TRPM-2* and *RP8* and their products are probably important in regulating apoptosis, although their exact functions are uncertain [24,25].

Active cell death is regulated by positive and negative factors. Hepatotropic factors such as epithelial growth factor, hepatocyte growth factor, transforming growth factor-α (TGF-α) and others, probably exert survival factor activity [25]. The accumulation of HBV surface antigen (HBsAg) in the cytoplasm is associated with increased expression of TGF-α [34,35]. Extracellular survival factors are usually mitogens acting on specific receptors. Nutrients can also directly or indirectly rescue cells from death. Recent results suggest that the Akt protein bridges the gap between extracellular and intracellular survival signals [30,36].

Positive signals that favour active cell death (death signal factors) participate in the selective elimination of damaged cells; these factors include the TGF-β–activin–inhibin family, the Fas (CD95 or Apo1) ligand and the tumour necrosis factor (TNF) family (Fig. 3) [25]. In addition, other death factors including interferon-γ (IFN-γ) exist [37]. The TGF-β family seems to be involved predominantly in the control of tissue homeostasis and the elimination of excessive cells, whereas the Fas family mainly seems to eliminate damaged cells [38]. The effects of TGF-$\beta_1$ and related peptides have been studied extensively in the liver. It has been found that TGF-$\beta_1$ induces apoptosis of hepatocytes both *in vitro* and *in vivo* [39]. Hepatocytes preparing for apoptosis are positive for pre-TGF-$\beta_1$ ('autocrine suicide') [40]. Additionally, TGF-$\beta_1$ might affect apoptosis in a paracrine fashion because non-parenchymal cells also synthesize TGF-$\beta_1$ [41]. Increased expression of TGF-$\beta_1$ was detected at the interface of the portal area and parenchyma and has been correlated with the activity of CH [42].

Another signal system involved in the induction of apoptosis is the Fas receptor and its ligand (Fig. 3) [24,25,27]. The Fas ligand–receptor system represents one of two known mechanisms of cell killing by CTLs; the second mechanism depends on perforin [27]. In patients with CH-C, Fas antigen has been

**Figure 4.** Fas expression on the membrane of a hepatocyte in a HCV-infected liver

**Figure 5.** Close contact between CD8⁺ CTLs and hepatocytes at the interface of the parenchyma and portal area in chronic hepatitis

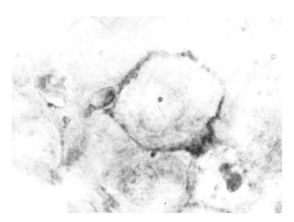

Immunoperoxidase staining for Fas.

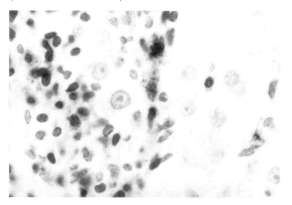

Immunoperoxidase staining; CTLs stain dark.

found to be expressed in the liver, particularly at the advancing edges of piecemeal necrotic tissue (Fig. 4; [43]). Piecemeal necrosis at the interface between parenchyma and connective tissue in inflammatory liver disease seems to reflect apoptotic cell death triggered by T cells (Fig. 5). In another study, Fas expression was low in intact liver tissue, but elevated in tissues derived from patients with cirrhosis and acute liver failure associated with HBV infection [44] and in HCV infection. By these mechanisms, damaged cells that are potentially dangerous because of their antigenic or infectious contents can be eliminated via apoptosis. This process may occur normally to remove virus-infected cells, but if exaggerated, may lead to fulminant hepatitis [44].

## VIRAL ANTIGENS IN THE LIVER

The different forms and patterns of expression of viral antigens during hepatitis have been extensively studied [45]. Hepadnavirus core and envelope polypeptides are integral constituents of hepatocyte membranes during the course of acute and chronic hepatitis [46].

### Hepatitis B virus

The early hypothesis that the immune response determines the morphological presentation and course of the non-cytopathic HBV infection has gained acceptance [45]. Although it is generally agreed that HBV is not directly cytotoxic [2], it does appear to cause cell death under certain circumstances. In an *in vitro* study, the accumulation of capsid proteins proved to be cytotoxic to HepG2 (human hepatoma) cells [47]. It has also been shown that overexpression of the large envelope protein of HBV can be directly cytotoxic to hepatocytes in transgenic mice [48]. Another example of direct cytotoxicity is in liver transplantation, after which re-infection of the graft can be characterized by the rapid accumulation of large amounts of HBsAg and HBV core antigen (HBcAg) and by damage to hepatocytes [49].

Specific antibodies have been used to visualize the viral proteins in HBV-infected liver tissue. HBcAg is localized mainly in the hepatocyte nuclei (Fig. 6a) and to a lesser degree in the cytoplasm and/or in close association with the cell membrane [45]. Excess accumulation of core particles can be observed in routinely stained sections, as 'sanded' nuclei [45]. Nuclear HBcAg probably represents accumulation of empty nucleocapsids, whereas the presence of cytoplasmic HBcAg is thought to indicate active virus replication as viral DNA can be detected by *in situ* hybridization

**Figure 6.** Hepatitis B infection

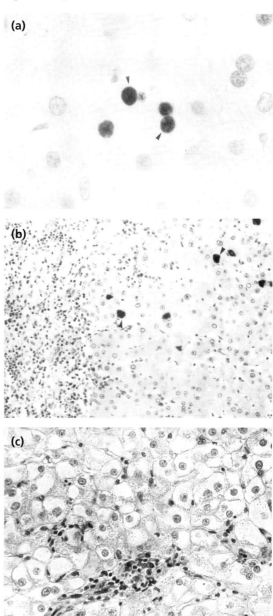

(a) HBV core antigen in hepatocyte nuclei (arrow). Immunoperoxidase staining. (b) HBV surface antigen in the cytoplasm of hepatocytes (arrow) in chronic active hepatitis. Immunoperoxidase staining. (c) Ground-glass hepatocytes in a HBV carrier. Stained with haematoxylin and eosin.

in such liver cells [45].

HBsAg expression can be visualized by immunohistochemical analysis of tissue sections (Fig. 6b), and can be detected in different cellular regions, including the membrane and cytoplasm using specific stains (such as

Shikata's Orcein, Aldehyde Fuchsin and Victoria Blue). Membrane staining for HBsAg on hepatocytes is a sensitive and specific marker for active HBV replication [50]. Excess accumulation of HBsAg in the hepatocyte cytoplasm gives it a characteristic homogeneous 'ground-glass' appearance (Fig. 6c; [45]). These ground-glass hepatocytes show a marked proliferation of endoplasmic reticulum with typical filaments of 22 nm in diameter containing HBsAg within the cisternae [51]. The presence of intracisternal HBsAg probably indicates accumulation of protein that cannot be secreted by the cell and represents a chronic elimination deficiency for this antigen [45].

Bianchi and Gudat have grouped four basic reaction types (elimination type, generalized HBcAg, focal HBcAg and HBcAg-free HBsAg) in HBV infection in a dynamic model suggesting a natural evolution of CH-B [45]. The reaction patterns suggested by these authors are not sharply delineated entities, but characteristic types that can overlap. Transitions between the patterns may occur in any direction. Application and withdrawal of immunosuppressive and/or antiviral therapy could result in simultaneous transition of histological findings and viral expression patterns.

The mechanisms involved in HBV persistence are poorly understood, although they probably involve viral and host factors. A role of defective particles in viral persistence has been suggested for several viruses, including HBV [52].

## Hepatitis D virus

After the discovery of the delta agent by Rizetto and co-workers [53], it was demonstrated that HDV co-exists with, and depends on, replicating HBV infection. Immunohistochemical analysis shows that hepatitis D antigen (HDAg) is found mainly in hepatocyte nuclei, and has a staining pattern different from that seen with other hepatitis viruses [54]. The pathogenesis of hepatitis D is still unclear, despite considerable progress in our understanding of the molecular biology of the virus. In certain circumstances, HDV infection causes a mild disease, whereas in others it induces aggravated and accelerated disease, leading to more frequent and accelerated cirrhosis, especially in drug addicts or in hyperendemic regions. In other areas, a carrier state with low-grade HDV replication and lack of tissue damage has been found [53]. In contrast to HBV, HDV is cytotoxic, producing direct cellular damage, in addition to immunologically mediated cellular cytotoxicity.

## Hepatitis C virus

Several groups have demonstrated the presence of HCV antigens and genome in the liver. The structural and non-structural antigens of HCV have been detected in human biopsy samples by immunohistochemistry [55–63]. The HCV antigens were detected within the cytoplasm of hepatocytes, but not in the mononuclear cell infiltrates, bile duct epithelium or endothelial cells. A high proportion of hepatocytes were HCV-antigen positive (60–90%), but the staining intensity was variable [55–63]. The amount of HCV antigens in the liver appeared to be predictive of the response to IFN-α therapy [56]. Identification and immunostaining of proteins encoded by the HCV genome suggests that most of them reside in the endoplasmic reticulum and that only NS3 and NS5a are soluble [62,63]. The observed location of the core protein and, to some extent, the NS5 protein suggests that viral assembly occurs in the cytoplasm. Recent *in vitro* and *in vivo* studies demonstrated that the HCV core protein co-localized with apolipoprotein AII at the surface of lipid droplets in the cytoplasm [6]. These data suggest a relationship between the expression of core protein and lipid metabolism in the hepatocytes [6]. Other results suggest that the HCV core protein has a role in immune-mediated liver injury, because intracellular expression of the core antigen sensitizes hepatocytes to Fas-mediated apoptosis [64].

Several groups report the detection of HCV RNA by *in situ* hybridization with varying results [65–69]. HCV RNA has also been detected in hepatocytes using the polymerase chain reaction (PCR) [70,71] and its presence correlates with the effects of interferon therapy [70].

## HOST IMMUNE RESPONSE

Liver injury in viral hepatitis is mainly a consequence of the cytotoxic host immune response directed against virus-encoded products, rather than the result of a direct cytopathic effect [45]. The predominance of activated T cells in inflammatory periportal infiltrates and the strong expression of human leukocyte antigen (HLA) class I and class II molecules on hepatocytes and T cells in CH suggest that the hepatic injury is mediated by viral antigen-specific immune reactions [45].

Cytokines released by activated T cells could be crucial for the development of CH [72]. These cytokines have many effects, including direct cytotoxicity, maturation of precursor cells, induction of the expression of HLA molecules, the activation of bystander cells and increasing the cellular susceptibility to natural killer cells [72]. It has been reported that local production of IFN-γ maintains a liver-specific inflammatory disease in transgenic mouse models [73].

It has been suggested that the central core of the portal inflammation in CH-B represents a B cell zone, and that the peripheral invading front of the piecemeal necrosis corresponds to a T cell zone, as in lymph nodes [45,74]. Lymphoid follicle formation is seen quite frequently at the centre of the portal and peri-portal infiltrate, especially in CH-C infection [75]. *In situ* immunophenotyping has shown that the lymphoid follicles with activated B cells in germinal centres are surrounded by a follicular dendritic cell network [75]. A T-cell zone composed of $CD4^+$ helper and $CD8^+$ suppressor/cytotoxic T cells is seen at the periphery of the nodules (Fig. 5; [75]).

Others have found that the intrahepatic lymphoid follicles are mainly primary, without germinal centres, and contain a very low number of follicular dendritic cells [76]. These studies also raise the possibility that intrahepatic lymphoid aggregates represent a site of viral replication [76], based on the observation that HCV can infect mononuclear cells in the peripheral blood [77]. It has been suggested that CTLs have direct and immediate access to the target hepatocytes, and have the potential to kill, because of the unique microanatomy of the sinusoids, which contain a discontinuous endothelium and lack a basement membrane [78].

The T-cell response to viruses could have two opposing effects. It could be critical for protection, either directly through CTLs, or indirectly through $CD4^+$ T cells, which help B cells to produce neutral-izing antibodies [79]. Conversely, T cells (mainly CTLs) may damage infected tissues while attempting to clear the virus [79].

$CD4^+$ and $CD8^+$ T cells recognize antigens as peptides bound to the major histocompatibility complex (MHC) class I and class II molecules on the surface of antigen-presenting cells. Using a model in which HBsAg-specific CTLs caused an acute necro-inflammatory liver disease in HBsAg-transgenic mice, it has been demonstrated that MHC class I-restricted disease pathogenesis is a multistep process that involves direct and indirect consequences of CTL acti-vation [78]. Direct consequences could be apoptosis; indirect consequences could be secretion of cytokines that damage hepatocytes. This hypothesis solves the problem that apoptosis itself is usually not a pro-inflammatory event. Ando *et al.* suggest that the second and third steps in their model are responsible for the inflammatory reactions and can be considered as independent indirect functions of the CTLs that are

mediated by IFN-γ and other currently unidentified cytokines [78].

Less information is available on CH-C and HLA expression. Hepatocellular HLA-A, -B and -C expression before treatment has been shown to be significantly higher in HCV patients who do not subsequently respond to IFN treatment than in responders [80]. It had been suggested that the higher hepatocellular expression of HLA class I molecules in non-responder cases could reflect a different viral effect on hepatocytes that is induced by different HCV genotypes or levels of viraemia [80]. It has also been proposed that HCV sequence variation leads to escape from cellular immune recognition and contributes to the development of persistent HCV infection.

Co-expression of HLA and adhesion molecules, such as intercellular adhesion molecule-1 (ICAM-1), is necessary to obtain hepatocyte and T-cell contact [81]. Normally ICAM-1 molecules are detected in sinusoidal cells and vascular endothelium; hepato-cytes and bile duct cells are negative [81]. In diseased liver, however, an increased intensity of immunos-taining of both HLA and ICAM-1 was observed on hepatocyte membranes. Double immunofluorescence has shown that hepatocytes containing viral antigens were also positive for ICAM-1 and HLA-A, -B and -C [81]. Viral persistence is associated with the devel-opment of mechanisms for avoiding viral recognition by host CTLs. Downregulation of HLA-A, -B, -C and ICAM-1 molecules are well-documented escape mechanisms of hepatic and non-hepatic viruses [81].

To summarize, the pathogenic mechanisms respon-sible for the final outcome of a hepatotropic viral infection are still not clear. Several variables, including viral factors (including the genotype and mutations), virus–host cell interactions, expression of viral proteins, the host immune response and antigen recognition are responsible for the liver injury and inflammation that leads to the characteristic morpho-logical alterations diagnosed as viral hepatitis.

## ACKNOWLEDGEMENTS

The work has been partly funded by National Science Foundation (OTKA) grants T 016077 and T 023579 and AKP 96/2-4393,2.

## REFERENCES

1. Scheuer PJ, Krawczynski K & Dhillon AP. Histopathology and detection of hepatitis C virus in liver. *Springer Seminars in Immunopathology* 1997; **19**:27–45.

2. Scheuer PJ. Viral hepatitis. In *Pathology of the Liver*. 3rd edn 1994; pp. 243–267. Edited by RNM MacSween, PP Anthony, PJ Scheuer, AD Burt & BC Portmann. New York: Churchill Livingstone.

3. Popper H, Paronetto F & Schaffner F. Immune processes in the pathogenesis of liver disease. *Annals of the New York Academy of Sciences* 1965; **124:** 781–799.

4. Kerr JFR, Searle J, Halliday WJ, Roberts I, Cooksley WGE, Halliday JW, Holder L, Burnett W & Powell LW. The nature of piecemeal necrosis in chronic active hepatitis. *Lancet* 1979; **ii:**827–828.

5. Schaff ZS, Szepesi Á & Jármay K. Histopathological features specific for chronic viral hepatitis B, D and C. *XVI European Congress of Pathology*. Maastricht, The Netherlands, August 31–September 4 1997.

6. Barba G, Harper F, Harada T, Kohara M, Goulinet S, Matsuura Y, Eder G, Schaff ZS, Chapman MJ, Miyamura T & Brechot C. Hepatitis C virus core protein shows a cytoplasmic localization and associates to cellular lipid storage droplets. *Proceedings of the National Academy of Sciences, USA* 1997; **94:** 1200–1205.

7. De Groote J, Gedigk P, Popper H, Scheuer PJ, Thaler H, Desmet VJ, Korb G, Poulsen H, Schmid M, Uehlinger E & Wepler W. A classification of chronic hepatitis. *Lancet* 1968; **ii:**626–628.

8. Desmet VJ, Gerber M, Hoofnagle JH, Manns M & Scheuer PJ. Classification of chronic hepatitis: diagnosis, grading and staging. *Hepatology* 1994; **19:**1513–1520.

9. Knodell RG, Ishak KG, Black WC, Chen TS, Craig R, Kaplowitz N, Kiernan TW & Wollman J. Formulation and application of a numerical scoring system for assessing histological activity in asymptomatic chronic active hepatitis. *Hepatology* 1981; **1:**431–435.

10. Ishak K, Baptista A, Bianchi L, Callea F, De Groote J, Gudat F, Denk H, Desmet V, Korb G, MacSween RNM, Phillips MJ, Portmann BG, Poulsen H, Scheuer PJ, Schmid M & Thaler H. Histological grading and staging of chronic hepatitis. *Journal of Hepatology* 1995; **22:**696–699.

11. Scheuer PJ. Scoring of liver biopsies: are we doing it right? *European Journal of Gastroenterology and Hepatology* 1996; **8:**1141–1143.

12. Scheuer PJ. Chronic hepatitis: what is activity and how should it be assessed? *Histopathology* 1997; **30:** 103–105.

13. Scheuer PJ, Davies SE & Dhillon AP. Histopathological aspects of viral hepatitis. *Journal of Viral Hepatitis* 1997; **3:**277–283.

14. Bedossa P & Poynard T. The METAVIR cooperative study group. An algorithm for the grading of activity in chronic hepatitis C. *Hepatology* 1996; **24:** 289–293.

15. Goldin RD, Goldin JG, Burt AD, Dhillon PA, Hubscher S, Wyatt J & Patel N. Intra-observer and inter-observer variation in the histopathological assessment of chronic viral hepatitis. *Journal of Hepatology* 1996; **25:** 649–654.

16. Booth JCL, Foster GR, Levine T, Thomas HC, & Golding RD. The relationship of histology to genotype in chronic HCV infection. *Liver* 1997; **17:**144–151.

17. Rossini A, Ravaggi A, Agostinelli E, Bercich L, Gazzola GB, Radaeli E, Callea F & Cariani E. Virological characterization and liver histology in HCV-positive subjects with normal and elevated ALT levels. *Liver* 1997; **17:**133–138.

18. Guido M, Rugge M, Thung SN, Chemello L, Leandro G, Alberti A, Cecchetto A, Pontisso P, Cavalletto L & Ninfo V. Hepatitis C virus serotypes and liver pathology. *Liver* 1996; **16:**353–357.

19. Mihm S, Fayyazi A, Hartmann H & Ramadori G. Analysis of histopathological manifestations of chronic hepatitis C virus infection with respect to virus genotype. *Hepatology* 1997; **25:**735–739.

20. Dusheiko G, Schumilovitz-Weiss H, Brown D, McOmish F, Yap PL, Sherlock S, Mcintyre N & Simmonds P. Hepatitis C virus genotypes: An investigation of type-specific differences in geographic origin and disease. *Hepatology* 1994; **19:**13–18.

21. Benvegnu L, Pontisso P, Cavalletto D, Noventa F, Chemello L & Alberti A. Lack of correlation between hepatitis C virus genotypes and clinical course of hepatitis C virus-related cirrhosis. *Hepatology* 1997; **25:**211–215.

22. Cathomas G, McGandy CE, Terracciano LM, Gudat F & Bianchi L. Detection and typing of hepatitis cRNA in liver biopsies and its relation to histopathology. *Virchows Archives* 1996; **429:**353–358.

23. Tsujimoto Y. Apoptosis and necrosis: Intracellular ATP level as a determinant for cell death modes. *Cell Death and Differentiation* 1997; **4:**420–434.

24. Patel T & Gores GJ. Apoptosis and hepatobiliary disease. *Hepatology* 1995; **21:**1725–1741.

25. Schulte-Hermann R, Grasl-Kraupp B & Bursch W. Active cell death (apoptosis) in liver biology and disease. In *Progress in Liver Disease*, vol. 13 1995; pp. 1–35. Edited by JL Boyler & RK Ockner. Philadelphia: WB Saunders & Co.

26. Shi L, Kraut RP, Aebersold R & Greenberg AH. A natural killer cell granule protein that induces DNA fragmentation and apoptosis. *Journal of Experimental Medicine* 1992; **175:**553–566.

27. Nagata S. Apoptosis by death factor. *Cell* 1997; **88:** 355–365.

28. Chen R-H & Chang T-Y. Involvement of caspase family proteases intransforming growth factor-ß-induced apoptosis. *Cell Growth and Differentiation* 1997; **8:**821–827.

29. Kumar S. & Lavin MF. The ICE family of cysteine proteases as effectors of cell death. *Cell Death and Differentiation* 1996; **3:**255-267.

30. del Peso L, Gonzalez-Garcia M, Page C, Herrera R & Nuñez G. Interleukin-3-induced phosphorylation of BAD through the protein kinase Akt. *Science* 1997; **278:**687–689.

31. Hockenbery D, Nunez G, Milliman C, Schreiber RD & Korsmeyer SJ. Bcl-2 is an inner mitochondrial membrane protein that blocks programmed cell death. *Nature* 1990; **348:**334–336.

32. Charlotte F, L'Herminé A, Martin N, Geleyn Y, Nollet M, Gaulard P & Zafrani ES. Immunohistochemical detection of bcl-2 protein in normal and pathological human liver. *American Journal of Pathology* 1994; **144:**460–465.

33. Alnemri E, Robertson N, Fernandes T, Croce C & Liwack G. Overexpression full-length human Bcl-2 extends the survival of baculovirus-infected SF9 insect cells. *Proceedings of the National Academy of Sciences, USA* 1992; **89:**7295–7299.

34. Hsia CC, Axiotis CA, Di Bisceglie A & Tabor E. Transforming growth factor-alpha in human hepatocellular carcinoma and co-expression with hepatitis B surface antigen in adjacent liver. *Cancer* 1992; **70:** 1049–1056.

35. Schaff ZS, Hsia CC, Sárosi I & Tabor E. Overexpression of TGF-α in benign and malignant liver

tumors from European patients. *Human Pathology* 1994; **25**:644–651.

36. Datta SR, Dudek H, Tao X, Masters S, Fu H, Gotoh Z & Greenberg ME. Akt phosphorylation of BAD couples survival signals to the cell-intrinsic death machinery. *Cell* 1997;**91**:231–241.

37. Gilles PN, Guerrette DL, Ulevitch RJ, Schreiber RD & Chisari FV. HBsAg retention sensitizes the hepatocyte to injury by physiological concentrations of interferon-γ. *Hepatology* 1992;**16**:655–663.

38. Peter ME, Kischkel FC, Hellbardt S, Chinnaiyan AM, Krammer PH & Dixit VM. CD95 (APO-1/FAS)-associating signalling proteins. *Cell Death and Differentiation* 1996; **3**:161–170.

39. Oberhammer F, Bursch W, Tiefenbacher R, Froschl G, Pavelka M, Purchio T & Schulte-Hermann R. Apoptosis is induced by transforming growth factor-beta 1 within 5 hours in regressing liver without significant fragmentation of the DNA. *Hepatology* 1993; **18**: 1238–1246.

40. Bursch W, Oberhammer F, Jirtle RL, Askari M, Sedivy R, Grasl-Kraupp B, Purchio AF & Schulte-Hermann R. Transforming growth factor beta 1 as a signal for induction of cell death by apoptosis. *British Journal of Cancer* 1993; **67**:531–536.

41. Fausto N & Mead JE. Regulation of liver growth: protooncogenes and transforming growth factors. *Laboratory Investigation* 1989; **60**:4–13.

42. Nagy P, Schaff Z & Lapis K. Immunohistochemical detection of transforming growth factor β1 in fibrotic liver diseases. *Hepatology* 1991; **14**:269–273.

43. Hiramatsu N, Hayashi N, Katayama K, Mochizuki K, Kawanishi Y, Kasahara A, Fusamoto H & Kamada T. Immunohistochemical detection of Fas antigen in liver tissue of patients with chronic hepatitis C. *Hepatology* 1994; **19**:1354–1359.

44. Galle PR, Hoffmann WJ, Walczak H, Schaller H, Otto G, Stremmel W, Krammer PH & Runkel L. Involvement of the CD95 (APO-1/Fas) receptor and ligand in liver damage. *Journal of Experimental Medicine* 1995; **182**:1223–1230.

45. Bianchi L & Gudat F. Chronic hepatitis. In *Pathology of the Liver*. 3rd edn 1994; pp. 349–395. Edited by RNM MacSween, PP Anthony, PJ Scheuer, AD Burt & BC Portmann. New York: Churchill Livingstone.

46. Michalak TI & Lin B. Molecular species of hepadnavirus core and envelope polypeptides in hepatocyte plasma membrane of woodchucks with acute and chronic viral hepatitis. *Hepatology* 1994; **20**:275–286.

47. Roingeard P, Romet-Lemonne J-L, Leturq D, Goudeau A & Essex M. Hepatitis B virus core antigen (HBcAg) accumulation in an HBV non-producer clone of HepG2-transfected cells is associated with cytopathic effect. *Virology* 1990; **179**:113–120.

48. Chisari FV. Hepatitis B virus biology and pathogenesis. *Molecular and Genetic Medicine* 1992; **2**:67–104.

49. Davies SE, Portmann BC, O'Grady JG, Aldis PM, Chaggar K, Alexander GJ, & Williams R. Hepatic histological findings after transplantation for chronic hepatitis B virus infection, including a unique pattern of fibrosing cholestatic hepatitis. *Hepatology* 1991; **13**: 150–157.

50. Chu CM, Liaw YF. Membrane staining for hepatitis B surface antigen on hepatocytes: a sensitive and specific marker of active viral replication in hepatitis B. *Journal of Clinical Pathology* 1995;**48**:470–473.

51. Schaff ZS & Lapis K. Fine structure of hepatocytes during the etiology of several common pathologies.

52. Rosmorduc O, Petit M-A, Pot S, Capel F, Bortolotti F, Berthelot P, Brechot C & Kremsdorf D. *In vivo* and *in vitro* expression of defective hepatitis B virus particles generated by spliced hepatitis B virus RNA. *Hepatology* 1995; **21**:10–19.

53. Rizetto M & Durazzo M. Hepatitis delta virus (HDV) infections. Epidemiological and clinical heterogeneity. *Journal of Hepatology* 1991; **13**:S116–118.

54. Negro F, Pacchioni D, Bussolati G & Bonino F. Hepatitis delta virus heterogeneity: a study by immuno-fluorescence. *Journal of Hepatology* 1991; **13**: S125–129.

55. Blight K, Lesniewiski RR, Labrooy JT & Gowans EJ. Detection and distribution of hepatitis C-specific antigens in naturally infected liver. *Hepatology* 1994; **20**:553–557.

56. Di Bisceglie A, Hoofnagle JH & Krawczynski K. Changes in hepatitis C virus antigen in liver with antiviral therapy. *Gastroenterology* 1993; **105**: 858–862.

57. Haruna Y, Hayashi N, Kamada T, Hytiroglou P, Thung SN & Gerber MA. Expression of hepatitis C virus in hepatocellular carcinoma. *Cancer* 1994; **73**: 2253–2258.

58. Hiramatsu N, Hayashi N, Haruna Y, Kasahara A, Fusamoto H, Mori C, Fuke I, Okayama H & Kamada T. Immunohistochemical detection of hepatitis C virus-infected hepatocytes in chronic liver disease with monoclonal antibodies to core, envelope and NS3 regions of the hepatitis C virus genome. *Hepatology* 1992; **16**:306–311.

59. Komminoth P, Adams V, Long AA, Roth J, Saremaslani P, Flury R, Schmid M & Heitz U. Evaluation of methods for hepatitis C virus detection in archival liver biopsies. *Pathology Research and Practice* 1994; **190**:1017–1025.

60. Krawczynski K, Beach MJ, Bradley DW, Kuo G, Di Bisceglie AM, Houghton M, Reyes GR, Kim JP, Choo Q-L & Alter MJ. Hepatitis C virus antigen in hepatocytes immunomorphologic detection and identification. *Gastroenterology* 1992; **103**:622–629.

61. Sansonno D & Dammacco F. Hepatitis C virus c100 antigen in liver tissue from patients with acute and chronic infection. *Hepatology* 1993; **18**:240–245.

62. Selby MJ, Choo Q-L, Berger K, Kuo G, Glazer E, Eckart M, Lee C, Chien D, Kuo C & Houghton M. Expression, identification and subcellular localization of the proteins encoded by the hepatitis C viral genome. *Journal of General Virology* 1993; **74**:1103–1113.

63. Tsutsumi M, Urashima S, Takada A, Date T & Tanaka Y. Detection of antigens related to hepatitis C virus RNA encoding the NS5 region in the livers of patients with chronic type C hepatitis. *Hepatology* 1994; **19**: 265–272.

64. Ruggieri A, Harada T, Matsuura Y & Miyamura T. Sensitization to fas-mediated apoptosis by hepatitis C virus core protein. *Virology* 1997; **229**:68–76.

65. Lamas E, Baccarini P, Housset C, Kremsdorf D & Brechot C. Detection of hepatitis C virus (HCV) RNA sequences in liver tissue by in situ hybridisation. *Journal of Hepatology* 1992; **16**:219–223.

66. Tanaka Y, Enomoto N, Kojima S, Tang L, Goto M, Marumo F & Sato C. Detection of hepatitis C virus RNA in the liver by in situ hybridisation. *Liver* 1993; **13**:203–208.

67. Cho SW, Hwang SG, Han DC, Jin SY, Lee MS, Shim CS & Lee DW. In situ detection of hepatitis C virus RNA

*Journal of Electron Microscopy* 1990; **14**:179–207.

in liver tissue using a digoxigenin-labelled probe created during a polymerase chain reaction. *Journal of Medical Virology* 1996; **48**:227–233.

68. Kojima S, Tanaka Y, Enomoto N, Marumo F & Sato C. Distribution of hepatitis C virus RNA in the liver and its relation to histopathological changes. *Liver* 1996;**16**:55–60.

69. Negro F, Pacchioni D, Shimizu Y, Miller RH, Bussolati G, Purcell RH & Bonino F. Detection of intrahepatic replication of hepatitis C virus RNA by in situ hybridization and comparison with histopathology. *Proceedings of the National Academy of Sciences, USA* 1992; **89**:2247–2251.

70. Diamond DA, Davis GL, Qian KP & Lau JYN. Detection of hepatitis C viral sequences in formalin-fixed, paraffin-embedded liver tissue: Effect of interferon alpha therapy. *Journal of Medical Virology* 1994;**42**:294–298.

71. Savage K, Dhillon AP, Smilivitz-Weiss H, El-Batanony M, Brown DD & Scheuer PJ. Detection of HCV-RNA in paraffin-embedded liver biopsies from patients with autoimmune hepatitis. *Journal of Hepatology* 1995; **22**:27–34.

72. Löhr HF, Schlaak JF, Gerken G, Fleischer B, Dienes H-P & Meyer K-H. Phenotypical analysis and cytokine release of liver-infiltrating and peripheral blood T lymphocytes from patients with chronic hepatitis of different etiology. *Liver* 1994; **14**:161–166.

73. Toyonaga T, Hino O, Sugai S, Wakasugi S, Abe K, Shichiri M & Yamamura K-I: Chronic active hepatitis in transgenic mice expressing interferon-γ in the liver. *Proceedings of the National Academy of Sciences, USA* 1994; **91**:614–618.

74. Desmet VJ. Liver lesions in hepatitis B viral infection. *Yale Journal of Biology and Medicine* 1988; **61**:61–83.

75. Mosnier J-F, Degott C, Marcellin P, Hénin D, Erlinger S & Benhamou J-P. The intraportal lymphoid nodule and its environment in chronic active hepatitis C: an immunohistochemical study. *Hepatology* 1993; **17**:366–371.

76. Freni MA, Artuso D, Gerken G, Spanti C, Marafioti T, Alessi N, Sparado A, Ajello A & Ferrau O. Focal lymphotic aggregates in chronic hepatitis C: occurrence, immunohistochemical characterization, and relation to markers of autoimmunity. *Hepatology* 1995; **22**:389–394.

77. Bouffard P, Hayashi PH, Acevedo R, Levy N & Zeldis JB: Hepatitis C virus is detected in a monocyte/macrophage subpopulation of peripherial blood mononuclear cells of infected patients. *Journal of Infectious Diseases* 1992; **166**:1276–1280.

78. Ando K, Moriyama T, Guidotti LG, Wirth S, Schreiber RD, Schlicht HJ, Huang S & Chisari FV: Mechanisms of class I restricted immunopathology a transgenic mouse model of fulminant hepatitis. *Journal of Experimental Medicine* 1993; **178**:1541–1554.

79. Botarelli P, Brunetto MR, Minutello MA, Calvo P, Unutmaz D, Weiner AJ, Choo Q-L, Shuster JR, Kuo G, Bonino F, Houghton M & Abrignani S. T-lymphocyte response to hepatitis C virus in different clinical courses of infection. *Gastroenterology* 1993; **104**:580–587.

80. Ballardini G, Groff P, Giostra F, Francesconi R, Zauli D, Bianchi G, Lenzi M, Cassani F & Bianchi F. Hepatocellular expression of HLA-A, B, C molecules predicts primary response to interferon in patients with chronic hepatitis C. *American Journal of Clinical Pathology* 1994; **102**:746–751.

81. Ballardini G, Groff P, Pontisso P, Giostra F, Francesconi R, Lenzi M, Zauli D, Alberti A & Bianchi FB. Hepatitis C virus (HCV) genotype, tissue HCV antigens, hepatocellular expression of HLA-A,B,C, and intercellular adhesion-1 molecules. *Journal of Clinical Investigation* 1995; **95**:2067–2075.

# 10 Hepatitis delta virus: molecular biology, pathogenesis and immunology

## John L Casey

## INTRODUCTION

Hepatitis delta virus (HDV) is a unique subviral pathogen that causes significant acute and chronic liver disease in association with hepatitis B virus (HBV), which provides hepatitis B surface antigen (HBsAg) for the HDV envelope [1,2]. HDV typically exacerbates the severity of disease associated with HBV infection: incidences of fulminant hepatitis, chronic active hepatitis and cirrhosis are greater in HDV–HBV co-infected individuals than in those infected with HBV alone [3,4]. The pattern of HDV infection and disease varies in different epidemiologic settings [5,6]. Endemicity is low in the United States, where transmission is often related to intravenous drug use, but is higher in parts of Greece and Italy, where familial transmission predominates [5,6]; in developing countries, 20% or more of HBsAg carriers are infected with HDV. Some studies have suggested that variations in disease severity may be influenced by the HDV genotype [7–9]. Currently there is no generally accepted therapy for chronic HDV infection.

This review will cover recent developments in our understanding of HDV biology and disease, with particular emphasis on advances in the molecular biology, immunology and pathogenesis of HDV that might provide insights for therapeutic approaches.

## MOLECULAR BIOLOGY OF HDV

The HDV particle is made up of the viral RNA, hepatitis delta antigen (HDAg), which is the sole viral protein, and HBsAg, which forms the envelope and is provided by the helper virus, HBV [10–13]. Both HDV RNA and HDAg possess numerous functional elements that play essential roles in the viral replication cycle.

## Functional elements of HDV RNA

The HDV genome is a 1.7 kilobase (kb) single-stranded circular RNA [14], and is the smallest known animal virus genome. There are no known animal RNA viruses related to HDV, but the RNA and its mechanism of RNA replication are similar in some ways to plant viroid and virusoid agents [15]. The circular RNA possesses intramolecular complementarity such that about 70% of the nucleotides are base-paired in an unbranched rod structure [14]. Two small segments of the unbranched rod structure have been shown to play essential roles in the HDV replication cycle: one encompasses an RNA-editing site [16], the other, which is at one end of the rod, may be a site for the initiation of transcription [17]. The strong conservation of the entire rod structure among isolates suggests that it is important for HDV replication [8,9,14,18]. The specific roles played by other segments of this structure in the HDV replication scheme are not known.

Two unique features of HDV RNA are central to its rolling circle replication mechanism [19]. The first is its transcription by a host RNA polymerase [20,21]. There is no known RNA-dependent RNA polymerase in humans, the only known natural host of HDV. It is likely that HDV corrupts the normal function of RNA polymerase II, the DNA-dependent RNA polymerase involved in transcription of cellular mRNAs, allowing it to act on an RNA template [20,21]. The mechanism by which this is achieved has not yet been defined. Some studies have suggested that transcription begins at one end of the rod-shaped RNA and can occur without HDAg in nuclear extracts [17]. However, the mechanisms by which this transcription occurs and the specific roles of HDAg, HDV RNA structures and additional host factors remain to be determined. The second unique feature of HDV RNA is its autocatalytic cleavage activity, which is required for the processing of linear transcripts to circular replication products. The genomic and antigenomic RNAs both contain autocatalytic RNA segments (ribozymes) that have been isolated and examined *in vitro* [22]. Although these elements are similar in function to the virusoid 'hammerhead' ribozymes, they are structurally and mechanistically distinct. Site-directed mutagenesis data give strongest support to a pseudoknot structure for the HDV ribozyme, but other models have also been proposed (reviewed in [22]).

Unlike the viroids, HDV produces a single protein, HDAg, which is encoded by an antigenomic-sense mRNA (approximately 800 nucleotides long) derived from one side of the rod-like RNA [23,24]. The mRNA is polyadenylated, and the antigenome includes a requisite AAUAAA polyadenylation signal [24]. Adenosine-to-inosine RNA editing on the RNA antigenome allows the virus to make two forms of HDAg (HDAg-S and HDAg-L; indicating 'short' and 'long', respectively) that differ minimally in size, but substantially in function [25,26]. Prior to editing, the antigenome contains A at position 1012, which is within the UAG termination codon of HDAg-S (the amber/W site). As a result of editing (and subsequent transcription) the A is changed to G, hence the codon is changed from UAG to UGG (Trp) and an additional 19 amino acids are added to the C terminus of HDAg, changing its function. For genotype I, efficient editing requires a base-paired structure that is consistent with the unbranched rod structure of HDV RNA [16]; a cellular enzyme, double-stranded RNA adenosine deaminase (ADAR1; formerly dsRAD), has been suggested as a likely candidate for catalysing the reaction [25]. The HDV antigenome is one of only a handful of RNAs that are known to be specifically edited by adenosine deamination; all other examples are host mRNAs that are expressed and edited in the brain [27].

## Functional elements of HDAg

HDAg-S and HDAg-L differ by the presence of an additional 19–20 amino acids at the C terminus of HDAg-L. The two forms of HDAg, which are present in similar amounts in virions, have distinct and partly opposed functions in the HDV RNA replication cycle [26]. HDAg-S is required for HDV RNA replication; HDAg-L inhibits RNA replication and is required for virion formation.

Dissection of the functional features of HDAg has identified several essential elements: a nuclear local-

ization signal [28], which is required for maximal replication activity (HDV RNA replication occurs in the nucleus); a coiled-coil domain that mediates formation of HDAg dimers [29,30]; arginine-rich motifs that are necessary for HDV RNA-binding activity [31]; and an isoprenylation signal sequence at the C terminus of HDAg-L [32]. Highly conserved elements of no known function include a glutamic acid stretch at amino acids 125–130 and a glycine/proline rich segment near the C terminus of HDAg-S [33]. The RNA-binding domain and the dimerization domains are essential for the support of RNA replication by HDAg-S [30]. Virion formation is mediated by an interaction between HDAg-L and HBsAg [34,35]. The mechanism of this interaction has not yet been determined, but it has been shown to require isoprenylation of HDAg-L at a highly conserved sequence motif at the C terminus [32,36].

## Replication

HDV replication occurs via a rolling circle mechanism [18]. In this replication scheme, circular genomic RNA serves as a template for transcription of multimeric linear antigenome RNA transcripts which undergo autocatalytic cleavage at the ribozyme sites. Ligation of ends created by autocatalytic cleavage yields circular antigenome monomers that then serve as templates for transcription of genomic RNA. Whereas the RNA requires no additional factors for ribozyme cleavage to occur *in vitro*, ligation occurs inefficiently and only under unusual conditions *in vitro* [37]; thus the ligation reaction is likely to involve a host RNA ligase. Because HDAg-L inhibits replication, only genomes encoding HDAg-S (about 70%) are likely to replicate upon entering a cell. The mRNA produced from such genomes would initially encode HDAg-S, which supports RNA replication. During the replication process, up to 30% of the HDV RNA is edited to produce HDAg-L, which inhibits RNA replication and is required for virion formation. Thus the virus switches from a replication mode to a packaging mode. Clearly, editing at the amber/W site must be regulated in some manner since complete editing at this site would result in viral genomes that could no longer produce HDAg-S, which is absolutely required for replication [38]. The observed ability of HDAg to inhibit amber/W editing in a concentration-dependent manner suggests a role for HDAg in this regulation [39].

## HDV genotypes

Genetic analysis of HDV isolates from around the

world has indicated that there are at least three phylogenetically distinct genotypes with different geographic distributions and associated disease patterns. The most geographically widespread is genotype I [8,33], which has been identified in isolates from North America, Europe, Africa, east and west Asia, and the south Pacific, and is associated with a broad spectrum of chronic disease [8]. Genotype II has been found only in east Asia, and may be responsible for some of the milder forms of HDV disease in that region [7,40]. Genotype III is exclusively found in northern South America, where HDV infection is associated with particularly severe disease [9,41,42]. Sequence divergence among the genotypes is as high as 40% over the entire RNA genome and 35% for the amino acid sequence of HDAg [9]. Recent analyses of HDV genotypes I and III in transfected cells have indicated that these genotypes differ functionally as well as genetically, suggesting that these might be referred to as separate types of HDV (HDV-I, HDV-II and HDV-III) rather than simply genotypes [43].

## PATHOGENESIS

The patterns of disease associated with chronic HDV infection vary in different epidemiological settings. It has been noted that a more slowly progressing stable disease pattern appears to predominate in some areas where HDV infection is endemic, such as southern Italy, the Greek island of Rhodes and American Samoa [44]. In these areas, and in areas where HDV infection is not endemic, such as northern Europe and North America, the most severe forms of type D hepatitis frequently occur among intravenous drug users. A very different pattern is found in northern South America: although HDV infection is endemic in some communities, disease frequently follows a rapidly progressive course and is associated with significant morbidity and mortality [45]. These varying patterns of disease could be related to a number of factors, including HDV viral genetics, characteristics of the HBV helper, variable responses in the host immune system, infection with other viruses and substance abuse. The suggested association of genotypes II and III, respectively, with mild and severe forms of type D hepatitis have been particularly intriguing [7,9,41]. Additional clinical, epidemiologic and laboratory investigation of these genotypes will prove valuable in determining whether these associations are definitively related to the HDV genotype, and also in the elucidation of disease mechanisms.

The pathogenesis of HDV remains poorly understood and it is not clear to what extent immunolog-ical and directly cytotoxic mechanisms contribute to disease. The immunological basis of HBV disease has been well established and intensively studied [46], and immunopathogenesis is also likely to play an important role in type D hepatitis. During acute HDV infection, disease is temporally associated with the developing immune response and a concomitant decrease in HDV levels [2]. The presence of classical necroinflammatory disease in chronic type D hepatitis is also consistent with a major role for immunopathogenesis. However, it is not yet clear whether immunopathogenesis in type D hepatitis is due to the response to HBV antigens, HDAg, or both. The experience of the transplant setting would suggest that HBV-related immunopathogenesis is predominant, because necroinflammation is absent until the reappearance of HBV antigens in the liver [47]. Investigations of the potential direct cytotoxicity of HDV in model systems have generally yielded negative results. Transgenic mice expressing HDV exhibit no particular liver pathology [48], nor do mice experimentally infected with HDV [49]. A study suggesting cytotoxic effects of HDAg on cell growth in stably transfected cells has not been confirmed in other laboratories [50]. Perhaps the most intriguing data regarding potential direct cytopathic effects of HDV are the observations of microvesicular steatosis in epidemics of severe HDV infection in northern South America and in some transplant patients who exhibit HDV infection in the graft prior to the reappearance of HBV [47,51]. The former effect could be related to the distinct genotype of HDV that is characteristic of northern South America, the latter to the unique setting of HDV re-infection following transplantation.

## IMMUNOLOGY

The role of the immune system in HDV disease and clearance has not been fully explored. HDV infection of chronic HBV carriers typically results in chronic HDV infection. Analogous to the immune system response to HBV core antigen (HBcAg), antibodies to HDAg are probably not protective, most probably because HDAg is an internal component of the virion. Indeed, chronic infection is typically accompanied by high titres of anti-HDAg immunoglobulin G (IgG); the presence of high anti-HDAg IgM titres typically indicates either acute disease or active chronic disease [52]. Thus, containment of viral spread in chronic infection is likely to involve T cell responses, which may also be responsible for cytotoxic effects in the infected liver. That such responses exist was suggested by observations of low levels of viraemia and disease following experimental reinfection of chimpanzees chronically infected with HBV that had recovered from previous HDV infection [53]. Consistent with a role for T cells in containment of HDV, Nisini *et al.* directly detected T-cell responses to HDAg in peripheral blood mononuclear cells isolated from individuals chronically infected with HDV, and showed that the T-cell response was correlated with a reduction in active disease [54].

Attempts to successfully prevent HDV infection by vaccination in a woodchuck hepatitis virus (WHV) model have had limited success [55–59]. (Woodchucks chronically infected with WHV, which is closely related to HBV, can be experimentally infected with HDV.) Approaches taken thus far have included vaccination of WHV-infected woodchucks with recombinant HDAg, conjugated peptides, or recombinant vaccinia virus expressing HDAg. Again, consistent with a predominant role of T cell immunity, limited protection (relatively lower levels of viraemia) was observed following challenge with infectious HDV, even in the absence of detectable anti-HDAg antibodies. Perhaps it will be possible to manipulate such T-cell responses to develop a therapeutic or prophylactic vaccine.

## DISCUSSION

HDV remains a serious health problem, even as the development of therapeutic approaches for the management of its helper, HBV, advance at a rapid pace. There is currently no widely accepted therapy for HDV infection or disease; the only option is liver transplantation. Although it might be expected that control of HBV infection would also control HDV, it is not certain that this would be the case. The only HBV function on which HDV depends is HBsAg, which is present at very high levels even in the face of many highly effective anti-HBV treatments. Indeed, in

a study of the effects of lamivudine in HDV-infected patients, neither HDV viraemia nor liver disease activity were reduced [60].

Perhaps a reduction of HBV in carriers to the point of minimal HBsAg levels remains the most attractive approach for the elimination of HDV in chronically infected individuals. However, it may be that even low levels of HBsAg will be sufficient to maintain HDV infection and that ultimately the most effective therapies will include specific anti-HDV as well as anti-HBV agents. Analysis of HDV molecular biology has led to the identification of several functional elements and processes that could be targeted for inhibition. These are included in Table 1. Current experimental systems for analysing the effectiveness of potential antiviral approaches include: specific *in vitro* assays using purified components (ribozymes and editing, for example); assays of virus replication and particle formation in transfected culture cells; and experimentally infected woodchucks.

## ACKNOWLEDGEMENTS

This work was supported by NIAID contract NO1-AI-45179.

## REFERENCES

1. Rizzetto M, Hoyer B, Canese MG, Shih JW, Purcell RH & Gerin JL. Delta agent: association of delta antigen with hepatitis B surface antigen and RNA in serum of delta-infected chimpanzees. *Proceedings of the National Academy of Sciences, USA* 1980; **77**: 6124–6128.
2. Rizzetto M, Canese MG, Gerin JL, London WT, Sly DL & Purcell RH. Transmission of the hepatitis B virus-associated delta antigen to chimpanzees. *Journal of Infectious Diseases* 1980; **141**:590–602.
3. Smedile A, Farci P, Verme G, Caredda F, Cargnel A, Caporaso N, Dentico P, Trepo C, Opolon P, Gimson A, Vergani D, Williams R & Rizetto M. Influence of delta infection on severity of hepatitis B. *Lancet* 1982; ii: 945–947.
4. Rizzetto M. The delta agent. *Hepatology* 1983; **3**:729–737.
5. Rizzetto M, Hadziyannis S, Hansson BG, Toukan A & Gust I. Hepatitis delta virus infection in the world: epidemiological patterns and clinical expression. *Gastroenterology International* 1992; **5**:18–32.
6. Rizzetto M & Durazzo M. Hepatitis delta virus (HDV) infections. Epidemiological and clinical heterogeneity. *Journal of Hepatology* 1991; **13**:116–118.
7. Wu JC, Choo KB, Chen CM, Chen TZ, Huo TI & Lee SD. Genotyping of hepatitis D virus by restriction-fragment length polymorphism and relation to outcome of hepatitis D. *Lancet* 1995; **346**:939–941.
8. Niro GA, Smedile A, Andriulli A, Rizzetto M, Gerin JL & Casey JL. Predominance of hepatitis delta virus genotype I among chronically infected Italian patients. *Hepatology* 1997; **25**:728–734.

**Table 1**. Potential targets for anti-HDV agents

| Target |
| --- |
| HBsAg |
| Ribozyme activity |
| RNA editing |
| RNA-dependent RNA polymerase activity of RNA polymerase II |
| Isoprenylation of HDAg-L |
| Interaction between HBsAg and HDAg-L |
| HDAg dimerization |
| HDAg–RNA binding |

9. Casey JL, Brown TL, Colan EJ, Wignall FS & Gerin JL. A genotype of hepatitis D virus that occurs in northern South America. *Proceedings of the National Academy of Sciences, USA* 1993; **90**:9016–9020.

10. Bergmann KF & Gerin JL. Antigens of hepatitis delta virus in the liver and serum of humans and animals. *Journal of Infectious Diseases* 1986; **154**:702–706.

11. Bonino F, Hoyer B, Ford E, Shih JW, Purcell RH & Gerin JL. The delta agent: HBsAg particles with delta antigen and RNA in the serum of an HBV carrier. *Hepatology* 1981; **1**:127–131.

12. Bonino F, Hoyer B, Shih JW, Rizzetto M, Purcell RH & Gerin JL. Delta hepatitis agent: structural and antigenic properties of the delta-associated particle. *Infection and Immunity* 1984; **43**:1000–1005.

13. Bonino F, Heermann KH, Rizzetto M & Gerlich WH. Hepatitis delta virus: protein composition of delta antigen and its hepatitis B virus-derived envelope. *Journal of Virology* 1986; **58**:945–950.

14. Wang KS, Choo QL, Weiner AJ, Ou JH, Najarian RC, Thayer RM, Mullenbach GT, Dannision KJ, Gerin JL & Houghton M. Structure, sequence and expression of the hepatitis delta viral genome. *Nature* 1986; **323**:508–514.

15. Lai MM. The molecular biology of hepatitis delta virus. *Annual Review of Biochemistry* 1995; **64**:259–286.

16. Casey JL, Bergmann KF, Brown TL & Gerin JL. Structural requirements for RNA editing in hepatitis delta virus: evidence for a uridine-to-cytidine editing mechanism. *Proceedings of the National Academy of Sciences, USA* 1992; **89**:7149–7153.

17. Beard MR, MacNaughton TB & Gowans EJ. Identification and characterization of a hepatitis delta virus RNA transcriptional promoter. *Journal of Virology* 1996; **70**:4986–4995.

18. Makino S, Chang MF, Shieh CK, Kamahora T, Vannier DM, Govindarajan S & Lai MM. Molecular cloning and sequencing of a human hepatitis delta virus RNA. *Nature* 1987; **329**:343–346.

19. Robertson HD. Replication and evolution of viroid-like pathogens. *Current Topics in Microbiology and Immunology* 1992; **176**:213–219.

20. Fu TB & Taylor J. The RNAs of hepatitis delta virus are copied by RNA polymerase II in nuclear homogenates. *Journal of Virology* 1993; **67**:6965–6972.

21. MacNaughton TB, Gowans EJ, McNamara SP & Burrell CJ. Hepatitis delta antigen is necessary for access of hepatitis delta virus RNA to the cell transcriptional machinery but is not part of the transcriptional complex. *Virology* 1991; **184**:387–390.

22. Been MD. Cis- and trans-acting ribozymes from a human pathogen, hepatitis delta virus. *Trends in Biochemical Sciences* 1994; **19**:251–256.

23. Weiner AJ, Choo QL, Wang KS, Govindarajan S, Redeker AG, Gerin JL & Houghton M. A single antigenomic open reading frame of the hepatitis delta virus encodes the epitope(s) of both hepatitis delta antigen polypeptides p24 delta and p27 delta. *Journal of Virology* 1988; **62**:594–599.

24. Hsieh SY, Chao M, Coates L & Taylor J. Hepatitis delta virus genome replication: a polyadenylated mRNA for delta antigen. *Journal of Virology* 1990; **64**:3192–3198.

25. Polson AG, Bass BL & Casey JL. RNA editing of hepatitis delta virus antigenome by dsRNA-adenosine deaminase. *Nature* 1996; **380**:454–456.

26. Chao M, Hsieh SY, Luo GX & Taylor J. Role of two forms of hepatitis delta virus antigen: evidence for a mechanism of self-limiting genome replication. *Journal of Virology* 1990; **64**:5066–5069.

27. Bass BL. RNA editing and hypermutation by adenosine deamination. *Trends in Biochemical Sciences* 1997; **22**:157–162.

28. Xia YP, Yeh CT, Ou JH & Lai MM. Characterization of nuclear targeting signal of hepatitis delta antigen: nuclear transport as a protein complex. *Journal of Virology* 1992; **66**:914–921.

29. Wang JG & Lemon SM. Dimeric and multimeric forms of hepatitis delta virus antigen are present in infected woodchuck liver. *Progress in Clinical and Biological Research* 1993; **382**:61–67.

30. Lazinski DW & Taylor JM. Relating structure to function in the hepatitis delta virus antigen. *Journal of Virology* 1993; **67**:2672–2680.

31. Lee CZ, Lin JH, Chao M, McKnight K & Lai MM. RNA-binding activity of hepatitis delta antigen involves two arginine-rich motifs and is required for hepatitis delta virus RNA replication. *Journal of Virology* 1993; **67**:2221–2227.

32. Glenn JS, Watson JA, Havel CM & White JM. Identification of a prenylation site in delta virus large antigen. *Science* 1992; **256**:1331–1333.

33. Shakil AO, Hadziyannis S, Hoofnagle JH, DiBisceglie AM, Gerin JL & Casey JL. Geographic distribution and genetic variability of hepatitis delta virus genotype I. *Virology* 1997; **234**:160–167.

34. Hwang SB & Lai MM. Isoprenylation mediates direct protein–protein interactions between hepatitis large delta antigen and hepatitis B virus surface antigen. *Journal of Virology* 1993; **67**:7659–7662.

35. Ryu WS, Bayer M & Taylor J. Assembly of hepatitis delta virus particles. *Journal of Virology* 1992; **66**:2310–2315.

36. Hwang SB, Lee CZ & Lai MM. Hepatitis delta antigen expressed by recombinant baculoviruses: comparison of biochemical properties and post-translational modifications between the large and small forms. *Virology* 1992; **190**:413–422.

37. Sharmeen L, Kuo MY & Taylor J. Self-ligating RNA sequences on the antigenome of human hepatitis delta virus. *Journal of Virology* 1989; **63**:1428–1430.

38. Kuo MY, Chao M & Taylor J. Initiation of replication of the human hepatitis delta virus genome from cloned DNA: role of delta antigen. *Journal of Virology* 1989; **63**:1945–1950.

39. Polson AG, Ley HL 3rd, Bass BL & Casey JL. Hepatitis delta virus RNA editing is highly specific for the amber/W site and is suppressed by hepatitis delta antigen. *Molecular and Cellular Biology* 1998; **18**: 1919–1926.

40. Wu JC, Chen CM, Sheen IJ, Lee SD, Tzeng HM & Choo KB. Evidence of transmission of hepatitis D virus to spouses from sequence analysis of the viral genome. *Hepatology* 1995; **22**:1656–1660.

41. Casey JL, Niro GA, Engle RE, Vega A, Gomez H, McCarthy M, Watts DM, Hyams KC & Gerin JL. Hepatitis B virus (HBV)/hepatitis D virus (HDV) coinfection in outbreaks of acute hepatitis in the Peruvian Amazon Basin: the roles of HDV genotype III and HBV genotype F. *Journal of Infectious Diseases* 1996; **174**: 920–926.

42. Maynard JE, Hadler SC, Fields HA. Delta hepatitis in the Americas: an overview. *Progress in Clinical and Biological Research* 1987; **234**:493–505.

43. Casey JL & Gerin JL. Genotype-specific complementation of hepatitis delta virus RNA replication by hepatitis delta antigen. *Journal of Virology* 1998; **72**:

2806–2814.

44. Rizzetto M, Ponzetto A & Forzani I. Hepatitis delta virus as a global health problem. *Vaccine* 1990; **8** (Supplement):10–14.

45. Hadler SC, De MM, Ponzetto A, Anzola E, Rivero D, Mondolfi A, Bracho A, Francis DP, Gerber MA, Thung S *et al*. Delta virus infection and severe hepatitis. An epidemic in the Yucpa Indians of Venezuela. *Annals of Intern Medicine* 1984; **100**:339–344.

46. Chisari FV & Ferrari C. Hepatitis B virus immunopathogenesis. *Annual Review of Immunology* 1995; **13**:29–60.

47. David E, Rahier J, Pucci A, Andorno E, Fassi L, Fortunato M, Fabiano A, Molla F & Rizetto M. Recurrence of hepatitis D (delta) in liver transplants: histopathological aspects. *Gastroenterology* 1993; **104**:1122–1128.

48. Polo JM, Jeng KS, Lim B, Govindarajan S, Hofman F, Sangiorgi F & Lai MM. Transgenic mice support replication of hepatitis delta virus RNA in multiple tissues, particularly in skeletal muscle. *Journal of Virology* 1995; **69**:4880–4887.

49. Netter HJ, Kajino K & Taylor JM. Experimental transmission of human hepatitis delta virus to the laboratory mouse. *Journal of Virology* 1993; **67**:3357–3362.

50. Cole SM, Gowans EJ, Macnaughton TB, Hall PD & Burrell CJ. Direct evidence for cytotoxicity associated with expression of hepatitis delta virus antigen. *Hepatology* 1991; **13**:845–851.

51. Popper H, Thung SN, Gerber MA, Hadler SC, de Monzon M, Ponzetto A, Anzola E, Rivera D, Mondolfi A, Bracho A *et al*. Histologic studies of severe delta agent infection in Venezuelan Indians. *Hepatology* 1983; **3**:906–912.

52. Farci P, Gerin JL, Aragona M, Lindsey I, Crivelli O, Balestrieri A, Smedile A, Thomas HC & Rizetto M Diagnostic and prognostic significance of the IgM antibody to the hepatitis delta virus. *Journal of the American Medical Association* 1986; **255**:1443–1446.

53. Negro F, Shapiro M, Satterfield WC, Gerin JL & Purcell RH. Reappearance of hepatitis D virus (HDV) replication in chronic hepatitis B virus carrier chimpanzees rechallenged with HDV. *Journal of Infectious Diseases* 1989; **160**:567–571.

54. Nisini R, Paroli M, Accapezzato D, Bonino F, Rosina F, Sanantonio T, Sallustra F, Amoroso A, Houghton M & Banaba V. Human CD4+ T-cell response to hepatitis delta virus: identification of multiple epitopes and characterization of T-helper cytokine profiles. *Journal of Virology* 1997; **71**:2241–2251.

55. Karayiannis P, Saldanha J, Jackson AM, Luther S, Goldin R, Monjardino J & Thomas HC. Partial control of hepatitis delta virus superinfection by immunisation of woodchucks (*Marmota monax*) with hepatitis delta antigen expressed by a recombinant vaccinia or baculovirus. *Journal of Medical Virology* 1993; **41**:210–214.

56. Karayiannis P, Saldanha J, Monjardino J, Goldin R, Main J, Luther S, Easton M, Ponzetto A & Thomas HC Immunization of woodchucks with recombinant hepatitis delta antigen does not protect against hepatitis delta virus infection. *Hepatology* 1990; **12**:1125–1128.

57. Bergmann KF, Casey JL, Tennant BC & Gerin JL. Modulation of hepatitis delta virus infection by vaccination with synthetic peptides: a preliminary study in the woodchuck model. *Progress in Clinical and Biological Research* 1993; **382**:181–187.

58. Eckart MR, Dong C, Houghton M, D'Urso N & Ponzetto A. The effects of using recombinant vaccinia viruses expressing either large or small HDAg to protect woodchuck hepadnavirus carriers from HDV superinfection. *Progress in Clinical and Biological Research* 1993; **382**:201–205.

59. Ponzetto A, Eckart M, D'Urso N, Negro F, Silvestro M, Bonino F, Wang KS, Chien D, Choo QL & Houghton M. Towards a vaccine for the prevention of hepatitis delta virus superinfection in HBV carriers. *Progress in Clinical and Biological Research* 1993; **382**:207–210.

60. Honkoop P, de Man RA, Niesters HGM, Heijtink RA & Schalm SW. Lamivudine treatment in patients with chronic hepatitis delta infection. *Hepatology* 1997; **24** (Supplement):1219.

# 11

# Molecular cloning and disease associations of hepatitis G virus

## Jungsuh P Kim*, Kirk E Fry and John Wages Jr for The HGV Study Group

## SUMMARY

We have cloned an RNA virus, designated hepatitis G virus (HGV), from a patient with chronic post-transfusion hepatitis. The virus is a novel member of the family *Flaviviridae* and is most closely related to hepatitis C virus (HCV) and GB virus (GBV) types A, B and C. The HGV genome is 9392 nucleotides and encodes a single polyprotein of 2893 amino acids, which appears to be cleaved into at least five non-structural proteins. The HGV open reading frame (ORF) contains zinc protease motifs in NS2b, serine protease and helicase motifs in NS3; and RNA-dependent RNA polymerase motifs in NS5b. HGV appears to be associated with 0.3% of cases of viral hepatitis and is present in around 1.5% of blood donors in the USA. The virus is transmitted by transfusion and probably also by intravenous drug use. There are some data for an association of HGV with several diseases, including post-transfusion hepatitis, acute hepatitis, cryptogenic liver diseases, hepatitis-associated aplastic anaemia and common variable immunodeficiency. Further study is required to clarify the diseases caused by this virus, and to establish practical diagnostic tests to screen potential blood donors.

## INTRODUCTION

Although sensitive and specific tests for detecting the known hepatitis viruses are available, the aetiology of a significant fraction of post-transfusion and community-acquired hepatitis cases remains unclear [1,2], which suggests the existence of additional infectious agents associated with hepatitis. In an attempt to search for such viruses, we have recently identified an RNA virus, tentatively designated hepatitis G virus (HGV) [3].

## CLONING OF HGV

Using an immunoscreening approach, we isolated a clone, 470-20-1, from a cDNA library derived from the plasma of a patient (PNF2161) who developed

chronic hepatitis after transfusion. Genomic PCR using primers from the 470-20-1 clone suggested that it contained a novel sequence exogenous to the *Escherichia coli*, *Saccharomyces cerevisiae* and human genomes (Fig. 1a), and a reverse transcriptase (RT)–PCR assay demonstrated that it was present in the serum of patient PNF2161 (Fig. 1b). The exogenous nature of the 470-20-1 clone was further confirmed by its failure to hybridize to Southern blots containing human and *E. coli* genomic DNAs (data not shown).

To confirm that the RNA sequences amplified from patient PNF2161 were associated with viral particles, fractions obtained after the ultracentrifugation of a plasma sample in a 10–60% sucrose density gradient were assayed by RT–PCR. The presence of HCV in the plasma of this patient provided an internal control for the behaviour of an enveloped virus. In addition, the plasma specimen was spiked with hepatitis A virus (HAV) as a representative non-enveloped RNA virus. Gradient fractions were analysed by RT–PCR for HAV, HCV and 470-20-1 sequences. The peak 470-20-1 RT–PCR signal was reproducibly found in fractions corresponding to a density of 1.11 $g/cm^3$ (Fig. 2); the peak HCV PCR signal was observed in the same fractions. The peak signal for the non-enveloped HAV was found in fractions of much greater density (1.25 $g/cm^3$). These data suggest that the 470-20-1 sequence is associated with enveloped viral particles [4,5].

Starting from an immunoreactive cDNA clone, overlapping sequences from the 470-20-1 clone were obtained by anchor PCR, and the 5′ and 3′ ends of the viral sequences were isolated by modified rapid amplification of cDNA ends (RACE).

## MOLECULAR CHARACTERISTICS

The HGV genome consists of 9392 nucleotides, which encode a single polyprotein of 2893 amino acids [3]. We have sequenced a second isolate from a patient (R10291), which has a 9103 nucleotide sequence. The

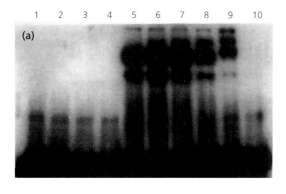

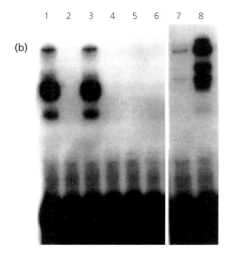

**Figure 1.** Molecular characterization of the 470-20-1 clone

**(a)** Determination of the exogenous nature of the 470-20-1 clone. To evaluate whether or not the cloned 470-20-1 sequence was exogenous to the human, *E. coli* and *S. cerevisiae* genomes, PCR was performed using primers 77F (5'-CTCTTTGTGGTAGTAGCCGA-GAGAT) and 211R (5'-CGAATGAGTCAGAGGACGGGGTAT). All PCR products were hybridized in solution to the 152F probe (5'-TCGGT-TACTGAGAGCAGCTCAGATGAG) specific to the 470-20-1 sequence. Hybridization products were electrophoresed on 10% polyacrylamide gels and detected by autoradiography. The template DNAs used were 100 ng of *E. coli* DNA (lane 1), 1 µg of human DNA (lane 2), 100 ng of *Sanguinus mystax* DNA (lane 3) and 100 ng of *S. cerevisiae* DNA (lane 4). Lanes 5–10 contain the hybridized products from PCR amplification using a 10-fold dilution series of a plasmid control template ($10^5$–0 copies, respectively).

**(b)** Detection of the 470-20-1 sequence in patient PNF2161. To demonstrate the presence of the 470-20-1 sequence in the cloning source, 125 µl of plasma from patient PNF2161 was ultracentrifuged (Beckman 70.1 Ti rotor at 40 000 r.p.m. for 1 h). RNA was extracted from the pellet [31] and subjected to RT–PCR analysis, using RNA corresponding to the equivalent of 50 µl of plasma per reaction. Reverse transcription and PCR analyses were performed as described previously [3]. Lanes 1 and 3 contain PCR products from patient PNF2161; lanes 2 and 5 contain results from PCR negative control reactions; lanes 4 and 6 contain results of RT–PCR from normal human sera; and lanes 7 and 8 contain the hybridized products from the amplification of plasmid control template (10 and 100 copies, respectively).

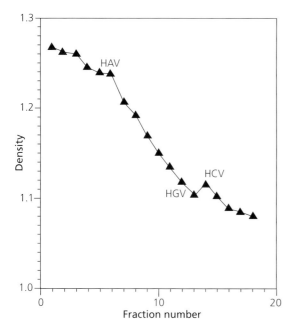

**Figure 2.** Demonstration that the 470-20-1 sequence is derived from RNA of an enveloped virus-like particle

Plasma from patient PNF2161 (25 µl), containing HCV as well as HGV, was spiked with HAV culture supernatant. Continuous 10–60% sucrose (Life Technologies) gradients were overlaid with the samples and centrifuged for 18 h at 40 000 r.p.m. in a Beckman SW 40 rotor. Fractions of 0.55–0.60 ml were collected, and densities were determined. RNA was prepared from gradient fractions by a salt precipitation method using the PureScript RNA isolation kit according to the manufacturer's suggested protocol for extraction from plasma and serum (Gentra Systems). RNA prepared from gradient fractions was then analysed by RT–PCR using the primers described in Fig. 1(a) for HGV. To detect HCV and HAV, the following primers were used: HCV: UTR-1 (5'-TTCACGCAGAAAGCGTCTAGC-CAT) and UTR-2 (5'-TCGTCCTGGCAATTCCGGTGTACT); HAV: F1 (5'-GATTGGAAATCTGATCCGTCCC) and R1 (5'-GTTGACCAACT-GAGTCTGAAGC). Fractions containing the peak RT–PCR signals for each viral RNA were determined by ethidium bromide agarose gel electrophoresis and confirmed by solution hybridization analysis using appropriate specific 5'-[$^{32}$P]-labelled probes.

**Table 1.** Global amino acid sequence identity comparison of hepatitis-associated and other viruses in the family *Flaviviridae*

| | Sequence identity (%) | | | | | | |
|---|---|---|---|---|---|---|---|
| | HGV | HCV | GBV-A | GBV-B | GBV-C | YFV | DEN1 |
| HCV | 25 | | | | | | |
| GBV-A | **45** | 24 | | | | | |
| GBV-B | 25 | 29 | 23 | | | | |
| GBV-C | **95** | 26 | **44** | 25 | | | |
| YFV | 15 | 14 | 15 | 13 | 15 | | |
| DEN1 | 15 | 14 | 13 | 14 | 15 | **45** | |
| HoCV | 16 | 17 | 15 | 17 | 16 | 15 | 16 |

Viruses were optimally aligned pairwise using the ALIGN program (version 1.6b) of the FASTA suite (version 1.7) of programs by Pearson. Percentage identities were determined by counting exact amino acid matches and dividing by the total number of nucleotides. The default parameters and scoring matrix (PAM250) were used [32]. Bold denotes a high degree of sequence identity. HCV, hepatitis C virus; HGV, hepatitis G virus; GBV-A and GBV-B, non-human primate flavi-like virus; YFV, yellow fever virus; DEN1, dengue 1 virus; HoCV, hog cholera virus.

PNF2161 and R10291 isolates had 90.5% identity at the nucleotide level and 97.5% at the amino acid level. The ORF derived from R10291 was slightly larger (2910 amino acids) than that from PNF2161.

ORF analysis shows that HGV belongs to the *Flaviviridae* family (Table 1). The viruses most closely related to HGV are other flavi-like viruses associated with hepatitis: HCV and GBV-C in humans [6] and GBV-A and GBV-B in animals [7]. Sequence analysis has suggested that HGV and GBV-C are different isolates of the same species of virus (85% identity at the RNA level and 95% identity at the amino acid level). However, there is little significant primary sequence conservation in both the structural proteins and untranslated control regions (UTRs) between HGV, HCV, GBV-A and GBV-B (Table 2), suggesting that these four viruses are different species of the family *Flaviviridae*. Phylogenetic analysis is also consistent with this conclusion (Fig. 3).

Motif searches using the MACAW [8] and BLASTP [9] programs identified sequence motifs associated with four ORFs in HGV: a zinc protease motif in the HGV NS2b ORF [10], a chymotrypsin-like serine protease motif in NS3, a helicase motif in NS3 and an RNA-dependent RNA polymerase motif in NS5b [11]. The zinc protease motif, which was originally identified (and confirmed by site-directed mutagenesis) in HCV, was identified by primary sequence similarity in HGV, GBV-A and GBV-B. The genomic structure of HGV is shown in Figure 4.

To study the polyprotein processing of HGV, a full cDNA and smaller constructs were expressed in vaccinia virus or baculovirus expression systems. The immuno-precipitation and Western blot data suggested that at least five non-structural proteins are cleaved from the polyprotein [12]. Preliminary results have also shown that the E2 protein is cleaved, translocated and glycosy-

**Table 2.** Global amino acid sequence identity between HGV and related viruses in structural and non-structural regions

| | Sequence identity with HGV (%) | | | |
|---|---|---|---|---|
| Region | HCV | GBV-A | GBV-B | GBV-C |
| Global | 25 | 45 | 25 | 95 |
| Structural | 17 | 35 | 16 | 92 |
| Non-structural | 28 | 47 | 28 | 97 |

The junctions between structural and non-structural regions were determined by primary similarity analysis. The structural and non-structural regions were then aligned as described for Table 1. HCV, hepatitis C virus; GBV-A and GBV-B, non-human primate flavi-like virus.

**Figure 3.** Phylogenetic relationships of HGV based on helicase-encoding gene

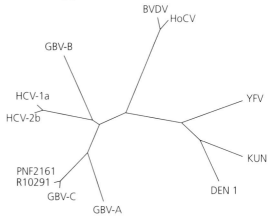

The tree is based on the conserved motifs found in the helicase-encoding gene. Tree and branch lengths were determined by the CLUSTALV program using the neighbour joining method. YFV, yellow fever virus; KUN, Kunjin virus, DEN1, dengue 1 virus; BVDV, bovine viral diarrhoea virus; HogCV, hog cholera virus; HCV-1a, HCV-2b, hepatitis C virus subtypes 1a and 2b; PNF2161, R10291, GBV-C, isolates of HGV; GBV-A, non-human primate flavi-like virus; GBV-B, non-human primate hepatitis flavi-like virus.

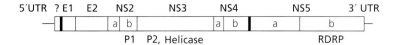

**Figure 4.** Location of HGV ORFs, as determined by similarity comparison, location of hydrophobic leader regions and *in vivo* processing in vaccinia virus and baculovirus expression systems

P1, zinc protease motif in NS2b; P2 chymotrypsin-like serine protease motif; RDRP, RNA-dependent RNA polymerase; UTR, untranslated region. The polyprotein is about 3000 amino acids long. Data from [12,13].

lated using a predicted signal sequence [13].

RT–PCR has been used to assess the sequence variation among different isolates of HGV from serum samples collected worldwide. Multiple sequence alignments demonstrated that the 5′ UTR contains blocks of highly conserved sequences. These data enabled us to optimize RT–PCR assays using primers from the conserved regions [14]. A single nucleotide deletion/substitution in the 5′ end of the genome introduces a frame shift, resulting in at least three distinct sizes of the putative capsid protein [15]. Therefore, it is possible that the capsid protein is missing or defective in HGV. The initiation site of the HGV polyprotein has not been clearly demonstrated.

## EPIDEMIOLOGY AND DISEASE ASSOCIATIONS

Testing of patients with community-acquired non-A, non-B hepatitis demonstrated that HGV can cause persistent viraemia for up to 9 years and that HGV is associated with 0.3% of cases of viral hepatitis [16]. HGV infection can be transmitted by transfusion, as shown by the demonstration of HGV RNA detection by PCR only after transfusion [17–19], by donor–recipient linkages and by the low frequency of HGV infection in non-transfused control groups [17]. Transfusion-associated HGV-induced hepatitis can become chronic at a very low frequency. Co-infection of HGV with HBV or HCV occurs frequently [20]. HGV appears to be associated with cryptogenic liver disease [21–23] and, in these patients, HGV is the only identifiable viral marker. The high frequency of HGV infection observed in multiply transfused patients, haemophiliacs and intravenous drug users is consistent with a parenterally transmitted agent [3].

To determine the prevalence of HGV among volunteer blood donors in the USA, we have used RT–PCR to screen plasma from accepted blood donors and from rejected volunteers with alanine aminotransferase levels >45 IU/ml. The HGV infection rates among accepted and rejected donors were 1.7% and 1.5%, respectively [3], with no significant difference in HGV RNA detec-

tion rate between the two groups. These observed infection rates among blood donors were much higher than the rate of transfusion-associated hepatitis cases in the recipients. Clearly, about 75% of transfusion recipients of HGV-containing blood do not appear to acquire hepatitis immediately [17].

So far, there have been numerous reports suggesting an association of HGV with acute hepatitis, cryptogenic liver diseases (with or without liver transplantation), hepatitis-associated aplastic anaemia [24], common variable immunodeficiency [25] and post-transfusion hepatitis. There are contradictory reports of a possible association of HGV with fulminant hepatitis [26–28]. To establish clear associations between HGV and disease, an organized effort among clinicians is necessary to define criteria and to select control groups for epidemiological studies.

If a clear disease association is established, it will be necessary to develop a practical screening assay to exclude HGV infection from the donor population. Currently, diagnostic assays based on nucleic acids [3,29,30] are available. If HGV proves to cause acute and chronic liver disease, development of therapies against the virus might be possible by targeting the viral NS2b and NS3 protease activities with inhibitors. Site-directed mutagenesis has been used to confirm that these HGV proteases are active *in vivo* (A Belyaev *et al.*, personal communication).

Many areas of research remain, including the identification of immunodominant epitopes, large-scale prevalence studies, immune response over time, causal relationship between HGV and liver disease (and possibly other diseases), site of replication, genotype studies, quasispecies studies, *in vitro* propagation and animal transmission studies. Answers to these questions are just beginning to emerge.

This article originally appeared in *Antiviral Therapy* 1996; **1** (Supplement 3):33–38. A list of recent references is included at the end of the paper.

# REFERENCES

1. Alter HJ, Purcell RH, Shih JW, Melpolder JC, Houghton M, Choo QL & Kuo G. Detection of antibody to hepatitis C virus in prospectively followed transfusion recipients with acute and chronic non-A, non-B hepatitis. *New England Journal of Medicine* 1989; **321**:1494–1500.

2. Alter MJ, Margolis HS, Krawczynski K, Judson FN, Mares A, Alexander WJ, Hu PY, Miller JK, Gerber MA, Sampliner RE, Meeks EL & Beach MJ. The natural history of community-acquired hepatitis C in the United States. *New England Journal of Medicine* 1992; **327**:1899–1905.

3. Linnen J, Wages J Jr, Zhang-Keck Z-Y, Fry KE, Krawczynski KZ, Alter HJ, Koonin E, Gallagher M, Alter M, Hadziyannis S, Karayiannis P, Fung K, Nakatsuji Y, Shih JW, Young L, Piatak M, Jr, Hoover C, Fernandez J, Chen S, Zou J-C, Morris T, Hyams KC, Ismay S, Lifson JD, Hess G, Foung SKF, Thomas H, Bradley D, Margolis H & Kim JP. Molecular cloning and disease association of hepatitis G virus: a transfusion-transmissible agent. *Science* 1996; **271**:505–508.

4. Hijikata M, Shimizu YK, Kato H, Iwamoto A, Shih JW, Alter HJ, Purcell RH & Yoshikura H. Equilibrium centrifugation studies of hepatitis C virus: evidence for circulating immune complexes. *Journal of Virology* 1993; **67**:1953–1958.

5. Kanto T, Hayashi N, Takehara T, Hagiwara H, Mita E, Naito M, Kasahara A, Fusamoto H & Kamada T. Buoyant density of hepatitis C virus recovered from infected hosts: two different features in sucrose equilibrium density-gradient centrifugation related to degree of liver inflammation. *Hepatology* 1994; **19**:296–302.

6. Leary TP, Muerhoff AS, Simmons JN, Pilot-Matias TJ, Erker JC, Chalmers ML, Schlauder GG, Dawson GJ, Desai SM & Mushahwar IK. Sequence and genomic organization of GBV-C: a novel member of the *Flaviviridae* associated with human non-A–E hepatitis. *Journal of Medical Virology* 1996; **48**:60–67.

7. Muerhoff AS, Leary TP, Simons JN, Pilot-Matias TJ, Dawson GJ, Erker JC, Chalmers ML, Schlauder GG, Desai SM & Mushahwar IK. Genomic organization of GBV-A and GBV-B: two new members of the *Flaviviridae* associated with GB-agent hepatitis. *Journal of Virology* 1995; **69**:5621–5630.

8. Schuler GD, Altschul SF & Lipman DJ. The workbench for multiple alignment construction and analysis. *Proteins* 1991; **9**:180–190.

9. Altschul SF, Gish W, Miller W, Myers EW & Lipman DJ. Basic local alignment search tool. *Journal of Molecular Biology* 1990; **215**:403–410.

10. Reed KE, Grakoui A & Rice CM. Hepatitis C virus-encoded NS2-3 protease: cleavage-site mutagenesis and requirements for bimolecular cleavage. *Journal of Virology* 1995; **69**:4127–4136.

11. Koonin EV & Dolja VV. Evolution and taxonomy of positive-strand RNA viruses: implications of comparative analysis of amino acid sequences. *Critical Reviews in Biochemistry and Molecular Biology* 1993; **28**:375–430.

12. Zhang YF, Belyaev AS, Zhang-Keck ZY, Chong S, Linnen J, Fung K, Yarbough PO, Lim M & Kim JP. Proteolytic processing of the hepatitis G virus polyprotein. *9th Triennial International Symposium on Viral Hepatitis and Liver Disease*, Rome, Italy, 21–24 April 1996. p 251.

13. Belyaev AS, Chong C, Wages J, Hoover C, Linnen J & Kim JP. Model of translocation and cleavage of the hepatitis G virus polyprotein. *Hepatology* 1995; **22**:182A.

14. Linnen JM, Fung K, Wages J, Zhang-Keck Z-Y, Hoover C, Fernandez J, Foung S, Hadziyannis S, Thomas H, Fry KE & Kim JP. Sequence variation of the 5′ terminus of hepatitis G virus. *9th Triennial International Symposium on Viral Hepatitis and Liver Disease*, Rome, Italy, 21–24 April 1996. p. 250.

15. Kim J, Linnen J, Wages J, Zhang-Keck Z-Y, Belyaev A, Zhang Y, Fung K, Krawczynski K, Alter M, Koonin E, Lim M, Hadlock K, Young L, Hoover C, Fernandez J, Piatak M, Chong S, Karayiannis P, Thomas H, Hadziyannis S, Hess G, Bradley D, Foung S, Margolis H, Shih J, Alter H & Fry K. Molecular cloning and characterization of hepatitis G virus (HGV). *9th Triennial International Symposium on Viral Hepatitis and Liver Disease*, Rome, Italy, 21–24 April 1996. p. 34.

16. Alter MJ, Gallagher M, Morris T, Moyer L, Krawczynski K, Khudyakov Y, Fields H, Kim J & Margolis H. Epidemiology of non-A, non-E hepatitis. *9th Triennial International Symposium on Viral Hepatitis and Liver Disease*, Rome, Italy, 21–24 April 1996. p. 34.

17. Alter, HJ, Nakatsuji Y, Shih JW-K, Melpolder J, Kiyosawa K, Wages J & Kim J. Transfusion-associated hepatitis G virus infection. *9th Triennial International Symposium on Viral Hepatitis and Liver Disease*, Rome, Italy, 21–24 April 1996. p. 34.

18. Mosley JW, Kim JP, Dawson GF, Aach RD, Hollinger FB, Stevens CE, Barbosa LH, Nemo GF & Nowicki MJ. HGV/GBV-C cases among blood recipients and controls. *9th Triennial International Symposium on Viral Hepatitis and Liver Disease*, Rome, Italy, 21–24 April 1996. p. 35.

19. Feinman SV, Kim JP, Sooknanen R, Blajchman M, Herst R, Minuk G & Schroeder MI. Hepatitis G virus infection in post-transfusion hepatitis (PTH). *9th Triennial International Symposium on Viral Hepatitis and Liver Disease*, Rome, Italy, 21–24 April 1996. p. 281.

20. Hess G, Kim J, Karayiannis P, Thomas HC & Hadziyannis S. The interaction of HCV with HGV. *9th Triennial International Symposium on Viral Hepatitis and Liver Disease*, Rome, Italy, 21–24 April 1996. p. 35.

21. Pessoa MG, Terrault NA, Ferrel L, Kim JP, Kolberg J, Detmer J, Collins M, Yun A, Lake J, Roberts J, Ascher N & Wright TL. Detection and quantitation of hepatitis G virus (HGV) in patients with cryptogenic liver disease undergoing liver transplantation (OLT). *American Association for the Study of Liver Disease/American Gastroenterological Association*, Rome, Italy, 21–24 April 1996. Abstr. 26.

22. Di Bisceglie AM, Bacon BR, Neuschwander-Tetri BA, Yun A & Kim JP. Role of hepatitis G virus in cryptogenic liver disease. *9th Triennial International Symposium on Viral Hepatitis and Liver Disease*, Rome, Italy, 21–24 April 1996. p. 255.

23. Watts DM, Kim J, Barham B, Wages J, Figueroa R, Hayes C & Hyams K. Chronic liver disease associated with hepatitis G virus in Peru. *9th Triennial International Symposium on Viral Hepatitis and Liver Disease*, Rome, Italy, 21–24 April 1996. p. 251.

24. Byrnes JJ, Banks AT, Piatak M & Kim JP. Hepatitis G-associated aplastic anemia. *Lancet* 1996; **348**:472

25. Webster ADB, Morris A, Wang Y, Deacock S, Dusheiko GM & Harrison TJ. HGV/GBV-C in patients with pri-

mary immunodeficiency. *9th Triennial International Symposium on Viral Hepatitis and Liver Disease*, Rome, Italy, 21–24 April 996. p. 260.

26. Moaven L, Angus P, Bowden DS, Kim J, Wages J, Jr, Yun A, McCaw R, Revill P & Locarnini SA. No apparent association of hepatitis G virus with non A–E fulminant hepatitis in a small cohort study. *9th Triennial International Symposium on Viral Hepatitis and Liver Disease*, Rome, Italy, 21–24 April 1996. p. 256.

27. Sallie R, Shaw J & Mutimer D. GBV-C virus and fulminant hepatic failure. *Lancet* 1996; **347:**1552–1552.

28. Yoshiba M, Okamoto H & Mishiro S. Detection of the GBV-C hepatitis virus genome in serum from patients with fulminant hepatitis of unknown aetiology. *Lancet* 1995; **346:**1131–1132.

29. Schlueter V, Schmolke S, Engel AM, Babiel R, Hess G & Ofenloch-Haehnle B. A sensitive RT–PCR assay for the detection of hepatitis G virus, a new virus associated with human hepatitis. *9th Triennial International Symposium on Viral Hepatitis and Liver Disease*, Rome, Italy, 21–24 April 1996. p. 251.

30. Terrault NA, Piatak M, Kim JP, Kolberg J, Collins M, Detmer J, Yun A, Lake JR, Roberts JP, Ascher NL & Wright T. New method for hepatitis G virus (HGV) RNA quantitation in liver transplantation (OLT) recipients with HBV/HGV coinfection. *American Association for the Study of Liver Disease/American Gastroenterological Association*, Rome, Italy, 21–24 April 1996. Abstr. 833.

31. Chomczynski, P. A reagent for the single-step simultaneous isolation of RNA, DNA and proteins from cell and tissues samples. *Biotechniques* 1993; **15:**532–537.

32. Pearson WR & Lipman DJ. Improved tools for biological sequence comparison. *Proceedings of the National Academy of Sciences, USA* 1988; **85:**2444–2448.

# RECENT REFERENCES

## Molecular virology

Simons JN, Desai SM, Schultz DE, Lemon SM & Mushahwar IK. Translation initiation in GB viruses A and C: evidence for internal ribosome entry and implications for genome organization. *Journal of Virology* 1996; **70:**6126–6135.

Belyaev AS, Chong S, Novikov A, Kongpachith A, Masiarz F, Lim M & Kim JP. Hepatitis G virus encodes protease activities which can affect processing of the virus putative nonstructural proteins. *Journal of Virolology* 1997; **72:**868–872.

Kim J, Linnen J, Wages J, Zhang-Keck Z-Y, Belyaev A, Zhang Y, Fung K, Krawczynski K, Alter M, Lim M, Hadlock K, Young L, Hoover C, Frenandez J, Piatak M, Chong S, Karayinnis P, Thomas H, Hadziyannis S, Hess G, Bradley D, Foung S, Margolis H, Shih J, Alter H & Fry K. Molecular cloning and characterization of hepatitis G virus (HGV). In *Viral Hepatitis and Liver Disease*, 1997; pp. 340–346, Edited by M Rizzetto, RH Purcell, JL Gerin & G Verne. Torino: Edizioni Minerva Medica.

Lim MY, Fry K, Yun A, Chong S, Linnen J, Fung K & Kim JP. Sequence variation and phylogenetic analysis of envelope glycoprotein of hepatitis G virus. *Journal of General Virology* 1997; **78:**2771–2777.

Linnen JM, Fung K, Fry KE, Mizokami M, Ohba K, Wages JM Jr, Zhang-Keck Z-Y, Song K & Kim JP. Sequence variation and phylogenetic analysis of the 5′ terminus of hepatitis G virus. *Journal of Viral Hepatitis* 1997; **4:**293–302.

Muerhoff AS, Smith DB, Leary TP, Erker JC, Desai SM & Mushahwar IK. Identification of GB virus C variants by phylogenetic analysis of 5′-untranslated and coding region sequences. *Journal of Virology* 1997; **71:**6501–6508.

Pickering JM, Thomas HC & Karayiannis P. Genetic diversity between hepatitis G virus isolates: analysis of nucleotide variation in the NS3 and putative 'core' peptide genes. *Journal of General Virology* 1997; **78:**53–60.

## Animal studies

Bukh J, Kim JP, Govindarajan S, Apgar CL, Foung SKH, Wages J Jr, Yun A, Shapiro M, Emerson SU & Purcell RH. Experimental infection of chimpanzees with hepatitis G virus and genetic analysis of the virus. *Journal of Infectious Diseases* 1998; **177:**855–862.

## HGV replication

Ikeda M, Sugiyama K, Mizutani T, Tanaka T, Tanaka K, Shimotohno K & Kato N. Hepatitis G virus replication in human cultured cells displaying susceptibility to hepatitis C virus infection. *Biochemical and Biophysical Research Communications* 1997; **235:**505–508.

Laskus T, Radkowski M, Wang L-F, Vargas H & Rakela J. Lack of evidence for hepatitis G virus replication in the livers of patients coinfected with hepatitis C and G viruses. *Journal of Virology* 1997; **71:**7804–7806.

Madejón A, Fogeda M, Bartolomé J, Pardo M, González C, Cotonat T & Carreño V. GB virus C RNA in serum, liver, and peripheral blood mononuclear cells from patients with chronic hepatitis B, C, and D. *Gastroenterology* 1997; **113:**573–578.

## Antibodies

Pilot-Matias TJ, Carrick RJ, Coleman PF, Leary TP, Surowy TK, Simons JN, Muerhoff AS, Buuk SL, Chalmers ML, Dawson GJ, Desai SM & Mushahwar IK. Expression of the GB virus C E2 glycoprotein using the Semliki Forest virus vector system and its utility as a serologic marker. *Virology* 1996; **225:**282–292.

Tacke M, Kiyosawa K, Stark K, Schlueter V, Ofenloche-Haehnle B & Hess G. Detection of antibodies to a putative hepatitis G virus envelope protein. *Lancet* 1997; **349:**318–320.

Tacke M, Schmolke S, Schlueter V, Sauleda S, Esteban JI, Tanaka E, Kiyosawa K, Alter HJ, Schmitt U, Hess G, Ofenloch-Haehnle B, & Engel AM. Humoral immune response to the E2 protein of hepatitis G virus is associated with long-term recovery from infection and reveals a high frequency of hepatitis G virus exposure among healthy blood donors. *Hepatology* 1997; **26:**1626–1633.

## Disease association

Alter HJ, Nakatsuji Y, Melpolder J, Wages J, Wesley R, Shih JWK & Kim JP. Incidence and disease implications of transfusion-associated hepatitis G virus infection. *New England Journal of Medicine* 1997; **336**:747–754.

Alter MJ, Gallagher M, Morris T, Moyer LA, Meeks EL, Krawczynski K, Kim JP & Margolis HS. Acute non-A, non-E hepatitis in the United States: clinical and epidemiologic characteristics and the role of hepatitis G virus infection. *New England Journal of Medicine* 1997; **336**:741–746.

Brown KE, Wong S & Young NS. Prevalence of GBV-C/HGV, a novel 'hepatitis' virus, in patients with aplastic anemia. *British Journal of Haematology* 1997; **97**:492–496.

Hoofnagle JH, Lombardero M, Wei Y, Everhart J, Wiesner R, Lake J, Zetterman R, Yun A, Yang L & Kim JP. Hepatitis G virus infection before and after liver transplantation. *Liver Transplantation and Surgery* 1997; **3**:578–585.

Kiem HP, Myerson D, Storb R, McDonald GB, Spurgeon CL & Leisenring W. Prevalence of hepatitis G virus in patients with aplastic anemia. *Blood* 1997; **90**:1335–1336.

Tameda Y, Kosaka Y, Tagawa S, Takase K, Sawada N, Nakao H, Tsuda F, Tanaka T, Okamoto H, Miyakawa Y & Mayumi M. Infection with GB virus (GBV-C) in patients with fulminant hepatitis. *Journal of Hepatology* 1996; **25**:842–847.

## Review

Cheung RC, Keefe EB & Greenberg HB. Hepatitis G virus; is it a hepatitis virus? *West Journal of Medicine* 1997; **167**:23–33.

# Section III

## GENETICS AND VIRAL DIAGNOSIS

# 12 Molecular tools for the treatment of hepatitis C

## Jean-Michel Pawlotsky and David R Gretch*

## INTRODUCTION

Hepatitis C virus (HCV) infects over 300 million individuals worldwide. In about 20% of cases, chronic HCV infection leads to cirrhosis, which predisposes the patient to hepatocellular carcinoma. It has been established that hepatocellular injury is associated with active HCV replication, since eradication of viral replication is almost always associated with normalization of serum biochemical markers of hepatitis and improvement of histological findings on liver biopsy [1,2]. Therefore, the treatment of chronic hepatitis C should be aimed at eliminating viral replication in order to prevent further evolution towards clinically significant complications.

Today, chronic hepatitis C treatment is based on the use of interferon (IFN)-α, which is usually administered at the dose of 3 MU three times per week for 6 to 12 months [3]. A sustained virological response, defined by normalization of serum alanine aminotransferase (ALT) levels and sustained elimination of HCV RNA from serum (detected by PCR) 6 months after treatment withdrawal, is obtained in 8 to 12% of cases after 6 months, and in about 25% of cases after 12 months of treatment at this dose [3]. New treatments with better expected efficacy are currently being evaluated. One promising therapeutic approach is combination therapy with IFN plus ribavirin, a drug which seems to potentiate the rate of sustained response to IFN by unknown mechanisms [4]. A second potential approach is more aggressive dosing with IFN, such as induction therapy with high doses (up to 10 MU) and daily administration. Evidence supporting this approach comes from recent findings of an IFN dose effect with HCV genotype 1 [5]. Finally, direct antiviral drugs, such as HCV protease, helicase or polymerase inhibitors, will become available in the next few years.

The availability of several therapeutic options for chronic HCV infection emphasizes the need for accurate markers to predict and monitor the response to therapy, which would help clinicians to tailor treatment of chronic hepatitis C in the future. In addition, understanding the molecular mechanisms underlying the resistance of HCV to antiviral drugs is necessary to improve further the clinical results of hepatitis C treatment. Several virological tests are now available which can be of help in these goals if properly employed. Virological parameters include HCV genotype, qualitative viraemia, quantitative viral load and the characteristics of HCV 'quasispecies' heterogeneity.

## CLINICAL VIROLOGY PARAMETERS

### HCV replication

Although extra-hepatic replication sites, such as peripheral blood mononuclear cells, have been suggested [6], it is assumed that HCV is mainly produced in the liver. The mechanisms of HCV replication remain poorly understood, mainly because there is no efficient cell culture system. Infectious full-length cDNA clones have recently been obtained [7,8], and it is anticipated that transfection of infectious HCV clones into eukaryotic cells may ultimately facilitate the production of mature virions *in vitro*. By analogy with other members of the family *Flaviviridae* [9], HCV is thought to replicate in the cytoplasm via the synthesis of a negative HCV RNA strand (replicative intermediate), which is used as a template for the synthesis of new positive-strand RNAs. Positive-strand RNAs may then be used as mRNAs for viral protein synthesis or may be encapsidated as genomic RNAs to form infectious HCV particles. The synthesis of both negative- and positive-strand RNAs is presumably performed by a viral RNA-dependent RNA polymerase encoded by the non-structural (NS) 5B gene of the HCV genome. Other HCV non-structural proteins (NS2, NS3, NS4, NS5A) probably play important roles in HCV replication, and as such represent potential targets for antiviral therapy (reviewed in [10]).

*Corresponding author

# HCV genetic heterogeneity: genotypes and quasispecies

One of the most important characteristics of HCV genomes is their genetic variability, a feature they have in common with many other RNA viruses such as human immunodeficiency virus (HIV) [11–13]. Viral heterogeneity primarily results from a high error rate of the RNA-dependent RNA polymerase (with misincorporation frequencies averaging about $10^{-4}$ to $10^{-5}$ per base site), and the apparent absence of any proofreading mechanism [11]. Most mutant viral particles are replication-deficient, but some genetic variants are efficiently propagated and selected for under specific host conditions. Throughout the genome, most nucleotide changes are 'silent'; that is, they do not affect the encoded amino acid sequence. This likely reflects constraints upon the extent to which proteins may vary in sequence and yet remain functional (for discussion, see [14]).

The accumulation of mutations, the selection of 'most fit' viral sequences, and transmission of the corresponding genomes over time within specific geographical areas or epidemiological groups, led to the progressive divergence of HCV genotypes from the common ancestor virus, following a classical Darwinian process [14]. Some viral genotypes initially restricted to geographically isolated human groups are thought to have spread widely because of population mixing and the emergence of efficient routes of infection. Blood transfusion indeed appears to be responsible for the worldwide spread of HCV genotype 1b, a genotype that may have originated from Western or Central Africa, while intravenous drug use is clearly associated with transmission of genotype 3a in most industrialized countries, a genotype possibly originating from the Indian subcontinent or South-East Asia [14,15]. Based on phylogenetic analysis, HCV types, subtypes and isolates can be distinguished on the basis of average sequence divergence rates of approximately 30%, 20% and 10%, respectively [16,17]. Six main HCV types have been recognized (numbered 1 to 6), which are themselves subdivided into more than 80 subtypes, identified by lower-case letters (1a, 1b, 1c, and so on). Figure 1 shows the present worldwide distribution of HCV genotypes [15,18].

In addition, HCV exists within the human host as a pool of genetically distinct, but closely related variants referred to as a quasispecies [19,20]. The quasispecies nature of HCV probably confers a significant survival advantage, since the simultaneous presence of multiple variant genomes and the high rate at which new variants are generated allow rapid selection of mutants better suited to new environmental conditions. The 'fittest' infectious particles are

**Figure 1.** Geographical distribution of genotypes of HCV

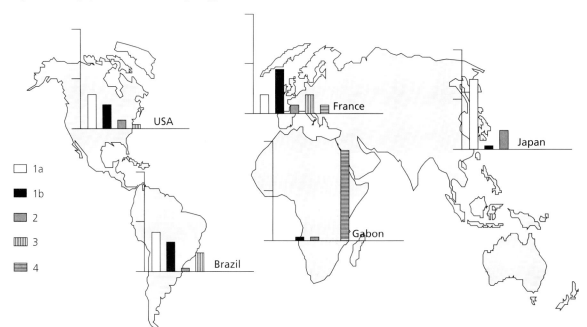

Adapted from [15,18].

continuously selected in a given patient on the basis of their replication capacities and especially by the selective pressure exerted through interactions with host cell proteins and the immune response, which targets regions encoding both cytotoxic and neutralizing epitopes [21–26]. It is noteworthy that the HCV quasispecies characteristics in a given patient is influenced by the rate of accumulation of mutations, which itself depends on: (i) the level of fidelity of the viral RNA polymerase (which may itself be altered by a variety of mutations in the genome); (ii) viral replication kinetics; and (iii) selection pressures, which are different for each patient and may vary from one genomic region to another [11]. During the chronic stage of infection, viral quasispecies are in a state of equilibrium at any given time point. Their composition may, however, be slightly or dramatically altered by any modification of the environment in which the quasispecies behaves. These changes can be spontaneous, related to complex metabolic interactions in the host, or triggered by external factors, such as associated infections, drug intakes, and so on. As discussed

below, antiviral treatments may dramatically alter the environment in which the virus behaves by exerting strong pressures on various HCV genomic regions. These modifications may induce profound HCV quasispecies modifications that could play a major role in HCV resistance to therapy [27,28].

## HCV viraemia and viral load

HCV viraemia is defined as the presence of HCV RNA in serum or plasma as detected by qualitative assays, usually based on PCR. HCV viraemia is recognized as a reliable marker of active HCV replication in the liver, since detection of HCV viraemia correlates strongly with the presence of disease on liver biopsy [29,30]. Quantitative assays allow the measurement of HCV viral load – the amount of circulating genomes per volume of serum or plasma – which provides an estimate of the amount of circulating viral particles. It has recently been shown that HCV viral load is at steady state in the chronic phase; viral load does not vary to a significant degree over a

**Figure 2.** Changes in HCV RNA at different intervals

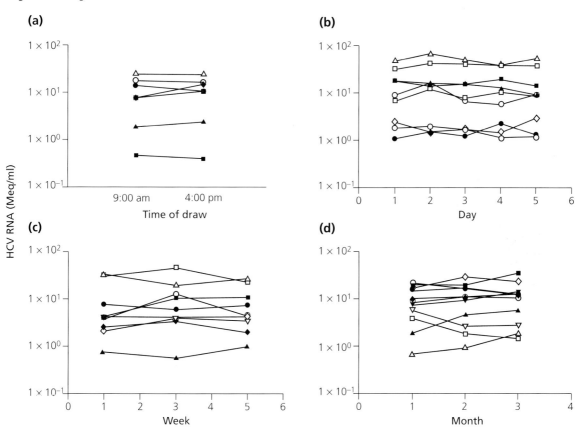

(a) Hourly; (b) daily; (c) weekly; (d) monthly. HCV RNA was quantified with bDNA assay. Reproduced with permission from N'guyen *et al.* [31]; *Journal of Viral Hepatitis* 1996; **3**:75–78. ©1996 Blackwell Science Ltd.

period of months to years (Fig. 2) [31]. Recent data based on mathematical modelling of HCV replication kinetics during treatment has suggested that viral load provides an accurate estimate of the rate of virion production in the liver, i.e. the level of HCV replication [5]. Based on the kinetics model, the minimum daily production rate of HCV was estimated to be $10^{12}$ virions per day, with a maximum virion half-life in serum of 3 hours (AU Neumann, NP Lam, H Dahari, DR Gretch, TJ Layden and AS Perelson, unpublished results). It must be stressed that HCV viral load is a global quantitative measurement which does not take into account the quasispecies distribution of HCV (the presence in the same individual of mixed viral populations of various sizes which may have different biological properties).

## METHODS

### Genotype determination

The reference method for HCV genotype determination is genome sequence analysis, followed by sequence alignments and phylogenetic analysis [16–18]. Although full-length sequence analysis appears to be the most reliable method, it has been shown that analysis of more limited regions of the genome (especially the E1 and NS5B genes) allows for reliable classification into the various HCV genotypes [16–18]. However, sequence analysis is labour-intensive and expensive and is not readily applicable in clinical settings.

From a practical standpoint, two categories of techniques can be used to determine the HCV genotype in patient sera: molecular biology-based techniques (genotyping techniques) and serological techniques (serotyping techniques). Several rapid PCR-based genotyping techniques have been described which allow for efficient identification of genotype-specific mutations in various regions of the genome (discussed in [32,33]). Such methods include: (i) nested PCR analysis of the HCV core gene using genotype-specific primers [34]; (ii) restriction fragment length polymorphism (RFLP) analysis of the highly conserved 5′ non-coding region [35]; (iii) reverse hybridization analysis using genotype-specific probes of 5′ non-coding region sequences (INNO-LiPA; Innogenetics, Gent, Belgium) [36] or of 5′ non-coding and core sequences (Gen.Eti.K DEIA HCV; Sorin Biomedica, Saluggia, Italy) [37]. The RFLP and reverse hybridization methods can both characterize genotypes and subtypes. They appear to be comparable in clinical performance, although minor differences are observed in some populations (reviewed in [32]).

Serotyping techniques are based on the detection of antibodies directed to genotype-specific HCV epitopes, which are usually chosen in the NS4 or core proteins. Several assays have been developed, based on competitive ELISA, such as the Murex HC1-6 Serotyping Assay (Murex Diagnostics, Dartford, UK) [38], or on immunoblot, such as the RIBA HCV Serotyping Assay (Chiron Diagnostics, Emeryville, Calififornia, USA) [39]. The potential advantages are low cost and ease of testing compared with molecular genotyping assays. In addition, HCV RNA-negative specimens can be serotyped but not genotyped. However, to date, HCV serotyping assays have not been able to discern different HCV subtypes. In HCV RNA-positive patients, the sensitivity of the Murex HC1-6 assay is about 90% relative to genotyping assays, but may be much lower in special populations such as immunocompromised or haemodialysed patients. The concordance between serotyping and genotyping assays is about 95% for typeable samples [40].

### Qualitative HCV RNA detection

HCV RNA can be detected in patient serum by means of highly sensitive tests such as reverse transcription–PCR (RT–PCR). Many variations in the HCV PCR assay have been described in the literature, and standardization of such in-house assays has been difficult [41,42]. Numerous factors contribute to RT–PCR assay variability, including specimen handling and storage conditions, correct design of amplification primers, variability of biochemical reactions, DNA product contamination and efficiency of post-amplification systems (discussed in [32]).

A standardized RT–PCR assay has been introduced for qualitative detection of HCV RNA in patient serum (Amplicor HCV, Roche Molecular Systems) [43]. This assay is designed to be used in any clinical laboratory equipped for molecular biology. However, rigorous training of technologists and repeated quality controls are needed to optimize the performance of any molecular biology diagnostic kit. When used in trained research laboratories, the modified Amplicor HCV assay has excellent analytical sensitivity (estimated to about 100 genome copies/ml; D Gretch, unpublished results) and a specificity of 97% to 99% [32]. This second-generation version of the Amplicor HCV assay is currently under Phase III clinical trial. Alternative technologies, such as an RT–PCR test based on LCx technology (Abbott Laboratories), are also currently under evaluation.

## Viral load

Currently, HCV RNA can be quantified by two types of methods: target amplification- and signal amplification-based techniques. In target amplification-based assays, large amounts of copies of viral RNA are synthesized in a cyclic enzymatic reaction, in competition with an internal standard present in known amounts (RNA or DNA transcript). In-house techniques based on competitive RT–PCR have been developed for research purposes [44,45]. As far as standardization among the techniques is concerned, they raise the same issues as in-house qualitative PCR assays.

The large-scale routine use of HCV RNA quantification for clinical purposes necessitates commercial, highly standardized assays. To date, the only commercially available target amplification-based assay is the Amplicor HCV Monitor kit (Roche Molecular Systems). Another test based on four separate competitive PCR amplifications, each terminating at different cycle numbers, is performed at the National Genetics Institute (Superquant HCV, National Genetics Institute, Culver City, California, USA) [46]. This assay appears to be more sensitive than the first-generation Monitor, but the samples must be sent to the manufacturer for testing, and the general performance of the technique has not yet been evaluated by independent investigators. Finally, the nucleic acid sequence-based amplification test (NASBA HCV, Organon Teknika, Boxtel, The Netherlands) appears to give adequate performance for HCV RNA quantification, but is not commercially available [47].

Signal amplification-based techniques are exclusively represented, today, by branched DNA (bDNA) technology, the second generation of which is commercially available (Quantiplex HCV RNA 2.0, Chiron Diagnostics). This assay involves specific capture of HCV genomes onto microwell plates and subsequent detection by hybridization and signal amplification. Signal amplification is achieved by hybridizing multiple alkaline phosphatase-conjugated oligonucleotide probes to a bDNA amplifier molecule [48].

The performance and limitations of current tests for HCV RNA quantification have recently been reviewed in detail [49,50]. New PCR-based assays are currently being evaluated: they include the second-generation Amplicor HCV Monitor, which has been modified in order to reach better sensitivity and to quantify equally HCV genotypes, and a new competitive RT–PCR assay, based on the use of LCx technology (Abbott Diagnostics). Significant improvement in HCV RNA quantification (especially sensitivity and linear ranges of quantification) could be provided by

real-time quantitative PCR, a technology which is still in developmental stages.

## Quasispecies

Most studies to date describing HCV quasispecies have focused on the viral hypervariable region 1 (HVR1), located at the 5′ end of the second envelope (E2) gene of HCV [19]. The hypervariable nature of the corresponding E2 glycoprotein domain is presumed to result from variant-specific neutralizing antibody pressure and tolerance to amino acid substitution in this region. However, it is important to note that HCV quasispecies heterogeneity can and does exist throughout the genome, and may vary in specific regions according to pressures [27,28]. Whatever the genomic region of interest, the reference method for HCV quasispecies analysis is to generate a series of molecular clones from a given specimen after PCR amplification, and to perform nucleotide sequence analysis [51]. It has been calculated that 20 clones should be analysed to obtain a 95% level of confidence that all major variants within a quasispecies population have been sampled [11,51]. Various parameters can then be measured from sequence data, such as: (i) genetic complexity, defined as the total number of genetic variants within a quasispecies population; (ii) quasispecies entropy, defined as the probability of different nucleotide or amino acid sequences or clusters of sequences appearing at a given time point; entropy provides expanded information regarding quasispecies repertoire, including number of variants and their relative proportion; (iii) genetic diversity, defined as the average genetic distance between the variants in a quasispecies population; and (iv) phylogenetic analysis, which assesses evolutionary relationships between specific variants of a quasispecies population [27,52]. These parameters are used to characterize HCV quasispecies in various genomic regions.

Because cloning and sequencing are labour-intensive and expensive, rapid methods have been developed for the study of HCV quasispecies, including direct sequencing and polymorphism analysis [53], heteroduplex analysis by temperature gradient gel electrophoresis (TGGE) [54], heteroduplex gel-shift technology [55], and single-strand conformation polymorphism (SSCP) analysis [56,57]. Heteroduplex gel-shift technology includes the homoduplex tracking assay, which proved to be useful for estimating both quasispecies genetic complexity and genetic diversity, and for studying the evolution of patient quasispecies over time, and clonal frequency analysis, which has been used to estimate genetic complexity and to select among numerous clones for sequencing [52,55]. SSCP proved to be useful for estimating quasispecies genetic complexity, for studying the evolution of patient HCV quasispecies over time, and for clonal frequency analysis [27,57,58]. Quasispecies technology can be used to study numerous aspects of HCV pathobiology, including persistence, pathogenesis, transmission, compartmentalization and response of HCV to therapy (see below).

## THERAPEUTIC APPLICATIONS

### Predicting the response to therapy

In patients with chronic hepatitis C, it has been demonstrated that several pretreatment parameters, including epidemiological, clinical and virological ones, are independent predictors of the responses to IFN therapy (reviewed in [59]). Various host factors have been associated with favourable response to IFN therapy, including female sex, younger age, a history of intravenous drug use or an unknown source of infection, shorter disease duration, low serum aspartate aminotransferase activity, low γ-glutamyl transpeptidase activity, low serum iron or ferritin, mild chronic hepatitis, and absence of fibrosis or cirrhosis on liver biopsy. However, not all of these factors remain significant after multivariate analysis. It must be stressed that the pretreatment parameters associated with early or end-of-treatment responses may be different from those associated with sustained responses [60]. The following paragraphs focus on the role of HCV viral load, genotype and quasispecies heterogeneity for predicting sustained responses to IFN treatment.

A low pretreatment viral load has been shown to be independently associated with sustained biochemical and/or virological response to IFN [48,60–62]. When reviewing the data on 652 patients from 11 published studies, Davis and Lau [59] observed that 50.5% of patients with a viral load lower than $10^6$ genome equivalents/ml achieved a sustained biochemical response, versus only 17.3% of the patients with a viral load higher than $10^6$ genome equivalents/ml. The lack of standardization among HCV RNA quantification assays does not allow for defining precisely the HCV RNA titre with the best predictive value in all cases, which could be on the order of 1 to $5\times10^6$ genome equivalents/ml when using a second-generation bDNA assay (reviewed in [49]). HCV genotype 1 (including subtypes 1a and 1b) has also been shown to be an independent predictor of a poor sustained response to therapy, whereas genotypes 2 and 3 were associated with a significantly better rate of response [59,61,63].

In 15 studies analysed by Davis and Lau [59], a sustained biochemical response was achieved in only 18.1% of 536 patients with genotype 1, whereas 54.9% of the 288 patients with genotypes 2 or 3 had a sustained response. In 100 patients with HCV genotype 4 infection, response rates to IFN appeared to be closer to those observed for genotype 1 than genotypes 2 and 3 [64].

As stated earlier, the most commonly studied HCV genetic region when analysing HCV quasispecies has been the E2 gene HVR1. A relationship between the genetic complexity of HVR1 quasispecies and the sustained response to IFN-α treatment has been suggested in several studies. In two studies, multivariate analysis showed that low HVR1 genetic complexity is an independent predictor of sustained virological response to a standard dose of IFN-α [57,65]. Other studies indicate that high pretreatment quasispecies diversity is associated with non-response [66].

Recently, a second genetic region of HCV has been called into question with regard to being important in determining response to IFN therapy. A consensus stretch of amino acids located within the central region of the NS5A gene of genotype 1b isolates was suggested to be associated with IFN resistance in Japan [67,68]. However, this finding is presently controversial, because some studies have not found a strong association, raising real concerns regarding methodological differences in studies. It was recently found that five genotype 1b-infected patients with sustained response to IFN had significantly lower entropy in the NS5A central region in pre-treatment quasispecies compared to eight non-responders ($P<0.02$), a result in keeping with the observations in HVR1 [27].

Recent studies have also suggested a role for HCV RNA testing during therapy in predicting nonresponse to a standard (3–5 MU three times per week) course of IFN [46,69–71]. Specifically, persistence of HCV RNA at 1 and 3 months after initiation of therapy is strongly predictive of failure in eliminating HCV replication over a 6–12 month treatment course. Alternatively, clearance of HCV RNA (conversion to PCR-negative) at months 1 or 3 has only a weak predictive value for sustained virological response due to breakthrough or relapse [46,69–71].

To date, the predictive role of clinical virology parameters on the sustained response to therapy has been studied only in patients receiving a standard dosage of IFN-α, 3 MU three times per week for 6 to 12 months. Recent unpublished data suggested that low viral load and a HCV genotype other than 1 could also be associated with a better response to combination therapy with IFN plus ribavirin, both in naive patients and in responder–relapsers to previous IFN treatment (Schering-Plough, personal communication). It is now apparent that the predictive role of pretreatment virological parameters should be prospectively determined for any new therapies of chronic hepatitis C.

## Selecting optimum therapy

IFN-α, 3 MU three times per week for 6 to 12 months, is presently the only approved treatment for chronic hepatitis C. Since only one therapeutical schedule has been authorized until now, the question arises as to whether clinical virology tools could be used to make the decision to treat or not to treat. As summarized by Davis and Lau [59], the optimum candidate for IFN therapy is a young patient without cirrhosis, genotype 1 or high levels of viraemia. By using this algorithm, 79% of their patients would have been excluded from treatment, which would have dramatically lowered the costs of treatment, while increasing the sustained response rate to 100%. However, treatment would have been denied to 60% of the sustained responders. As emphasized by these authors, "when the prevalence of the factor with the higher response rate is low, the greater number of responders may be in the group without the factor even though their rate of response is lower" [59]. In this context, molecular virology tools must not be used to deny treatment to any HCV-infected patient in the absence of absolute contraindication to IFN therapy.

In the future, pretreatment patient characteristics will almost certainly be used to tailor treatment as soon as multiple therapeutic options are available, in order to improve cost–efficacy ratios. For example, it now appears that pretreatment genotype and viral load may be useful for selecting duration of IFN plus ribavirin combination therapy. The problem is that, to date, clinical virology parameters such as viral load, genotype or genetic complexity of HCV quasispecies have only been identified as predictors of sustained response to a standard IFN regimen and to the combination of IFN plus ribavirin in specific subgroups. Two steps are now necessary before these parameters can be confidently used to decide which treatment will give the best chance of response to each individual patient. First, the predictors of sustained response to new treatment schedules need to be defined in large-scale prospective studies; it is especially important to determine whether genotype, viral load and quasispecies heterogeneity prior to therapy are still associated with different outcomes. Second, how to use these parameters to tailor treatment must be estab-

lished in large-scale prospective, randomized controlled trials.

## Therapeutic monitoring

Today, the virological response to IFN is assessed by qualitative, non-quantitative PCR, which is the most sensitive available HCV RNA detection technique. The end-of-treatment and the sustained virological responses are defined by normal ALT activity and negative HCV RNA by PCR at the end of treatment and 6 months later, respectively. It must be stressed, however, that the best sensitivity cut-off for predicting definitive viral elimination is not known, and that it could be below the lower cut-off of currently available PCR assays. In the future, qualitative assays will probably be replaced in their current indications by quantitative assays provided that they reach comparable levels of sensitivity. Real-time quantitative PCR is an interesting candidate technique for reaching the goal of a high sensitivity quantitative test, since it has been shown to be considerably more sensitive and more accurate than classical PCR techniques while having a significantly broader linear range of quantification [72].

As stated earlier, the lack of HCV RNA clearance during the early stages of treatment is highly predictive of non-response to IFN therapy. HCV RNA assessment during treatment could prove to be useful in the decision to maintain or to stop therapy, or to switch to another treatment schedule, although it is still unclear what is the best time point to make such a decision. It is therefore conceivable to tailor hepatitis C treatment not only to pretreament parameters, but also to the evolution of HCV viral load during therapy. For example, viral load monitoring is currently effectively used in managing HIV infection to allow clinicians to tailor treatment to the actual effect of antiviral drugs on viraemia. This, in addition to the recent introduction of new HIV polymerase and protease inhibitors, has led to a significant improvement in the results of HIV therapy [73]. For HCV, several therapeutic options are now under study and even more will be available in the next few years. Thus, it is hopeful that development of new drugs and efficient use of laboratory methods will greatly improve therapeutic outcome for hepatitis C. Prospective randomized controlled clinical trials should address both points with equal vigour: optimization of therapeutic regimens, and optimization of laboratory markers for assessment of treatment response, tailoring therapy and maximizing cost benefit. Owing to the large number of patients needed for such trials, large-scale international multicentre studies should certainly be encouraged.

## UNDERSTANDING THE MECHANISMS UNDERLYING HCV RESISTANCE TO ANTIVIRAL TREATMENT

With appropriate study design, molecular virology methods can also be used to obtain deeper insight into the mechanisms underlying HCV resistance to antiviral drugs. So far, data are available only for HCV resistance to a standard dosage of IFN-α. For instance, recent findings based on mathematical modelling of viral replication suggested that the direct antiviral effect of IFN, at least on HCV genotype 1, is dose-dependent [5], and that the current recommended IFN schedule might not be optimum for this HCV genotype since the daily production rate of HCV virions appears to be very rapid (AU Neumann, NP Lam, H Dahari, DR Gretch, TJ Layden and AS Perelson, unpublished results). Insufficient IFN pressure on HCV replication might therefore account for the observed high rates of therapeutic resistance, which can be characterized by a lack of response, a transient response followed by a relapse after therapy, or a transient response followed by a breakthrough during therapy. In keeping with the significant association between high levels of replication and non-response to IFN, patients with rapid viral replication kinetics would be predicted to respond less well to low doses of IFN in the first days/weeks of treatment.

In addition, the predictive roles of a low genetic complexity of HVR1 [57,65] and a low entropy of the NS5A central region [27] on sustained HCV RNA clearance suggest that a small quasispecies repertoire at the time treatment is started is necessary to achieve HCV RNA clearance at the currently used dose of IFN. As a possible mechanism, a large quasispecies repertoire at initiation of treatment might increase the probability that minor, 'poorly fit' variants would be selected based on better fitness in the presence of IFN-induced environmental changes. Indeed, in patients who do not clear HCV RNA, IFN treatment induces profound qualitative modifications of HCV quasispecies in various genomic regions, characterized by the selection and later diversification of minor pretreatment variants (Fig. 3) [27,28,58].

It has been suggested that the presence of specific HCV genome nucleotide and amino acid sequences prior to therapy could confer sensitivity or resistance to IFN-α therapy [68]. In fact, recent data suggested that there is no absolute 'interferon sensitivity determining region' in the central region of the NS5A gene [27,28,74]. However, it is possible that sequences located in various genomic regions play a major role in the modulation of HCV replication during treatment and, as a consequence, in viral elimination. For

**Figure 3.** Heteroduplex tracking analysis of HCV quasi-species during interferon therapy

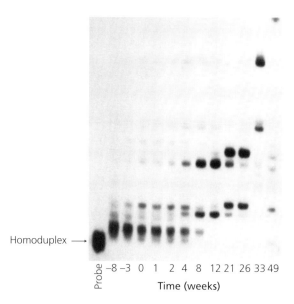

Heterogeneous HVR1 PCR products were obtained from the serum of an HCV-infected patient receiving IFN therapy (3 MU three times per week for 24 weeks) at different intervals during therapy. PCR products were hybridized to a clonal radiolabelled HVR1 probe and separated by electrophoresis on a non-denaturing polyacrylamide gel. The extent of the gel shift relative to the homoduplex probe increases over time, indicating that progressive evolution of the HVR1 occurred during IFN therapy in this patient.

instance, amino acid sequences in the central region of the NS5A protein were shown to interact with the IFN-induced double-stranded RNA-dependent protein kinase (PKR) and to inhibit its antiviral action *in vitro* [75]. This property was abolished by as few as two point mutations in the NS5A sequence [76] Whether PKR–NS5A interaction plays a role in HCV resistance to IFN therapy *in vivo* remains to be proven. It is nevertheless possible that genotype-dependent differences in viral sequences involved in interactions between HCV and IFN-induced defence mechanisms may explain the different rates of response among the various genotypes. These hypotheses are currently under investigation. It is clear that molecular virology tools will be particularly useful for improving our understanding of the mechanisms of HCV resistance to IFN.

## CONCLUSIONS

It has been a decade since the historic discovery of HCV as the aetiological agent of chronic hepatitis C by Houghton and colleagues [77]. Based on exciting new advances, we are now witnessing the co-evolution of parallel tools for fighting the clinically important disease of chronic hepatitis C: (i) development of a wide spectrum of new drugs designed to possess potent direct antiviral activity; and (ii) development of sensitive, specific and versatile molecular techniques for accurately assessing virological dynamics during therapy. Carefully controlled clinical trials are now mandated to enhance our ability to learn to use these tools. Ultimately, the clinician will be well armed to guide the patients through the battle with chronic hepatitis C.

# ACKNOWLEDGEMENTS

We thank Stephen J Polyak and Cindy Kurosu for assistance with preparation of the manuscript.

# REFERENCES

1. Chemello L, Cavalletto L, Casarin C, Bonetti P, Bernardinello E, Pontisso P, Donada C, Belussi F, Martinelli S, Alberti A & the TriVeneto Viral Hepatitis Group. Persistent hepatitis C viremia predicts late relapse after sustained response to interferon-α in chronic hepatitis C. *Annals of Internal Medicine* 1996; **124**:1058–1060.

2. Marcellin P, Boyer N, Gervais A, Martinot M, Pouteau M, Castelnau C, Kilani A, Areias J, Auperin A, Benhamou JP, Degott C & Erlinger S. Long-term histologic improvement and loss of detectable intrahepatic HCV RNA in patients with chronic hepatitis C and sustained response to interferon-α therapy. *Annals of Internal Medicine* 1997; **127**:875–881.

3. Lindsay KL. Therapy of hepatitis C: overview. *Hepatology* 1997; **26** (Supplement 1):71S–77S.

4. Reichard O, Norkrans G, Frydén A, Braconier JH, Sönnerborg A & Weiland O. Randomised, double-blind, placebo-controlled trial of interferon alpha-2b with and without ribavirin for chronic hepatitis C. *Lancet* 1998; **351**:83–87.

5. Lam NP, Neumann AU, Gretch DR, Wiley TE, Perelson AS & Layden TJ. Dose-dependent acute clearance of hepatitis C virus genotype 1 virus with interferon alfa. *Hepatology* 1997; **26**:226–231.

6. Lerat H, Berby F, Trabaud MA, Vidalin O, Major M, Trépo C & Inchauspé G. Specific detection of hepatitis C virus minus strand RNA in hematopoietic cells. *Journal of Clinical Investigation* 1996; **97**:845–851.

7. Kolykhalov AA, Agapov EV, Blight KJ, Mihalik K, Feinstone SM & Rice CM. Transmission of hepatitis C by intrahepatic inoculation with transcribed RNA. *Science* 1997; **277**:570–574.

8. Yanagi M, Purcell RH, Emerson SU & Bukh J. Transcripts from a single full-length cDNA clone of hepatitis C virus are infectious when directly transfected into the liver of a chimpanzee. *Proceedings of the National Academy of Sciences, USA* 1997; **94**:8738–8743.

9. Chambers TJ, Hahn CS, Galler R & Rice CM. Flavivirus genome organization, expression, and replication. *Annual Review of Microbiology* 1990; **44**:649–688.

10. Major ME & Feinstone SM. The molecular virology of hepatitis C. *Hepatology* 1997; **25**:1527–1538.

11. Domingo E. Biological significance of viral quasispecies. *Viral Hepatitis Reviews* 1996; **2**:247–261.

12. Delwart EL, Sheppard HW, Walker BD, Goudsmit J & Mullins JI. Human immunodeficiency virus type 1 evolution in vivo tracked by DNA heteroduplex mobility assays. *Journal of Virology* 1994; **68**:6672–6683.

13. Wolinsky SM, Korber BTM, Neumann AU, Daniels M, Kunstman KJ, Whetsell AJ, Furtado MR, Cao Y, Ho DD, Safrit JT & Koup RA. Adaptive evolution of human immunodeficiency virus-type 1 during the natural course of infection. *Science* 1996; **272**:537–542.

14. Simmonds P & Smith DB. Investigation of the pattern of diversity of hepatitis C virus in relation to times of transmission. In *Hepatitis C Virus: Genetic Heterogeneity and Viral Load*, 1997; pp. 37–43. Edited by the Groupe Français d'Etudes Moléculaires des Hépatites. Paris: John Libbey Eurotext.

15. Pawlotsky JM, Tsakiris L, Roudot-Thoraval F, Pellet C, Stuyver L, Duval J & Dhumeaux D. Relationship between hepatitis C virus genotypes and sources of infection in patients with chronic hepatitis C. *Journal of Infectious Diseases* 1995; **171**:1607–1610.

16. Simmonds P. Variability of hepatitis C virus. *Hepatology* 1995; **21**:570–583.

17. Bukh J, Miller RH & Purcell RH. Genetic heterogeneity of hepatitis C virus: quasispecies and genotypes. *Seminars in Liver Disease* 1995; **15**:41–63.

18. Maertens G & Stuyver L. Genotypes and genetic variation of hepatitis C virus. In *The Molecular Medicine of Viral Hepatitis*, 1997; pp. 183–233. Edited by TJ Harrison & AJ Zuckerman. New York: John Wiley.

19. Weiner AJ, Brauer MJ, Rosenblatt J, Richman KH, Tung J, Crawford K, Bonino F, Saracco G, Choo QL & Houghton M. Variable and hypervariable domains are found in the regions of HCV corresponding to the flavivirus envelope and NS1 proteins and the pestivirus envelope glycoproteins. *Virology* 1991; **180**:842–848.

20. Martell M, Esteban JI, Quer J, Genesca J, Weiner A, Esteban R, Guardia J & Gomez J. Hepatitis C virus (HCV) circulates as a population of different but closely related genomes: quasispecies nature of HCV genome distribution. *Journal of Virology* 1992; **66**:3225–3229.

21. Farci P, Alter HJ, Wong DC, Miller RH, Govindarajan S, Engle R, Shapiro M & Purcell RH. Prevention of hepatitis C virus infection in chimpanzees after antibody-mediated in vitro neutralization. *Proceedings of the National Academy of Sciences, USA* 1994; **91**:7792–7796.

22. Koziel MJ, Dudley D, Afdhal N, Choo QL, Houghton M, Ralston R & Walker BD. Hepatitis C virus (HCV)-specific cytotoxic T-lymphocytes recognize epitopes in the core and envelope proteins of HCV. *Journal of Virology* 1993; **67**:7522–7532.

23. Weiner AJ, Geysen HM, Christopherson C, Hall JE, Mason TJ, Saracco G, Bonino F, Crawford K, Marion CD, Crawford KA, Brunetto M, Barr PJ, Miyamura T, McHutchison J & Houghton M. Evidence for immune selection of hepatitis C virus (HCV) putative envelope glycoprotein variants: potential role in chronic HCV infections. *Proceedings of the National Academy of Sciences, USA* 1992; **89**:3468–3472.

24. Higashi Y, Kakumu S, Yoshioka K, Wakita T, Mizokami M, Ohba K, Ito Y, Ishikawa T, Takayanagi M & Nagai Y. Dynamics of genome change in the E2/NS1 region of hepatitis C virus in vivo. *Virology* 1993; **197**:659–668.

25. Kato N, Sekiya H, Ootsuyama Y, Nakazawa T, Hijikata M, Ohkoshi S & Shimotohno K. Humoral immune response to hypervariable region 1 of the putative envelope glycoprotein (gp70) of hepatitis C virus. *Journal of Virology* 1993; **67**:3923–3930.

26. Ziebert A, Schreier E & Roggendorf M. Antibodies in human sera specific to hypervariable region 1 of hepatitis C virus can block viral attachment. *Virology* 1995;

208:653–661.

27. Pawlotsky JM, Germanidis G, Neumann AU, Pellerin M, Frainais PO & Dhumeaux D. Interferon resistance of hepatitis C virus genotype 1b: relationship with non structural 5A (NS5A) gene quasispecies mutations. *Journal of Virology* 1998; **72**:2795–2805.

28. Polyak SJ, McArdle S, Liu SL, Sullivan DG, Chung M, Hofgärtner WT, Carithers RL, McMahon BJ, Mullins JI, Corey L & Gretch DR. Evolution of hepatitis C virus quasispecies in hypervariable region 1 and the putative interferon sensitivity-determining region during interferon therapy and natural infection. *Journal of Virology* 1998; **72**:4288–4296.

29. Alberti A, Morsica G, Chemello L, Cavalletto D, Noventa F, Pontisso P & Ruol A. Hepatitis C viraemia and liver disease in symptom-free individuals with anti-HCV. *Lancet* 1992; **340**:697–698.

30. Lok ASF & Gunaratnam NT. Diagnosis of hepatitis C. *Hepatology* 1997; **26** (Supplement 1):48S–56S.

31. N'guyen T, Sedghi-Vaziri A, Wilkes L, Mondala T, Pockros P, Lindsay K & McHutchison J. Fluctuations in viral load (HCV RNA) are relatively insignificant in untreated patients with chronic HCV infection. *Journal of Viral Hepatitis* 1996; **3**:75–78.

32. Gretch DR. Diagnostic tests for hepatitis C. *Hepatology* 1997; **26** (Supplement 1):43S–47S.

33. Pawlotsky JM. HCV viral load, genotypes, and HCV IgM: clinical relevance. In *Hepatitis C 1997: Essays and Expert Opinions on its Natural History, Epidemiology, Diagnosis and Therapy*, 1997; pp. 116–121. Edited by R Decker & H Troonen. Wiesbaden: Abbott Diagnostics Educational Services.

34. Okamoto H, Kobata S, Tokita H, Inoue T, Woodfield GD, Holland PV, Al-Knawy BA, Uzunalimoglu O, Miyakawa Y & Mayumi M. A second-generation method of genotyping hepatitis C virus by the polymerase chain reaction with sense and antisense primers deduced from the core gene. *Journal of Virological Methods* 1996; **57**:31–45.

35. Davidson F, Simmonds P, Ferguson JC, Jarvis LM, Dow BC, Follett EAC, Seed CRG, Krusius T, Lin C, Medgyesi GA, Kiyokawa H, Olim G, Duraisamy G, Cuypers T, Saeed AA, Teo D, Conradie J, Kew MC, Lin M, Nuchaprayoon C, Ndimbie OK & Yap PL. Survey of major genotypes and subtypes of hepatitis C virus using RFLP of sequences amplified from the 5′ non-coding region. *Journal of General Virology* 1995; **76**:1197–1204.

36. Stuyver L, Rossau R, Wyseur A, Duhamel M, Vanderborght B, Van Heuverswyn H & Maertens G. Typing of hepatitis C virus isolates and characterization of new subtypes using a line probe assay. *Journal of General Virology* 1993; **74**:1093–1102.

37. Biasin MR, Fiordalisi G, Zanella I, Cavicchini A, Marchelle G & Infantolino D. A DNA hybridization method for typing hepatitis C virus genotype 2c. *Journal of Virological Methods* 1997; **65**:307–315.

38. Battacherjee V, Prescott LE, Pike I, Rodgers B, Bell H, El-Zayadi AR, Kew MC, Conradie J, Lin CK, Marsden H, Saeed AA, Parker D, Yap PL & Simmonds P. Use of NS-4 peptides to identify type-specific antibody to hepatitis C virus genotypes 1, 2, 3, 4, 5 and 6. *Journal of General Virology* 1995; **76**:1737–1748.

39. Dixit V, Quan S, Martin P, Larson D, Brezina M, DiNello R, Sra K, Lau JYN, Chien D, Kolberg J, Tagger A, Davis G, Polito A & Gitnick G. Evaluation of a novel serotyping system for hepatitis C virus: strong correlation with standard genotyping methodologies. *Journal of Clinical Microbiology* 1995; **33**:2978–2983.

40. Pawlotsky JM, Prescott L, Simmonds P, Pellet C, Laurent-Puig P, Labonne C, Darthuy F, Rémiré J, Duval J, Buffet C, Etienne JP, Dhumeaux D & Dussaix E. Serological determination of hepatitis C virus genotype: comparison with a standardized genotyping assay. *Journal of Clinical Microbiology* 1997; **35**:1734–1739.

41. Zaaijer HL, Cuypers HTM, Reesink HW, Winkel IN, Gerken G & Lelie PN. Reliability of polymerase chain reaction for detection of hepatitis C virus. *Lancet* 1993; **341**:722–724.

42. French Study Group for the Standardization of Hepatitis C Virus PCR. Improvement of hepatitis C virus RNA polymerase chain reaction through a multicentre quality control study. *Journal of Virological Methods* 1994; **49**:79–88.

43. Wolfe L, Tamatsukuri S, Sayada C & Ryff JC. Detection of HCV RNA in serum using a single-tube, single-enzyme PCR in combination with a colorimetric microwell assay. In *Hepatitis C Virus: New Diagnostic Tools*, 1994; pp. 83–94. Edited by the Groupe Français d'Etudes Moléculaires des Hépatites. Paris: John Libbey Eurotext.

44. Gretch DR, dela Rosa C, Carithers RL, Willson RA, Williams B & Corey L. Assessment of hepatitis C viremia using molecular amplification technologies: correlations and clinical implications. *Annals of Internal Medicine* 1995; **123**:321–329.

45. Roth WK, Lee JH, Rüster B & Zeuzem S. Comparison of two quantitative hepatitis C virus reverse transcriptase PCR assays. *Journal of Clinical Microbiology* 1996; **34**:261–264.

46. Tong MJ, Blatt LM, McHutchison JG, Co RL & Conrad A. Prediction of response during interferon alfa 2b therapy in chronic hepatitis C patients using viral and biochemical characteristics: a comparison. *Hepatology* 1997; **26**:1640–1645.

47. Melsert R, Damen M, Cuypers T, Boele S, van Deursen P, Ehren R, Frantzen I, Sillekens P & Lens P. Combined quantitation and genotyping of hepatitis C virus RNA using NASBA. In *Hepatitis C Virus: Genetic Heterogeneity and Viral Load*, 1997; pp. 79–88. Edited by the Groupe Français d'Etudes Moléculaires des Hépatites. Paris: John Libbey Eurotext.

48. Urdea MS. Quantification of hepatitis C virus RNA: clinical applications of the branched DNA assay. In *Hepatitis C Virus: Genetic Heterogeneity and Viral Load*, 1997; pp. 73–78. Edited by the Groupe Français d'Etudes Moléculaires des Hépatites. Paris: John Libbey Eurotext.

49. Pawlotsky JM. Measuring hepatitis C viremia in clinical samples: can we trust the assays? *Hepatology* 1997; **26**:1–4.

50. Gretch DR, dela Rosa C, Corey L & Carithers RL. Assessment of hepatitis C viremia using molecular amplification technologies. *Viral Hepatitis Reviews* 1996; **2**:85–96.

51. Gretch DR & Polyak SJ. The quasispecies nature of hepatitis C virus: research methods and biological implications. In *Hepatitis C Virus: Genetic Heterogeneity and Viral Load*, 1997; pp. 57–72. Edited by the Groupe Français d'Etudes Moléculaires des Hépatites. Paris: John Libbey Eurotext.

52. Gretch DR, Polyak SJ, Wilson JJ, Carithers RL, Perkins JD & Corey L. Tracking hepatitis C virus quasispecies major and minor variants in symptomatic and asymptomatic liver transplant recipients. *Journal of Virology* 1996; **70**:7622–7631.

53. Odeberg J, Yun Z, Sönnerborg A, Uhlen M & Lundeberg J. Dynamic analysis of heterogeneous hepatitis C virus

populations by direct solid-phase sequencing. *Journal of Clinical Microbiology* 1995; **33**:1870–1874.

54. Lu M, Funsch B, Wiese M & Roggendorf M. Analysis of hepatitis C virus quasispecies populations by temperature gradient gel electrophoresis. *Journal of General Virology* 1995; **76**:881–887.

55. Wilson JJ, Polyak SJ, Day TD & Gretch DR. Characterization of simple and complex hepatitis C virus quasispecies by heteroduplex gel shift analysis: correlation with nucleotide sequencing. *Journal of General Virology* 1995; **76**:1763–1771.

56. Enomoto N, Kurosaki M, Tanaka Y, Marumo F & Sato C. Fluctuation of hepatitis C virus quasispecies in persistent infection and interferon treatment revealed by single-strand conformation polymorphism analysis. *Journal of General Virology* 1994; **75**:1361–1369.

57. Pawlotsky JM, Pellerin M, Bouvier M, Roudot-Thoraval, Germanidis G, Bastie A, Darthuy F, Rémiré J, Soussy CJ & Dhumeaux D. Genetic complexity of the hypervariable region 1 (HVR1) of hepatitis C virus (HCV): influence on the characteristics of the infection and responses to interferon alfa therapy in patients with chronic hepatitis C. *Journal of Medical Virology* 1998; **54**:256–264.

58. Pawlotsky JM, Bouvier M, Bastie A, Lefrere JJ, Da Costa I, Germanidis G, Pellerin M, Zafrani ES & Dhumeaux D. What is the real effect of interferon alfa on hepatitis C virus replication and quasispecies and the liver in patients with chronic hepatitis C? *Hepatology* 1997; **26**:367A.

59. Davis GL & Lau JYN. Factors predictive of a beneficial response to therapy of hepatitis C. *Hepatology* 1997; **26** (Supplement 1):122S–127S.

60. Pawlotsky JM, Roudot-Thoraval F, Bastie A, Darthuy F, Rémiré J, Métreau JM, Zafrani ES, Duval J & Dhumeaux D. Factors affecting treatment responses to interferon-α in chronic hepatitis C. *Journal of Infectious Diseases* 1996; **174**:1–7.

61. Martinot-Peignoux M, Marcellin P, Pouteau M, Castelnau C, Boyer N, Poliquin M, Degott C, Descombes I, Le Breton V, Milotova V, Benhamou JP & Erlinger S. Pretreatment HCV RNA levels and HCV genotype are the main and independent prognostic factors of sustained response to alpha interferon therapy in chronic hepatitis C. *Hepatology* 1995; **22**:1050–1056.

62. Nousbaum JB, Pol S, Nalpas B, Landais P, Berthelot P, Bréchot C & the Collaborative Study Group. Hepatitis C virus type 1b (II) infection in France and Italy. *Annals of Internal Medicine* 1995; **122**:161–168.

63. Mahaney K, Tedeschi V, Maertens G, DiBisceglie AM, Vergalla J, Hoofnagle JH & Sallie R. Genotypic analysis of hepatitis C virus in American patients. *Hepatology* 1994; **20**:1405–1411.

64. El-Zayadi A, Simmonds P, Dabbous H, Prescott L, Selim O & Ahdy A. Response to interferon-α of Egyptian patients infected with hepatitis C virus genotype 4. *Journal of Viral Hepatitis* 1996; **3**:261–264.

65. Toyoda H, Kumada T, Nakano S, Takeda I, Sugiyama K, Osada T, Kiriyama S, Sone Y, Kinoshita M & Hadama T. Quasispecies nature of hepatitis C virus and response to alpha interferon: significance as a predictor of direct response to interferon. *Journal of Hepatology* 1997; **26**:6–13.

66. Polyak SJ, Faulkner G, Carithers RL, Corey L & Gretch DR. Assessment of hepatitis C virus quasispecies heterogeneity by gel shift analysis: correlation with response to interferon therapy. *Journal of Infectious Diseases* 1997; **175**:1101–1107.

67. Enomoto N, Sakuma I, Asahina Y, Kurosaki M, Murakami T, Yamamoto C, Izumi N, Marumo F & Sato C. Comparison of full-length sequences of interferon-sensitive and resistant hepatitis C virus 1b. Sensitivity to interferon is conferred by amino acid substitutions in the NS5A region. *Journal of Clinical Investigation* 1995; **96**:224–230.

68. Enomoto N, Sakuma I, Asahina Y, Kurosaki M, Murakami T, Yamamoto C, Ogura Y, Izumi N, Marumo F & Sato C. Mutations in the nonstructural protein 5A gene and response to interferon in patients with chronic hepatitis C virus 1b infection. *New England Journal of Medicine* 1996; **334**:77–81.

69. Karino Y, Toyota J, Sugawara M, Higashino K, Sato T, Ohmura T, Suga T, Okuuchi Y & Matsushima T. Early loss of serum hepatitis C virus RNA can predict a sustained response to interferon therapy in patients with chronic hepatitis C. *American Journal of Gastroenterology* 1997; **92**:61–65.

70. Orito E, Mizokami M, Suzuki K, Ohba K, Ohno T, Mori T, Hayashi K, Kato K, Iino S & Lau JYN. Loss of serum HCV RNA at week 4 of interferon-alpha therapy is associated with more favorable long-term response in patients with chronic hepatitis C. *Journal of Medical Virology* 1995; **46**:109–115.

71. Gavier B, Martinez-Gonzalez MA, Riezu-Boj JI, Lasarte JJ, Garcia N, Civeira MP & Prieto J. Viremia after one month of interferon therapy predicts treatment outcome in patients with chronic hepatitis C. *Gastroenterology* 1997; **113**:1647–1653.

72. Gibson UEM, Heid CA & Williams PM. A novel method for real time quantitative RT–PCR. *Genome Research* 1996; **6**:995–1001.

73. Ho DD. Dynamics of HIV-1 replication in vivo. *Journal of Clinical Investigation* 1997; **99**:2565–2567.

74. Hofgärtner WT, Polyak SJ, Sullivan DG, Carithers RL & Gretch DR. Mutations in the NS5A gene of hepatitis C virus in North American patients infected with HCV genotype 1a or 1b. *Journal of Medical Virology* 1997; **53**:118–126.

75. Gale MJ, Korth MJ, Tang NM, Tan SL, Hopkins DA, Dever TE, Polyak SJ, Gretch DR & Katze MG. Evidence that hepatitis C virus resistance to interferon is mediated through repression of the PKR protein kinase by the nonstructural 5A protein. *Virology* 1997; **230**:217–227.

76. Gale M, Blakely CM, Kwieciszewski B, Tan SL, Dossett M, Tang NM, Korth MJ, Polyak SJ, Gretch DR and Katze MG. Control of the PKR protein kinase by the hepatitis C virus non-structural 5A protein: molecular mechanisms of kinase regulation. *Molecular and Cellular Biology* 1998; in press.

77. Choo Q, Kuo G, Weiner AJ, Overby LR, Bradley DW & Houghton M. Isolation of a cDNA clone derived from a blood-borne non-A, non-B viral hepatitis genome. *Science* 1989; **244**:359–362.

# 13 Utility of hepatitis virus nucleic acid assays in therapeutic drug trials

Maurice Rosenstraus*, Karen Gutekunst and Beverly Dale

## INTRODUCTION

Rapid, sensitive methods that accurately detect and quantitate viral nucleic acids have recently played an essential role in the development of more effective treatments for chronic viral infections. Because pathological changes or clinical endpoints may require invasive procedures to identify, or take years to develop, surrogate endpoints must be used to provide safe and timely information on the efficacy of therapeutic regimens. Traditionally, immunological or biochemical markers, such as CD4$^+$ cell count in HIV infection or serum alanine aminotransferase (ALT) in hepatitis infection, have served as early, but imperfect, indicators of a therapeutic response. Direct measurements of viral nucleic acid now allow clinicians to determine whether the infectious agent itself is being eradicated by the treatment. This information, used in conjunction with traditional surrogate endpoints, should provide a more rapid, accurate indication of therapeutic efficacy, allowing regulatory agencies to grant confidently accelerated or full approvals for promising new therapies.

Recent advances in HIV treatment dramatically illustrate the synergistic interplay between the development of improved viral therapies and nucleic acid-based diagnostics. First, quantitative tests for HIV-1 viral RNA provided basic insight into the natural history of HIV-1 infection, indicating the need for early introduction of antiviral therapy [1–4]. Second, viral RNA levels have prognostic value [5–11] and, thus, can be used to target expensive therapies having significant side-effects to those most likely to develop AIDS. Third, viral RNA levels have been used to monitor antiviral therapy [12–14] and have served as a surrogate end-point for assessing the utility of new drugs and combination treatment regimens [15–18]. At the same time, the large volume of data generated during drug trials indicates how viral nucleic assays can best be used for routine patient management and suggests strategies for taking a diagnostic test through the regulatory process. As a result of these synergies, HIV-1 viral load testing is now regarded as the standard of good medical practice for measuring the effectiveness of excellent new drugs and combination treatment regimens [19–25].

Although the success of viral nucleic acid tests in the management of HIV infection and disease has taken centre stage in the molecular diagnostics industry, the potential of molecular tests for hepatitis viruses could be even more impressive given the magnitude of disease distribution. More than 520 million people worldwide are at risk for developing cirrhosis or liver cancer caused by chronic viral hepatitis. Hepatitis B virus (HBV) is the most common cause of chronic viral hepatitis with an estimated 350 million carriers worldwide [26], including 1.25 million in the USA [27]. Hepatitis C virus (HCV) is the second principal cause of viral hepatitis with an estimated 170 million carriers worldwide [28], 3.9 million of whom reside in the USA (Centers for Disease Control, unpublished data, available at: http://www.cdc.gov/ncidod/diseases/hepatitis/heptab3.htm). In the USA, complications from chronic HBV and HCV infection cause approximately 6000 and 8000 to 10000 deaths each year, respectively (Centers for Disease Control, unpublished data, available at: http://www.cdc.gov/ncidod/diseases/hepatitis/heptab3.htm).

Treatment regimens for chronic hepatitis are less well developed than those for HIV-1, as is our understanding of how to use nucleic acid diagnostic tests to maximize therapeutic efficacy. In this review, we will focus on the following issues for both HCV and HBV: (i) what are the limitations of current treatments for chronic hepatitis that are being addressed in therapeutic drug trials?; (ii) how are nucleic acid diagnostics being used in addition to traditional surrogate markers in therapeutic drug trials?; and (iii) what improvements in molecular assay characteristics are most desirable in order to effectively answer drug efficacy questions?

## TREATMENT OF CHRONIC HEPATITIS

Here we provide a brief review of the current state of viral hepatitis therapeutics. Other chapters in this volume review existing and coming therapeutics in detail and the reader is referred to them for particulars.

Interferon α (IFN-α) is the only treatment of proven benefit to patients with chronic HBV and HCV, but its effectiveness is limited [29–36]. Recent clinical studies have evaluated new treatment schedules and dosing regimens [35,37–40], and have explored the efficacy of combining immunomodulatory interferon treatment with antiviral drugs: ribavirin (1-β-D-ribofuranosyl-1H-1,2,4-triazole-3-carboxamide; RTCA) for HCV [41–45] and lamivudine [(–)-β-L-2′,3′-dideoxy-3′-thiacytidine] for HBV [46–49]. These encouraging results have also led to the investigation of other nucleoside and nucleotide analogues for the treatment of chronic hepatitis B [50–52]. In addition to serving as a useful surrogate endpoint for demonstrating the efficacy of these enhanced therapies, the level of viral nucleic acid in serum appears to be an early indicator for the effectiveness of therapy [53–59]. Rapid, accurate viral load testing is being used to monitor the kinetics of viral replication in real time for the purpose of modifying treatment (such as daily dosing) or terminating it early (see section entitled *Utility of HCV RNA assays in therapeutic drug trials: virological response to therapy and test of cure*).

The limited effectiveness of interferon treatment, combined with its expense [60–63] and side-effects, makes it critical to target treatment to those who will benefit most and to modify treatment as early as possible in non-responsive patients. Nucleic acid diagnostics may help achieve these objectives. HCV genotype and viral RNA load are important, independent predictors of therapeutic success [37,39,64–68] as is a low concentration of HBV DNA in serum [53,69].

## SURROGATE MARKERS IN DRUG TRIALS FOR HEPATITIS ANTIVIRALS

ALT and HCV RNA levels in serum serve as the principal surrogate markers for evaluating therapy in patients with chronic HCV infection [53]. The efficacy of interferon α therapy is currently defined biochemically as normalization of serum ALT and virologically

as loss of serum HCV RNA, as measured by reverse transcriptase PCR (RT–PCR). Approximately 10% to 25% of interferon-treated patients exhibit a long-term response, which is defined as normalization of ALT and no detectable HCV RNA for at least six months after termination of therapy. Approximately 25% to 40% of patients exhibit a transient response to therapy; ALT normalizes and HCV RNA initially disappears, but both return within six months after termination of treatment. HCV RNA must be used as a surrogate marker along with ALT because approximately 20% of patients exhibit partial responses in which ALT normalizes but HCV RNA persists. These patients ultimately relapse, exhibiting elevated ALT levels more than one year after termination of treatment [53,70–72].

ALT, hepatitis B e antigen (HBeAg), hepatitis B s antigen (HBsAg) and HBV DNA in serum serve as surrogate markers for evaluating therapy in patients with chronic HBV infection. A beneficial response to therapy is defined as no detectable HBV DNA and HBeAg, and normal, or near-normal, ALT levels six months after termination of therapy [53]. HBsAg cannot serve as an early indicator of therapeutic success because it often persists long after treatment, even in patients exhibiting improved clinical outcome [69]. ALT levels eventually normalize in complete responders, but often exhibit a transient increase during interferon treatment [53]. While this early rise may be due to immunological destruction of infected hepatocytes [53], it means that ALT cannot, by itself, serve as an early indicator of therapeutic response. Both HBV DNA and HBeAg can serve as early indicators of a therapeutic response. Generally, all HBeAg-negative patients are also negative for HBV DNA [69]. One prospective study has demonstrated the utility of these two surrogate markers by showing that loss of HBeAg and HBV DNA results in better long-term clinical outcome [69]. It is not clear whether more accurate predictions of response can be achieved by following both, instead of one, of these markers. HBV DNA may provide an earlier indication of therapeutic success because it disappears before HBeAg in some patients [53,69]. Also, HBV DNA may provide a more accurate therapeutic indicator in rare patients who are HBeAg-negative due to outgrowth of a mutant virus [53,73–76]. Importantly, most of the studies to date used non-amplified hybridization assays to quantitate HBV DNA; preliminary data obtained using more sensitive, amplified assays suggest that HBV DNA quantitation will eventually play a more important role for monitoring therapy.

# HCV VIRAL RNA TESTING

Both qualitative and quantitative tests for HCV RNA have contributed to our understanding of the natural history of HCV infection. Quantitative tests are used to measure viral burden for patient identification and stratification, and to provide real-time information for modifying treatment. Less expensive, easier-to-perform qualitative tests may serve as a test of cure, where it may suffice to demonstrate that the viral RNA load falls below a critical threshold associated with long-term clinical benefit.

Based on our current knowledge of viral HCV RNA levels in plasma, a qualitative test should be highly sensitive and reliable, and a quantitative test should, in addition, have a broad dynamic range. Chronic HCV patients generally have viral RNA loads between $10^2$ and $> 10^7$ copies/ml of plasma [58,59,77]. Only 10% of chronic HCV patients have less than $10^2$ copies [58,59]. The ability to measure titres above $10^6$ copies/ml may not be useful because there is little difference in prognosis for viral RNA titres in excess of $10^5$ copies/ml [39,40,54,58,59,68].

Approximately one-third of chronic HCV patients are infected with genotypes other than genotype 1 [67,78–80]. In addition to being a substantial minority, these patients respond better to therapy than patients infected with genotype 1. Thus, it is important to design tests that accurately quantitate all HCV genotypes.

## Properties of HCV RNA tests

Two basic approaches have been used to detect and quantitate HCV RNA. The first utilizes a coupled RT-PCR to amplify minute quantities of RNA, whereas the second uses a signal amplification system to detect small quantities of RNA. Thorough, up-to-date descriptions of molecular tests for HCV are available [81]. Here, we will provide a brief description of the molecular tests for HCV RNA, with emphasis on commercially available RT-PCR assays, and focus on their current application to therapeutic drug trials. The properties of the commonly used assays are summarized in Table 1.

The Quantiplex test (Chiron Corporation, Emeryville, California, USA) uses the branched DNA technology to generate a readable signal from small quantities of RNA. Viral RNA is captured on a solid support by hybridization to a specific probe. A second set of probes hybridize specifically to the captured RNA, which then allows binding of the labelled branched DNA molecules. The Quantiplex assay has been shown to be highly reproducible and have a broad dynamic range. This assay was used to demonstrate the association between viral RNA load and disease prognosis. The relatively poor sensitivity of this assay limits its usefulness [64].

Qualitative and quantitative versions of RT-PCR tests are commercially available from Roche Diagnostics. Both the qualitative test and quantitative test (MONITOR) come in two formats: the manual AMPLICOR format, in which amplification products are detected on microwell plates, and the fully automated COBAS AMPLICOR format, in which the COBAS AMPLICOR system performs amplification, detection and results calculation without user intervention. All four of these tests are now available with Version 2.0 reagents, which provide improved sensitivity and more accurate quantitation of all genotypes compared to the Version 1.0 reagents that have been broadly available to date. The qualitative tests use an internal control to monitor the efficiency of specimen extraction and amplification and, by identifying specimens inhibitory to PCR, to provide assurance that negative test results are true-negative. In the quantitative tests, the internal control serves as an internal quantitation standard. The AMPLICOR tests provide standardized reagents, fixed procedures and well-defined performance characteristics. Such standardized tests are essential for comparing the efficacy of new therapeutic protocols evaluated in different test centres on different populations. In addition, all AMPLICOR tests incorporate contamination control systems to guard against contamination caused by carry-over of previously amplified DNA.

Despite efforts to simplify and standardize HCV molecular testing, the ability of laboratories to accurately perform various HCV RNA tests has been questioned by the results of two early proficiency studies [82,83]. A recent proficiency study conducted by World Viral Quality Control (VQA) program in 1997 suggests that laboratories now obtain more reproducible results, especially when using commercially available tests (N Lelie, Central Laboratory of the Netherlands Red Cross Blood Transfusion Service, personal communication). Manufacturers and users have the ongoing responsibility to provide educational and proficiency testing programs that will establish and maintain high confidence in HCV RNA test results.

## Performance characteristics of the Version 2.0 COBAS AMPLICOR and AMPLICOR HCV tests

The Version 1.0 COBAS AMPLICOR and AMPLICOR HCV tests had a sensitivity of 1000 RNA copies/ml of plasma. This sensitivity was enhanced by modifying the specimen processing procedure in the Version 2.0 tests to increase the specimen volume tested 10-fold, from the equivalent of 5 µl to the equivalent of 50 µl of plasma. An end-point titration experiment showed that this 10-fold increase in specimen volume produced a corresponding increase in sensitivity to 100 RNA copies/ml of plasma; samples containing as little as 100 copies/ml of plasma were detected in 9 out of 9 replicate tests (Table 2).

The COBAS AMPLICOR HCV MONITOR test exhibited excellent reproducibility when a panel of serial dilutions from a high-titre sample was evaluated in different laboratories (Fig. 1). The concentration measured by the test matched the input over the concentration range of $10^3$ to $10^6$ copies/ml of sample (Fig. 1). As the input concentration increased from $10^6$ to $10^{6.5}$ copies/ml, the measured concentration continued to increase, but underestimated the input concentration (Fig. 1). The COBAS AMPLICOR HCV MONITOR test equivalently amplified all genotypes (Fig. 2). The Version 2.0 AMPLICOR HCV MONITOR test uses the same reagents and has the same performance characteristics as the COBAS AMPLICOR HCV MONITOR test.

## Future assay enhancements

The next generation of commercially available PCR tests available from Roche Diagnostics will use a homogeneous, TaqMan 5′-nuclease assay format in which amplification and detection are performed simultaneously [84,85]. Such homogenous tests will generate results more rapidly than the current heterogeneous test formats by eliminating the need to detect products after amplification is completed. In addition, the homogenous tests combine exquisite sensitivity with an extremely broad dynamic range; the signal generated is linear over a target concentration range from 5 to $10^8$ copies per amplification reaction (Fig. 3). Furthermore, these assays yield quantitative data without requiring any extra effort by laboratory personnel. Thus, separate quantitative and qualitative assay formats will no longer be needed to choose between sensitivity and dynamic range, or to control costs.

## Utility of HCV RNA assays in therapeutic drug trials

Either the Roche AMPLICOR or the National Genetics Institute (NGI) home-brew (SuperQuant) quantitative RT-PCR assays, are the tests most frequently selected for use in ongoing HCV drug trials for new interferon formulations, dosing regimens and combination treatments. The Quantiplex Version 2.0 assay is unlikely to find broad application until its sensitivity is significantly improved. In the drug trials that resulted in USA Food and Drug Administration

**Table 1.** Comparison of HCV RNA tests

| | Quantitative | | | Qualitative |
|---|---|---|---|---|
| | AMPLICOR HCV MONITOR, Ver 2.0 | Quantiplex HCV RNA 2.0 Assay* | 'Home-brew' PCR | AMPLICOR HCV |
| Method | Target amplification | Signal amplification | Target amplification | Target amplification |
| Sensitivity | ~100 copies/ml | $2 \times 10^5$ copies/ml | Assay-dependent (~10–$10^3$ copies/ml) | 100 copies/ml |
| Dynamic range | $10^3$–$10^6$ copies/ml | $10^{5.3}$–$10^8$ copies/ml | Assay-dependent $10^2$–$10^{6.7}$ copies/ml [45] $10^3$–$10^{10}$ [81] | N/A |
| Internal control | Yes | N/A | Assay-dependent | Yes |
| Carry-over contamination control | Yes | N/A | Assay-dependent | Yes |
| Standardization | Yes | Yes | No | Yes |
| Automation | MWP format - Manual; COBAS format - Automated amplification, detection and calculation of results | Manual, automated calculation of results | Automated amplification | MWP format - manual; COBAS format - automated amplification, detection and calculation of results |

*The Quantiplex assay reports results in units of genome equivalents. These are approximately equivalent to copies of target DNA.
N/A, not applicable; MWP, microwell plate.

**Table 2.** Sensitivity of the 1st and 2nd generation AMPLICOR HCV tests

| HCV target level (copies/ml) | Positive replicates (positive/total) | |
| | 1st Generation (5 µl/PCR) | 2nd Generation (50 µl/PCR) |
| --- | --- | --- |
| 400 | 67% (6/9) | 100% (9/9) |
| 200 | 56% (5/9) | 100% (9/9) |
| 100 | 44% (4/9) | 100% (9/9) |
| 50 | 44% (4/9) | 89% (8/9) |

(FDA) approval for Amgen's recombinant interferon, INFERGEN, both ALT and HCV-RNA, as determined by 'a quantitative RT-PCR assay with a lower limit of sensitivity of 100 copies/ml', were used to monitor treatment success [86]. This product approval has probably set the 'gold standard' for HCV RNA testing sensitivity at 100 copies/ml, although the requirement for prognosis and monitoring has not been established.

In therapeutic drug trials, HCV RNA assays can be used for several purposes, as discussed below.

## Patient identification and stratification

The 1997 USA National Institutes of Health (NIH) Consensus Guidelines on Management of Hepatitis C state that a positive enzyme immunoassay (EIA) test is sufficient for diagnosis of hepatitis C in patients presenting with biochemical or clinical evidence of liver disease, but suggest that a qualitative HCV RNA test be used for confirmation [87]. Furthermore, as judgement of therapeutic efficacy will increasingly rely on disappearance of HCV RNA as well as normalization of ALT, a qualitative assay for confirmed diagnosis of viraemia is essential prior to initiating therapy.

Many clinical investigators recommend that patients also be tested with a quantitative HCV RNA assay prior to initiating therapy. RNA titres can be used to stratify patients into various treatment arms, as a large body of data has demonstrated that patients with lower levels of viraemia exhibit higher response rates when treated with interferon [87]. For the first generation AMPLICOR HCV-MONITOR test, patients with low viral titres ($<10^4$ RNA copies/ml of serum) exhibited a 3.5- to 6.5-fold higher long-term response rate than patients with high ($>10^5$ RNA copies/ml of serum, Table 3). In one study, patients with intermediate viral titres ($>10^4$ but $<10^5$ RNA copies/ml) exhibited an intermediate response rate of 32% [59]. Similar results were observed using a 'home-brew' competitive PCR or the Quantiplex assay, but the viral titre cut-offs indicating a higher response rate were $10^{5.3}$ RNA copies/ml and $10^{6.3}$ RNA copies/ml, respectively (Table 3).

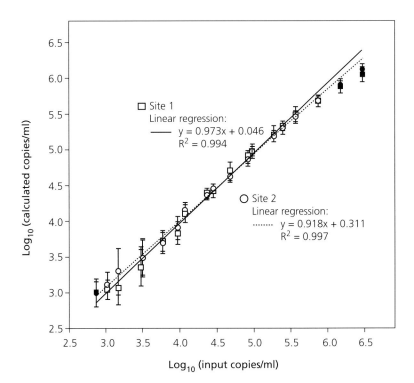

**Figure 1.** Reproducibility and linearity of the COBAS AMPLICOR HCV MONITOR test

Two laboratories independently tested a panel of serially diluted samples containing known amounts of HCV RNA. Each lab performed ten runs for each panel. The log of the calculated concentration was determined for each sample in each run and the mean log calculated concentration was plotted against the log of the input concentration. Error bars show the standard deviation. Linear regression analysis (solid and dashed lines) was performed for the set of samples within the linear range of the test (open symbols). Samples outside the linear range are shown (solid symbols), but not included in the regression analysis.

**Figure 2.** Relative amplification efficiency of different HCV genotypes in the COBAS AMPLICOR HCV MONITOR test

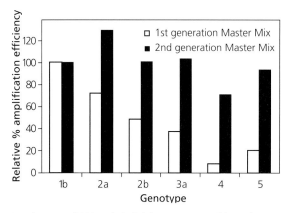

Equal amounts (1000 copies) of viral RNA were tested for each HCV genotype. Each genotype was tested using both the Master Mix from the first generation AMPLICOR HCV MONITOR test (open bars) and the Master Mix that is used in the COBAS AMPLICOR and second generation AMPLICOR HCV MONITOR tests (closed bars). The relative amplification efficiency for each genotype was determined by dividing the calculated copy number for the genotype by the calculated copy number for genotype 1b.

**Figure 3.** Relationship between target concentration and time to appearance of detectable signal in a homogeneous 5′-exonuclease PCR assay

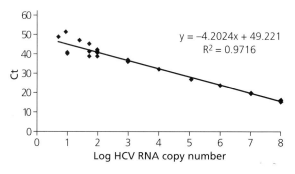

Various amounts of HCV RNA were amplified in separate reactions. The first amplification cycle number exhibiting a signal increase (Ct) was determined for each target concentration, plotted versus the log of the target concentration and analyzed by linear regression. These data were provided by Sue Tsang of Roche Molecular Systems.

While measurements of viral titre provide useful prognostic information, their positive and negative predictive values are not accurate enough for deciding whether to administer or withhold interferon treatment from an individual patient [64,87,88]. Treatment should not automatically be administered to patients with relatively low RNA titres since only 60 to 75% will benefit. It may be appropriate to withhold treatment in low titre patients if interferon treatment is contraindicated by other factors. Likewise, treatment should not be withheld from patients with a relatively high viral titre since as many as 20% could benefit from the therapy.

This limited prognostic value may, in part, reflect the fluctuation of RNA titres over time [64]. All of the studies to date have used a single pre-treatment measurement of viral titre, which may or may not have been representative of the patients' viral burden. Future studies may show that multiple measurements over a defined interval result in more accurate predictions. Also, even single measurements of pre-treatment RNA titres may prove more useful for making treatment decisions for new therapeutic regimens.

## Virological response to therapy and test of cure

Both serial ALT measurements and qualitative HCV RNA testing are recommended for monitoring patients undergoing antiviral therapy as loss of HCV RNA is regarded as a strong predictor of a sustained beneficial results [87]. The most conservative and widely accepted approach is to use a qualitative HCV RNA assay to measure virological response at the end of treatment (end-of-treatment response; ETR) and at six months post treatment (sustained response; SR); in both instances a response is defined as loss of detectable HCV RNA. An ETR determined with a sensitive assay may indicate that an SR will be achieved. In one study, 79% of patients exhibiting an ETR, as determined by AMPLICOR HCV MONITOR, ultimately exhibited an SR [60]. Also, during a 6 to 12 month course of interferon therapy, an assessment of serum ALT and HCV RNA three months into the treatment regimen is useful as abnormal ALT and detectable HCV RNA at this time point predicts non-response and suggests termination of the unsuccessful regimen [64,87].

Beyond the consensus recommendations stated above, HCV RNA assays may be useful for modifying therapies in response to changes in HCV RNA levels. In the future, switching to combination therapy in individuals exhibiting a minimal HCV RNA response may increase the chance of achieving long-term remission [88]. Also, it may prove possible to reduce the length of treatment or dose of interferon in patients exhibiting an early, strong HCV RNA response. In one study [57], patients who were HCV RNA negative after four months of therapy received a reduced (0.5×) interferon dose for four more months.

**Table 3.** Ability of pre-treatment HCV RNA level to predict response to interferon

| Test | Ref. | Low titre | | | High titre | | |
|------|------|-----------|---|---|-----------|---|---|
| | | Viral load | No. of patients | Responders (%) | Viral load | No. of patients | Responders (%) |
| AMPLICOR | 60 | $<10^{4.5}$ | 21 | 67 | $>10^{4.5}$ | 27 | 19 |
| | 61 | $<10^{4.0}$ | 69 | 71 | $>10^{5.0}$ | 175 | 11 |
| 'Home-brew' | 60 | $<10^{5.5}$ | 20 | 75 | $>10^{5.5}$ | 28 | 14 |
| | 61 | $<10^{5.3}$ | 69 | 62 | $>10^{6.3}$ | 127 | 6 |
| Quantiplex | 60 | $<10^{6.0}$ | 23 | 74 | $>10^{6.0}$ | 25 | 8 |
| | 61 | $<10^{5.7}$ | 100 | 61 | $>10^{6.0}$ | 137 | 4 |
| | 70 | $<10^{6.3}$ | 39 | 59 | $>10^{6.3}$ | 21 | 0 |

The SR rate in this study was similar to the response rate observed in patients receiving 12 months of full-dose therapy. Further studies are, however, required because this study did not include a control group who received the standard course of therapy; an even better SR rate may have been obtained had the dose been maintained.

## HBV VIRAL DNA TESTING

The role of amplified HBV DNA assays in the evaluation of new HBV antiviral therapies lags behind that of HCV RNA assays in the evaluation of new HCV therapies. The application of molecular assays to the study and treatment of HBV can be generally summarized as follows.

First, unlike HCV infection, serological assays for HBV infection (assays for three viral antigens and assays for their corresponding host antibodies) are mature and well understood, and serve as well-accepted hallmarks of viral activity and disease progression [89].

Second, patients with active HBV infection generally have very high titres of HBV DNA in plasma or serum. Thus, relatively insensitive, non-amplified hybridization assays have been useful for quantitating HBV replication and monitoring the response to antiviral therapy. Despite their low sensitivity, these non-amplified molecular methods were more sensitive than assays for HBeAg, the serological marker of active replication.

Third, highly sensitive, standardized commercially available PCR assays for HBV DNA have only recently become available for studying both the natural history of HBV infection and the antiviral activity of potential new therapies. Given this new ability to measure very low levels of HBV DNA, investigators must re-evaluate the definition of successful anti-HBV drug therapy. A recent review of clinical HBV disease provocatively states, "[i]ndeed, PCR has demonstrated the presence of HBV DNA after apparent clinical, biochemical, and serological resolution of infection, a phenomenon that challenges the clinical relevance and biological significance of a positive result with an assay of such exquisite sensitivity"[89].

## Properties of HBV DNA tests

Three basic approaches have been used to detect and quantitate HBV DNA. The first utilizes the PCR to amplify minute quantities of DNA, the second uses a signal amplification system to detect small quantities of DNA and the third uses nucleic acid hybridization to specifically capture HBV DNA from clinical specimens. The properties of the commonly used assays are summarized in Table 4.

With a sensitivity of 400 copies/ml, the quantitative AMPLICOR HBV MONITOR test is at least 1000-fold more sensitive than the Quantiplex test. The Quantiplex test is approximately 4-fold more sensitive than the Digene Hybrid-Capture System test and at least 40-fold more sensitive than the Abbott liquid hybridization test (see footnote in Table 4). Due to its much greater sensitivity, the AMPLICOR HBV MONITOR test should enable researchers to overcome many of the limitations of early studies, providing us with a more complete understanding of the relationship between HBV DNA load, prognosis and response to therapy.

The AMPLICOR HBV MONITOR test contains an internal control that monitors the efficiency of specimen extraction and amplification and serves as an internal quantitation standard. The AMPLICOR test also incorporates a contamination control system to guard against contamination caused by carry-over of previously amplified DNA.

Table 4. Comparison of quantitative HBV DNA tests

| | AMPLICOR HBV MONITOR* | Quantiplex HBV DNA Assay† | Hybrid Capture System HBV-DNA | Abbott HBV DNA Assay |
|---|---|---|---|---|
| Method | Target amplification | Signal amplification | Nucleic acid hybridization | Nucleic acid hybridization |
| Sensitivity | ~400 copies/ml | $7\times10^5$ copies/ml (2.5 pg DNA/ml) | 10 pg DNA/ml | 2 pg DNA/ml‡ |
| Dynamic range | $10^3$–$10^7$ copies/ml | $10^{5.8}$–$10^{9.7}$ copies/ml (2.5–17700 pg DNA/ml) | 10–2000 pg DNA/ml | 2≥2000 pg DNA/ml‡ |
| Internal control | Yes | N/A | N/A | N/A |
| Carry-over contamination control | Yes | N/A | N/A | N/A |
| Automation | Automated amplification | Manual, automated calculation of results | Manual | Manual |

*A fully automated COBAS AMPLICOR version of this test will be available in 1998.
†The Quantiplex assay reports results in units of genome equivalents. These are approximately equivalent to copies of target DNA.
‡These values may underestimate the actual DNA concentration in test samples and, thus, overestimate sensitivity. Concentrations calculated by the Abbott assay are approximately 40- to 100-fold and 35-fold lower than those obtained when the same sample is tested by the Quantiplex and Hybrid Capture System HBV-DNA assays, respectively [90,91].
N/A, not applicable.

## Characteristics of AMPLICOR HBV MONITOR test

In the AMPLICOR HBV MONITOR test, only one of the two primer oligonucleotides is biotinylated, enabling amplification products to be captured on streptavidin-coated microwell plates. The captured double-stranded DNA is then denatured. The DNA strand that contains the biotinylated primer remains bound to the plate while the DNA strand containing the non-biotinylated primer is released and washed away. The bound DNA is detected using labelled oligonucleotide probe. Separate probes are used to detect amplified target and the co-amplified internal control DNA.

HBV DNA is quantitated by determining the ratio of the HBV-specific signal to the internal control signal for each specimen. This ratio is converted into the input HBV concentration using a standard curve. A series of reactions containing known amounts of HBV DNA are included in each run to construct the standard curve. For this set of reactions, the ratios of HBV signal to the internal control signal are plotted versus the input HBV DNA concentrations. This format provides for accurate quantitation over a broad dynamic range of $10^3$ to $10^7$ copies/ml (Fig. 4).

## Utility of HBV DNA tests in clinical trials

The potential value of a sensitive HBV DNA test was illustrated by a recent study in which the AMPLICOR

HBV MONITOR test was used to follow patients receiving combination therapy. Patients who had failed interferon therapy were re-treated with a combination of interferon and lamivudine. The AMPLICOR test showed that the viral DNA was greatly reduced, but not eliminated (Fig. 5). The viral load rebounded one month after therapy was stopped, but a modest, stable reduction in viral load was induced by an additional 6 month treatment with lamivudine alone (Fig. 5).

Figure 4. Linearity of the AMPLICOR HBV test

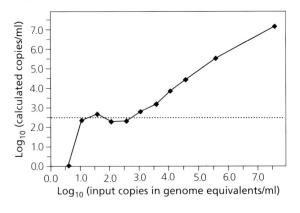

Samples of the CLB panel containing various concentrations of HBV DNA were tested by the AMPLICOR HBV MONITOR test. For each sample, the log of the calculated concentration was plotted against the log of the input concentration. The point on the x-axis represents a sample that gave a negative test result.

Figure 5. HBV DNA level in an individual with chronic hepatitis B who failed interferon therapy

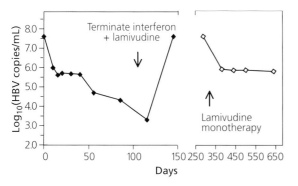

Lamivudine plus interferon combination therapy was initiated on Day 0 and terminated as indicated. Six months after the HBV DNA recovered, lamivudine monotherapy was initiated as indicated.

Figure 6. HBV DNA level in a liver transplant patient

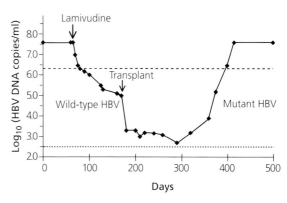

Lamivudine therapy was initiated and transplantation was performed as indicated. The long and short dashed lines represent the limit of detection for the Abbott DNA hybridization assay and the AMPLICOR HBV MONITOR test, respectively. Resistant, mutant virus was detected upon recovery of the HBV DNA titre.

Another recent study suggests that the AMPLICOR HBV MONITOR test may also prove useful for tracking HBV infection in liver transplant patients. Lamivudine was administered prior to and after transplantation in an attempt to prevent viral damage to the transplanted liver. Transplantation was delayed until the viral load was decreased substantially. In four of nine patients, HBV DNA was not detected at the time of transplant, but the other five had relatively low burdens. Seven of the nine patients were free of HBV DNA during follow-up. Two patients did relapse due to the appearance of lamivudine-resistant virus; the AMPLICOR test detected an increase in viral replication three months earlier than a less sensitive, conventional hybridization test (Fig. 6).

These studies suggest that highly sensitive PCR assays will contribute significantly to our understanding of the relationship between HBV replication and clinical outcome, and, thus, be useful for evaluating new drug treatments. HBV infection may prove to be somewhat different from HCV infection, where elimination of circulating virus is the therapeutic goal. PCR assays may reveal that there are 'acceptable' levels of HBV virus in arrested disease and that chronic therapies, more like those used for HIV infection, may be able to maintain health in the face of HBV infection.

## SUMMARY

Because of their unsurpassed sensitivity, PCR tests for HCV RNA and HBV DNA will provide new insights into the relationship between viral load and disease progression. This new knowledge should help us target therapies to those who have the highest probability of responding. We should also be able to identify better surrogate endpoints for evaluating new therapeutic regimens. Indeed, standardized, highly reproducible PCR tests may prove instrumental in comparing the efficacy of different drug combinations, doses and treatment schedules. As our knowledge increases, sensitive, quantitative HCV RNA and HBV DNA tests may, like HIV-1 RNA tests, become standard practice for monitoring antiviral therapy.

## ACKNOWLEDGEMENTS

We thank Sue Tsang for providing the TaqMan results. The lamivudine therapy studies in HBV-infected patients were conducted in collaboration with D Mutimer.

## REFERENCES

1. Piatak M Jr, Saag MS, Yang LC, Clark SJ, Kappes JC, Luk KC, Hahn BH, Shaw GM & Lifson JD. High levels of HIV-1 in plasma during all stages of infection determined by competitive PCR. *Science* 1993; **259**:1749–1754.
2. Ho DD, Neumann AU, Perelson AS, Chen W, Leonard JM & Markowitz M. Rapid turnover of plasma virions and CD4 lymphocytes in HIV-1 infection. *Nature* 1995; **373**:123–126.
3. Perelson AS, Neumann AU, Markowitz M, Leonard JM & Ho DD. HIV-1 dynamics in vivo: virion clearance rate, infected cell life-span, and viral generation time. *Science* 1996; **271**:1582–1586.
4. Havlir DV & Richman DD. Viral dynamics of HIV: implications for drug development and therapeutic strategies. *Annals of Internal Medicine* 1996; **124**:984–994.

5. Henrard DR, Phillips JF, Muenz LR, Blattner WA, Wiesner D, Eyster ME & Goedert JJ. Natural history of HIV-1 cell-free viremia. *Journal of the American Medical Association* 1995; **274**:554–558.

6. Lathey JL, Hughes MD, Fiscus SA, Pi T, Jackson JB, Rasheed S, Elbeik T, Reichman R, Japour A, D'Aquila RT, Scott W, Griffith BP, Hammer SM & Katzenstein DA for the AIDS Clinical Trials Group Protocol 175 Team. Variability and prognostic values of virologic and CD4 cell measures in Human Immunodeficiency Virus Type 1-infected patients with 200–500 CD4 cells/mm³. *Journal of Infectious Diseases* 1998; **177**:617–624.

7. Mellors JW, Kingsley LA, Rinaldo CR Jr, Todd JA, Hoo BS, Kokka RP & Gupta P. Quantitation of HIV-1 RNA in plasma predicts outcome after seroconversion. *Annals of Internal Medicine* 1995; **122**:573–579.

8. Mellors JW, Rinaldo CR Jr, Gupta P, White RM, Todd JA & Kingsley LA. Prognosis in HIV-1 infection predicted by the quantity of virus in plasma. *Science* 1996; **272**:1167–1170.

9. O'Brien WA, Hartigan PM, Martin D, Esinhart J, Hill A, Benoit S, Rubin M, Simberkoff MS & Hamilton JD. Changes in plasma HIV-1 RNA and CD4⁺ lymphocyte counts and the risk of progression to AIDS. Veterans Affairs Cooperative Study Group on AIDS. *New England Journal of Medicine* 1996; **334**:426–431.

10. Saksela K, Stevens CE, Rubinstein P, Taylor PE & Baltimore D. HIV-1 messenger RNA in peripheral blood mononuclear cells as an early marker of risk for progression to AIDS. *Annals of Internal Medicine* 1995; **123**:641–648.

11. Wong MT, Dolan MJ, Kozlow E, Doe R, Melcher GP, Burke DS, Boswell RN & Vahey M. Patterns of virus burden and T cell phenotype are established early and are correlated with the rate of disease progression in human immunodeficiency virus type 1-infected persons. *Journal of Infectious Diseases* 1996; **173**:877–887.

12. Fiscus SA, Hughes MD, Lathey JL, Pi T, Jackson JB, Rasheed S, Elbeik T, Reichman R, Japour A, Byington R, Scott W, Griffith BP, Katzenstein DA & Hammer SM for the AIDS Clinical Trials Group Protocol 175 Team. Changes in virologic markers as predictors of CD4 cell decline and progression of disease in human immunodeficiency virus type 1-infected adults treated with nucleosides. *Journal of Infectious Diseases* 1998; **177**:625–633.

13. Hughes MD, Johnson VA, Hirsch MS, Bremer JW, Elbeik T, Erice A, Kuritzkes DR, Scott WA, Spector SA, Basgoz N, Fischl MA & D'Aquila RT. Monitoring plasma HIV-1 RNA levels in addition to CD4⁺ lymphocyte count improves assessment of antiretroviral therapeutic response. ACTG 241 Protocol Virology Substudy Team. *Annals of Internal Medicine* 1997; **126**:929–938.

14. O'Brien WA, Hartigan PM, Daar ES, Simberkoff MS & Hamilton JD. Changes in plasma HIV RNA levels and CD4⁺ lymphocyte counts predict both response to antiretroviral therapy and therapeutic failure. VA Cooperative Study Group on AIDS. *Annals of Internal Medicine* 1997; **126**:939–945.

15. Eron JJ, Benoit SL, Jemsek J, MacArthur RD, Santana J, Quinn JB, Kuritzkes DR, Fallon MA & Rubin M. Treatment with lamivudine, zidovudine, or both in HIV-positive patients with 200 to 500 CD4⁺ cells per cubic millimeter. North American HIV Working Party. *New England Journal of Medicine* 1995; **333**:1662–1669.

16. Gulick RM, Mellors JW, Havlir D, Eron JJ, Gonzalez C, McMahon D, Richman DD, Valentine FT, Jonas L, Meibohm A, Emini EA & Chodakewitz JA. Treatment with indinavir, zidovudine, and lamivudine in adults with human immunodeficiency virus infection and prior antiretroviral therapy. *New England Journal of Medicine* 1997; **337**:734–739.

17. Myers MW, Montaner JSG & the INCAS Study Group. A randomized, double-blinded comparative trial of the effects of zidovudine, didanosine and nevirapine combinations in antiviral naïve, AIDS-free HIV-infected patients with CD4 counts 200–600/mm³. *XI International Conference on AIDS*. Vancouver, Canada, 7–12 July 1996; Abstract Mo B294.

18. Perelson AS, Essunger P, Cao Y, Vesanen M, Hurley A, Saksela K, Markowitz M & Ho DD. Decay characteristics of HIV-1-infected compartments during combination therapy. *Nature* 1997; **387**:188–191.

19. Carpenter CC, Fischl MA, Hammer SM, Hirsch MS, Jacobsen DM, Katzenstein DA, Montaner JS, Richman DD, Saag MS, Schooley RT, Thompson MA, Vella S, Yeni PG & Volberding PA. Antiretroviral therapy for HIV infection in 1996. Recommendations of an international panel. International AIDS Society-USA. *Journal of the American Medical Association* 1996; **276**:146–154.

20. Saag MS, Holodniy M, Kuritzkes DR, O'Brien WA, Coombs R, Poscher ME, Jacobsen DM, Shaw GM, Richman DD & Volberding PA. HIV viral load markers in clinical practice. *Nature Medicine* 1996; **2**:625–629.

21. Volberding PA. HIV quantification: clinical applications. *Lancet* 1996; **347**:71–73.

22. BHIVA Guidelines Co-ordinating Committee. British HIV Association guidelines for antiretroviral treatment of HIV seropositive individuals. *Lancet* 1997; **349**:1086–1092.

23. Office of Public Health and Science, Department of Health and Human Services. Guidelines for the use of antiretroviral agents in HIV-infected adults. *Federal Register* 1997; **62**:33417–33418.

24. Centers for Disease Control and Prevention. Public Health Service task force recommendations for the use of antiretroviral drugs in pregnant women infected with HIV-1 for maternal health and for reducing perinatal HIV-1 transmission in the United States. *Morbidity and Mortality Weekly Report* 1998; **47**(No. RR-2):1–39.

25. Centers for Disease Control and Prevention. Guidelines for the use of antiretroviral agents in pediatric HIV infection. *Morbidity and Mortality Weekly Report* 1998; **47**(No. RR-4): 1–51.

26. The Global Programme for Vaccines and Immunization, the Division of Child Health and Development & the Division of Reproductive Health (Technical Support) of the World Health Organization. Hepatitis B and breastfeeding. *Division of Child Health Update* November, 1996; **22** (available at: http://www.who.ch/chd/pub/newslet/update/updt-22.htm).

27. Shapiro CN, Mahoney FJ and Mast EE. Hepatitis B. In *Manual for the Surveillance of Vaccine-Preventable Diseases*, 1997; Edited by M Wharton & S Roush. Atlanta: Centers for Disease Control and Prevention.

28. World Health Organization. Hepatitis C: global prevalence. *Weekly Epidemiological Record* 1997; **72**:341–344.

29. Wong DK, Cheung AM, O'Rourke K, Naylor CD, Detsky AS & Heathcote J. Effect of alpha-interferon treatment in patients with hepatitis B e antigen-positive

chronic hepatitis B. A meta-analysis. *Annals of Internal Medicine* 1993; **119**:312–323.

30. Davis GL, Balart LA, Schiff ER, Lindsay K, Bodenheimer HC Jr, Perrillo RP, Carey W, Jacobson IM, Payne J, Dienstag JL, Van Thiel DH, Tamburro C, Lefkowitch J, Albrecht J, Meschievitz C, Ortego TJ & Gibas A. Treatment of chronic hepatitis C with recombinant interferon alfa. A multicenter randomized, controlled trial. Hepatitis Interventional Therapy Group. *New England Journal of Medicine* 1989; **321**:1501–1506.

31. Di Bisceglie AM, Martin P, Kassianides C, Lisker-Melman M, Murray L, Waggoner J, Goodman Z, Banks SM & Hoofnagle JH. Recombinant interferon alfa therapy for chronic hepatitis C. A randomized, double-blind, placebo-controlled trial. *New England Journal of Medicine* 1989; **321**:1506–1510.

32. Causse X, Godinot H, Chevallier M, Chossegros P, Zoulim F, Ouzan D, Heyraud JP, Fontanges T, Albrecht J, Meschievitz C & Trepo C. Comparison of 1 or 3 MU of interferon alfa-2b and placebo in patients with chronic non-A, non-B hepatitis. *Gastroenterology* 1991; **101**:497–502.

33. Marcellin P, Boyer N, Giostra E, Degott C, Courouce AM, Degos F, Coppere H, Cales P, Couzigou P & Benhamou JP. Recombinant human alpha-interferon in patients with chronic non-A, non-B hepatitis: a multicenter randomized controlled trial from France. *Hepatology* 1991; **13**:393–397.

34. Poynard T, Leroy V, Cohard M, Thevenot T, Mathurin P, Opolon P & Zarski JP. Meta-analysis of interferon randomized trials in the treatment of viral hepatitis C: effects of dose and duration. *Hepatology* 1996; **24**:778–789.

35. Poynard T, Leroy V, Mathurin P, Cohard M, Opolon P & Zarski JP. Treatment of chronic hepatitis C by interferon for longer duration than six months. *Digestive Diseases and Sciences* 1996; **41**(Supplement): 99S–102S.

36. Hoofnagle JH. Therapy of acute and chronic viral hepatitis. *Advances in Internal Medicine* 1994; **39**: 241–275.

37. Chemello L, Bonetti P, Cavalletto L, Talato F, Donadon V, Casarin P, Belussi F, Frezza M, Noventa F, Pontisso P, Benvegnu L, Casarin C & Albert A. Randomized trial comparing three different regimens of alpha 2a-interferon in chronic hepatitis C. The TriVeneto Viral Hepatitis Group. *Hepatology* 1995; **22**:700–706.

38. Lindsay KL, Davis GL, Schiff ER, Bodenheimer HC, Balart LA, Dienstag JL, Perrillo RP, Tamburro CH, Goff JS, Everson GT, Silva M, Katkov WN, Goodman Z, Lau JY, Maertens G, Gogate J, Sanghvi B & Albrecht J. Response to higher doses of interferon alfa-2b in patients with chronic hepatitis C: a randomized multicenter trial. Hepatitis Interventional Therapy Group. *Hepatology* 1996; **24**:1034–1040.

39. Rumi M, Del Ninno E, Parravicini ML, Romeo R, Soffredini R, Donato MF, Wilber J, Russo A & Colombo M. A prospective, randomized trial comparing lymphoblastoid to recombinant interferon alfa 2a as therapy for chronic hepatitis C. *Hepatology* 1996; **24**:1366–1370.

40. Manesis EK, Papaioannou C, Gioustozi A, Kafiri G, Koskinas J & Hadziyannis SJ. Biochemical and virological outcome of patients with chronic hepatitis C treated with interferon alfa-2b for 6 or 12 months: a 4-year follow-up of 211 patients. *Hepatology* 1997; **26**:734–739.

41. Chemello L, Cavalletto L, Bernardinello E, Guido M, Pontisso P & Alberti A. The effect of interferon alfa and ribavirin combination therapy in naive patients with chronic hepatitis C. *Journal of Hepatology* 1995; **23** (Supplement 2):8–12.

42. Brillanti S, Miglioli M & Barbara L. Combination antiviral therapy with ribavirin and interferon alfa in interferon alfa relapsers and non-responders: Italian experience. *Journal of Hepatology* 1995; **23** (Supplement 2):13–15.

43. Lai MY, Kao JH, Yang PM, Wang JT, Chen PJ, Chan KW, Chu JS & Chen DS. Long-term efficacy of ribavirin plus interferon alfa in the treatment of chronic hepatitis C. *Gastroenterology* 1996; **111**:1307–1311.

44. Schalm SW, Hansen BE, Chemello L, Bellobuono A, Brouwer JT, Weiland O, Cavalletto L, Schvarcz R, Ideo G & Alberti A. Ribavirin enhances the efficacy but not the adverse effects of interferon in chronic hepatitis C. Meta-analysis of individual patient data from European centers. *Journal of Hepatology* 1997; **26**:961–966.

45. Reichard O, Norkrans G, Fryden A, Braconier JH, Sonnerborg A & Weiland O. Randomised, double-blind, placebo-controlled trial of interferon alpha-2b with and without ribavirin for chronic hepatitis C. The Swedish Study Group. *Lancet* 1998; **351**:83–87.

46. Dienstag JL, Perrillo RP, Schiff ER, Bartholomew M, Vicary C & Rubin M. A preliminary trial of lamivudine for chronic hepatitis B infection. *New England Journal of Medicine* 1995; **333**:1657–1661.

47. Nevens F, Main J, Honkoop P, Tyrrell DL, Barber J, Sullivan MT, Fevery J, De Man RA & Thomas HC. Lamivudine therapy for chronic hepatitis B: a six-month randomized dose-ranging study. *Gastroenterology* 1997; **113**:1258–1263.

48. Rostaing L, Henry S, Cisterne JM, Duffaut M, Icart J, Durand D. Efficacy and safety of lamivudine on replication of recurrent hepatitis B after cadaveric renal transplantation. *Transplantation* 1997; **64**:1624–1627.

49. Dusheiko G, Whalley S, Manolakopoulos S, Davies S, Ling R, Harrison T, Grellier L & Brown D. Lamivudine treatment of advanced hepatitis B. *Second International Conference on Therapies for Viral Hepatitis*, Kona, Big Island, Hawaii, 15–19 December 1997; Abstract O32.

50. Trepo C, Atkinson GF & Boon RJ. Famciclovir treatment in chronic hepatitis B - predictors of response. *Second International Conference on Therapies for Viral Hepatitis*, Kona, Big Island, Hawaii, 15–19 December 1997; Abstract O33.

51. Virani-Ketter N. Adefovir dipivoxil for the treatment of chronic hepatitis B. *Second International Conference on Therapies for Viral Hepatitis*, Kona, Big Island, Hawaii, 15–19 December 1997; Abstract O34.

52. Bloomer J, Chan R, Sherman M, Ingraham P, De Hertog D & the -008 Study Group. Phase 1/2 study of oral lobucavir in adults with chronic hepatitis B infection. *Second International Conference on Therapies for Viral Hepatitis*, Kona, Big Island, Hawaii, 15–19 December 1997; Abstract O35.

53. Hoofnagle JH & Di Bisceglie AM. The treatment of viral hepatitis. *New England Journal of Medicine* 1997; **336**:347–356.

54. Lau JY, Davis GL, Kniffen J, Qian KP, Urdea MS, Chan CS, Mizokami M, Neuwald PD & Wilber JC. Significance of serum hepatitis C virus RNA levels in chronic hepatitis C. *Lancet* 1993; **341**:1501–1504.

55. Diodati G, Bonetti P, Noventa F, Casarin C, Rugge M,

Scaccabarozzi S, Tagger A, Pollice L, Tremolada F, Davite C, Realdi G & Ruol A. Treatment of chronic hepatitis C with recombinant human interferon-alpha 2a: results of a randomized controlled clinical trial. *Hepatology* 1994; **19**:1–5.

56. Magrin S, Craxi A, Fabiano C, Simonetti RG, Fiorentino G, Marino L, Diquattro O, Di Marco V, Loiacono O, Volpes R, Almasio P, Urdea MS, Neuwald P, Sanchez-Pescador R, Detmer J, Wilber JC & Pagliaro L. Hepatitis C viremia in chronic liver disease: relationship to interferon-alpha or corticosteroid treatment. *Hepatology* 1994; **19**:273–279.

57. Bonetti P, Chemello L, Antona C, Breda A, Brosolo P, Casarin P, Crivellaro C, Dona G, Martinelli S, Rinaldi R, Zennaro V, Santonastaso M, Urban F, Pontisso P & Alberti A. Treatment of chronic hepatitis C with interferon-alpha by monitoring the response according to viraemia. *Journal of Viral Hepatitis* 1997; **4**:107–112.

58. Ichijo T, Matsumoto A, Kobayashi M, Furihata K & Tanaka E. Quantitative measurement of HCV RNA in the serum: a comparison of three assays based on different principles. *Journal of Gastroenterology and Hepatology* 1997; **12**:500–506.

59. Shiratori Y, Kato N, Yokosuka O, Hashimoto E, Hayashi N, Nakamura A, Asada M, Kuroda H, Ohkubo H, Arakawa Y, Iwama A & Omata M. Quantitative assays for hepatitis C virus in serum as predictors of the long-term response to interferon. *Journal of Hepatology* 1997; **27**:437–444.

60. Bennett WG, Inoue Y, Beck JR, Wong JB, Pauker SG & Davis GL. Estimates of the cost-effectiveness of a single course of interferon-$\alpha$2b in patients with histologically mild chronic hepatitis C. *Annals of Internal Medicine* 1997; **127**:855–865.

61. Wong JB, Koff RS, Tine F & Pauker SG. Cost-effectiveness of interferon-alpha 2b treatment for hepatitis B e antigen-positive chronic hepatitis B. *Annals of Internal Medicine* 1995; **122**:664–675.

62. Koff RS. Therapy of Hepatitis C: cost-effectiveness analysis. *Hepatology* 1997; **26** (Supplement 1):152S–155S.

63. Kim WR, Poterucha JJ, Hermans JE, Therneau TM, Dickson ER, Evans RW & Gross JB. Cost-effectiveness of 6 and 12 months of interferon-$\alpha$ therapy for chronic hepatitis C. *Annals of Internal Medicine* 1997; **127**:866–874.

64. Fried MW. Clinical applications of hepatitis C virus genotyping and quantitation. *Clinics in Liver Disease* 1997; **1**: 631–645.

65. Tsubota A, Chayama K, Ikeda K, Yasuji A, Koida I, Saitoh S, Hashimoto M, Iwasaki S, Kobayashi M & Hiromitsu K. Factors predictive of response to interferon-alpha therapy in hepatitis C virus infection. *Hepatology* 1994; **19**:1088–1094.

66. Martinot-Peignoux M, Marcellin P, Pouteau M, Castelnau C, Boyer N, Poliquin M, Degott C, Descombes I, Le Breton V, Milotova V, Benhamou JP & Erlinger S. Pretreatment serum hepatitis C virus RNA levels and hepatitis C virus genotype are the main and independent prognostic factors of sustained response to interferon alfa therapy in chronic hepatitis C. *Hepatology* 1995; **22**: 1050–1056.

67. Nousbaum JB, Pol S, Nalpas B, Landais P, Berthelot P & Brechot C. Hepatitis C virus type 1b (II) infection in France and Italy. Collaborative Study Group. *Annals of Internal Medicine* 1995; **122**:161–168.

68. Yamada G, Takatani M, Kishi F, Takahashi M, Doi T, Tsuji T, Shin S, Tanno M, Urdea MS & Kolberg JA.

Efficacy of interferon alfa therapy in chronic hepatitis C patients depends primarily on hepatitis C virus RNA level. *Hepatology* 1995; **22**:1351–1354.

69. Niederau C, Heintges T, Lange S, Goldmann G, Niederau CM, Mohr L & Häussinger D. Long-term follow-up of HBeAg-positive patients treated with interferon alpha for chronic hepatitis B. *New England Journal of Medicine* 1996; **334**:1422–1427.

70. Lau JY, Mizokami M, Ohno T, Diamond DA, Kniffen J & Davis GL. Discrepancy between biochemical and virological responses to interferon-alpha in chronic hepatitis C. *Lancet* 1993; **342**:1208–1209.

71. Marcellin P, Boyer N, Degott C, Martinot-Peignoux M, Duchatelle V, Giostra E, Areias J, Erlinger S & Benhamou JP. Long-term histologic and viral changes in patients with chronic hepatitis C who responded to alpha interferon. *Liver* 1994; **14**:302–307.

72. Chemello L, Cavalletto L, Casarin C, Bonetti P, Bernardinello E, Pontisso P, Donada C, Belussi F, Martinelli S & Alberti A. Persistent hepatitis C viremia predicts late relapse after sustained response to interferon-alpha in chronic hepatitis C. TriVeneto Viral Hepatitis Group. *Annals of Internal Medicine* 1996; **124**:1058–1060.

73. Brunetto MR, Oliveri F, Rocca G, Criscuolo D, Chiaberge E, Capalbo M, David E, Verme G & Bonino F. Natural course and response to interferon of chronic hepatitis B accompanied by antibody to hepatitis B e antigen. *Hepatology* 1989; **10**:198–202.

74. Fattovich G, Farci P, Rugge M, Brollo L, Mandas A, Pontisso P, Giustina G, Lai ME, Belussi F, Busatto G, Balestrieri A, Ruol A & Alberti A. A randomized controlled trial of lymphoblastoid interferon-alpha in patients with chronic hepatitis B lacking HBeAg. *Hepatology* 1992; **15**:584–589.

75. Hadziyannis SJ. Hepatitis B e antigen negative chronic hepatitis B: from clinical recognition to pathogenesis and treatment. *Viral Hepatitis Reviews* 1995; **1**:7–15.

76. Kako M, Kanai K, Aikawa T, Iwabuchi S, Takehira Y, Kawasaki T, Tsubouchi H, Hino K, Tsuda F, Okamoto H, Miyakawa Y & Mayumi M. Response to interferon-alpha 2a in patients with e antigen-negative chronic hepatitis B. *Journal of Clinical Gastroenterology* 1997; **25**:440–445.

77. Schmidt WN, Wu P, Han JQ, Perion MJ, LaBrecque DR & Stapleton JT. Distribution of hepatitis C virus RNA in whole blood and blood cell fractions: plasma HCV RNA analysis underestimates circulating virus load. *Journal of Infectious Diseases*, 1997; **176**:20–26.

78. Dusheiko G, Schmilovitz-Weiss H, Brown D, McOmish F, Yap PL, Sherlock S, McIntyre N & Simmonds P. Hepatitis C virus genotypes: an investigation of type-specific differences in geographic origin and disease. *Hepatology* 1994; **19**:13–18.

79. Pol S, Thiers V, Nousbaum JB, Legendre C, Berthelot P, Kreis H & Brechot C. The changing relative prevalence of hepatitis C virus genotypes: evidence in hemodialyzed patients and kidney recipients. *Gastroenterology* 1995; **108**:581–583.

80. Lau JY, Davis GL, Prescott LE, Maertens G, Lindsay KL, Qian K, Mizokami M & Simmonds P. Distribution of hepatitis C virus genotypes determined by line probe assay in patients with chronic hepatitis C seen at tertiary referral centers in the United States. Hepatitis Interventional Therapy Group. *Annals of Internal Medicine* 1996; **124**:868–876.

81. Polyak SJ & Gretch DR. Molecular diagnostic testing

for viral hepatitis: methods and applications. In *Viral Hepatitis: Diagnosis - Treatment - Prevention*, 1997; pp.1–34. Edited by RA Willson. New York: Marcel Dekker, Inc.

82. Zaaijer HL, Cuypers HTM, Reesink HW, Winkel IN, Gerkin G & Lelie PN. Reliability of polymerase chain reaction for detection of hepatitis C virus. *Lancet* 1993; **341**:722–724.

83. Damen M, Cuypers HTM, Zaaijer HL, Reesink HW, Schaasberg WP, Gerlich WH, Niesters HGM & Lelie PN. International collaborative study on the second EUROHEP HCV-RNA reference panel. *Journal of Virological Methods* 1996; **58**:175–185.

84. Holland PM, Abramson RD, Watson R & Gelfand DH. Detection of specific polymerase chain reaction product by utilizing the 5′–3′ exonuclease activity of *Thermus aquaticus*. *Proceedings of the National Academy of Sciences, USA,* 1991; **88**:7276–7280.

85. Livak KJ, Flood SJA, Marmaro J, Giusti W & Deetz K. Oligonucleotides with fluorescent dyes at opposite ends provide a quenched probe system useful for detecting PCR product and nucleic acid hybridization. *PCR Methods and Applications* 1995; **4**:357–362.

86. Amgen Inc. *INFERGEN Package Insert*. 1997. Thousand Oaks, California: Amgen Inc.

87. NIH Consensus Statement Online 1997 March 24–26 [cited 98 May 07]; 15(3): in press. (available at http://odp.od.nih.gov/consensus/statements/cdc/105/10 5_stmt.html)

88. Davis GL & Lau JYN. Factors predictive of a beneficial response to therapy of hepatitis C. *Hepatology* 1997; **26** (Supplement 1):122S–127S.

89. Rogers SA, Dienstag JL & Liang TJ. Hepatitis B virus: clinical disease – prevention and therapy. In *Viral Hepatitis: Diagnosis - Treatment - Prevention*, 1997; pp.119–146. Edited by RA Willson. New York: Marcel Dekker.

90. Butterworth LA, Prior SL, Buda PJ, Faoagali JL & Cooksley WGE. Comparison of four methods for quantitative measurement of hepatitis B viral DNA. *Journal of Viral Hepatology* 1996; **24**:686–691.

91. Kapke GE, Watson G, Sheffler S, Hunt D & Frederick C. Comparison of the Chiron Quantiplex branched DNA (bDNA) assay and the Genostics solution hybridization assay for quantification of hepatitis B viral DNA. *Journal of Viral Hepatitis* 1997; **4**:67–75.

# 14 New developments in hepatitis C diagnostics and monitoring

## Judith C Wilber

## SUMMARY

Technological advances in tests for hepatitis C virus (HCV) have enabled their application to diagnosis, viral typing and monitoring the effects of antiviral therapy. One approach to testing is to detect antibodies to a range of HCV antigens, either by enzyme immunoassay or by strip immunoassay. Sensitivity continues to increase with increases in the number of viral antigens to which antibodies can be detected. These tests are most useful for diagnosis and viral serotyping. Tests have been devised to detect viral RNA itself, generally by reverse transcriptase–PCR, and to quantify HCV RNA, by branched DNA (bDNA) signal amplification technology or RT–PCR. These methods provide a more direct measurement of the progress of disease and enable monitoring of the effects of therapy.

## INTRODUCTION

The first diagnostic assay for HCV became widely available in 1990. Since then, there have been rapid advances in the number of tools available for the diagnosis and monitoring of HCV infection and in our understanding of the virus. This paper describes a few of the new tests that can aid in determining or improving the efficacy of antiviral therapy.

### Diagnosis

HCV infection is diagnosed and detected in the donor blood supply by the use of antibody testing. First-generation enzyme immunoassays (EIAs) were developed by Houghton *et al.* at Chiron [1] using the first recombinant antigen, c100 antigen (genomic region NS3 and NS4), which was produced from the expanded clone of HCV. This antibody test was first introduced into blood screening in 1990, and it led to a great reduction in the number of cases of transfusion-associated hepatitis [2]. Once the full sequence of the HCV genome was elucidated and new antigens were discov-

ered, the sensitivities of antibody tests were improved in the subsequent generation of assays. Second-generation antibody tests include antigens C22 (from the capsid region) and C33 (from the NS3 genomic region). The latest assays also include an antigen derived from the full NS5 region. Another technique available, called the RIBA strip immunoassay (RIBA SIA), is similar to a Western blot. Nitrocellulose strips with recombinant and synthetic antigens are incubated with the patient's serum to detect specific antibody reactions. RIBA SIA 3.0 uses epitopes designed for greater sensitivity and specificity and detects antibody to portions of the c100, C22, C33 and NS5 antigens.

Before seroconversion, the viral load is extremely high, reaching peak levels long before the serum alanine aminotransferase (ALT) peak is seen [3]. After seroconversion, virus levels can become extremely low in the serum, often falling below the detection limits of qualitative RT–PCR for HCV RNA. Therefore, if the serology tests (EIA and RIBA SIA) are positive, a negative RT–PCR result should not be used to rule out HCV infection and should be followed up by further testing at a later date. Positive antibody tests with repeatedly negative RNA tests might represent resolved infection, which occurs in only 10–20% of HCV cases.

### Typing

HCV genotypes vary in their global distribution, although type 1 is the most common [4]. HCV type 1 has also been found to be the most unresponsive to therapy. Currently available genotyping methods are based on the following techniques: amplification of the 5′ untranslated region (5′ UTR) or NS5 region, followed by digestion with restriction enzymes and restriction fragment length polymorphism (RFLP) analysis; amplification of the capsid region of the genome with genotype-specific primers; hybridization of genotype-specific probes to amplified products from the 5′ UTR or NS5; and serotyping by SIA or EIA [5–8]. Direct sequencing is often necessary to resolve subtypes.

## Monitoring therapy

HCV and hepatitis B virus (HBV) can be quantified directly from serum using a solid-phase nucleic acid hybridization assay based on bDNA signal amplification technology. Serum ALT and other liver enzyme tests are essentially surrogate markers, as they are markers of liver disease but not of viral activity. Quantification of viral load has the advantage of providing information on viral kinetics and provides a greater knowledge of the disease process, as it yields a direct measurement of viraemia.

The bDNA assay is a quantitative signal-amplification method based on a series of specific hybridization reactions and chemiluminescent detection of hybridized probes in a microwell format. It involves binding of HCV RNA to the surface of a microwell plate by a series of probes that are complementary to 'capture' probe on the plate, the other part of the probe being specific for HCV RNA. Another series of probes is added, designed to be complementary to the RNA and to bind to synthetic bDNA molecules. Each bDNA molecule has 15 arms, and each arm can bind three alkaline phosphatase molecules. This gives the potential for 45 alkaline phosphatase molecules to bind to each bDNA, and in the HCV assay 18 bDNA molecules are bound to each HCV RNA molecule. Part of the design of new probes has been to ensure that each of the HCV genotypes is detected with equal efficiency [9,10]. The overall clinical sensitivity is over 91% and reproducibility is excellent [11,12].

The relationship between the initial viral load and the patient's response to therapy has been extensively studied using the bDNA technology [13–16]. I and my colleagues have combined data from all the studies in which our laboratory had participated, which yielded HCV RNA baseline levels determined by bDNA from 482 patients treated with interferon (IFN) whose biochemical response to treatment was known. For this analysis, a sustained response was defined as normalization of serum ALT for at least 6 months after the discontinuation of therapy (biochemical sustained response). The long-term viral response was not known in all cases and was therefore not analysed. The results demonstrated that there was no significant difference in initial viral load between non-responders and responders who relapsed. The majority of sustained responders, however, had very low baseline viral load. Quantification of HCV RNA by bDNA assay as a predictor of sustained response to administration of interferon in an HCV-infected population illustrates that in the entire population, 19% will have a sustained response to therapy, with this figure increasing to as high as 49% as the viral load decreases (Fig. 1). Knowledge of the predicted response to IFN therapy could help to set expectations for the patient. It is possible that those with high virus levels might benefit from more aggressive therapy, resulting in better long-term response rates.

Viral load in chronically HCV-infected patients is generally stable. In a subset of patients, however, RNA and ALT levels can fluctuate considerably, becoming stable only after several years. Fluctuations are also seen more frequently after therapy is stopped. It is possible that improved treatment efficacy might be achieved if treatment or retreatment is initiated at a time point when a patient's viral load is at its lowest. In a small study conducted in Japan [17], therapy-naive individuals were grouped before initial treatment by their HCV RNA levels, as determined by the bDNA assay, into >10 million Eq/ml ($n=19$), 1–10 million Eq/ml ($n=22$), 0.5–1 million Eq/ml ($n=4$) and <0.5 million Eq/ml ($n=4$). All participants responded to therapy but eventually relapsed. Virus levels were noted at the time of retreatment, and, regardless of their pretherapy levels, the only patients who experienced a sustained response were those who had viral loads <10 million Eq/ml at the start of retreatment. The sustained response rates based on the viral load at the start of retreatment were 3/7 (42.9%) at <0.5 million Eq/ml; 2/7 (28.6%) at 0.5–1 million Eq/ml; 4/27 (14.8%) at 1–10 million Eq/ml; and 0/17 (0%) at >10 million Eq/ml. These results demonstrate that not only can accurate measurement of HCV RNA levels help predict a patient's response to therapy, it could also aid decisions about the timing of initiation of treatment or retreatment in HCV-infected individuals.

At the end of therapy, HCV RNA is often undetectable in the serum, even though many of these patients relapse. A preliminary study by Chien et al. [18] examined the potential clinical utility of measuring antibody titres to various antigens in predicting the long-term response to IFN therapy. Antibody profiles from ten responders and ten non-responders to IFN therapy were determined before and during IFN therapy (3 MU, three times weekly for 6 months), and again after discontinuation of therapy. Neither the absolute HCV antibody titres nor the antibody profile before therapy predicted the therapeutic outcome. No significant difference was detected in the NS4 (c100-3) and core (C22-3) antibody titres of responders and non-responders. There were some differences in antibody levels to products of the E2 region, but little dynamic change occurred with time. However, dynamic changes in HCV antibody titre to the non-structural antigens NS3 (C33) and NS5 (ns5) over the

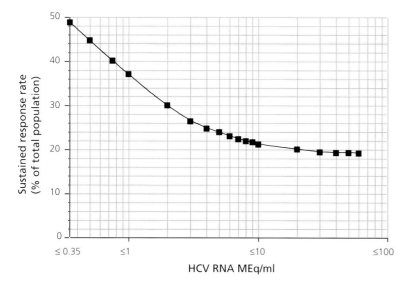

**Figure 1.** Quantification of HCV RNA using the bDNA assay as a predictor of sustained response to the administration of IFN in an HCV-infected population

Combined data from several studies, with a total of 482 patients. A sustained response was defined as the normalization of serum ALT levels for ≥6 months after therapy was stopped.

course of therapy significantly correlated ($P<0.001$) with sustained response to IFN therapy (undetectable serum HCV RNA and normalization of ALT levels for at least 1 year after treatment was stopped). Similar results have been obtained by measuring antibody levels to the same antigens in the RIBA format. Larger studies are needed to verify these findings in relation to genotype, viral load and histology.

Determining whether or not a patient has completely cleared the virus can be problematic, owing to residual viral replication in the liver. If a follow-up liver biopsy is performed to determine whether the histological appearance of the liver tissue has improved, examination of the liver biopsy material for HCV RNA could provide a way of determining the real response of a patient. A modification of the bDNA assay can be used to quantify HCV RNA in liver tissue, requiring only simple RNA extraction from liver biopsy samples, followed by the standard microplate assay [19]. As pure nucleic acid is not required for the bDNA procedure, the extraction procedure was optimized for RNA recovery, yielding results that reflected the concentration of the virus in the liver of the patient. In contrast, RT–PCR has been found to be inhibited by haem, which is present in high concentrations in liver tissue. This means that in this technique the RNA must be purified, which prevents the assay from being quantitative.

Finally, it is often noted that the bDNA assay is not as sensitive as target amplification methods. However, the achievable analytical sensitivity is as high as that of PCR. The bDNA procedure is similar to an EIA, as its sensitivity is also limited by the background signal.

To reduce non-specific hybridization, two new bases, iso-cytosine (iso-C) and iso-guanosine (iso-G), were synthesized and used in the development of new probes. These bases strongly base pair with each other, but as they are not naturally occurring bases they do not base pair with natural guanosine and cytosine. In this manner, non-specific hybridization between the bDNA amplifier and the capture probes has been reduced by substituting some cytosine and guanosine bases with iso-C and iso-G. This method has been used together with modifications in probe design and multisite pre-amplification molecules in a bDNA assay for HIV RNA, where the detection limit has been demonstrated to be 50 copies/ml.

## CONCLUSIONS

There are many questions that need to be answered in order to determine the best treatment for HCV-infected individuals, but there are several new tools to help guide decisions. To a great extent, the use of new diagnostic tools to optimize therapy awaits the development of better therapies and more choices in treatment regimens, but accurate measurement of viral load and other indicators of viral activity will help to define and refine antiviral therapy.

## REFERENCES

1. Houghton M, Weiner A, Han J, Kuo G & Choo Q-L. Molecular biology of the hepatitis C viruses: implications for diagnosis, development and control of viral disease. *Hepatology* 1991; **14:**381–388.
2. Alter HJ. Descartes before the horse: I clone, therefore

I am: the hepatitis C virus in current perspective. *Annals of Internal Medicine* 1991; **115**:644–649.

3. Alter HJ, Sanchez-Pescador R, Urdea MS, Wilber JC, Lagier RJ, Di Bisceglie AM, Shih JW & Neuwald PD. Evaluation of branched DNA signal amplification for the detection of hepatitis C virus RNA. *Journal of Viral Hepatitis* 1995; **2**:121–132.

4. Bukh J, Miller RH & Purcell RH. Genetic heterogeneity of hepatitis C virus: quasispecies and genotypes. *Seminars in Liver Disease* 1995; **15**:41–63.

5. Gish RG, Qian KP, Quan S, Xu YL, Pike I, Polito A, DiNello R & Lau JYN. Concordance between hepatitis C virus serotyping assays. *Journal of Viral Hepatitis* 1997; **4**:421–422.

6. Lau JYN, Davis GL, Prescott LE, Maertens G, Lindsay KL, Qian K, Mizokami M, Simmonds P & The Hepatitis Interventional Therapy Group. Distribution of hepatitis C virus genotypes determined by line probe assay in patients with chronic hepatitis C seen at tertiary referral centers in the United States. *Annals of Internal Medicine* 1996; **124**:868–876.

7. Simmonds P, Holmes EC, Cha T-A, Chan S-W, McOmish F, Irvine B, Beall E, Yap PL, Kolberg J & Urdea MS. Classification of hepatitis C virus into six major genotypes and a series of subtypes by phylogenetic analysis of the NS-5 region. *Journal of General Virology* 1993; **74**:2391–2399.

8. Simmonds P, Alberti A, Alter HJ, Bonino F, Bradley DW, Bréchot C, Brouwer JT, Chan S-W, Chayama K, Chen DS *et al.* A proposed system for the nomenclature of hepatitis C viral genotypes. *Hepatology* 1994; **19**:1321–1324.

9. Collins ML, Zayati C, Detmer JJ, Daly B, Kolberg JA, Cha T-A, Irvine BD, Tucker J & Urdea MS. Preparation and characterization of RNA standards for use in quantitative branched DNA hybridization assays. *Analytical Biochemistry* 1995; **226**:120–129.

10. Hawkins A, Davidson F & Simmonds P. Comparison of plasma virus loads among individuals infected with hepatitis C virus (HCV) genotypes 1, 2, and 3 by Quantiplex HCV RNA assay versions 1 and 2, Roche Monitor Assay, and an in-house limiting dilution method. *Journal of Clinical Microbiology* 1997; **35**:187–192.

11. Detmer J, Lagier R, Flynn J, Zayati C, Kolberg J, Collins M, Urdea M & Sanchez-Pescador R. Accurate quantification of hepatitis C virus (HCV) RNA from all HCV genotypes by using branched-DNA technology. *Journal of Clinical Microbiology* 1996; **34**:901–907.

12. Jacob S, Baudy D, Jones E, Lizhe X, Mason A, Regenstein F & Perrillo R. Comparison of quantitative HCV RNA assays in chronic hepatitis C. *American Journal of Clinical Pathology* 1997; **107**:362–367.

13. Lau JYN, Davis GL, Kniffen J, Qian K-P, Urdea MS, Chan CS, Mizokami M, Neuwald PD & Wilber JC. Significance of serum hepatitis C virus RNA levels in chronic hepatitis C. *Lancet* 1993; **341**:1501–1504.

14. Magrin S, Craxi A, Fabiano C, Simonetti RG, Fiorentino G, Marino L, Diquattro O, Di Marco V, Loiacono O, Volpes R, Almasio P, Urdea MS, Neuwald P, Sanchez-Pescador R, Detmer J, Wilber JC & Pagliaro L. Hepatitis C viremia in chronic liver disease: relationship to interferon-α or corticosteroid treatment. *Hepatology* 1994; **19**:273–279.

15. Yuki N, Hayashi N, Kasahara A, Hagiwara H, Takehara T, Oshita M, Katayama K, Fusamoto H & Kamada T. Pretreatment viral load and response to prolonged interferon-α course for chronic hepatitis C. *Journal of Hepatology* 1995; **22**:457–463.

16. Orito E, Mizokami M, Nakano T, Terashima H, Nojiri O, Sakakibara K, Mizuno M, Ogino M, Nakamura M, Matsumoto Y, Miyata K-I & Lau JYN. Serum hepatitis C virus RNA level as a predictor of subsequent response to interferon-a therapy in Japanese patients with chronic hepatitis C. *Journal of Medical Virology* 1994; **44**:410–414.

17. Arase Y, Kumada H, Chayama K, Naoya M, Tsubota A, Koida I, Kobayashi M, Suzuki Y, Ikeda K, Saitoh S & Kobayashi M. Usefulness of HCV-RNA counts by the method of HCV-bDNA probe in interferon retreatment for patients with HCV-RNA positive chronic hepatitis C. *International Hepatology Communications* 1995; **4**:19–25.

18. Chien DY, Tong MJ, Tabrizi-Wright A, Archangel P, Co RL, Sayadzadeh K, Ko E, Kuo C & Kuo G. Clinical usefulness of measuring antibody titers to hepatitis C virus non-structural NS3 and NS5 antigens in monitoring of the response to interferon therapy. *3rd International Meeting on Hepatitis C Virus and Related Viruses*, 1995, Gold Coast, Australia. Abstract C31.

19. Coehlo-Little E, Jeffers LJ, Bartholomew M, Reddy KR, Schiff ER & Dailey PJ. Correlation of HCV-RNA levels in serum and liver of patients with chronic hepatitis C. *Journal of Hepatology* 1995; **22**:248.

# 15 Genomic structure and variability of hepatitis C virus

Jens Bukh* and Robert H Purcell

## SUMMARY

Hepatitis C virus (HCV) is an important human pathogen that frequently causes chronic liver disease, including hepatocellular carcinoma. Its positive RNA genome has a single long open reading frame encoding at least ten proteins, some of which have been characterized by studies *in vitro*. Genetic analyses of the complete or partial genomic sequences of various HCV isolates have shown that the virus circulates as a quasispecies in the host, and that numerous genotypes with differing geographical distributions exist. Attempts to characterize these forms of HCV are taking place, using sequence analysis and other techniques.

## INTRODUCTION

Infection with HCV is common throughout the world and this virus is a major aetiological agent of acute and chronic hepatitis [1]. The acute infection is subclinical in the majority of HCV-infected individuals. However, more than 80% of the individuals acutely infected with HCV become chronically infected, and such chronic infection leads to the development of chronic liver diseases, including chronic hepatitis, liver cirrhosis and hepatocellular carcinoma. The RNA genome of HCV has been cloned and sequenced [2]. Further analysis of genomic sequence data obtained from multiple HCV isolates has demonstrated that HCV shows significant genetic heterogeneity (for a detailed review, see [3]). The extensive genetic variability of HCV is likely to have important implications for diagnosis, pathogenesis, treatment and vaccine development.

## GENOMIC ORGANIZATION

HCV is distantly related to the pestiviruses and flaviviruses [2,4–11], and was recently classified as a third genus of the family *Flaviviridae*, which has been provisionally named hepacivirus. HCV is also related to the recently discovered GB agents (GBV-A, GBV-B and GBV-C), which cause hepatitis in tamarins and humans [12–14]. These viral agents have not yet been classified.

Like all other members of the family *Flaviviridae*, HCV contains a single-stranded RNA genome of positive polarity [4–7,9–11]. The genome consists of a single, approximately 9 kb, open reading frame (ORF) that is enclosed by 5′ and 3′ non-coding (NC) regions. The 5′ NC region, which consists of ≤342 nucleotides, includes sequences with significant similarity to the 5′ NC sequences of members of the pestiviruses [4,15–17], as well as sequences with similarity to the 5′ NC sequence of the GBV-B virus [12]. The 3′ NC region consists of a short variable nucleotide sequence of <100 nucleotides followed by a poly(U) or poly(A) tract [4,7,9–11,15]. Recently, an additional 98 nucleotides were discovered 3′ of the poly(U) tract [18]. These nucleotides are presumably highly conserved among different HCV isolates. This additional sequence 3′ of the poly(U) tract also occurs in members of the pestiviruses [19], as well as in GB-B [12]. The single ORF of HCV encodes structural proteins (C, E1 and E2) and possible structural proteins (E2–p7 and p7) at its 5′ end and non-structural proteins (NS2, NS3, NS4A, NS4B, NS5A and NS5B) at its 3′ end. The predicted amino acid sequence of the polyproteins of HCV, pestiviruses, flaviviruses and the GB agents contain three collinear domains with significant similarity (serine proteases and nucleoside triphosphate-binding helicases in NS3; RNA-dependent RNA polymerase motifs in NS5B) [4,8,14]. Furthermore, the hydrophobicity plot of the HCV polyprotein is similar to that of the polyproteins of pestiviruses, flaviviruses and GB agents [4,7,11,14], indicating that these viruses have maintained a similar structure and function within the individual proteins. The genomic organization of the HCV genome is shown in Figure 1.

---

*Corresponding author

**Figure 1.** Genomic organization of HCV

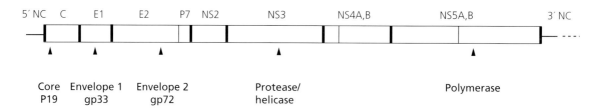

The single-stranded RNA genome of positive polarity consists of a single approximately 9 kb ORF that is enclosed by 5′ and 3′ non-coding (NC) regions. The 5′ NC region consists of ≤ 342 nucleotides. The 3′ NC region consists of a short variable nucleotide sequence of < 100 nucleotides followed 3′ by a poly(U) or a poly(A) tract and 98 additional nucleotides. The single ORF of HCV encodes structural proteins (C, E1 and E2) and possible structural proteins (E2–p7 and p7) at its 5′ end and non-structural proteins (NS2, NS3, NS4A, NS4B, NS5A and NS5B) at its 3′ end. The predicted functions of the HCV proteins are indicated.

## GENETIC HETEROGENEITY

Genetic heterogeneity of HCV has been found throughout the viral genome, although the degree of heterogeneity varies in different regions (reviewed in [3]). The most highly conserved sequences occur in the 5′ NC region, which contains several domains that are invariant among HCV isolates of the different genotypes [9,17,20]. Importantly, such conserved sequences have been used as the targets for the development of sensitive diagnostic reverse transcriptase–polymerase chain reaction (RT–PCR) assays [16,21,22]. The predicted nucleocapsid protein is the most highly conserved of the various viral proteins [9,10,23] and is an important part of current commercially available serological tests [24]. The envelope proteins are highly variable [9]. In particular, there is a short domain at the amino-terminal end of the E2 protein with extensive genetic heterogeneity [25,26]. This region was termed hypervariable region 1 (HVR1). Among the non-structural proteins the most conserved sequences were found in the NS3 and NS5B proteins.

## SPECTRUM OF GENETIC HETEROGENEITY

The genetic heterogeneity of HCV can be divided into two components: quasispecies and genotypes (reviewed in [3]). The term 'quasispecies' refers to the genetic diversity of a virus population that can be observed in a single infected individual owing to changes that have taken place during the course of the infection. In general, the sequences of a quasispecies genome population differ from each other by 1–2%. At any particular time, one quasispecies predominates within an infected host, but this dominant form might change or be replaced over time. In contrast, geno-types primarily result from the accumulation of mutations that have occurred during the long-term evolution of the virus. In general, isolates of the same genotype differ in sequence by 5–10% and isolates of different genotypes differ from each other by as much as 35%.

## QUASISPECIES

Changes that give rise to distinct quasispecies occur throughout the HCV genome, but a particularly high rate of nucleotide change, which often results in alterations in the predicted amino acid sequence of the coded viral proteins, has been observed in the HVR1 region. For example, genetic drift in the HVR1 region was demonstrated for HCV strain H in a chronically infected individual [27]. Interestingly, serum obtained from this patient in the chronic phase of the infection was found to contain antibodies that could neutralize the virus isolated in the acute phase of the infection [28,29]. However, the HVR1 sequence of the virus isolated from chronic phase sera was very different from that of the original isolate, suggesting that this virus had escaped neutralization. In fact, it has been demonstrated that the sequence changes observed in HVR1 could alter the antigenicity of epitopes within this region such that they became unrecognizable by pre-existing antibodies [30–33]. Such observations have supported the theory that the existence of quasispecies could be one mechanism by which HCV escapes immune surveillance and establishes persistent infection in the majority of infected individuals. It might also influence the outcome of some antiviral therapies. For example, some studies suggest that individuals with a homogeneous HCV sequence population respond better to interferon therapy than those with a relatively heterogeneous population [3,34].

## GENOTYPES

So far, genetic analyses of the full-length sequences of 21 HCV isolates have been reported (reviewed in [3]). These sequences represent three major genetic groups, with differences of 30–35% in their nucleotide sequences. These major groups are each divided into subgroups (subtypes 1a, 1b and 1c for group 1; subtypes 2a and 2b for group 2; and subtypes 3a and 3b for group 3) with differences of 20–25% between their sequences. Within each of these subgroups there are different isolates with differences among their

**Figure 2.** Phylogenetic tree showing the calculated evolutionary relationships between the nucleotide sequences of the entire ORF of the 21 HCV isolates for which the full-length sequence has been determined

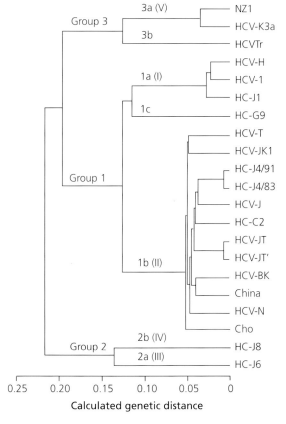

This phylogenetic tree was constructed by the unweighted pair-group method with arithmetic mean, using the computer software package 'GeneWorks' from IntelliGenetics (Campbell, California, USA). The lengths of the horizontal lines connecting the sequences are proportional to the estimated genetic distances between the sequences. Genotype designations of HCV isolates are indicated. The Roman numeral genotype designations originally proposed by Okamoto and co-workers [9,10] are shown in parentheses. See [3] for a list of relevant references.

nucleotide sequences of < 10%. A phylogenetic analysis of the full-length sequences of HCV is shown in Figure 2. We constructed this phylogenetic tree by the unweighted pair-group method with arithmetic mean using the computer software package GeneWorks from IntelliGenetics (Campbell, California, USA), [3].

The analysis of the full-length sequences might not, however, reflect the full extent of the genetic diversity of HCV because genetic analysis of partial genomic sequences has identified several additional major genetic groups and subgroups [17,20,23,35–38]. Overall, at least ten major genetic groups and more than 50 subgroups have now been reported [3,37].

The clinical implications of the existence of multiple HCV genotypes are unclear. However, some genotypes (in particular genotype 1b) were found to be associated with rapid progression of liver disease in liver-transplant recipients [39]. In addition, patients infected with genotype 1b were found to respond less well to interferon therapy than patients infected with other genotypes (reviewed in [3]). However, a recent report indicates that the outcome of interferon therapy might also vary among different isolates of genotype 1b, depending on the occurrence of mutations in the NS5A protein [40].

## WORLDWIDE GENETIC HETEROGENEITY OF HCV

The classification of all forms of HCV worldwide required the study of the genomic sequences of viral isolates from many locations. Initially, we tested serum samples from 114 anti-HCV-positive individuals from 12 countries around the world for HCV RNA, using the RT–PCR assay and primers from the 5′ NC region [16]. A total of 89 individuals infected with HCV were identified. Sequence analysis of the 5′ NC region of these HCV isolates subsequently revealed significant heterogeneity and clustering of the sequences for this region, which allowed the isolates to be divided into multiple genetic groups [17].

The sequences of the E1 and core genes were then determined for 51 and 52 isolates, respectively [20,23]. The analysis of the E1 gene sequences suggested that the isolates could be grouped into six major groups and 12 subgroups. Group 1 had subtypes 1a and 1b, group 2 had subtypes 2a, 2b and 2c, group 3 had a single subtype (3a), group 4 had four different subtypes (4a–d), and groups 5 and 6 each had a single subtype (5a and 6a, respectively). The differences in the nucleotide sequences between these groups were 30–45%, while those among the subtypes were equivalent to a difference in the genomic nucleotide sequences of 20–30%, and those among isolates within a subtype were less than 10%. Analysis of the core-gene sequences also allowed the isolates to be grouped into six major groups. Slight variations in the genetic distances between different gene regions were observed. For example, the differences between subtypes within group 2 were equivalent to those between the major groups 1 and 4 in the analysis of the core gene sequences. Additional subtypes have now been identified by other investigators in genotypes 1–6, and isolates of additional major genetic groups (groups 7–10) have been identified in Asia [3,35–38].

Demographic analysis has revealed some differences in the geographical distributions of genotypes (reviewed in [3]). Overall, genotype 1 is common in North America, Europe and Asia. Genotype 1a seems to predominate in North America, whereas subtypes 1a and 1b have similar prevalences in Europe. Genotype 1b is the predominant genotype in Japan. Genotypes 2 and 3 are found in significant numbers of cases in North America, Europe and Asia. However, other genotypes predominate in Africa: genotype 4 is the predominant form in North and Central Africa, and genotype 5 accounts for the majority of isolates in South Africa. These genotypes are only sporadically elsewhere. Genotype 6 constitutes about 20% of infections in Hong Kong and is also found frequently in Vietnam.

The classification of the many genotypes of HCV is the subject of continuing debate. Furthermore, as more sequence data become available, it is becoming increasingly difficult to classify them based only on data collected unsystematically. The final classification will require analysis of the complete genomic sequences of isolates representative of the various genotypes of HCV.

The recently discovered GB agents are related to HCV; however, these viruses do not represent HCV genotypes. An analysis of the nucleotide sequences of the NS3 helicase from some of the major genotypes of HCV [3] and from the various GB agents [12–14] is shown in Figure 3. Even in this conserved region, the GB agents differ more from HCV and from each other than the differences observed among isolates of the major genetic groups of HCV.

## DETERMINATION OF HCV GENOTYPES

Only some subtypes of HCV genotypes 1, 2 and 3 have been completely sequenced. For isolates of the other genotypes, analysis has usually been restricted to the 5′ end of the HCV genome (5′ NC, C and E1) and/or parts of the NS5B gene domain. This is an

**Figure 3.** Phylogenetic tree showing the calculated evolutionary relationships of the nucleotide sequences of the NS3 helicases from some of the major genotypes of HCV (genotypes 1, 2, 3 and 5) and the various GB agents (GBV-A, GBV-B and GBV-C [12-14])

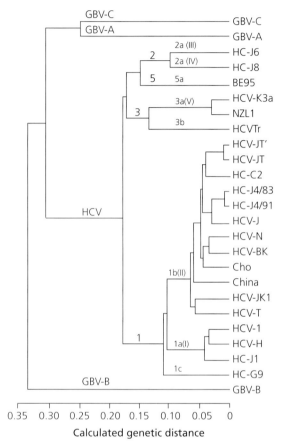

Further details of the methods used are given in the legend to Fig. 2.

important limitation because partial sequence analysis might not provide the data required to classify viral forms definitively. For example, the short 222 nucleotide sequence of NS5B recommended by an international group of researchers [35] might be too short to give an accurate indication of the genotype of viral isolates [36,38]. Furthermore, it is now well established that the genotype cannot be determined by analysis of the 5′ NC sequences alone [3]. Nevertheless, complete sequence analysis is expensive and time consuming, and partial sequence analysis is often the only viable option. However, the region chosen for such sequence analysis should include sequences from which reference data are available for most of the recognized genotypes, such as core–E1 and NS5B sequences.

Many researchers have attempted to devise alternatives to nucleotide sequence analysis for the determination of viral genotypes. The options evaluated included PCR followed by a second PCR with type-specific primers [41], restriction length polymorphism [42], hybridization with type-specific probes [43] or study of type-specific antibody responses [44,45]. However, all these approaches are limited in that they depend on a small number of specific sequence changes and require very precise experimental conditions. For these reasons, sequence analysis is likely to remain the most useful approach to the determination of genetic diversity of HCV.

This article originally appeared in *Antiviral Therapy* 1996; **1** (Supplement 3):39–45.

# REFERENCES

1. Alter HJ & Seeff LB. Transfusion-associated hepatitis. In *Viral Hepatitis: Scientific Basis and Clinical Management*. Edited by AJ Zuckerman & HC Thomas. 1993; pp. 467–499. Edinburgh: Churchill Livingstone.
2. Choo Q-L, Kuo G, Weiner AJ, Overby LR, Bradley DW & Houghton M. Isolation of a cDNA clone derived from a blood-borne non-A, non-B viral hepatitis genome. *Science* 1989; **244**:359–362.
3. Bukh J, Miller RH & Purcell RH. Genetic heterogeneity of hepatitis C virus: quasispecies and genotypes. *Seminars in Liver Disease* 1995; **15**:41–63.
4. Choo Q-L, Richman KH, Han JH, Berger K, Lee C, Dong C, Gallegos C, Coit D, Medina-Selby A, Barr PJ, Weiner AJ, Bradley DW, Kuo G & Houghton M. Genetic organization and diversity of the hepatitis C virus. *Proceedings of the National Academy of Sciences, USA* 1991; **88**:2451–2455.
5. Houghton M, Han J, Kuo G, Choo Q-L & Weiner AJ. Structure and molecular virology. In *Viral Hepatitis: Scientific Basis and Clinical Management*. Edited by AJ Zuckerman & HC Thomas. 1993; pp 229–240. Edinburgh: Churchill Livingstone.
6. Inchauspe G, Zebedee S, Lee D-H, Sugitani M, Nasoff M & Prince AM. Genomic structure of the human prototype strain H of hepatitis C virus: comparison with American and Japanese isolates. *Proceedings of the National Academy of Sciences, USA* 1991; **88**:10292–10296.
7. Kato N, Hijikata M, Ootsuyama Y, Nakagawa M, Ohkoshi S, Sugimura T & Shimotohno K. Molecular cloning of the human hepatitis C virus genome from Japanese patients with non-A, non-B hepatitis. *Proceedings of the National Academy of Sciences, USA* 1990; **87**:9524–9528.
8. Miller RH & Purcell RH. Hepatitis C virus shares amino acid sequence similarity with pestiviruses and flaviviruses as well as members of two plant virus supergroups. *Proceedings of the National Academy of Sciences, USA* 1990; **87**:2057–2061.
9. Okamoto H, Kurai K, Okada S-I, Yamamoto K, Iizuka H, Tanaka T, Fukuda S, Tsuda F & Mishiro S. Full-length sequence of a hepatitis C virus genome having poor homology to reported isolates: comparative study of four distinct genotypes. *Virology* 1992; **188**:331–341.
10. Sakamoto M, Akahane Y, Tsuda F, Tanaka T, Woodfield DG & Okamoto H. Entire nucleotide sequence and characterization of a hepatitis C virus of genotype V/3a. *Journal of General Virology* 1994; **75**:1761–1768.
11. Takamizawa A, Mori C, Fuke I, Manabe S, Murakami S, Fujita J, Onishi E, Andoh T, Yoshida I & Okayama H. Structure and organization of the hepatitis C virus genome isolated from human carriers. *Journal of Virology* 1991; **65**:1105–1113.
12. Simons JN, Pilot-Matias TJ, Leary TP, Dawson GJ, Desai SM, Schlauder GG, Muerhoff AS, Erker JC, Buijk SL, Chalmers ML, Van Sant CL & Mushahwar IK. Identification of two flavivirus-like genomes in the GB hepatitis agent. *Proceedings of the National Academy of Sciences, USA* 1995; **92**:3401–3405.
13. Simons JN, Leary TP, Dawson GJ, Pilot-Matias TJ, Muerhoff AS, Schlauder GG, Desai SM & Mushahwar IK. Isolation of novel virus-like sequences associated with human hepatitis. *Nature Medicine* 1995; **1**:564–569.
14. Muerhoff AS, Leary TP, Simons JN, Pilot-Matias TJ, Dawson GJ, Erker JC, Chalmers ML, Schlauder GG, Desai SM & Mushahwar IK. Genomic organization of GB viruses A and B: two new members of the *Flaviviridae* associated with GB agent hepatitis. *Journal of Virology* 1995; **69**:5621–5630.
15. Han JH, Shyamala V, Richman KH, Brauer MJ, Irvine B, Urdea MS, Tekamp-Olson P, Kuo G, Choo Q-L & Houghton M. Characterization of the terminal regions of hepatitis C viral RNA: identification of conserved sequences in the 5′ untranslated region and poly(A) tails at the 3′ end. *Proceedings of the National Academy of Sciences, USA* 1991; **88**:1711–1715.
16. Bukh J, Purcell RH & Miller RH. Importance of primer selection for the detection of hepatitis C virus RNA with the polymerase chain reaction assay. *Proceedings of the National Academy of Sciences, USA* 1992; **89**:187–191.
17. Bukh J, Purcell RH & Miller RH. Sequence analysis of the 5′ noncoding region of hepatitis C virus. *Proceedings of the National Academy of Sciences, USA* 1992; **89**:4942–4946.
18. Tanaka T, Kato N, Cho M-J & Shimotohno K. A novel sequence found at the 3′ terminus of hepatitis C virus genome. *Biochemical and Biophysical Research Communications* 1995; **215**:744–749.
19. Deng R & Brock KV. 5′ and 3′ untranslated regions of pestivirus genome: primary and secondary structure analyses. *Nucleic Acids Research* 1993; **21**:1949–1957.
20. Bukh J, Purcell RH & Miller RH. At least 12 genotypes of hepatitis C virus predicted by sequence analysis of the putative E1 gene of isolates collected worldwide. *Proceedings of the National Academy of Sciences, USA* 1993; **90**:8234–8238.
21. Cha T-A, Kolberg J, Irvine B, Stempien M, Beall E, Yano M, Choo Q-L, Houghton M, Kuo G, Han JH & Urdea MS. Use of a signature nucleotide sequence of hepatitis C virus for detection of viral RNA in human serum and plasma. *Journal of Clinical Microbiology* 1991; **29**:2528–2534.
22. Okamoto H, Okada S, Sugiyama Y, Tanaka T, Sugai Y, Akahane Y, Machida A, Mishiro S, Yoshizawa H, Miyakawa Y & Mayumi M. Detection of hepatitis C virus RNA by a two-stage polymerase chain reaction

with two pairs of primers deduced from the 5′-noncoding region. *Japanese Journal of Experimental Medicine* 1990; **60**:215–222.

23. Bukh J, Purcell RH & Miller RH. Sequence analysis of the core gene of 14 hepatitis C virus genotypes. *Proceedings of the National Academy of Sciences, USA* 1994; **91**:8239–8243.

24. Kuo G, Choo Q-L, Alter HJ, Gitnick GL, Redeker AG, Purcell RH, Miyamura T, Dienstag JL, Alter MJ, Stevens CE, Tegtmeier GE, Bonino F, Colombo M, Lee W-S, Kuo C, Berger K, Shuster JR, Overby LR, Bradley DW & Houghton M. An assay for circulating antibodies to a major etiologic virus of human non-A, non-B hepatitis. *Science* 1989; **244**:362–364.

25. Hijikata M, Kato N, Ootsuyama Y, Nakagawa M, Ohkoshi S & Shimotohno K. Hypervariable regions in the putative glycoprotein of hepatitis C virus. *Biochemical and Biophysical Research Communications* 1991; **175**:220–228.

26. Weiner AJ, Brauer MJ, Rosenblatt J, Richman KH, Tung J, Crawford K, Bonino F, Saracco G, Choo Q-L, Houghton M & Han JH. Variable and hypervariable domains are found in the regions of HCV corresponding to the flavivirus envelope and NS1 proteins and the pestivirus envelope glycoproteins. *Virology* 1991; **180**:842–848.

27. Ogata N, Alter HJ, Miller RH & Purcell RH. Nucleotide sequence and mutation rate of the H strain of hepatitis C virus. *Proceedings of the National Academy of Sciences, USA* 1991; **88**:3392–3396.

28. Farci P, Alter HJ, Wong DC, Miller RH, Govindarajan S, Engle R, Shapiro M & Purcell RH. Prevention of hepatitis C virus infection in chimpanzees after antibody-mediated *in vitro* neutralization. *Proceedings of the National Academy of Sciences, USA* 1994; **91**:7792–7796.

29. Shimizu YK, Hijikata M, Iwamoto A, Alter HJ, Purcell RH & Yoshikura H. Neutralizing antibodies against hepatitis C virus and the emergence of neutralization escape mutant viruses. *Journal of Virology* 1994; **68**:1494–1500.

30. Kato N, Sekiya H, Ootsuyama Y, Nakazawa T, Hijikata M, Ohkoshi S & Shimotohno K. Humoral immune response to hypervariable region 1 of the putative envelope glycoprotein (gp70) of hepatitis C virus. *Journal of Virology* 1993; **67**:3923–3930.

31. Kato N, Ootsuyama Y, Sekiya H, Ohkoshi S, Nakazawa T, Hijikata M & Shimotohno K. Genetic drift in hypervariable region 1 of the viral genome in persistent hepatitis C virus infection. *Journal of Virology* 1994; **68**:4776–4784.

32. Taniguchi S, Okamoto H, Sakamoto M, Kojima M, Tsuda F, Tanaka T, Munekata E, Muchmore EE, Peterson DA & Mishiro S. A structurally flexible and antigenically variable N-terminal domain of the hepatitis C virus E2/NS1 protein: implication for an escape from antibody. *Virology* 1993; **195**:297–301.

33. Weiner AJ, Geysen HM, Christopherson C, Hall JE, Mason TJ, Saracco G, Bonino F, Crawford K, Marion CD, Crawford KA, Brunetto M, Barr PJ, Miyamura T, McHutchinson J & Houghton M. Evidence for immune selection of hepatitis C virus (HCV) putative envelope glycoprotein variants: potential role in chronic HCV infections. *Proceedings of the National Academy of Sciences, USA* 1992; **89**:3468–3472.

34. Okada S-I, Akahane Y, Suzuki H, Okamoto H & Mishiro

S. The degree of variability in the amino terminal region of the E2/NS1 protein of hepatitis C virus correlates with responsiveness to interferon therapy in viremic patients. *Hepatology* 1992; **16**:619–624.

35. Simmonds P, Holmes EC, Cha T-A, Chan S-W, McOmish F, Irvine B, Beall E, Yap PL, Kolberg J & Urdea MS. Classification of hepatitis C virus into six major genotypes and a series of subtypes by phylogenetic analysis of the NS-5 region. *Journal of General Virology* 1993; **74**:2391–2399.

36. Stuyver L, Van Arnhem W, Wyseur A, Hernandez F, Delaporte E & Maertens G. Classification of hepatitis C viruses based on phylogenetic analysis of the envelope 1 and nonstructural 5B regions and identification of five additional subtypes. *Proceedings of the National Academy of Sciences, USA* 1994; **91**:10134–10138.

37. Stuyver L, Wyseur A, Van Arnhem W, Lunel F, Laurent-Puig P, Pawlotsky J-M, Kleter B, Bassit L, Nkengasong J, Van Doorn L-J & Maertens G. Hepatitis C virus genotyping by means of 5′-UR/core line probe assays and molecular analysis of untypeable samples. *Virus Research* 1995; **38**:137–157.

38. Tokita H, Okamoto H, Tsuda F, Song P, Nakata S, Chosa T, Iizuka H, Mishiro S, Miyakawa Y & Mayumi M. Hepatitis C virus variants from Vietnam are classifiable into the seventh, eighth, and ninth major genetic groups. *Proceedings of the National Academy of Sciences, USA* 1994; **91**:11022–11026.

39. Féray C, Gigou M, Samuel D, Paradis V, Mishiro S, Maertens G, Reynés M, Okamoto H, Bismuth H & Bréchot C. Influence of the genotypes of hepatitis C virus on the severity of recurrent liver disease after liver transplantation. *Gastroenterology* 1995; **108**:1088–1096.

40. Enomoto N, Sakuma I, Asahina Y, Kurosaki M, Murakami T, Yamamoto C, Ogura Y, Izumi N, Marumo F & Sato C. Mutations in the nonstructural protein 5A gene and response to interferon in patients with chronic hepatitis C virus 1b infection. *New England Journal of Medicine* 1996; **334**:77–81.

41. Okamoto H, Sugiyama Y, Okada S, Kurai K, Akahane Y, Sugai Y, Tanaka T, Sato K, Tsuda F, Miyakawa Y & Mayumi M. Typing hepatitis C virus by polymerase chain reaction with type-specific primers: application to clinical surveys and tracing infectious sources. *Journal of General Virology* 1992; **73**:673–679.

42. Nakao T, Enomoto N, Takada N, Takada A & Date T. Typing of hepatitis C virus genomes by restriction fragment length polymorphism. *Journal of General Virology* 1991; **72**:2105–2112.

43. Stuyver L, Rossau R, Wyseur A, Duhamel M, Vanderborght B, Van Heuverswyn H & Maertens G. Typing of hepatitis C virus isolates and characterization of new subtypes using a line probe assay. *Journal of General Virology* 1993; **74**:1093–1102.

44. Machida A, Ohnuma H, Tsuda F, Munekata E, Tanaka T, Akahane Y, Okamoto H & Mishiro S. Two distinct subtypes of hepatitis C virus defined by antibodies directed to the putative core protein. *Hepatology* 1992; **16**:886–891.

45. Simmonds P, Rose KA, Graham S, Chan S-W, McOmish F, Dow BC, Follett EAC, Yap PL & Marsden H. Mapping of serotype-specific, immunodominant epitopes in the NS-4 region of hepatitis C virus (HCV): use of type-specific peptides to serologically differentiate infections with HCV types 1, 2, and 3. *Journal of Clinical Microbiology* 1993; **31**:1493–1503.

# 16

# A line probe assay for hepatitis B virus genotypes

Caroline Van Geyt, Sija De Gendt, Annelies Rombout, Ann Wyseur, Geert Maertens, Rudi Rossau and Lieven Stuyver*

## INTRODUCTION

Hepatitis B virus (HBV) is the prototype member of the *Hepadnaviridae* and is the aetiological agent of a widespread form of acute and chronic liver disease which is distributed throughout the world. The genome of HBV consists of four open reading frames S, C, P and X encoding the envelope [pre-S1, pre-S2 and surface antigen (HBsAg)], core (precore precursor protein and HBeAg, and HBcAg), polymerase (HBV pol), and X proteins [1,2], respectively.

Historically, HBV variability has been assessed by means of monoclonal antibodies against HBsAg and classified into serological subtypes. The latter are defined by two mutually exclusive determinant pairs *d/y, w/r* and a common 'a' determinant [3,4]. By further subdivision of the four major subtypes, a total of nine different subtypes has been identified: *adw1, ayw1, ayw2, ayw3, ayw4, adwyq⁻, adrq+, adrq⁻* and *ayr* [5].

Based on the entire nucleotide sequence of HBV genomes, a genetic classification system has been established. Six genomic groups named A, B, C, D, E and F, showing an intergroup divergence of 8% or more with reference to the complete nucleotide sequence, were described [6]. The correlation between the nine serological subtypes and the six different genotypes was proven [7]. Apart from the fact that genotyping can be used for tracing the route of HBV transmission and the geographical migration of HBV carriers [8,9], the clinical value of genotyping and serological subtyping remains to be further investigated. However, some observations point towards clinical relevance: (i) a Japanese study showed that liver disease is more common in carriers with genotype C as compared to the other genotypes [10]; (ii) another report indicated that patients infected with genotype A respond better to interferon therapy than those with non-A types [11]; and (iii) genotype A is found to circulate rarely as an HBeAg-negative mutant (in contrast to genotype D

which is the most frequent viral genotype among the precore-negative mutants in Western countries) [12].

In order to further investigate the possible influence of the viral genotype on HBV pathogenesis and epidemiology, a genetic typing system based on the reverse hybridization line probe assay (LiPA) technology, was developed. LiPA HBV genotyping has already been described for the HBV preS1 region [13], but is now further developed for the HBsAg region. Here we report an epidemiological study showing the genetic distribution of the different genotypes in different parts of the world.

## MATERIALS AND METHODS

### Collection of serum samples

A total of 939 serum samples originating from 25 countries on four continents were analysed. The sera were collected in Europe ($n=577$), Africa ($n=174$), Asia ($n=155$), and South America ($n=33$) and stored at –20°C until use.

### HBV DNA extraction

HBV DNA was extracted from serum samples with the High Pure PCR Template Preparation Kit (Boehringer Mannheim). A nested set of PCR primers was designed, allowing the amplification of the relevant HBsAg region generating a 341 bp fragment (outer sense primer HBPr 134: 5′-TGCTGCTATGCCT-CATCTTC-3′; outer antisense primer HBPr 135: 5′–CA(A/G)AGACAAAAGAAAATTGG-3′; nested sense primer HBPr 75: 5′–CAAGGTATGTTGCCCGTTTG-TCC-3′; nested antisense primer HBPr 94: 5′-GGTA-(A/T)AAAGGGACTCA(C/A)GATG-3′). All primers were tagged with a biotin group at the 5′ end. Outer PCR amplified the DNA over 40 cycles (30 s at 95°C;

**Figure 1.** Nucleotide sequence alignment of the LiPA probe target regions

```
           328         337   339     360   365  374      381 390                 408        417                   438                   473          483      547       567   574    608    619
            •           •     •       •     •    •         •                       •          •                     •                     •            •        •         •     •      •      •
Cons.  ATTCCAGGAT  AACACA     ATGCAA       CGACTCCT  CAACTCTATGTTTCCCTCA  TACAAAACCTACGGATGGAAAT   TCGCAAAATAC       TTCCGTAGG   TGTTTGGC   CAAGACTGTGACA

3076A  --G-------  ------ -------   ------  ------  -------  -------  -------------------  ----------------------    -----------     ----------  ---------   --------  -------  ----------
29466A -----------------193  -------   ------  ------  T------  -------  ---------------140  ----------------------  -------148      ----------  ---------  --------  -------  ---T---
29661A C---------  C----- -------   C-----  ------  -------  -------  -------------------  ----------------------  -------148      ----------  ---------  --------  -------  ---T--C---
29670A C-------  ------ -------   C-----  ------  -------  -------  -------A-------140  -------T--              -------          ----------  ---------  --------  -------  --RT---
29915A -----------------193  -------   ------  --G---  -------  -------  ---------------140  ----------------------  -------148      ----------  ---------  --------  -------  ---T---
29987A -----------------193  -------   ------  --G---  -------  -------  ---------------140  -------T--  -------T--  -------148      ----------  ---------  --------  -------  ---T---

3073B  -------- A153 -T----  ------   ------  -A----  G-------  G-C----  -----------C78  --------  ----------C78          ------  ----------148     ---------  ----T--  --C---239  ----T---
29742B  -------- A153 -T----  ------   ------  -AG---  -------  A-C----  -----------C78  ---------  ----------C78          --G-T-204  ----------148  ---------  ----T--  --C---239  ----T---
29751B  -------- A153 -T--C  -T-G--   ------  ------  -------  A-C----  -----------C78          --G-T-204  ----------148  ---------  ----T--  --C---239  ----T---
29757B  -------- A153 -T--C  ------   ---G--  ------  -------  A-C----  -----------C78          --G-T-204  ----------148  ---------  ----T--  --C---239  ----T---
29758B  -------- A153 -T--C  ------   ---G--  ------  -------  A-C----  -----------C78          --G-T-204  ----------148  ---------  ----T--  --C---239  ----T---
29762B  -------- A153 -T--C  ------   ---G--  ------  -------  A-C----  -----------C78          --G-T-204  ----------148  ---------  ----T--  --C---239  ----T---

3074C  C-------  -T--T  ------   ------  ---G--  -------  A-C----  -----------80  -T-------  -----C----  --G-T-  ---------  ---------  ----T--
29218C  C-------  -T--T  ------   ------  ---G--  -------  A-C----  -----------80  -C------  -----C----  --G-T-  ---------  ---------  ----T--
29258C  C-------  -T-G-T -------   ------  ------  -------  A-C----  -----------80  -T------  -----C----  --G-T-  ---------  ---------  ----T--
29260C  C-------  -T--T  C-----   ------  --T---154  A-C----  -----------80  -T-------  -----C----  --G-T-  ---------  ---------  ---TTT--
29299C  C-------  -T--T  ------   ------  --T---154  A-C----  -----------80  -T-------  -----C----  --G-T-  ---------  ---------  ----T--
29706C  C-------  -T--T  ------   ------  ------  -------  A-C----  ----------C80  -T-------  ----------  --G-T-204  -------C  ---------  ----T--

3075D  --------  CT----C  ----CG   C---CG172  ------  A-C----  -----------80;208  C----  -A------C165  C-------  ------  ---G--  --C---239  ----T--
27492D  --------  TT----C  ----CG   C---CG172  ---A--  A-C----  -----------80;208  C----  --CA---  ----------  --G--  ---------  --C---239  --NT---
27499D  --------  -T----C  ----CG   C---CG172  ------  A-C----  -----------C  -T-----  -A---C165  C-------  ------  ---G--  --C---239  ----T--
29651D  --------  CT----C  ----CG   C---CG172  ------  A-C----  -----------80;208  C----  -A---C165  C-------  ------  ---G--  --C---239  ---TTT--
29678D  --------  CT----C  ----CG   C---CG172  ------  A-C----  -----------80;208  C----  -A---C165  C-------  ------  ---G--  --C---239  ---AT--N---
29681D  --------  GT----C  -----G   C---CG172  ------  A-C----  -----------C  -T-----  -A---C165  C-------  ------  ---G--  --C---239  ----T--

3077E  --------  -T----C  ------   ------  -T----  A-C----  -----------80;177  -T---  ------  --G-T-  --CC--213  --C---239  ---T--
29494E  --------  -T----C  ------   ------  -T----  A-C----  -----------80;177  -T---  ------  --G-T-  --CC--213  --C---239  --TTT--
29511E  --------  -T----C  ---G   ------  -T----  A-C----  -----------80;177  -T---  ------  --G-T-  --CC--213  --C---239  --TTT--
29535E  --------  -T----C  ---G   ------  -T----  A-C----  -----------80;177  -T---  ------  --G-T-  --CC--213  --C---239  --TTT--
29539E  --------  -T----C  ------   ------  -T----  A-C----  -----------80;177  -T---  ------  --G-T-  --CC--213  --C---239  ---T--

22298F  C-------C216  C-G-C  C------   C-----  -A--T-  -C-------C  -T-C----  -----C219  -A-G----  -G--C  --C---  --AT---G-186
29165F  -T-G-C  T--G-C  -------   ------  -A--T-  A--------  -T------C  -----C  -A-G----  -G----  --C---  --AT---G-186
29974F  C-G--C216  C-G--C  -----G   ------  -A--T-  -T-C----  -----C219  -A-G----  -G----  --C---  --AT---G-186
29976F  C-G--C216  C-G--C  -----G   ------  -A--T-  -T-C----  -----C219  -A-G----  -G----  --C---  --AT---G-186
29979F  C-G--C216  C-G--C  -------   ------  -A----  -C------  -----C219  -A-G----  -G----  --C---  --AT---G-186
29981F  C-G--C216  C-G--C  -------   ------  -A--T-  -C-CT----C  -----C219  -A-G----  -G----  --C---  --AT---G-186
```

Only relevant regions showing sufficient variability were retained, while the conserved areas were deleted and are represented here as a gap. The nucleotide positions are indicated above the sequence, starting from the ATG of HBsAg. The sequences are grouped according to the genotype, shown on the right of the strain number. A number shown to the right of a target sequence indicates a positive reaction with that particular probe on the LiPA.

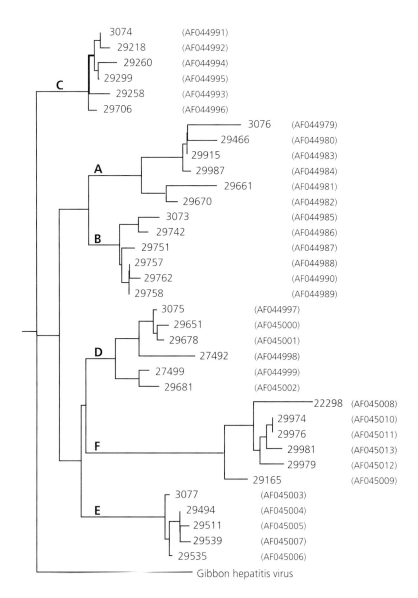

**Figure 2.** Phylogenetic tree of the HBsAg region

Thirty-five sequences from 6 different genotypes (codons 109 to 207) are included. The genotype is indicated above the branch of each genotype cluster; reference samples are not included in this tree, but the genotype assignment is based on the co-localization of the reference strains described by Norder et al. [15]. The gibbon hepatitis B virus sequence (U46935) was included as the outgroup.

30 s at 45°C; 30 s at 72°C). Samples negative in first round PCR were further amplified with nested PCR primers for 35 cycles with the same thermal profile.

## Probe design

A total of 18 genotype-specific probes was designed. The target regions for the relevant probes are indicated on the nucleotide sequence alignment shown in Figure 1.

## LiPA strips, preparation and test performance

After enzymatic addition of a poly d(T) tail, the selected oligonucleotide probes were applied as hori-

zontal lines on nitrocellulose membranes. One line of biotinylated DNA was applied alongside as a positive control. The assay was essentially carried out as described for the HCV line probe assay [14]. Briefly, biotinylated PCR product was mixed with an equal volume (10 μl each) of denaturation solution, and incubated at room temperature for 5 min, after which 2 ml of prewarmed (37°C) hybridization solution was added. Hybridization with probes on LiPA was allowed to proceed for 1 h at 50°C±0.5°C in a shaking waterbath. The strips were washed twice at room temperature for 20 s and once at 50°C for 30 min. Following stringent washing, the strips were incubated with an alkaline phosphatase/streptavidin conjugate for 30 min at room temperature. Strips were then washed twice, and colour development was initiated by addition of 5-bromo-4-chloro-3-indolylphosphate and nitroblue tetrazolium. The colour reaction was stopped by aspiration of the substrate buffer and addition of distilled water. After drying, the strips were immediately interpreted by eye.

## Recombinant DNA cloning protocol

HBsAg PCR was performed using the nested primer set HBPr 104: 5'-CAAGGTATGTTGCCCGTTT-GTCC-3' and HBPr 105: 5'-GGTA(A/T)AAAGGG-ACTCA(C/A)GATG-3'. PCR fragments were ligated into the pGEM-T plasmid vector (pGEM-T Vector Systems, Promega). After transformation into DH5α F', plasmid DNA was prepared (High Pure Plasmid Isolation Kit; Boehringer Mannheim) and recombinant clones were selected by restriction enzyme analysis.

## Sequence analysis and phylogenetic tree construction

Sequencing was performed on an automated DNA sequencer Model 373A (Applied Biosystems), using fluorescence-labelled dideoxynucleotide chain terminators (Prism Ready Reaction Dye Deoxy Terminator Cycle Sequencing Kit with AmpiTaq FS; Applied Biosystems). The primers used for sequencing were (i) for PCR products HBPr 75-T7 and HBPr94; and (ii) for plasmid material SP6 and T7. Sequences obtained from a recombinant clone are indicated with a four-digit number; and sequences from a population-based sequencing protocol (direct sequence of a PCR fragment) are indicated with a five-digit number (Figs 1 and 2). Sequences were brought into alignment, and a phylogenetic tree was constructed using the PHYLIP program, as was described for HCV [14].

## Nucleotide sequence accession numbers

HBsAg sequences used in Figure 1 received the GenBank Accession numbers AF044979 to AF045013.

## RESULTS

### LiPA for HBsAg genotyping

Figure 1 shows the relatedness between 35 sequences

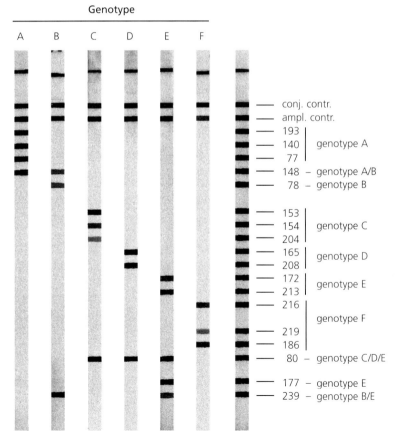

**Figure 3.** Examples of the HBsAg genotyping LiPA

From left to right: strips incubated with PCR fragments of a representative isolate of each. Strip A: isolate 29466; strip B: isolate 29234; strip C: isolate 29749; strip D: isolate 29710; strip E: isolate 29210; strip F: isolate 29979. Right: LiPA strip showing the positions of all probes applied; the numbering of the probes corresponds to those given in Fig. 2. Conj. contr.: conjugate control; ampl. contr.: amplification control (probe reacting with all genotypes, located in conserved area).

**Table 1.** Geographical distribution of the HBV genotypes

| Region | HBV genotypes | | | | | | |
| --- | --- | --- | --- | --- | --- | --- | --- |
| | A | B | C | D | E | F | Total |
| *Europe* | | | | | | | |
| France | 248 | 3 | 63 | 137 | 7 | 2 | 460 |
| Belgium | 63 | 2 | 1 | 35 | 2 | 3 | 106 |
| Russia | | | | 6 | 1 | | 7 |
| Bosnia | 1 | 1 | | | | | 2 |
| Czechoslovakia | | 1 | | 1 | | | 2 |
| Total | 312 | 7 | 64 | 179 | 10 | 5 | 577 |
| *Africa* | | | | | | | |
| Burkino Faso | 1 | | | 7 | 90 | 1 | 99 |
| Guinea | 3 | | | | 18 | | 21 |
| Somalia | 11 | 1 | | 3 | | | 15 |
| Central African Republic | 4 | | | | 8 | | 12 |
| Morocco | 1 | | | 5 | | | 6 |
| Tunisia | 1 | | | 4 | | | 5 |
| Ivory Coast | | | | | 4 | | 4 |
| Senegal | 1 | | | | 3 | | 4 |
| Cameroon | 2 | | | | | | 2 |
| Congo | 2 | | | | | | 2 |
| Mali | | | | | 2 | | 2 |
| Total | 26 | 1 | 0 | 19 | 125 | 1 | 172 |
| *Asia* | | | | | | | |
| Saudi Arabia | 2 | 1 | | 79 | 14 | | 96 |
| Vietnam | 2 | 39 | 12 | 1 | | | 54 |
| Laos | | 3 | | | | | 3 |
| Thailand | 1 | | 1 | | | | 2 |
| Total | 5 | 43 | 13 | 80 | 14 | 0 | 155 |
| *South America* | | | | | | | |
| Brazil | 9 | | | | | 5 | 14 |
| Venezuela | 3 | 1 | | | | 7 | 11 |
| Guadeloupe | 1 | | | 5 | | | 6 |
| Guyana | | | | 2 | | | 2 |
| Colombia | 2 | | | | | | 2 |
| Total | 15 | 1 | 0 | 7 | 0 | 12 | 35 |

obtained from a set of representative clinical samples from different geographical areas. Prior to the construction of this tree, sequences of reference strains for the six different genotypes were retrieved from the database [15], and compared with the sequences included in this tree. From this analysis, it became clear that the degree of variability found in the carboxy-terminal part of the HBsAg open reading frame (codon 109 to codon 207) allows for reliable grouping of the isolates into the six different genotypes, A through F. Based on this phylogenetic tree, a multiple nucleotide sequence alignment was created (Figure 2). In the HBsAg region between nucleotide positions 328 and 619, we were able to recognize 10 variable regions containing sufficient variability for the design of a genotyping assay. For these variable regions, a total of 18 specific probes were designed: three probes for genotype A (probes 193, 140, 77), one for genotype B (probe 78), three for genotype C (probes 153, 154, 204), two for genotype D (probes 165, 208), three for genotype E (probe 172, 213, 177), three for genotype F (probes 216, 219, 186); and generic probes for genotype A and B (probe 148), genotypes C, D and E (probe 80), and genotype B and E (probe 239). These 18 probes were applied together on a strip and their specific reactivity was assessed with the cloned reference panel and with randomly selected clinical samples. Figure 3 shows the result of some representative samples after hybridization of the PCR product to the probes on LiPA.

## Geographical distribution of HBV genotypes

A collection of 939 clinical samples with HBV infection from a total of 25 different countries was genotyped using the LiPA shown in Figure 3. The combination of the type-specific probes with the generic probes allowed in all cases the resolution of the genotype. In Table 1, the genotypes of infection in the different countries are presented. Genotype A has a global distribution, while other genotypes are more or less regionally restricted: genotype B and C in South-East Asia, genotype D in Europe, genotype E in Africa, and genotype F in South America.

## CONCLUSIONS

A selection of LiPA probes covering variability in the carboxy-terminal region of HBsAg permitted the genotyping of HBV-infected samples collected worldwide. Of the samples listed in Table 1, at least 200 were previously genotyped with LiPA in the preS1 region ([13]; and data not shown). Genotyping results in preS1 and HBsAg were 100% concordant, indicating the absence of recombinant or mosaic viruses in the HBV large surface antigen.

Genotyping HBV isolates in the HBsAg region has several advantages over using preS1: (i) the test results also allow for immediate and relevant comparison with the serotype determination [7]; (ii) the epidemiologically important drug vaccine escape mutants [16] are located in the same PCR fragment and can be detected with an additional set of specific LiPA probes; and (iii) the overlapping reading frame for HBV *pol* covers the clinically important drug-resistance motifs described previously [17]. The latter resistance motifs (HBV *pol* mutations) are reducing the susceptibility of these virus strains to drugs like lamivudine and famciclovir, and these mutations again can be detected with a set of LiPA probes.

With the availability of a rapid and convenient genotyping system, studies investigating: (i) the differential outcome of the disease; (ii) the influence of genotypes on the selection pressure for mutants in the precore promoter, the precore open reading frame, the core region, and the serological HBe antigenaemia; (iii) the influence on response rate in interferon treatment trials; and (iv) the influence of genotypes on the magnitude

and duration of response and the emerging resistance patterns in antiviral treatment, can be performed.

## ACKNOWLEDGEMENTS

We thank C Fretz, F Lunel, C Trépo, G Leroux-Roels, F Zoulim, E Moreaux, F Pujol, AA Saeed, B Vanderborght, P Swenson, R Schinazi, and N Naoumov for providing us with serum samples.

## REFERENCES

1. Ganem D & Varmus HE. The molecular biology of hepatitis viruses. *Annual Review of Biochemistry* 1987; **56**:651–693.
2. Lau JYN & Wright TL. Hepatitis B virus: molecular virology and pathogenesis. *Lancet* 1993; **342**: 1335–1340.
3. Lebouvier GL. The heterogeneity of Australia antigen. *Journal of Infectious Diseases* 1971; **123**:671–675.
4. Bancroft WH, Mundon FK & Russell PK. Detection of additional antigenic determinants of hepatitis B antigen. *Journal of Immunology* 1972; **109**:842–848.
5. Couroucé AM, Holland PV, Muller JY & Soulier JP. HBs Antigen subtypes. *Bibliotheca Haematologica* 1976; no. 42. Karger, Basel.
6. Okamoto H, Tsuda F, Sakugawa H, Sastrosoewignjo RI, Imai M, Miyakawa Y & Mayumi. Typing hepatitis B virus by homology in nucleotide sequence: comparison of surface antigen subtypes. *Journal of General Virology* 1988; **69**:2575–2583.
7. Blitz L, Pujol FH, Swenson PD, Porto L, Atencio R, Araujo M, Costa L, Monsalve CD, Torres JR, Fields HA, Lambert S, Van Geyt C, Norder H, Magnius LO, Echevarría JM & Stuyver L. Antigenic diversity of hepatitis B virus strains within genotype F in Amerindian and other populaion groups from Venezuela. *Journal of Clinical Microbiology* 1998; **36**: 648–651.
8. Alter HJ, Seeff LB, Kaplan PM, McAuliffe VJ, Wright EC, Gorin JL, Purcell RH, Holland PV & Zimmerman HJ. Type B hepatitis: the infectivity of blood positive for e-antigen and DNA polymerase after accidental needlestick exposure. *New England Journal of Medicine* 1976; **295**:909–913.
9. Couroucé-Pauty AM, Plancon A & Soulier JP. Distribution of HBsAg subtype in the world. *Vox Sanguinis* 1983; **44**:197–211.
10. Shiina S, Fujino H, Uta Y, Tagawa K, Unuma T, Yoneyama M, Ohmori T, Suzuki S, Kurita M & Ohashi Y. Relationship of HBsAg subtypes with HBeAg/anti-HBe status and chronic liver disease. Part I: analysis of 1744 HBsAg carriers. *American Journal of Gastroenterology* 1991; **86**:866–871.
11. Zhang X, Zoulim F, Habersetzer F, Xiong S & Trépo C. Analysis of hepatitis B virus genotypes and pre-core region variability during interferon treatment of HBe antigen negative chronic hepatitis B. *Journal of Medical Virology* 1996; **48**:8–16.
12. Li JS, Tong SP, Wen YM, Zhang Q & Trépo C. Hepatitis B virus genotype A rarely circulates as an Hbe-minus mutant: possible contribution of a single nucleotide in the precore region. *Journal of Virology* 1993; **67**:5402–5410.
13. Stuyver L, Rossau R & Maertens G. Line probe assays for the detection of hepatitis B and C virus. *Antiviral*

*Therapy* 1996; **1** (Supplement 3):53–57.

14. Stuyver L, Wyseur A, van Arnhem W, Hernandez F & Maertens G. Second-generation line probe assay for hepatitis C virus genotyping. *Journal of Clinical Microbiology* 1996; **34**:2259–2266.

15. Norder H, Couroucé AM & Magnius LO. Complete genomes, phylogenetic relatedness, and structural proteins of six strains of the hepatitis B virus, four of which represent two new gentypes. *Virology* 1994; **189**:489–503.

16. Carman WF, Van Deursen FJ, Mimms LT, Hardie D, Coppola R, Decker R & Sanders R. The prevalence of surface antigen variants of hepatitis B virus in Papua New Guinea, South Africa, and Sardinia. *Hepatology* 1997; **26**:1658–1666.

17. Bartholomeusz A & Locarnini S. Mutations in the hepatitis B virus polymerase gene that are associated with resistance to famciclovir and lamivudine. *International Antiviral News* 1997; **5**:123–124.

# Section IV

ANIMAL MODELS FOR
HEPATITIS B AND C

# 17 Hepatitis C and hepatitis B animal models

## Shlomo Dagan*, Ehud Ilan and Raymond F Schinazi

## INTRODUCTION

Hepatitis B virus (HBV) infection presents a major public health problem worldwide. Approximately 5% of the world's population is chronically infected with HBV. About 25–40% of these chronic patients develop progressive necroinflammatory changes in the liver, which can result in cirrhosis and/or hepatocellular carcinoma [1]. Likewise, hepatitis C virus (HCV) has a prevalence of about 1% in most developed countries and a much higher prevalence in most developing countries, as determined by the presence of anti-HCV antibodies [2]. HCV has been defined as the most important aetiological agent of parenterally transmitted non-A, non-B (NANB) hepatitis and, as with HBV, it is also a major cause of chronic liver disease and hepatocellular carcinoma [3–5]. Although significant progress has been achieved in characterization and identification of the two viruses and their components, the development of therapies has been hampered by the lack of adequate, simple and low-cost animal models. At present, chimpanzees provide good HBV and HCV animal models for evaluation of vaccines and therapeutic agents [6–8]. Nonetheless, the limited availability and the high cost of these primates severely restrict their use for such purposes. This brief review will, therefore, focus primarily on viable, and preferably small, HBV and HCV animal models. The main HBV and HCV animal models currently available are shown in Figure 1.

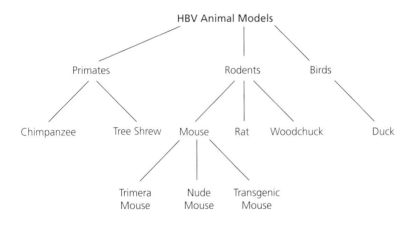

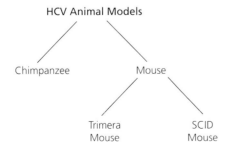

**Figure 1.** The main HBV and HCV experimental animal models

---

*Corresponding author

# HCV ANIMAL MODELS

## Essential role of the chimpanzee model in understanding HCV

Since NANB hepatitis was recognized as a distinct entity from hepatitis A and B [9], attempts have been made to transmit the disease to other non-human primate species, including the chimpanzee, with inocula of proven infectivity. For reasons that are unclear, early attempts were unsuccessful [7]. In 1978, four independent groups almost simultaneously reported the transmission of NANB hepatitis to chimpanzees [10–13], and demonstrated serial transmission to other animals [13,14]. Several other groups [15–19] subsequently confirmed these observations. A variety of different inocula were used for successful transmissions, including acute phase and chronic phase serum or plasma from individuals with post-transfusion or community-acquired NANB hepatitis, clinical specimens from implicated blood donors, clotting factor VIII and IX, and fibrinogen [20]. Both acute and chronic hepatitis were observed in the chimpanzees [21–24]. The course of primary infection, acute phase of the disease, development of the host immune response and long-term sequelae of HCV infection in chimpanzees mimic very closely the clinical and immunological observations in humans [6]. In fact, the chimpanzee has proved to be an excellent animal model for HCV.

The term $CID_{50}$/ml (50% chimpanzees infectious dose per ml), widely used for showing the infectious titre of several clinical samples implicated in the transmission of the disease, evolved from experiments performed by injection of dilutions of virus-containing samples into chimpanzees. The endpoint titre of infectivity is defined as the greatest dilution of the inocula at which 50% of the animals become infected [25,26]. Titrated inocula were then used for characterization of the virus [3], development of diagnostic methods, such as the detection of circulating HCV antibody [4], and for evaluating the sensitivity of novel PCR techniques [27–29].

The chimpanzee model also permitted studies of the physicochemical properties of the virus. For example, it was found that HCV is an enveloped virus by showing that it was inactivated by lipid solvents [30,31]. Its size was found to be 30–60 nm in diameter by using differential microfiltration [32], and its density determined as very low by ultracentrifugation [33]. The model was also used for evaluating a number of procedures for inactivating the virus in biological products, including formalin [34,35], chloroform [30,31], heat [34–36], β-propiolactone and UV irradiation [37].

Perhaps the greatest current use of the chimpanzee HCV model is as one of the most suitable sources for biological amplification of the virus. From litres of pooled chimpanzee plasma with an unusually high infectious titre [38], Houghton and colleagues [3] constructed the cDNA library of infectious material and obtained a single positive cDNA clone, 5-1-1, that expressed a virus-specific immunogenic peptide confirmed by the sera from patients with blood transfusion-associated NANB hepatitis. Using overlapping clones, the entire sequence of the HCV genome was subsequently obtained. Thus, HCV represents the first virus in the history of virology that was characterized primarily by molecular means without virus isolation in culture, and before visualization by immunoelectron microscopy [6].

Because of their phylogenetic closeness to humans [39], chimpanzees will clearly continue to be important for HCV research. In the absence of a useful cell culture system to propagate HCV, the chimpanzee will continue to provide a means for biological amplification of rare or interesting strains of HCV. The most important role for the chimpanzee HCV model will most likely be its employment for vaccine development. This will not be an easy task, as the genetic heterogeneity of HCV [40] will make the development of a broadly effective HCV vaccine difficult [7].

## Other HCV primate models

Several groups reported that both the F strain and H strain of HCV have been successfully transmitted and serially passaged in marmosets (tamarins) [25,41–43], indicating that certain species of marmoset are susceptible to human NANB hepatitis agents and could serve as a useful animal model. However, the results obtained were not consistent. The susceptibility of the marmosets to HCV appeared to be less than that of chimpanzees and the incubation periods were irregular in length [7,25].

Five other different species of primates (cynomolgus monkey, rhesus monkey, green monkey, Japanese monkey and doguera baboon) were tested and found not to be susceptible to HCV [44].

## Transgenic and *in vivo* gene transfer HCV models

A strategy of using an HCV transgenic mouse model similar to that used for HBV could be adopted. However, no work on an HCV transgenic animal model has yet been reported.

It is interesting that Hayashi and colleagues reported a new animal model with the expression of

HCV genome in adult rat liver [45]. They transfected the gene *in vivo* by retrograde biliary injection of HCV DNA complex with cationic liposomes. The cationic liposome-coated DNA has a net positive charge and facilitates the interaction with the negatively charged target cell surface, and thus gives optimal gene transfection. Retrograde biliary injection brings the DNA complex proximate to hepatocytes, which directly face the biliary canaliculi. Two days after retrograde biliary injection, the presence of HCV transcripts was confirmed in rat liver by RT–PCR analysis. A small number of HCV core-positive hepatocytes were found scattered in the lobules, resembling human HCV infection. The authors considered that the *in vivo* gene transfer model has advantages over the transgenic model for analysis of immune pathogenesis, owing to the presence of a developed adult immune system in the former model. However, HCV expression is transient in this system, as both the HCV transcripts and the HCV core proteins were not observed on day 7 after transfection.

## HCV SCID mouse model

Homozygous mutation of the SCID (severe combined immunodeficient) locus in SCID mice disrupts both B- and T-cell lymphoid development, resulting in low serum immunoglobulin (Ig) levels and the lack of functional T cells [46]. SCID mice are valuable animals for the study of a variety of physiological and disease processes. Their capacity to support multiple tissue xenografts allows these mice to be used as intermediate models for fastidiously host-specific organisms for which a small animal model has not been previously available. Using this system (SCID-hu), several virus infections have been investigated for replication and *in vivo* pathogenesis, as well as for antiviral testing. For example, Epstein–Barr virus [47,48], human cytomegalovirus [49], herpes simplex virus [50], adenovirus [51] and human immunodeficiency virus [52–55] infections in SCID mice have been reported.

We have obtained preliminary results for the first step in the creation of a model for HCV infection in SCID mice (RF Schinazi, unpublished results). Adult human liver fragments from a biopsy of a patient without hepatitis were transplanted either subcutaneously or intraperitoneally into SCID mice. Microscopic examination demonstrated that the implants survived 4–5 weeks after implantation, showing proliferation of the bile ductules and ductular epithelium. The typical architecture of the hepatic lobules was less obvious. The biliary elements could be differentiated from the presumed stem cell located at terminal ductules in the transplanted liver

tissue, but the stem cells should also have the potential to differentiate into hepatocytes [56,57]. Additionally, a group of mice were injected with PK15 cells (a swine kidney cell line), which have been proven to be relatively susceptible to *in vivo* HCV infection by Beach *et al.* [58]. Intraperitoneal injections produced tumours. These were confirmed to be of pig origin by FACS and histological examination.

Recently, Schinazi *et al.* [59] demonstrated that fragments of HCV-infected human liver tissue implanted subcutaneously in the backs of SCID mice were still HCV-positive, as determined by PCR, 10 weeks after engraftment. In addition, mouse livers from the engrafted animals presented a morphology consistent with mild hepatitis on the paraffin-embedded specimens taken 1–15 weeks after implantation. This work provides the foundation for an HCV animal model appropriate for extended immunological and antiviral studies.

## HCV-Trimera mouse model

Lubin and coworkers have developed a human–mouse radiation chimera in which normal mice, preconditioned by lethal split-dose total body irradiation and reconstituted with SCID mouse bone marrow cells, are permissive for engraftment of human haematopoietic cells and tissues [60–64]. This human–mouse model, which comprises three genetically disparate sources of tissue, is termed Trimera [65]. Eren *et al.* [66] have adapted the Trimera mouse, engrafted with human peripheral blood lymphocytes, for the successful generation of human monoclonal antibodies. Similarly, Galun *et al.* [62] have utilized transplantation of Trimera mice with HCV-infected human liver tissue for the development of an HCV infection model.

Recently, Trimera studies were extended to develop and optimize murine models for both HBV and HCV infection [67]. In these models, named HBV-Trimera and HCV-Trimera, a relatively long-term viraemia can be induced and readily detected. The generation of the HBV- and HCV-Trimera models is portrayed in Figure 2. CB6F1 mice, lethally irradiated and radioprotected with SCID mouse bone marrow cells, are transplanted under the kidney capsule or in the ear pinna with *ex vivo* HBV- or HCV-infected human liver fragments. Engraftment of the liver fragments, as evaluated by haematoxylin–eosin histological staining (Fig. 2), was observed in 85% of the transplanted animals 1 month after transplantation. The presence of human serum albumin-encoding mRNA in the grafted tissues indicates that viable and functional hepatocytes are maintained in these mice.

**Figure 2.** Preparation of the HBV- and HCV-Trimera models

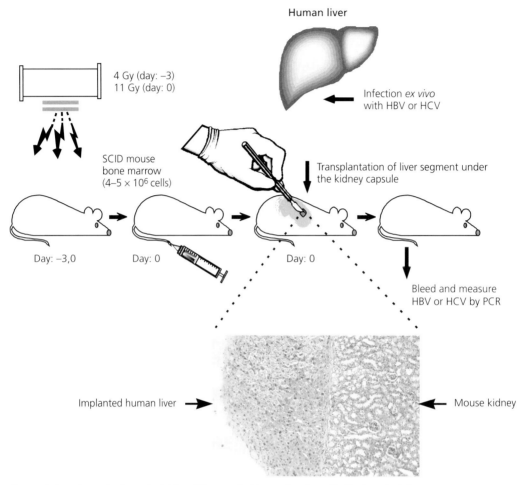

The micrograph shows haematoxylin–eosin staining of the engrafted human liver 1 month after transplantation.

Induction of viraemia in sera of HCV-Trimera mice was determined by RT–PCR followed by dot-blot hybridization. HCV RNA sequences can be detected 8 days after liver transplantation and their levels peak between days 18 and 25, by which time the percentage of infected mice reaches 80% (Fig. 3a). Replicative form of the virus (negative-strand RNA) could be detected in the engrafted liver up to a few weeks post-implantation, indicating virus replication within the graft. Thus, the HCV-Trimera mouse offers a means for simulating human HCV infection and for evaluating the *in vivo* efficacy of potential anti-HCV agents.

## HEPATITIS B ANIMAL MODELS

### HBV primate models

Presently, two useful HBV primate models exist: the chimpanzee and the tree shrew *Tupaia belangeri*. As with HCV infection, the chimpanzee model has played an important role in understanding of HBV replication, the characterization of HBV viral constituents, the development of serological tests and in molecular cloning [68–70]. The HBV chimpanzee model has also contributed significantly to preclinical testing of antiviral drugs, such as anti-HBs antibodies and small molecules [71–73], and to the development of vaccines [74,75].

The second HBV primate model, the tree shrew *T. belangeri*, can be experimentally infected with HBV by inoculation with human serum positive for HBV. Yan *et al.* [76] have shown that the experimental infection rate is 55% and that successive infections can be passed through five generations of tree shrews inoculated with HBV-positive sera. They also demonstrated that experimental infection of tree shrews with HBV may be prevented by immunization with hepatitis B vaccine. Walter *et al.* [77] have shown that the *in vivo* inoculation of tupaias with HBV-positive human sera can cause only a transient HBV infection and that viral replication and gene expression in tupaia livers are rather low. Yan *et al.* [78] were able to induce hepatocellular carcinoma in tupaias exposed to HBV and/or aflatoxin B1. Their results suggest that exposure to HBV and aflatoxin B1 may play a synergistic role in the development of hepatocellular carcinoma. The aforementioned results establish the tree shrew as a model for research on HBV infection and its relationship to hepatocarcinogenesis.

## HBV avian models

The avian hepatitis B viruses include duck hepatitis B virus (DHBV) and heron hepatitis B virus, which belong to the same DNA virus family as human HBV. Of these two, domestic ducks (Pekin ducks) infected with DHBV serve as a practical animal model for chronic HBV infection in preclinical studies and other situations [79–81]. Ducks can either be congenitally infected with DHBV or experimentally infected by intravenous inoculation of DHBV into duck embryos or very young ducklings [82,83]. Considering that as many as 10% of ducks from commercial flocks might be congenitally infected with DHBV and that the methods for experimental infection produce high titre viraemia in at least 80% of the inoculated animals [82], the use of both congenitally and experimentally infected ducks as an HBV model is quite common [79,83–85]. Owing to its low cost, the duck HBV model is used in many studies involving the *in vivo* assessment of antiviral drugs, including nucleoside analogues and interferons [79,85–88].

It should be noted that ducks appear to be less sensitive to toxic drug effects than other model animals or humans [8,89]. This is a serious disadvantage of the duck model, as the testing of HBV antiviral activity of certain drugs in the model cannot predict severe side-effects that become apparent only when clinical trials are performed [8]. The duck model is also used to study mechanisms of carcinogenesis [90] and viral replication [91,92].

## HBV rodent models

The discovery of HBV-related animal viruses designated hepadnaviruses [93] in woodchucks, ground squirrels, tree squirrels, ducks and herons offers new

**Figure 3.** Time course of viraemia in HCV- and HBV-Trimera mice

**(a)**

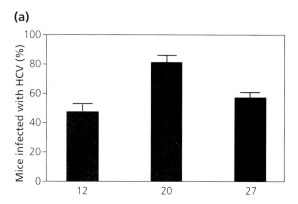

**(b)**

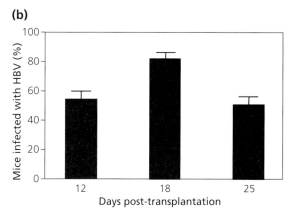

(a) HCV-Trimera mice; (b) HBV-Trimera mice. The percentage of infected animals is expressed as mean±SEM.

possibilities to test potential anti-HBV agents. Among these animal viruses, the woodchuck hepatitis virus (WHV) is the most closely related to HBV [94]. The natural courses of WHV and human HBV chronic hepatitis are comparable, including the progression to hepatocellular carcinoma [95]. Because of this similarity, the woodchuck model is used in many studies aimed at the development of new vaccines, immunotherapeutics and antiviral agents [96–99]. The woodchuck system is also used for investigating mechanisms of the viral replication cycle, carcinogenesis and cell infection [100–104].

Another member of the hepadnavirus family is the arctic squirrel hepatitis virus (ASHV). ASHV-infected ground squirrels may serve as a model to analyse the contribution of hepadnavirus and host-specific determinants to liver pathology and tumorigenesis [105].

Attempts to induce HBV infection in rats to study cellular functions and the role of immune and inflammatory responses by transfection of human HBV

DNA into rat livers have been described [106–108]. In these models, low levels of viraemia could be detected only during the first 3 days after transfection, indicating an inability to establish a model in which HBV could replicate.

Experimental models to study the effects of drugs on *in vivo* HBV replication were described using nude mice [109,110]. These mice were inoculated with HBV-transfected hepatoma cell lines. The resulting models are suitable to study tumour formation rather than chronic HBV infection.

Chisari and colleagues [111–114] developed transgenic mice that overproduce the HBV large envelope polypeptide. These mice accumulate toxic quantities of HBsAg within hepatocytes and consequently develop severe prolonged hepatocellular injury. This initiates a programmed response within the liver, characterized by inflammation, regenerative hyperplasia, and transcriptional deregulation. Similarly, Yamamura *et al.* [115] developed transgenic mice in which HBV DNA was expressed specifically in liver and kidney tissues. The normal process of HBV replication, inducing the packaging of the pregenome 3.5 kb RNA into a nucleocapsid, the reverse transcription of the complete negative-strand DNA, and the release of Dane particles into the serum before the completion of synthesis of the posititve strand, occurs in the liver of these mice. This model suggests that the species specificity of HBV infection is not due to the inability to replicate in the non-natural host, but to the lack of receptors or factors needed for virus absorption and internalization. These transgenic mice show no clinical or pathological changes, suggesting that HBV itself is not cytopathic.

The transgenic mouse models for HBV infection were used to study immunopathogenesis of viral hepatitis [116], mechanisms of tumorigenesis [117,118], antiviral agents [119], inflammatory processes and responses during HBV infection [120–123], and the role of the major histocompatibility complex class I-restricted cytotoxic T lymphocyte response [116].

Among the various HBV small animal models, the HBV-Trimera mouse is remarkable in its ability to adequately simulate human HBV infection. This stems from the ability of human HBV to replicate within human viable hepatocytes in the engrafted liver tissue. Viraemia levels are determined in these mice by measuring serum HBV DNA using PCR followed by dot-blot hybridization. HBV DNA is first detected 8 days after liver transplantation. As with the HCV-Trimera model, viraemia peaks between days 18 and 25, when HBV infection is observed in 85% of the transplanted animals (Fig. 3b). The HBV-Trimera

model was used to evaluate the therapeutic effects of human polyclonal anti-HBs antibodies (Hepatect; Biotest Pharma, Dreieich, Germany), human monoclonal anti-HBs antibodies (generated by Eren *et al.* [66]) and the reverse transcriptase inhibitor β-L-5-fluoro-2′,3′-dideoxycytidine (β-L-5FddC). Treatment of HBV-Trimera mice with these drugs effectively reduced both the percentage of infected animals and the viral load in their sera (Fig. 4a). Treatment cessation resulted in rebound of viral load, indicating HBV replication upon drug withdrawal. HBV-Trimera mice were also given two treatment courses with β-L-5FddC. Figure 4b shows a considerable reduction in the infection rate after the first treatment. A few days after treatment cessation a rebound of the infection rate was observed. A second treatment course again

Figure 4. Use of the HBV-Trimera model for evaluation of drugs

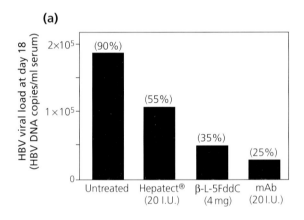

(a)

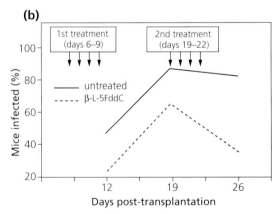

(b)

(a) Use of the HBV-Trimera model for evaluation of the therapeutic effects of polyclonal (Hepatect) and monoclonal (mAb) anti-HBs antibodies, and the reverse transcriptase inhibitor β-L-5FddC. Mice were treated at days 14–17 post-transplantation (total doses per mouse and percentages of infected mice in each group are given in parentheses). (b) Two treatment courses of HBV-Trimera mice with β-L-5FddC.

resulted in a significant reduction of the infection rate. These results show that the HBV-Trimera model represents a novel experimental tool for simulating human HBV infection and evaluating potential anti-HBV therapeutic agents.

## CONCLUSIONS

The need for reliable and reproducible animal models for HBV and HCV is critical for the development of novel therapeutic agents and combined modalities. Validation of a model can only be confirmed when agents found to be active in it are also found to be effective in humans. Since there is a paucity of effective agents against HBV infections in humans [124], and only interferon for HCV infection, it is unlikely that a correlation between animal models and studies in humans can be made at the present time. However, recent studies in woodchucks, ducks and HBV-Trimera mice treated with lamivudine indicate that these models can be good prognosticators for what will happen in humans [125] (S Dagan, unpublished results). It should be noted that lamivudine was found to be effective in humans before it was evaluated in animal models for HBV. Furthermore, the pharmacokinetics, drug distribution and metabolism can be different in woodchucks and ducks when compared with humans. For example, lamivudine is phosphorylated to low levels in woodchucks relative to human liver homogenates [126]. Nevertheless, these and related models provide powerful tools for examining the ability of the agent or modality to maximize antiviral efficacy, delay the development of hepatocarcinogenesis [127], prevent the emergence of resistant variants and predict toxicity with prolonged chronic exposure. Thus, these models should provide insights on ways to control viral replication, manage chronic carriers of HBV and HCV, and perhaps eradicate these viruses from all liver cells and extrahepatic reservoirs.

## ACKNOWLEDGEMENTS

This work was supported in part by NIH Public Health Service, NIH grant number 1R01-AI-41980 (RFS). In addition, we gratefully acknowledge Amy Juodawlkis for her editorial points.

## REFERENCES

1. Brown N & Rubin M. Lamivudine therapy for hepatitis B: current worldwide results. *Second International Conference on Therapies for Viral Hepatitis*, Kona, Hawaii, December 15–19 1997, Abstract O2.

2. Purcell RH. Hepatitis viruses: changing patterns of human disease. *Proceedings of the National Academy of Sciences, USA* 1994; **91**:2401–2406.

3. Choo QL, Kuo G, Weiner AJ, Overby LR, Bradley DW & Houghton M. Isolation of a cDNA clone derived from a blood-borne non-A, non-B viral hepatitis genome. *Science* 1989; **244**:359–362.

4. Kuo G, Choo QL, Alter HJ, Stevens CE, Tegtmeter GE, Bonino F, Colombo M, Lee WS, Kou C, Berger K, Shuster JR, Overby LR, Bresley DW & Houghton M. An assay for circulating antibodies to a major etiologic virus of human non-A, non-B hepatitis. *Science* 1989; **244**:362–364.

5. Mast EE & Alter MJ. Epidemiology of viral hepatitis: an overview. *Seminars in Virology* 1993; **4**:277–283.

6. Farci P, London WT, Wong DC, Dawson GJ, Vallari DS, Engle R & Purcell RH. The natural history of infection with hepatitis C virus (HCV) in chimpanzees: comparison of serologic responses measured with first- and second-generation assays and relationship to HCV viremia. *Journal of Infectious Diseases*, 1992;**165**:.1006–1011.

7. Purcell RH. Hepatitis C virus: historical perspective and current concepts. *FEMS Microbiology Reviews* 1994; **14**:181–192.

8. Caselmann WH. HBV and HDV replication in experimental models: effect of interferon. *Antiviral Research* 1994; **24**:121–129

9. Feinstone SM, Kapikian AZ & Purcell RH. Transfusion-associated hepatitis not due to viral hepatitis A or B. *New England Journal of Medicine* 1975; **292**:767–770.

10. Alter HJ, Purcell RH, Holland PV & Popper H. Transmissible agent in non-A, non-B hepatitis. *Lancet* 1978; i:459–463.

11. Hollinger FB, Gitnick GL, Arch RD, Szmuness W, Mosley JW, Stevens CE, Peters RL, Weiner JM, Werch JB & Lander JJ. Non-A, non-B hepatitis transmission in chimpanzees: a project of the transfusion-transmitted virus study group. *Intervirology* 1978; **10**:60–68.

12. Prince AM, van der Ende MC, Richardson L & Kellner A. Non-A, non-B hepatitis: identification of a virus-specific antigen and antibody: a preliminary report. In *Viral Hepatitis*, 1978; pp. 633–640. Edited by GN Vyas, SN Cohen & R Schmid. Philadelphia: Franklin Institute Press.

13. Tabor E, Gerety RJ, Drucker JA, Seeff LB, Hoofnagle JH, Jackson DR, April M, Barker LF & Pineda-Tamondong G. Transmission of non-A, non-B hepatitis from man to chimpanzee. *Lancet* 1978; i:463–466.

14. Tabor E, April M, Seeff LB & Gerety RJ. Acquired immunity to human non-A, non-B hepatitis: cross-challenge of chimpanzees with three infectious human sera. *Journal of Infectious Diseases* 1979; **40**:789–793.

15. Bradley DW, Cook EH, Maynard JE, McCaustland KA, Ebert JW, Dolana GH, Petzel RH, Kantor RJ, Heilbrunn A, Feilds HA & Murphy BL. Experimental infection of chimpanzees with anti-hemophilic (factor VIII) materials: recovery of virus-like particles associated with non-A, non-B hepatitis. *Journal of Medical Virology* 1979; **3**:253–269.

16. Wyke RJ, Tsiquaye KN, Thornton A, White Y, Portmann B, Das PK, Zuckerman AJ & Williams R. Transmission of non-A, non-B hepatitis to chimpanzees by factor IX concentrations after fatal complications in patients with chronic liver disease. *Lancet* 1979; i:520–524.

17. Yoshizawa H, Akahane Y, Itoh Y, Iwarkiri S, Kitajima K, Morita M, Tanaka A, Nojiri T, Suimizu M,

Miyakawa Y & Mayami M. Virus-like particles in a plasma fraction (fibrinogen) and in the circulation of apparently healthy blood donors capable of inducing non-A, non-B hepatitis in humans and chimpanzees. *Gastroenterology* 1980; **79**:512–520.

18. Tsiquaye KN & Zuckerman AJ. New human hepatitis virus. *Lancet* 1979; i:1135–1136.

19. Eder G, Gudat F & Bianchi L. Transmission of non-A, non-B hepatitis to chimpanzees. In *Virus Hepatitis – 1981 International Symposium*, 1982; p. 665. Edited by W Szmuness, HJ Alter & JE Maynard. Philadelphia: Franklin Institute Press.

20. Dienstag JL. Non-A, non-B hepatitis. II. Experimental transmission, putative virus agents and markers, and prevention. *Gastroenterology* 1983; **85**:743–768.

21. Bradley DW, Maynard JE, Popper H, Ebert JW, Cook EH, Fields HA & Kemler BJ. Persistent non-A, non-B hepatitis in chimpanzees. *Journal of Infectious Diseases* 1981; **143**:210–218.

22. Shimizu YK, Weiner AJ, Rosenblatt J, Wong DC, Shapiro M, Popkin T, Houghton M, Alter HJ & Purcell RH. Early events in hepatitis C virus infection of chimpanzees. *Proceedings of the National Academy of Sciences, USA* 1990; **87**:6441–6444.

23. Negro F, Pacchioni D, Shimizu Y, Miller RH, Bussolati G, Purcell RH & Bonino F. Detection of intrahepatic replication of hepatitis C virus RNA by in situ hybridization and comparison with histopathology. *Proceedings of the National Academy of Sciences, USA* 1992; **89**:2247–2251.

24. Erickson AL, Houghton M, Choo QL, Weiner AJ, Ralston R, Muchmore E & Walker CM. Hepatitis C virus-specific CTL responses in the liver of chimpanzees with acute and chronic hepatitis. *Journal of Immunology* 1993; **151**:4189–4199.

25. Feinstone SM, Alter HJ, Dienes HP, Shimizu Y, Popper H, Blackmore D, Sly Dl, London WT & Purcell RH. Non-A, non-B hepatitis in chimpanzees and marmosets. *Journal of Infectious Diseases* 1981; **144**:588–598.

26. Tabor E, Purcell RH & Gerety RJ. Primate animal models and titrated inocula for the study of human hepatitis A, hepatitis B, and non-A, non-B hepatitis. *Journal of Medical Primatology* 1983; **1**:305–318.

27. Cristiano K, Di Bisceglie AM, Hoofnagle JH & Feinstone SM. Hepatitis C viral RNA in serum of patients with chronic non-A, non-B hepatitis: detection by polymerase chain reaction using multiple primer sets. *Hepatology* 1991; **14**:51–55.

28. Farci P, Alter HJ, Wong D, Miller RH, Shih JW, Jett B & Purcell RH. A long-term study of hepatitis C virus replication in non-A, non-B hepatitis. *New England Journal of Medicine* 1991; **325**:98–104.

29. Bukh J, Purcell RH & Miller RH. Importance of primer selection for the detection of hepatitis C virus RNA with the polymerase chain reaction assay. *Proceedings of the National Academy of Sciences, USA* 1992; **89**:187–191.

30. Feinstone SM, Mihalik KB, Kamimura T, Alter HJ, London WT & Purcell RH. Inactivation of hepatitis B virus and non-A, non-B hepatitis by chloroform. *Infection and Immunity* 1983; **41**:816–821.

31. Bradley DW, Maynard JE, Popper H, Cook EH, Ebert JW, McCaustland KA, Schable CA & Fields HA. Posttransfusion non-A, non B hepatitis: physicochemical properties of two distinct agents. *Journal of Infectious Diseases* 1983; **148**:254–265.

32. He LF, Alling D, Popkin T, Shapiro M, Alter HJ & Purcell RH. Non-A, non-B hepatitis virus: detemina-tion of size by filtration. *Journal of Infectious Diseases* 1987; **156**:634–640.

33. Bradley DW, Krawcynski K, Beach M & Purdy M. Non-A, non-B hepatitis: toward the discovery of hepatitis C and E viruses. *Seminars in Liver Disease* 1991; **11**:128–146.

34. Tabor E & Gerety RJ. Inactivation of an agent of human non-A, non-B hepatitis by formalin. *Journal of Infectious Diseases* 1980;**142**:767–770.

35. Yoshizawa H, Itoh Y, Iwakiri S, Kitajima K, Tanaka A, Tachibana T, Nakamura T, Miyakawa Y & Mayumi M. Non-A, non-B (type 1) hepatitis agent capable of inducing tubular ultrastructures in the hepatocyte cytoplasm of chimpanzees: inactivation of formalin and heat. *Gastroenterology* 1982; **82**:502–506.

36. Purcell RH, Gerin JL, Popper H, London WT, Cicmance J, Eichberg JW, Newman J & Hrinda M. Hepatitis B virus, hepatitis non-A, non-B virus and hepatitis delta virus in lyophilized antihemophilic factor: relative sensitivity to heat. *Hepatology* 1985; **5**:1091–1099.

37. Heinrich D, Kotitshke R & Berthold H. Clinical evaluation of the hepatitis safety of a β-propiolactone/ultraviolet treated factor IX concentrate (PPSB). *Thrombosis Research* 1982; **28**:75–83.

38. Bradley DW. The agents of non-A, non-B viral hepatitis. *Journal of Medical Virology* 1985; **10**:307–319.

39. King MC & Wilson AS. Evolution at two levels in human and chimpanzees. *Science* 1975; **188**:107–118.

40. Bukh J, Purcell RH & Miller RH. At least 12 genotypes of hepatitis C virus predicted by sequence analysis of the putative E1 gene of isolates collected worldwide. *Proceedings of the National Academy of Sciences, USA* 1993; **90**:8234–8238.

41. Feinstone SM, Alter HJ, Dienes HP, Shimizu Y, Popper H, Blackmore D, Sly D, London WT & Purcell RH. Non-A, non-B hepatitis in chimpanzees and marmosets. *Journal of Infectious Diseases* 1981; **144**:588–598.

42. Karayiannis P, Scheuer PJ, Bamber M, Cohn D, Hurn BA & Thomas HC. Experimental infection of tamarins with human non-A, non-B hepatitis virus. *Journal of Medical Virology* 1983; **11**:251–256.

43. Watanabe T, Katagiri J, Kojima H, Kamimura T, Ichida F, Ashida M, Hamada C & Shibayama T. Studies on transmission of human non-A, non-B hepatitis to marmosets. *Journal of Medical Virology* 1987; **22**: 143–156.

44. Abe K, Kurata T, Teramoto Y, Shiga J & Shikata T. Lack of susceptibility of various primates and woodchucks to hepatitis C virus. *Journal of Medical Primatology* 1993; **22**:433–434.

45. Takahara T, Hayashi N, Miyamoto Y, Yamamoto M, Mita E, Fusamoto H & Kamada T. Expression of the hepatitis C virus genome in rat liver after cationic liposome-mediated in vivo gene transfer. *Hepatology* 1995; **21**:746–751.

46. Bosma GC, Custer RP & Bosma MJ. A severe combined immunodeficiency mutation in the mouse. *Nature* 1983; **301**:527–530.

47. Nakamine H, Masih AS, Okano M, Taguchi Y, Pirruccello SJ, Davis JR, Mahloch ML, Beisel KW, Kleveland K, Sanger WG *et al.* Characterization of clonality of Epstein–Barr virus-induced human B lymphoproliferative disease in mice with severe combined immunodeficiency. *American Journal of Pathology* 1993; **142**:139–147.

48. Blanc-Brunat N, Laurin D, Vivier G, Touraine JL, Sergeant A & Gamier JL. Epstein–Barr virus

lymphoblastoid cell lines from transplanted patients induced B lymphomas in SCID/hu mice: study of EBV replication. *Transplant Proceedings* 1995; **27**:1776.

49. Mocarski ES, Bonyhadi M, Salimi S, McCune JM & Kaneshima H. Human cytomegalovirus in SCID-hu mouse: thymic epithelial cells are prominent targets of viral replication. *Proceedings of the National Academy of Sciences, USA* 1993; **90**:104–108.

50. Neyts J, Jahne G, Andrei G, Snoeck K, Winkler & De Clercq E. In vivo antiherpesvirus activity of N-7-substituted acyclic nucleoside analog 2-amino-7-[(1,3-dihydroxy-2-propoxyl)methyl]purine. *Antimicrobial Agents and Chemotherapy* 1995; **39**:56–60.

51. Pilewski JM, Engelhardt JF, Bavaria JE, Kaiser LR, Wilson JM & Albelda SM. Adenovirus-mediated gene transfer to human bronchial submucosal glands using xenografts. *American Journal of Physiology* 1995; **268**:657–665.

52. McCune J, Kaneshima H, Krowka J, Namikawa R, Outzen H, Peault B, Rabin L, Shih CC, Yee E, Lieberman M *et al*. The SCID-hu mouse: a small animal model for HIV infection and pathogenesis. *Annual Review of Immunology* 1991; **9**:399–420.

53. Mosier DE, Gulizia RJ, MacIsaac PD, Torbett BE & Levy JA. Rapid loss of CD⁺ T cells in human-PBL-SCID mice by noncytopathic HIV isolates. *Science* 1993; **260**:689–692.

54. Mosier DE, Gulizia RJ, MacIsaac PD, Corey L & Greenberg PD. Resistance to human immunodeficiency virus 1 infection of SCID mice reconstituted with peripheral blood leukocytes from donors vaccinated with vaccinia gp 160 and recombinant gp 160. *Proceedings of the National Academy of Sciences, USA* 1993; **90**:2443–2447.

55. Gauduin MC, Safrit JT, Weir R, Fung MS & Koup RA. Pre- and postexposure protection against human immunodeficiency virus type 1 infection mediated by a monoclonal antibody. *Journal of Infectious Diseases* 1995; **171**:1203–1209.

56. Sigal S, Brill S, Fiorino A & Reid L. The liver as a stem cell and lineage system. *American Journal of Physiology* 1992; **263**:139–148.

57. Thorgeirsson S. Hepatic stem cells. *American Journal of Pathology* 1993; **142**:1331–1333.

58. Beach MJ, Nichols BL, Gallagher M, Hou Z, Humphrey C, Goldsmith C, Meeks L, Wang W, Hagedom CH, Krawczynski K & Bradley DW. Characterization of hepatitis C virus propagated in tissue culture. *2nd International Meeting on Hepatitis C and Related Viruses*, San Diego, July 31–August 5 1994; pp. 35.

59. Schinazi RF, Hough LM, Yao X, Lloyd RL, Fallon M, Sommadossi J-P, Fried MW & Mead JR. Hepatitis C infection in SCID mice using xenografted human livers. *Second International Conference on Therapies for Viral Hepatitis*, Kona, Hawaii, December 15–19 1997; Abstract P33.

60. Lubin I, Faktotowich Y, Lapidot T, Gan Y, Eshhar Z, Gazit E, Levite M & Reisner Y. Engraftment and development of human T and B cells in mice after bone marrow transplantation. *Science* 1991; **252**:427–431.

61. Lubin I, Segall H, Marcus H, David M, Kulova L, Steinitz M, Erlich P, Gan J & Reisner Y. Engraftment of human peripheral blood lymphocytes in normal strains of mice. *Blood* 1994; **83**:2368–2381.

62. Galun E, Burakova T, Ketzinel M, Lubin I, Shezen E, Kahana Y, Eid A Ilan Y, Rivkind A, Pizov G *et al*. Hepatitis C virus viremia in SCID→BNX mouse chimera.

*Journal of Infectious Diseases* 1995; **172**:25–30.

63. Dekel B, Burakova T, Marcus H, Shezen E, Polack S, Canaan A, Passwell J & Reisner Y. Engraftment of human kidney tissue in SCID/rat radiation chimera I. A new model of human kidney allograft rejection. *Transplantation* 1997; **64**:1541–1550.

64. Dekel B, Burakova T, Ben-Hur H, Marcus H, Oren R, Laufer J & Reisner Y. Engraftment of human kidney tissue in SCID/rat radiation chimera II. Human fetal kidney display reduced immonugenicity to adoptively transferred human PBMC and exhibit rapid growth and development. *Transplantation* 1997; **64**:1550–1558.

65. Reisner Y & Dagan S. The Trimera mouse: a novel system for the generation of human monoclonal antibodies and animal models for human diseases. *Trends in Biotechnology* 1998; **16**:242–246.

66. Eren R, Lubin I, Terkieltaub D, Ben Moshe O, Zauberman A, Uhlmann R, Tzahor T, Moss S, Ilan E, Shouval D, Galun E, Daudi N, Marcus H, Reisner Y & Dagan S. Human monoclonal antibodies specific to hepatitis B virus generated in a human/mouse radiation chimera: the Trimera system. *Immunology* 1998; **93**:154–161.

67. Ilan E, Nussbaum O, Eren R, Ben-Moshe O, Arazi Y, Berr S, Lubin I, Shouval D, Galun E, Reisner Y & Dagan S. The Trimera mouse system: a mouse model for hepatitis B and hepatitis C infection and evaluation of therapeutic agents. *Second International Conference on Therapies for Viral Hepatitis*, Kona, Hawaii, December 15–19 1997; Abstract P46.

68. Thung SN, Gerber MA, Purcell RH, London TW, Mihalik KB & H Popper. Chimpanzee carriers of hepatitis B virus. *American Association for Pathology* 1981; **105**:328–332.

69. Soike KF, Rangan SR & Gerone PJ. Viral disease models in primates. *Advances in Veterinary Science and Comparative Medicine* 1984; **28**:151–199.

70. Purcell RH, Satterfield WC, Bergmann KF, Smedile A, Ponzetto A & Gerin JI. Experimental hepatitis delta virus infection in the chimpanzee. *Progress in Clinical and Biological Research* 1987; **364**:27–36.

71. Iwarson S, Tabor E, Thomas HC, Godall A, Waters J, Snoy P, Shih JWK & Gerety R. Neutralization of hepatitis B virus infectivity by a murine monoclonal antibody: an experimental study in the chimpanzee. *Journal of Medical Virology* 1985; **16**:89–96.

72. Ogata N, Ostberg L, Ehrlich PH, Wong DC, Miller RH & Purcell RH. Markedly prolonged incubation period of hepatitis B in a chimpanzee passively immunized with human monoclonal antibody to the α determinant of hepatitis B surface antigen. *Proceedings of the National Academy of Sciences, USA* 1993; **90**:3014–3018.

73. Sawada H, Iwasa S, Nishimura O & Kitano K. Efficient production of anti-(hepatitis B virus) antibodies and their neutralizing activity in chimpanzees. *Applied Microbiology and Biotechnology* 1995; **43**:445–451.

74. Emini EA, Ellis RW, Miller WJ, McAleer WJ, Scolnick EM & Gerety RJ. Production and immunological analysis of recombinant hepatitis B vaccine. *Journal of Infection* 1986; **13**:3–9.

75. Ellis RW. Recombinant-derived hepatitis B vaccine – a paradigm for other subunit vaccine. In *AIDS Vaccine: Research and Clinical Trials*, 1990; pp. 381. Edited by S Putney & D Bolognesi. New York: Marcel Dekker.

76. Yan RQ, Su JJ, Huang DR, Gan YC, Yang C & Huang GH. Human hepatitis B virus and hepatocellular carcinoma I. Experimental infection of tree shrews with

hepatitis B virus. *Journal of Cancer Research and Clinical Oncology* 1996; **122**:283–288.

77. Walter E, Keist R, Niederost B, Pult I & Blum HE. Hepatitis B virus infection of Tupaia hepatocytes in vitro and in vivo. *Hepatology* 1996; **24**:1–5.

78. Yan RQ, Su JJ, Huang DR, Gan YC, Yang C & Huang GH. Human hepatitis B virus and hepatocellular carcinoma. II. Experimental induction of hepatocellular carcinoma in tree shrews exposed to hepatitis B virus and aflatoxin B1. *Journal of Cancer Research and Clinical Oncology* 1996; **122**:289–295.

79. Mason WS, Cullen J, Saputelli J, Wu TT, Liu C, London WT, Lustbader E, Schaffer P, O'Connell AP, Fourel I *et al.* Characterization of the antiviral effects of 2′carbodeoxyguanosine in ducks chronically infected with duck hepatitis B virus. *Hepatology* 1994; **19**:398–411.

80. Deva AK, Vickery K, Zou J, West RH, Harris JP & Cossart YE. Establishment of an in-use testing method for evaluating disinfection of surgical instruments using the duck hepatitis B model. *Journal of Hospital Infections* 1996; **33**:119–130.

81. Howe AY, Robins MJ, Wilson JS & Tyrrell DL. Selective inhibition of the reverse transcription of duck hepatitis B virus by binding of 2′,3′-dideoxyguanosine 5′-triphosphate to the viral polymerase. *Hepatology* 1996; **23**:87–96.

82. Mason WS, Halpern MS, England JM, Seal G, Egan J, Coates L, Aldrich C & Summers J. Experimental transmission of duck hepatitis B virus. *Virology* 1983; **131**:375–384.

83. Zoulim F, Dannaoui E, Borel C, Hantz O, Lin TS, Liu SH, Trepo C & Cheng YC. 2′,3′-dideoxy-beta-L-5-fluorocytidine inhibits duck hepatitis B virus reverse transcription and suppresses viral DNA synthesis in hepatocytes, both in vitro and in vivo. *Antimicrobial Agents and Chemotherapy* 1996; **40**:448–453.

84. Nicoll AJ, Angus PW, Chou ST, Luscombe CA, Smallwood RA & Locarnini SA. Demonstration of duck hepatitis B virus in bile duct epithelial cells: implications for pathogenesis and persistent infection. *Hepatology* 1997; **25**:463–469.

85. Colledge D, Luscombe C, Lin E, Wang Y, Pedersen J & Locarnini S. Pathogenic effects of antiviral therapy in chronic hepatitis B: efficacy of penciclovir versus toxicity of ganciclovir. *Second International Conference on Therapies for Viral Hepatitis*, Kona, Hawaii, December 15–19 1997; Abstract P40.

86. Niu J, Wang Y, Dixon R, Bowden S, Qiao M, Einck L & Locarnini S. The use of ampligen alone and in combination with genciclovir and coumermycin A1 for the treatment of ducks congenitally-infected with duck hepatitis B virus. *Antiviral Research* 1993; **21**: 155–171.

87. Dean J, Bowden S & Locarnini S. Reversion of duck hepatitis B virus DNA replication in vivo following cessation of treatment with the nucleoside analogue ganciclovir. *Antiviral Research* 1995; **27**:171–178.

88. Dean J & Locarnini S. Characterization of the relapse phenomenon in duck hepatitis B virus infection postpenciclovir and ganciclovir therapy. *Second International Conference on Therapies for Viral Hepatitis*, Kona, Hawaii, December 15–19 1997; Abstract P41.

89. Cova L, Fourel I, Vitvitski L, Lambert V, Chassot S, Hantz O & Trepo C. Animal models for the understanding and control of HBV and HDV infections. *Journal of Hepatology* 1993; **17** (Suppl. 3):143–148.

90. Seawright AA, Snowden RT, Olubuyide IO, Riley J, Judah DJ & Neal GE. A comparison of the effects of aflatoxin B1 on the livers of rats and duck hepatitis B

virus-infected and noninfected ducks. *Hepatology* 1993; **18**:188–197.

91. Summers J, Smith PM & Horwich AL. Hepadnaviral envelope proteins regulate covalently closed circular DNA amplification. *Journal of Virology* 1990; **64**:2819–2824.

92. Seeger C & Mason W. Hepadnavirus replication and approaches to antiviral therapy. In *Virus Strategies*, 1993; vol. 4. Edited by W Doerfler & P Bohm. Weinheim: Wiley-VCH.

93. Ganem D & HE Varmus. The molecular biology of the hepatitis B viruses. *Annual Review of Biochemistry* 1987; **56**:651–693.

94. Hantz O, Ooka T, Vitvitski L & Trepo C. Comparison of properties of woodchuck hepatitis virus and human hepatitis B virus endogenous DNA polymerases. *Antimicrobial Agents and Chemotherapy* 1984; **25**: 242–246.

95. Roggendorf M & Tolle TK. The woodchuck: an animal model for hepatitis B virus infection in man. *Intervirology* 1995; **38**:100–112.

96. Fourel I, Hantz O, Watanabe KA, Jaquet C, Chomel B, Fox JJ & Trepo C. Inhibitory effects of 2′-fluorinated arabinosyl-pyrimidine nucleosides on woodchuck hepatitis virus replication in chronically infected woodchucks. *Antimicrobial Agents and Chemotherapy* 1990; **34**:473–475.

97. Schinazi RF, Liotta DC, Hurwitz SJ, Painter G, Furman P, Barry D, Korba BE & Tennant B. Dose response of oral (–)-β-2′,3′-dideoxy-5-fluoro-3′-thiacytidine [(–)-FTC] in carriers of infected woodchuck hepatitis virus (WHV). *Second International Conference on Therapies for Viral Hepatitis*, Kona, Hawaii, December 15–19 1997; Abstract P26.

98. Furman PA, Szczech G, Cleary DG, Korba B, Sommadossi J-P & Schinazi RF. Development of novel HBV inhibitors. *Second International Conference on Therapies for Viral Hepatitis*, Kona, Hawaii, December 15–19 1997; Abstract O26.

99. Cheng Y-C, Chu CK, Peek SF, Tennant BC, Korba BE & FD Boudinot. Preclinical investigation of L-FMAU (clevudine): chemistry, biochemistry and in vivo woodchuck studies. *Second International Conference on Therapies for Viral Hepatitis*, Kona, Hawaii, December 15–19 1997; Abstract O27.

100. Pardoe IU & Michalak TI. Detection of hepatitis B and woodchuck hepatitis viral DNA in plasma and mononuclear cells from heparinized blood by the polymerase chain reaction. *Journal of Virological Methods* 1995; **51**:277–288.

101. Cote PJ & Gerin JL. In vitro activation of woodchuck lymphocytes measured by radiopurine incorporation and interleukin-2 production: implications for modeling immunity and therapy in hepatitis B virus infection. *Hepatology* 1995; **22**:687–699.

102. Li DH, Newbold JE & Cullen JM. Natural populations of woodchuck hepatitis virus contain variant precore and core sequences including a premature stop codon in the epsilon motif. *Virology* 1996; **220**: 256–262.

103. Menne S, Maschke J, Tolle TK, Lu M & Roggendorf M. Characterization of T-cell response to woodchuck hepatitis virus core protein and protection of woodchucks from infection by immunization with peptides containing a T-cell epitope. *Journal of Virology* 1997; **71**:65–74.

104. Shanmuganathan S, Waters JA, Karayiannis P, Thursz M & Thomas HC. Mapping of the cellular immune responses to woodchuck hepatitis virus core antigen

epitopes in chronically infected woodchucks. *Journal of Medical Virology* 1997; **52**:128–135.

105. Testut P, Renard CA, Terradillos O, Vitvitski-Trepo L, Tekaia F, Degott C, Blake J, Boyer B & Buendia MA. A new hepadnavirus endemic in arctic ground squirrels in Alaska. *Journal of Virology* 1996; **70**: 4210–4219.

106. Kato K, Kaneda Y, Sakurai M, Nakanishi M & Okada Y. Direct injection of hepatitis B virus DNA into liver induced hepatitis in adult rats. *Journal of Biological Chemistry* 1991; **266**:22071–22074.

107. Takahashi H, Fujimoto J & Hans S. Acute hepatitis in rats expressing human hepatitis B virus transgenes. *Proceedings of the National Academy of Sciences, USA* 1995; **92**:1470–1474.

108. Wang Y, Chen H, Wang F, Li Q, Chen G & Feng B. Rat as an animal model carrying human hepatitis B virus in hepatocytes. *Chinese Medical Journal* 1996; **109**:674–679.

109. Zhai W, Gabor G, Acs G & Paronetto F. A nude mouse model for the in vivo production of hepatitis B virus. *Gastroenterology* 1990; **98**:470–477.

110. Yao Z, Zhou Y, Feng X, Chen C & Guo J. In vivo inhibition of hepatitis B viral gene expression by antisense phosphorothioate oligodeoxynucleotides in athymic nude mice. *Journal of Viral Hepatitis* 1996; **3**:19–22.

111. Chisari FV, Klopchin K, Moriyama T, Pasquinelli C, Dunsford H, Sell S, Pinkert CA, Brinster RL & Palmiter RD. Molecular pathogenesis of hepatocellular carcinoma in hepatitis B virus transgenic mice. *Cell* 1989; **59**:1145–1156.

112. Chisari FV. Hepatitis B virus transgenic mice: insights into the virus and the disease. *Hepatology* 1995; **22**: 1316–1325.

113. Guidotti LG & Chisari FV. To kill or to cure: options in host defense against viral infection. *Current Opinions in Immunology* 1996; **8**:478–483.

114. Chisari FV. Hepatitis B virus transgenic mice: models of viral immunobiology and pathogenesis. *Current Topics in Microbiology and Immunology* 1996; **206**:149–173.

115. Yamamura K, Araki K, Hino O, Miyazaki J & Matsubara K. HBV production in transgenic mice. *Gastroenterologia Japonica* 1990; **25** (Supplement 2): 49–52.

116. Ando K, Moriyama T, Guidotti LG, Wirth S, Schreiber RD, Schlicht HJ, Huang SN & Chisari FV. Mechanisms of class I restricted immunopathology. A transgenic mouse model of fulminant hepatitis. *Journal of Experimental Medicine* 1993; **178**:1541–1554.

117. Farza H, Dragani TA, Metzler T, Manenti G, Tiollais P, Della Porta G & Pourcel C. Inhibition of hepatitis B virus surface antigen gene expression in carcinogen-induced liver tumors from transgenic mice. *Molecular Carcinogenesis* 1994; **9**:185–192.

118. Kirby GM, Chemin I, Montesano R, Chisari FV, Lang MA & Wild CP. Induction of specific cytochrome P450s involved in aflatoxin B1 metabolism in hepatitis B virus transgenic mice. *Molecular Carcinogenesis* 1994; **11**:74–80.

119. Morrey JD, Sidwell RW, Korba BE, Guidotti LG & Chisari FV. HBV transgenic mice as a chemotherapeutic model for HBV infection. *Second International Conference on Therapies for Viral Hepatitis*, Kona, Hawaii, December 15–19 1997; Abstract O193.

120. Guidotti LG, Guilhot S & Chisari FV. Interleukin-2 and alpha/beta interferon down-regulate hepatitis B virus gene expression in vivo by tumor necrosis factor-dependent and -independent pathways. *Journal of Virology* 1994; **68**:1265–1270.

121. Wirth S, Guidotti LG, Ando K, Schlicht HJ & Chisari FV. Breaking tolerance leads to autoantibody production but not autoimmune liver disease in hepatitis B virus envelope transgenic mice. *Journal of Immunology* 1995; **154**:2504–2515.

122. Guidotti LG, Ishikawa T, MV Hobbs, Matzke B, Schreiber R & Chisari FV. Intracellular inactivation of the hepatitis B virus by cytotoxic T lymphocytes. *Immunity* 1996; **4**:25–36.

123. Cavanaugh VJ, Guidotti LG & Chisari FV. Interleukin-12 inhibits hepatitis B virus replication in transgenic mice. *Journal of Virology* 1997; **71**:3236–3243.

124. Schinazi RF. Impact of nucleosides on hepatitis viruses. In *Proceedings of the IX Triennial International Symposium on Viral Hepatitis and Liver Disease*, 1997; pp. 736–742. Edited by R Purcell, J Gerin, G Verme & M Rizzetto. Torino: Minerva Medica.

125. Tennant BC, Baldwin BH, Hornbuckle WE, Korba BE, Cote PJ and Gerin JL. Animal models in the preclinical assessment of therapy for viral hepatitis. *Antiviral Therapy* 1996; **1** (Suppl. 4):47–52.

126. Schinazi RF, Hough L, Juodawlkis A, Marion P & Tennant B. Comparative activation of 2′-deoxycytidine and antiviral oxathiolane cytosine nucleosides by different mammalian liver extracts. *Antiviral Research* 1997; **34**:A65.

127. Peek SF, Toshkov IA, Erb HN, Schinazi RF, Korba BE, Cote PJ, Gerin JL & Tennant BC. 3′-Thiacytidine delays development of hepatocellular carcinoma in woodchucks with experimentally induced chronic woodchuck hepatitis virus infection. Preliminary results of a lifetime study. *American Association for the Study of Liver Diseases*, Chicago, Ill., USA, November 7–11, 1997, Abstract 957.

# 18 Transgenic mice as a chemotherapeutic model for hepatitis B virus infection

## John D Morrey*, Brent E Korba and Robert W Sidwell

## INTRODUCTION

The development of the transgenic mouse model carrying the infectious hepatitis B virus (HBV) genome has been motivated in part by the expense and minimal availability of the chimpanzee HBV model and the absence of more convenient, non-primate small animal models that can be infected with HBV. Much of the knowledge about HBV has been extrapolated from the infection of natural hosts with non-human hepatitis viruses that possess characteristics similar to those of HBV. The respective animal hepatitis virus infections of ducks, woodchucks and squirrels [1] have been enormously important in formulating much of our knowledge of HBV infection, however, small animal models carrying the human virus have not been available prior to HBV-transgenic mice because of the limited host range of HBV.

## TRANSGENIC MICE CARRYING PORTIONS OF THE HBV GENOME

The limitation of the host range of viruses can be overcome partially by genetically engineering animals to possess viral genomes. This approach has been demonstrated with human immunodeficiency virus [2,3], papillomavirus [4], and human HBV [5–10]. Many different lines of transgenic mice have been generated over the last 10 years that contain either the complete HBV genome or portions of it (Table 1). Before the generation of transgenic mice that had high levels of viral replication, highlighted later in this chapter, transgenic mice expressing specific genes either under the control of the HBV promoter [11,12] or heterologous promoter sequences [13–16] provided large amounts of information regarding immune-induced hepatitis [17–19], HBV surface antigen (HBsAg) storage disease [16,19], hepatocellular carcinoma (HCC) as promoted by HBx protein [11,20], and immunotolerance to surface [15], precore [21], or core [13] antigens. Many of the HBV proteins are not cytopathic by themselves in transgenic mice [14,22,23] unless the large surface antigen is expressed in large amounts and subsequently sequestered in hepatocytes [16,19]. Also, a number of transgenic mice have been generated to express the X protein [11,20,24], but only one study reported the spontaneous development of HCC [11] due the X protein (Table 1). The availability of these various transgenic mice could potentially provide the opportunity to evaluate cancer drugs or therapies anticipated to protect against injurious immune-induced hepatitis. These transgenic mice have not been used, overall, to evaluate therapeutics; rather, they have effectively been used to define mechanisms of pathogenesis. A transgenic mouse model was needed that completed the HBV replication cycle to a sufficient extent that it produced quantifiable levels of infectious virus so that antiviral drugs could be evaluated.

## TRANSGENIC MICE CARRYING COMPLETE HBV GENOME

Prior to 1995, transgenic mice had been reported in the literature that harboured the complete HBV genome, but did not replicate high-levels of HBV (Table 1). Two transgenic lines were reported in 1989 with the complete genome. Transgenic line 1.2HB-BX10 expressed some HBV RNA species and HBV proteins, but did not possess appreciable levels of HBV DNA replicative intermediates [10,25]. The other transgenic line (PC21), microinjected with an HBV dimer, did possess HBV DNA replicative intermediates, RNA species and HBV proteins [20,25], but it did not yield appreciable levels of infectious virions in the serum. Transgenic line pFC80-219 [12], reported in 1992, contained four tandem-copy repeats of the HBV genome. Unfortunately, it did not possess appreciable HBV DNA replicative intermediates. Nevertheless, this strain was used by Frank

---

**Table 1.** Summary of hepatitis B virus mouse models

| Type | Composition (transgenic identification number) | High-level virus replication* | Human virus used (HBV) | Drug evaluation performed | DNA replicative intermediates in liver† | RNA species in liver‡ | Antigens in liver and/or serum§ | Pathology¶ | Reference |
|---|---|---|---|---|---|---|---|---|---|
| Transgenic: complete HBV genome | Greater than unit length, (1.3.32, 1.3.46) | + | + | + | +, Except cccDNA | +, All | +, All | +, Inducible | 5,30,48–50 |
| | Greater than unit length, (1.1, 1.2) | – | + | NT** | +, Low level | +, Low level | +, Low level | NT | 5 |
| | HBV dimer (PC21) | ± Trace | + | – | +, NT cccDNA | +, 3.5 kb, 2.1 kb | + | NT | 8 |
| | 4 Tandem HBV copies (pFC80-219) | – | + | + | – | +, Only 2.1 kb | +, HBsAg | +, Inducible | 12,26,31,32,50 |
| | 1.2 Genome copies (1.2HB-BX10) | – | + | + | – | +, Some | + | NT | 10,25 |
| Transgenic: partial HBV genome | HBV small s/promoter | – | + | – | – | +, 2.1 kb | +, HBsAg | +, CTL-induced | 7,9,12,23,26,28,51 |
| | Large and small s, HBV or heterologous promoters | – | + | – | – | +, 2.4 and 2.1 kb | +, large and small s antigen | +, HCC, inducible hepatitis, HBsAg storage disease†† | 11,15, 17–19,52 |
| | HBx protein | – | + | – | – | – | +, HBxAg | +, HCC‡‡ | 11 |
| | HBx protein | – | + | – | – | – | +/– | no HCC | 20,24 |
| | Precore | – | + | – | – | + | +, HBeAg | – | 14,21 |
| | Core | – | + | – | – | + | +, HBcAg | – | 13,22 |
| Non-HBV transgenic | Woodchuck liver cell implant in uPA/RAG-2 knock-out mice§§ | + | –, WHV¶¶ | + | + | + | +, all WHV antigens | +, HCC | 29 |

* Indicated by viraemia of $10^4$–$10^7$ genome equivalents/ml in serum.
† Includes relaxed circular (rc), double-stranded linear (ds), and single-stranded (ss) HBV DNAs.
‡ Includes 3.5 kb, 2.4 kb and 2.1 kb HBV RNAs.
§ Includes HBsAg (surface), HBeAg (precore), and HBcAg (core).
¶ Any liver pathology such as hyperplasia, hepatitis or carcinoma. 'Inducible' implies that liver disease is induced by liver damage, cytokines, and cytotoxic T cell transfer.
‖ Involves adoptive immune cell transfer and immune tolerance.
** Not tested.
†† Development of the various pathologies depended on which transgenic founder was used.
‡‡ Hepatocellular carcinoma.
§§ Transplanted woodchuck hepatocytes into liver of mice that contained the urokinase-type plasminogen activator transgene (uPA) and lacked mature B and T cells due to a recombination activation gene 2 (RAG-2) gene knockout.
¶¶ Woodchuck hepatitis virus.

Chisari's group (Scripps Institute, La Jolla, California) to demonstrate that transgenic mice possessing the complete genome, and expressing the HBsAg, could be induced to develop hepatitis by HBV-specific cytotoxic T cells (CTLs) [26]. Moreover, this transgenic line was used to show that CTLs could also inhibit viral replication. It had been determined that the antiviral effects of CTLs in HBV transgenic mice not only included direct killing of HBV-infected cells, but also involved the secretion of soluble, diffusable cytokines [6,27]. A panel of cytokines was then evaluated in the pFC80-219 transgenic line (Table 2), thereby demonstrating the utility of HBV transgenic mice at least for the evaluation some cytokines as anti-HBV agents. A comprehensive categorization and descriptions of these various transgenic mice can be found in other review papers [6,27,28].

## WOODCHUCK HEPATITIS VIRUS MOUSE MODEL

Another mouse model for viral hepatitis was recently reported ([29]; Table 1). Woodchuck hepatocytes were transplanted into the livers of mice that contained the urokinase-type plasminogen activator transgene (uPA) and knockout recombination activation gene 2 (RAG-2), which lack mature B and T cells. Normal adult woodchuck hepatocytes colonized up to 90% of the mouse liver. These mice can be infected de novo with the woodchuck hepatitis virus (WHV) and can produce very high levels of infectious virus in the serum (up to $10^{11}$ virions/ml). Pre-cancerous woodchuck liver cells were also clonally expanded by transplantation of the cells into these mice to yield HCC. The therapeutic efficacy of interferon α (IFN-α) was also demonstrated in these WHV-infected mice (Table 2). The advantage of this mouse model is the de novo infection of mice with WHV, high-level production of virus, clonal expansion of pre-cancerous cells to yield HCC and the use of mice instead of woodchucks. The potential disadvantages with this model are the use of a non-human virus, a technically involved protocol for establishing the mice, and potential variability in the reconstitution of woodchuck liver cells and virus production.

## TRANSGENIC MICE WITH HIGH-LEVEL HBV REPLICATION

Transgenic lines (1.3.32 and 1.3.46) were reported in 1995 [5] to replicate virus in the liver and produce high levels of HBV in the serum (Table 1), comparable to levels found in chronically infected human patients. HBV DNA replicative intermediates (relaxed circular, double-stranded linear and single-stranded) were iden-

tified in liver. Since these intermediates are normally produced in assembled virions as a part of the HBV replication cycle, such data indicates that virus assembly was occurring in these mice. Indeed, virus particles with infectious Dane particle-like morphology were identified by electron microscopy [5]. RNA species (3.5 kb, 2.4 kb and 2.1 kb) in proportions comparable to those found in chronically infected human liver were also identified. HBV antigens found in infected human subjects were also found in these mice, namely, HBsAg and HBV e antigen (HBeAg) in the serum and liver, and HBV core antigen (HBcAg) in the liver [5].

Previously generated transgenic mice carrying either dimer [20], four tandem [12] or 1.2 [25] copies of the HBV genome did not yield high levels of virus replication. The 1.3 greater-than-genome length construct [5] appeared to be the determining factor in generating mice expressing large amounts of virus, presumably because of the need for certain redundant sequences during transgenic virus replication. From the downstream to upstream direction, the microinjected DNA consisted of the 3′ terminus at nucleotide position 1, 982 nucleotides downstream of the polyadenylation signal, through the entire length of the genome, plus a terminally redundant section of the nucleocapsid promoter, enhancer II, X promoter and enhancer I.

## DRUG THERAPY STUDIES

Five studies [10, 29–32] have previously reported the efficacy of cytokines and one nucleoside analogue in reducing viral parameters in mouse models of viral hepatitis (Table 2).

### Woodchuck hepatitis virus mouse model

As mentioned previously, viraemia was inhibited in woodchuck liver cell-transplanted mice infected with WHV by IFN-α2b (once daily intramuscular injection with 135 000 IU/kg for 15 days) (Table 2). This demonstrated the utility of this transgenic mouse as a model for antiviral therapy.

### Transgenic mice with little or no viraemia

Because of the observation that the antiviral effects of CTLs in HBV transgenic mice not only included direct killing of HBV-infected cells, but also involved the secretion of soluble cytokines [6,27], a panel of cytokines was then evaluated in the pFC80-219 transgenic line [31,32] (Table 2). Since these mice only produced HBsAg, the corresponding mRNA was the only viral parameter monitored in these studies. It was deter-

**Table 2.** Summary of drug therapy studies performed in viral hepatitis mouse models

| Type | Composition | Identification* | Drug | Route | Dosage | Outcome | Ref. |
|---|---|---|---|---|---|---|---|
| Transgenic: complete HBV genome | High viraemia, 1.3 unit-length genome | 1.3.32 [5] | Lamivudine (3TC) | Oral | 100–25 mg/kg/day, bid†, 21 days | Reduced virus load in dose-responsive manner, reduced liver and serum HBV DNA titres, viraemia rebounded after cessation of treatment | In text |
| | High viraemia, 1.3 unit-length genome | 1.3.32 | Zidovudine (AZT) | Oral | 22 mg/kg/day, 21 days | Not effective on any viral parameters | In text |
| | High viraemia, 1.3 unit-length genome | 1.3.32 | Interferon-α B/D | i.p. | $5\times10^6$, $5\times10^5$ IU/kg, once every other day, 21 days | Reduced viraemia below detectable levels in most male mice, but not females | in text |
| | High viraemia, 1.3 unit-length genome | 1.3.46 | Interleukin-12 | i.p. | 1 ng to 1 µg/mouse, qd‡ up to 14 days | Reduced viraemia, HBV DNA replicative intermediates in liver and kidney, liver HBcAg, did not inhibit HBV RNA (expression), liver toxicity at high dosages | 30 |
| | No viraemia, tandem HBV copies | pFC80-219 | Murine interleukin-2 | i.p. | 100000–400000 U, once only | Reduced HBV mRNA in liver by post-transcriptional modification | 31 |
| | No viraemia, tandem HBV copies | pFC80-219 | Human interferon-α A/D | i.p. | 500000 U, qd, 6 days | Reduced HBV mRNA in liver | 32 |
| | No viraemia, tandem HBV copies | pFC80-219 | Murine interferon-β | i.p. | 500000 U, qd, 6 days | Reduced HBV mRNA in liver | 32 |
| | No viraemia, tandem HBV copies | pFC80-219 | Mouse interferon-γ | i.p., single for 1 or 6 days | 100000–500000 U, | No effect | 32 |
| | No viraemia, tandem HBV copies | pFC80-219 | Human interleukin-1α | i.p. once only | 200000–1000000 U, | No effect | 32 |
| | No viraemia, tandem HBV copies | pFC80-219 | Murine interleukin-3 | i.p. 1 or 6 days | 45000 U, single for | No effect | 32 |
| | No viraemia, tandem HBV copies | pFC80-219 | Human interleukin-6 | i.p. 1 or 6 days | 500000 U, single for | No effect | 32 |
| | No viraemia, tandem HBV copies | pFC80-219 | Murine TNF-β | i.p. once only | 50000–500000 U, | No effect | 32 |
| | No viraemia, tandem HBV copies | pFC80-219 | Human TGF-β | i.p. | 5 µg, once only | No effect | 32 |
| | No viraemia, tandem HBV copies | pFC80-219 | Murine GM-CSF | i.p. once only | 250–4000 U, | No effect | 32 |
| | No viraemia, tandem HBV copies | pFC80-219 | rTNF-α | i.p. once only | $3.2\times10^5$–$2\times10^6$ U | Reduced HBV 2.1 kb RNA in liver | 32 |
| | No viraemia, 1.2 unit-length genome | 1.2HB-BS10 | Oxetanocin G, nucleoside analogue | i.p. | 15 mg/kg/inj., bid, 7 days | Reduced HBV DNA in liver | 10 |
| | No viraemia, 1.2 unit-length genome | 1.2HB-BS10 | Mouse interferon-α | i.p. | 200000 IU, bid, 3 days (only 3 mice) | Reduced serum HBsAg, liver HBV DNA | 10 |
| | No viraemia, 1.2 unit-length genome | 1.2HB-BS10 | Adenine arabinoside (Ara-A) | p.o. | 100 mg/kg, bid, 7 days (only 2 mice) | No effect | 10 |
| Non-transgenic HBV mice | High WHV§ viraemia, woodchuck hepatocyte transplantation | uPA/RAG-2¶ | Interferon-α2b | i.m. | 135000 IU/kg, qd, 15 days | Reduced viraemia | 29 |

* Transgenic mouse number.
† bid, twice each day.
‡ qd, once each day.
§ Woodchuck hepatitis virus (WHV).
¶ Transplanted woodchuck hepatocytes into liver of mice that contained the urokinase-type plasminogen activator transgene (uPA) and lacked mature B and T cells due to a recombination activation gene 2 (RAG-2) gene knockout.

mined that murine interleukin-2 (IL-2) [31,32], human IFN-α [32], and murine IFN-β [32] reduced HBV mRNA in the liver. The antiviral effect of IL-2 was through post-transcriptional modification and probably not through repression of transcriptional activation [31]. The effect was mediated by induction of tumour necrosis factor α. Other cytokines, with mostly single injections, were found not to reduce this viral parameter (Table 2). However, other treatment schedules would need to be performed and larger numbers of animals replicating high-levels of HBV would need to be used to conclude that these cytokines could have no anti-HBV effect.

Another transgenic mouse line (1.2HB-BS10) [10] was used to demonstrate the efficacy of murine IFN-α and a nucleoside analogue (oxetanocin G) to inhibit liver HBV DNA replicative intermediates. The IFN-α also appeared to reduce serum HBsAg, but larger numbers of mice would be required in order to confirm this observation.

## Transgenic mice with high-level HBV replication

Interest in using HBV transgenic mice for antiviral studies has increased since the development of mice that replicate high levels of virus (lines 1.3.32 and 1.3.46) [5]. The use of these mice for antiviral evaluations is described in more detail below along with information on the safety issues of working with these mice, and detection of HBV DNA by PCR.

### Safety issues

The safety classification of the HBV is biosafety level 2 or 3 (BSL-2 or -3), depending on the potential for droplet or aerosol production [33,34]. However, when more than two-thirds of infectious viral genomes are used to generate transgenic animals, the recommendation is to increase the containment conditions [35]. Francis Chisari's group has confirmed the infectivity of the transgenic viral particles by transferring the virus to the chimpanzee model (personal communication). The biosafety level for the transgenic mice of this review (lines 1.3.32 and 1.3.46) [5], containing the infectious virus, is BSL3-N where the N denotes additional precautions for animals. In our laboratory, all personnel who handle the animals are require to receive the commercially available hepatitis B vaccination (Engerix-B, SmithKline Beecham Pharmaceuticals). Vaccinated individuals are monitored for seroconversion by the local health department to verify that personnel are protected. The personnel receive special training on blood-borne pathogen handling by our institution's Environmental Health and Safety Office.

### HBV DNA detection by PCR

Since antiviral therapy can significantly lower HBV serum DNA levels, PCR-based analysis can be valuable to accurately follow the progress of viraemia as illustrated in a chemotherapeutic study described in a subsequent section. The DNA primers utilized for these analyses were: 5′-CATTGTTCACCTCACCATACTGCAC-3′ ('forward primer', initiation site 2041) and 5′-GATTGA-GACCTTCGTCTGCGAG-3′ ('backward primer', initiation site 2411). HBV DNA was prepared for amplification by extraction using GeneReleaser matrix (Bioventures) by following manufacturer's instructions. Following the lysis incubation procedure, the remaining components of the PCR reaction mixture were added [36], and the reaction tubes were subjected to the following amplification programme: 94°C for 2 min; then 39 cycles of 94°C for 1 min followed by 55°C for 1 min and then 72°C for 1 min. The completed reaction was then held at 4°C. Following PCR amplification, the contents were applied to nitrocellulose membranes using a 96-well dot-blot manifold and hybridized to a [32]P-labelled, 3.2 kb cloned HBV DNA fragment as previously described [37]. HBV DNA content in the mouse sera was quantified by comparison with a dilution series of chronic HBV carrier chimpanzee serum that contained a previously determined concentration of HBV DNA. The sensitivity of this HBV DNA detection procedure was approximately 500 HBV genome equivalents/ml serum.

## Gender variability of viral parameters

HBV surface antigens in transgenic mice have been found to be regulated by sex steroids and glucocorticoids [7]. This raised the possibility that the female murine values might vary due to hormone fluctuations and therefore female transgenic mice may not be suitable for initial antiviral experiments. HBeAg, HBsAg and HBV DNA in the serum (as an indicator of viraemia) were measured in a population of female and male transgenic mice (line 1.3.32) (Table 3). The means and variability of serum HBV DNA and HBsAg levels were essentially the same for male and female mice, indicating that females are as suitable for HBV chemotherapeutic studies as males, in terms of variability. The usability of females is fortuitous because they do not need to be housed in separate cages, as do the males. The biological significance of female mice possessing significantly lower serum HBeAg titres, as compared to male mice, is not known, but this observation

Table 3. Comparing variability of serum HBV DNA and serum viral antigen titres between male and female transgenic mice

| HBV marker | Males | Females |
|---|---|---|
| HBV DNA* | 5.4±1.0 | 5.2±0.7 |
| HBsAg† | 0.90±0.82 | 1.0±0.85 |
| HBeAg† | 0.62±0.22 | 0.39±0.15‡ |

*Mean $\log_{10}$ HBV DNA (genome equivalents/ml)±SD.
†Mean optical density (1/30 dilution)±SD.
‡$P<0.01$ as compared with male values.

does not preclude the use of female mice in such chemotherapeutic studies.

## Efficacy of IFN-$\alpha$ therapy and gender-dependent response

As indicated above, there is no difference in the mean and variability of serum HBV DNA levels between untreated male or female mice. The sexes may, however, respond differently to specific drug therapies to yield differing viral outcomes. We found this to be the case with IFN-$\alpha$ treatment; female mice did not respond as well as male mice to IFN-$\alpha$ treatment to reduce virus load. The methods and results from this study are considered below.

### Drugs

Recombinant IFN-$\alpha$ B/D was obtained from David Gangemi (Clemson University) who obtained it from Novartis (formerly CIBA-Gigy) Pharmaceuticals. IFN-$\alpha$ was prepared in sterile pyrogen-free water and stored at 4°C until use. Intraperitoneal (i.p.) dosages $5\times10^6$ or $5\times10^5$ IU/kg in a volume of 0.1 ml was given every other day (e.o.d.).

### Experimental design

A group of 14 transgenic male mice and 13 female mice were treated with the highest dosage of IFN-$\alpha$ ($5\times10^6$ IU). Thirteen male mice were treated with saline. Treatment occurred on days 0, 2, 4, 6, 8, 10, 12, 14, 16, 18 and 20. All mice were tail-bled for serum collection on the day of treatment (day 0) and every week thereafter (days 7, 14, 21, 28, 35 and 42).

### Results

Intraperitoneally administered IFN-$\alpha$ ($5\times10^6$ IU/kg) was efficacious in reducing virus titres in the sera of both male and female mice, but the responsiveness of female mice was less than that of the males (Fig. 1). As early as day 7 after the initial treatment, the mean reduction in virus load in male mice was nearly 3 $\log_{10}$, but the reduction in female mice was less than 1 $\log_{10}$. The day after the last treatment (day 21) male titres had dropped 5 $\log_{10}$; those of females had only dropped about 1 $\log_{10}$. After cessation of treatment, titres in both genders rebounded. The clinical relevance, if any, is not known, but these results do illustrate that there can be gender-dependent responses to therapies which can be accommodated with appropriate experimental design.

## Studies with lamivudine and zidovudine

In nearly all earlier transgenic studies chemotherapeutic agents were used to address basic virological events and not primarily to develop a well-defined chemotherapeutic model. The following experiment was to help develop a well-defined model. HBV and all retroviruses have reverse transcriptase activities, so nucleoside analogues functional against one of these viruses could conceivably be efficacious for both these groups of viruses. However, the nucleoside analogue, zidovudine (3′-azido-3′-deoxythymidine), does not inhibit HBV infection in man, but it is highly efficacious for reducing human immunodeficiency virus (HIV) titres in humans [38], and retrovirus titres in mice [39,40] and in other animal species [41,42]. The nucleoside analogue, lamivudine [(–)2′-deoxy-3′-thiacytidine] has previously been shown to be effective for both treatment of HBV [43,44] and HIV infections [38,45]. Therefore, we tested the validity of the transgenic model expressing high levels of virus (line 1.3.32) by using it to evaluate both zidovudine and lamivudine.

### Drug experimental design

Lamivudine (courtesy of Bud Tennant, Cornell University, Ithaca, New York) was prepared in sterile physiological saline. Zidovudine (Glaxo-Wellcome) was prepared in sterile double-distilled water at a concentration of 0.2 mg/ml. Both compounds were stored at 4°C until use. Transgenic mice were treated *per os* (p.o.) twice a day for 21 days with lamivudine (100mg/kg/day). The zidovudine was administered *ad libitum* via the drinking water, which was changed daily. Previous studies [46] indicated that the mice would drink sufficient water to achieve a dosage of about 22mg/kg/day. A group of 8 to 13 mice were included in each treatment. Blood was collected from the tails weekly for 4 weeks. As a control, transgenic mice treated p.o. with saline were studied in parallel. The viral parameters for individual mice were recorded so that the effect of drug could be monitored over time for each animal.

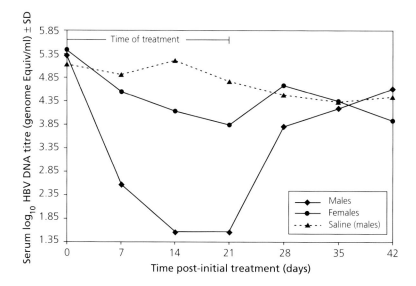

**Figure 1.** Comparison of the effect of intraperitoneal interferon-$\alpha$ B/D ($5 \times 10^6$ IU/kg) on female and male transgenic mice

The range of SD of interferon-treated male or female mice was 0.7 to 1.7. The range of SD of saline-treated mice was 0.3 to 1.1.

## Results

There was a dose-responsive reduction in virus load (serum HBV DNA) on days 14 and 21 post-initial treatment (Fig. 2). Moreover, titres were reduced in a time-dependent manner at all three dosages of lamivudine. The virus load rebounded to at least the original levels after cessation of treatment on day 20. Zidovudine was administered in parallel with the lamivudine at a concentration shown to be highly efficacious in Friend virus-infected mice [39,46]. As might be predicted, however, zidovudine treatment did not affect HBV DNA titres in transgenic mice (Fig. 3) when the titres were compared to the values at day 0 of the same group or with titres from lamivudine-treated animals (Fig. 4). These results were the predicted outcome based on human studies using lamivudine against HIV [45] and HBV [43,44].

## Efficacy studies with interleukin-12

One study [30] evaluating the efficacy of recombinant murine IL-12 described antiviral activity below toxic concentrations of the drug and yielded some information on the antiviral mechanism of Th1 response (Table 2). This study demonstrated that IL-12 had the ability to generate Th1 responses [47] and induce IFN-$\gamma$ [30]. Intraperitoneal treatment (100 ng, once daily for 14 days) reduced viraemia as determined by HBV DNA in the serum, HBV DNA replicative intermediates in the liver and kidney, and liver HBcAg. However, it did not reduce HBV RNA expression in the liver. The effect was mediated by induction of IFN-$\gamma$. It was hypothesized, in these transgenic mice, that either IL-12 prevented virion assembly or that it triggers the degradation of the nucleocapsid particles.

**Figure 2.** Effect of orally administered lamivudine (100, 50 and 25 mg/kg/day) on mean serum HBV DNA in transgenic mice

Treatment was twice daily for 21 days. Serum was assayed for HBV DNA by quantitative PCR every 7 days until day 35.

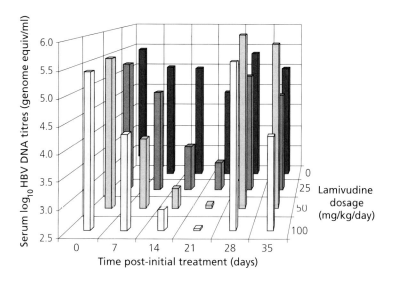

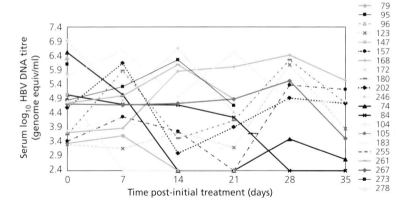

**Figure 3.** Effect of orally administered zidovudine (~22 mg/kg/day) on individual serum HBV DNA values in transgenic mice

Treatment was via drinking water *ad libitum* for 21 days in parallel to the lamivudine treatment shown in Fig. 4. The identification numbers for the mice are shown in the box in the figure. Some mice were sacrificed during the experiment, so partial data is shown for these mice with the following identification numbers: 79, 95, 96, 147, 172, 246, 104, 105, 255, 261, 278.

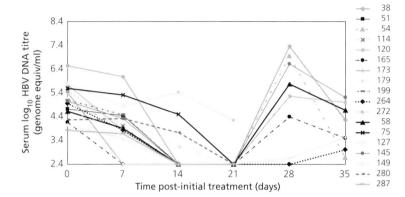

**Figure 4.** Effect of orally administered lamivudine (100 mg/kg/day) on individual serum HBV DNA values in transgenic mice

Treatment was twice daily for 21 days in parallel to the zidovudine treatment shown in Fig. 3. The identification numbers for the mice are shown in the box in the figure. Some mice were sacrificed during the experiment, so partial data is shown for these mice with the following identification numbers: 51, 78, 109, 127, 173, 179, 234, 272, 274, 280, 287.

## ADVANTAGES AND DISADVANTAGES OF THE HIGH-LEVEL EXPRESSING TRANSGENIC MODEL

This HBV transgenic mouse model does have some disadvantages as compared with the woodchucks, ducks and squirrels infected with their respective animal viruses, and with the other mouse models listed in Table 1. Some disadvantages include (i) no pathology or death is observed with these animals [5] unless it is induced by CTLs or cytokines [48]; and (ii) supercoiled DNA intermediate (cccDNA) is not present [5]. Some advantages of this model are: (i) this study demonstrated that the model is predictive for two nucleoside analogues and IFN-α; (ii) the transgenic mouse model uses the human virus [1]; (iii) mouse maintenance costs are relatively low; (iv) less drug is required for treatment of mice as compared with larger animals; (v) large numbers of the mice can be used to generate statistical power; and (vi) inbred mice have homogenous genetics for immunological and virological experimentation. These advantages indicate this to be a valuable therapeutic model for HBV.

One anticipates that as this high-level HBV transgenic-expressing mouse becomes more fully developed as a chemotherapeutic model, questions about the efficacy of different agents, routes of administration, synergy of antiviral combinations, and novel drug therapies will be answered.

## ACKNOWLEDGEMENTS

We thank Francis Chisari and Luca Guidotti (The Scripps Research Institute, La Jolla, California) for providing embryos from which to generate transgenic mice, and Brent A Korba (Division of Molecular Virology and Immunology, Georgetown University, Rockville, Maryland) for running assays. This work was supported by contract NO1-AI-65291 from the Virology Branch, National Institute of Allergy and Infectious Diseases, National Institutes of Health.

## REFERENCES

1. Ganem D. Hepadnaviridae and their replication. In *Field's Virology*, vol. 3 1996; pp. 2703–2727. Edited by BN Fields, DM Knipe & PM Howley. Philadelphia:

Lippencott-Raven.

2. Morrey JD, Bourn SM, Bunch TD, Jackson MK, Sidwell RW, Barrows LR, Daynes RA & Rosen CA. In vivo activation of human immunodeficiency virus type 1 long terminal repeat by UV light type-A (UV-A) plus psoralen and UV-B light in skin of transgenic mice. *Journal of Virology* 1991; **65**:5045–5051.

3. Leonard JM, Abramczuk JW, Pezen DS, Rutledge R, Belcher JH, Hakim F, Shearer G, Lamperth L, Travis W, Fredrickson T, Notkins AL & Martin MA. Development of disease and virus recovery in transgenic mice containing HIV proviral DNA. *Science* 1988; **242**:1665–1670.

4. Lacey M, Alpert S & Hanahan D. Bovine papillomavirus genome elicits skin tumours in transgenic mice. *Nature* 1986; **322**:609–612.

5. Guidotti LG, Matzke B, Schaller H & Chisari FV. High-level hepatitis B virus replication in transgenic mice. *Journal of Virology* 1995; **69**:6158–6169.

6. Chisari FV. Hepatitis B virus transgenic mice: insights into the virus and the disease. *Hepatology* 1995; **22**:1316–1325.

7. Farza H, Salmon AM, Hadchouel M, Moreau JL, Babinet C, Tiollais P & Pourcel C. Hepatitis B surface antigen gene expression is regulated by sex steriods and glucocorticoids in transgenic mice. *Proceedings of the National Academy of Sciences, USA* 1987; **84**:1187–1191.

8. Farza H, Hadchouel M, Scotto J, Tiollais P, Babinet C & Pourcel C. Replication and gene expression of hepatitis B virus in a transgenic mouse that contains the complete viral genome. *Journal of Virology* 1988; **62**:4144–4152.

9. DeLoia JA, Burk RD & Gearhart JD. Developmental regulation of hepatitis B surface antigen expression in two lines of hepatitis B virus transgenic mice. *Journal of Virology* 1989; **63**:4069–4073.

10. Nagahata T, Araki K, Yamamura K-I & Matsubara K. Inhibition of intrahepatic hepatitis B virus replication by antiviral drugs in a novel transgenic mouse model. *Antimicrobial Agents and Chemotherapy* 1992; **36**:2042–2045.

11. Kioke K, Moriya K, Iino S, Yotsuyanagi H, Endo Y, Miyamura T & Kurokawa K. High-level expression of hepatitis B virus HBx gene and hepatocarcinogenesis in transgenic mice. *Hepatology* 1994; **19**:810–819.

12. Gilles PN, Fey G & Chisari FV. Tumor necrosis factor alpha negatively regulates hepatitis B virus gene expression in transgenic mice. *Journal of Virology* 1992; **66**:3955–3960.

13. Milich DR, Jones JE, Hughes JL, Maruyama T, Price J, Melhado I & Jirik F. Extrathymic expression of the intracellular hepatitis B core antigen results in T cell tolerance in transgenic mice. *Journal of Immunology* 1994; **152**:455–466.

14. Guidotti LG, Matzke B, Pasquinelli C, Shoenberger JM, Rogler CE & Chisari FV. The hepatitis B virus (HBV) precore protein inhibits HBV replication in transgenic mice. *Journal of Virology* 1996; **70**:7056–7061.

15. Wirth S, Guidotti LG, Ando K, Schlicht H-J & Chisari FV. Breaking tolerance leads to autoantibody production but not autoimmune liver disease in hepatitis B virus envelope transgenic mice. *Journal of Immunology* 1995; **154**:2504–2515.

16. Chisari FV, Filippi P, McLachlan A, Milich DR, Riggs M, Lee S, Palmiter RD, Pinkert CA & Brinster RL. Expression of hepatitis B virus large envelope polypeptide inhibits hepatitis B surface antigen secretion in transgenic mice. *Journal of Virology* 1986; **60**:880–887.

17. Gilles PN, Guerrette DL, Ulevitch IJ, Schreiber RD & Chisari FV. Hepatitis B surface antigen retention sensitizes the hepatocyte to injury by physiologic concentrations of gamma interferon. *Hepatology* 1992; **16**:655–663.

18. Ando K, Moriyama T, Guidotti LG, Wirth S, Schreiber RD, Schlicht HJ, Huang SN & Chisari FV. Mechanisms of class I restricted immunopathology: a transgenic mouse model of fulminant hepatitis. *Journal of Experimental Medicine* 1993; **178**:1541–1554.

19. Moriyama T, Guilhot S, Klopchin K, Moss B, Pinkert CA, Palmiter RD & Brinster RL. Immunobiology and pathogenesis of hepatocellular injury in hepatitis B virus transgenic mice. *Science* 1990; **248**:361–364.

20. Perfumo S, Amicone I, Colloca S, Giorgio M, Pozzi I & Tripodi M. Recognition efficiency of the hepatitis B virus polyadenylation signals is tissue specific in transgenic mice. *Journal of Virology* 1992; **66**:6819–6823.

21. Milich DR, Jones JE, Hughes JL, Price J, Raney AK & McLachlan A. Is a function of the secretory hepatitis B e antigen to induce immunologic tolerance *in utero*?. *Proceedings of the National Academy of Sciences, USA* 1990; **87**:6599–6603.

22. Guidotti LG, Martinez V, Loh Y-T, Rogler CE & Chisari FV. Hepatitis B virus nucleocapsid particles do not cross the hepatocyte nuclear membrane in transgenic mice. *Journal of Virology* 1994; **68**:5469–5475.

23. Chisari FV, Pinkert CA, Miltch DR, Filippi P, McLachlan A, Palmiter RD & Brinster RL. A transgenic mouse model of the chronic hepatitis B surface antigen carrier state. *Science* 1985; **230**:1157–1160.

24. Lee T-H, Finegold MJ, Shen R-F, DeMayo JL, Woo SLC & Butel JS. Hepatitis B virus transactivator X protein is not tumorigenic in transgenic mice. *Journal of Virology* 1990; **64**:5939–5947.

25. Araki K, Miyazaki J, Hino O, Tomita N, Chisaka O, Matsubara K & Yamamura K-I. Expression and replication of hepatitis B virus genome in transgenic mice. *Proceedings of the National Academy of Sciences, USA* 1989; **86**:207–211.

26. Guidotti LG, Ando K, Hobbs MV, Ishikawa T, Runkel L, Schreiber RD & Chisari FV. Cytotoxic T lymphocytes inhibit hepatitis B virus gene expression by a noncytolytic mechanism in transgenic mice. *Proceedings of the National Academy of Sciences, USA* 1994; **91**:3764–3768.

27. Chisari FV. Hepatitis B virus transgenic mice: models of virus immunobiology and pathogenesis. *Current Topics in Microbiology and Immunology* 1996; **206**:149–173.

28. Chisari FV. Hepatitis B virus immunopathogenesis. *Annual Review of Immunology* 1995; **13**:29–60.

29. Petersen J, Dandri M, Gupta S & Rogler CE. Liver repopulation with xenogenic hepatocytes in B and T cell-deficient mice leads to chronic hepadnavirus infection and clonal growth of hepatocellular carcinoma. *Proceedings of the National Academy of Sciences, USA* 1998; **95**:310–315.

30. Cavanaugh VJ, Guidotti LG & Chisari FV. Interleukin-12 inhibits hepatitis B virus replication in transgenic mice. *Journal of Virology* 1997; **71**:3236–3243.

31. Guilhot S, Guidotti LG & Chisari FV. Interleukin-2 downregulates hepatitis B virus gene expression in transgenic mice by a posttranscriptional mechanism. *Journal of Virology* 1993; **67**:7444–7449.

32. Guidotti LG, Guilhot S & Chisari FV. Interleukin-2 and alpha/beta interferon down-regulate hepatitis B virus gene expression *in vivo* by tumor necrosis factor-dependent and -independent pathways. *Journal of Virology*

1994; **68**:1265–1270.

33. *Biosafety in Microbiological and Biomedical Laboratories*. 1993. US Government Printing Office: Washington, DC.

34. Appendix B-II-D. Class 2 viral, rickettsial, and chlamydial agents. In *Guidelines for Research Involving Recombinant DNA Molecules (NIH Guidelines)* (1994). United States Government: Washington, DC.

35. Section III-C-4. Experiments involving whole animals. In *Guidelines for Research Involving Recombinant DNA Molecules (NIH Guidelines)* (1994). United States Government: Washington, DC.

36. Kaneko S, Feinstone SM & Miller RH. Rapid and sensitive method for the detection of serum hepatitis B virus DNA using the polymerase chain reaction technique. *Journal of Clinical Investigation* 1989; **27**: 1930–1933.

37. Korba BE, Wells F, Tennant BC, Yoakum GH, Purcell RH & Gerin JL. Hepadnavirus infection of peripheral blood lymphocytes in vivo: woodchuck and chimpanzee models of viral hepatitis. *Journal of Virology* 1986; **58**:1–8.

38. Clumeck N. Current use of anti-HIV drugs in AIDS. *Journal of Antimicrobial Chemotherapy* 1993; **32** (Supplement A): 133–138.

39. Morrey JD, Warren RP, Burger RA, Okleberry KM, Johnston MA & Sidwell RW. Effects of zidovudine on Friend virus complex infection in Rfv-3r/s genotype-containing mice used as a model for HIV infection. *Journal of Acquired Immune Deficiency Syndromes* 1990; **3**:500–510.

40. Ruprecht RM, Chou T-C, Chipty F, Sosa MG, Mullaney S, O'Brain L & Rosas D. Interferon-α and 3′-azido-3′-deoxythymidine are highly synergistic in mice and prevent viremia after acute retrovirus exposure. *Journal of Acquired Immune Deficiency Syndromes* 1990; **3**:591–600.

41. Fazely F, Haseltine WA, Rodger RF & Ruprecht R. Postexposure chemoprophylaxis with ZDV combined with interferon-alpha: failure after inoculating rhesus monkeys with a high dose of SIV. *Journal of Acquired Immune Deficiency Syndromes* 1991; **4**:1093–1097.

42. Tavares L, Roneker C, Johnson K, Nusinoff-Lehrman S & de Noronha F. 3′-Azido-3′-deoxythymidine in feline leukemia and lymphocyte decline but not primary infection in feline immunodeficiency virus-infected cats: a model for therapy and prophylaxis of AIDS. *Cancer Research* 1997; **47**:3190–3194.

43. Schnittman SM & Pierce PF. Potential role of lamivudine (3TC) in the clearance of chronic hepatitis B virus infection in a patient coinfected with human immunodeficient virus type. *Clinical Infectious Diseases* 1996; **23**:638–639.

44. Ling R, Mutimer D, Ahmed M, Boxall EH, Elias E, Dusheiko GM & Harrison TJ. Selection of mutations in the hepatitis B virus polymerase during therapy of transplant recipients with lamivudine. *Hepatology* 1996; **24**:711–713.

45. Hart GJ, Orr DC, Penn CR, Figueiredo HT, Gray NM, Boehme RE & Cameron JM. Effects of (–)-2′-deoxy-3′-thiacytidine (3TC) 5′-triphosphate on human immunodeficiency virus reverse transcriptase and mammalian DNA polymerases alpha, beta, and gamma. *Antimicrobial Agents and Chemotherapy* 1992; **36**: 1688–1694.

46. Morrey JD, Okleberry KM & Sidwell RW. Early-initiated zidovudine therapy prevents disease but not low levels of presistent retrovirus in mice. *Journal of Acquired Immune Deficiency Syndromes* 1991; **4**:506–512.

47. Schreiber RD, Hicks LJ, Celada A, Buchmeier NA & Gray PW. Monoclonal antibodies to murine γ-interferon which differentially modulate macrophage activation and antiviral activities. *Journal of Immunology* 1985; **134**:1609–1618.

48. Guidotti LG, Ishikawa T, Hobbs MV, Matzke B, Schreiber R & Chisari FV. Intracellular inactivation of the hepatitis B virus by cytotoxic T lymphocytes. *Immunity* 1996; **4**:25–36.

49. Guidotti LG, Borrow P, Hobbs MV, Matzke B, Gresser I, Oldstone MBA & Chisari FV. Viral cross talk: intracellular inactivation of the hepatitis B virus during an unrelated viral infection of the liver. *Proceedings of the National Academy of Sciences, USA* 1996; **93**:4589–4594.

50. Tsui IV, Guidotti LG, Ishikawa T & Chisari FV. Posttranscriptional clearance of hepatitis B virus RNA by cytotoxic T lymphocyte-activated hepatocytes. *Proceedings of the National Academy of Sciences, USA* 1995; **92**:12398–12402.

51. Burk RD, DeLoia JA, El Awady MK & Gearhart JD. Tissue preferential expression of the hepatitis B virus (HBV) surface antigen gene in two lines of HBV transgenic mice. *Journal of Virology* 1988; **62**:649–654.

52. Phillips JW & Morgan WF. Illegitimate recombination induced by DNA double-strand breaks in a mammalian chromosome. *Molecular and Cellular Biology* 1994; **14**:5794–5803.

# 19 The woodchuck in preclinical assessment of therapy for hepatitis B virus infection

Bud C Tennant\*, Simon F Peek, Ilia A Tochkov, Betty H Baldwin, William E Hornbuckle, Brent E Korba, Paul J Cote and John L Gerin

## INTRODUCTION

The Eastern woodchuck (*Marmota monax*) is a rodent and a member of the family Sciuridae that includes squirrels, prairie dogs, chipmunks, and other marmots. The hepatitis B virus (HBV) is the prototype species of the family *Hepadnaviridae* and is classified in the genus *Orthohepadnavirus*. Orthohepadnaviruses have been shown to infect several members of the family Sciuridae [1] (Table 1). The hepadnavirus infecting woodchucks is the woodchuck hepatitis virus (WHV) [2]; that infecting the California ground squirrel has been called the ground squirrel hepatitis virus (GSHV) [3] and, recently, infection with the Arctic ground squirrel virus (AGSV) has been demonstrated in the Arctic ground squirrel [4].

The woodchuck is native to the eastern USA, most of Canada and eastern Alaska. Natural infection with WHV is hyperendemic in the mid-Atlantic states, including Pennsylvania, Maryland, Delaware, New Jersey, Virginia and North Carolina. The range of the California ground squirrel is from northern Mexico to southern Washington state and, as such, does not overlap with the range of the woodchuck. Infection with GSHV is said to have been demonstrated only in squirrels from the area near Palo Alto, California. The grey squirrel is native to the eastern half of the USA. To date, evidence for an hepadnavirus infection has come only from squirrels trapped in Philadelphia, Pennsylvania [5,6]. The Richardson's ground squirrel is found in western Canada, and in the northwestern USA. Hepadnavirus infection has been demonstrated in squirrels from two Canadian sites [7,8]. The Arctic ground squirrel is a native of Alaska. The extent of hepadnavirus infection in this species has not been thoroughly studied.

WHV, GSHV and AGSV have been well characterized virologically. Much less information is available regarding the hepatitis viruses of grey squirrels [5,6] and of Richardson's ground squirrels [7,8]. Infection with the Richardson's ground squirrel agent is associated with a disease remarkably similar to that caused by WHV in woodchucks [8].

The other recognized genus of hepadnaviruses, *Avihepadnavirus*, includes the duck hepatitis B virus (DHBV) [9] and the heron hepatitis virus (HHBV) [10]. DHBV has been well characterized, but less is known about the prevalence of the disease associated with HHBV infection.

## THE WOODCHUCK MODEL OF HBV INFECTION

The woodchuck model was developed following the observation that this species was naturally infected with a virus closely related to HBV [2]. Woodchucks trapped in the native habitat with chronic WHV infection were found to have chronic hepatitis, and many developed hepatocellular carcinoma (HCC). Initial experimental work showed that while acute WHV infection could be produced in susceptible adult woodchucks, the infection was characteristically self-limited. This

Table 1. Members of the family Sciuridae in which naturally occurring hepadnavirus infection has been demonstrated

| Scientific name | Common name |
| --- | --- |
| *Marmota monax* | Eastern woodchuck |
| *Spermophilus beecheyi* | California ground squirrel (Beechy ground squirrel) |
| *Sciurus carolinensis* | Grey squirrel (Tree squirrel) |
| *Spermophilus richardsonii* | Richardson's ground squirrel |
| *Spermophilus parryii* | Arctic ground squirrel |

\*Corresponding author

suggested that persistent WHV infection in the wild woodchuck population was the result of WHV infection early in life. If this were true, experimental studies of chronic WHV infection and HCC would require inoculation of WHV during the neonatal period and, for this, methods were required for breeding and maintaining woodchucks under laboratory conditions. Laboratory rearing of woodchucks was also required to control several diseases of wild woodchucks including infection with *Ackertia marmota* and *Cooperia* spp. that were associated with liver disease. Rabies is also an important infection of wildlife, including woodchucks. The racoon is a species of major importance in the current epidemic occurring in the northeastern USA. Racoons share burrows with woodchucks and may be a source of rabies in wild woodchucks.

## PATHOGENESIS OF EXPERIMENTAL WHV INFECTION

A woodchuck colony was established at Cornell University in 1979. It has been possible to produce woodchucks in the laboratory, to successfully infect neonatal woodchucks with WHV, and to produce woodchucks with persistent WHV infection for studies of pathogenesis. Two principal factors influence the outcome of experimental neonatal WHV infection. One factor is age. High rates of chronic WHV infection (50–70%) develop in woodchucks infected during the first week of life. In woodchucks infected with WHV at 2 months of age or older, however, chronic carrier rates of 10% or less are characteristically observed. Another factor determining outcome of neonatal infection has been the infectious dose of the WHV inoculum. In one study, 24 of 24 neonatal woodchucks inoculated with a standard dose of 100 µl of a $10^{-1}$ dilution of serum (5 million $WCID_{50}$) became infected based on development of antibodies to WHV core antigen (anti-WHc). Twenty-three of 24 became detectably viraemic, and 17 of the 24 became chronic carriers. At a dilution of $10^{-5}$, the same volume of inoculum resulted in WHV infection in 21 of 23 woodchucks. Ten of 21 woodchucks inoculated at the low dose became viraemic, but only 2 of 21 became chronic carriers. The difference in infectious dose altered the incubation period. At the high dose, the first serologic marker of WHV infection was detected at two months of age on average, and at the low dose was slightly more than three months. Because of the influence of age on the rate of chronicity, this difference in incubation period may be a relevant factor in determining the relationship between infectious dose and the rate of chronicity.

Following neonatal inoculation with WHV, there was characteristically no clinical evidence of acute illness. After one year, chronic WHV carriers had mild histological evidence of hepatitis. Thereafter, portal hepatitis became progressively more severe. In our studies, the median time to death in carriers was 29 months and the longest survivor lived for 56 months. The lifetime risk of developing HCC was virtually 100% in chronic WHV carriers. Woodchucks that resolved WHV infection and developed antibodies to WHV surface antigen (anti-WHs) also had a significantly reduced life expectancy. At 28 months of age when 50% of the chronic carriers had died of HCC, 80% of woodchucks with resolved WHV infection were alive. Fifty per cent survived for 60 months. The lifetime risk of developing HCC was 20% in woodchucks infected with WHV at birth and in which resolution of infection occurred based on development of anti-WHs. In uninfected, control woodchucks, raised under similar laboratory conditions, survival was 90% at 28 months and 60% at 60 months. HCC was not observed in uninfected control woodchucks.

## ANTIVIRAL STUDIES

Adult woodchucks with experimentally induced chronic WHV infection have been used for the evaluation of antiviral agents. Woodchucks are tested prior to initiation of therapy for serologic markers of WHV infection, and woodchucks positive for WHs antigen and anti-WHc antibody are used. Serum WHV DNA concentration is measured before treatment, at regular intervals during 4-, 12- or 24-week periods of treatment, and for a minimum of 12 weeks following drug withdrawal. Ultrasound-directed percutaneous liver biopsies are also obtained before treatment, after treatment is ended, and after post-treatment follow-up. The biopsies are examined histologically by routine light microscopy and histochemically for WHc and WHs antigens. Aliquots of the biopsies also are analyzed quantitatively for WHV nucleic acids.

Fifteen drugs have been tested for antiviral activity in woodchucks (Table 2). Of these, 13 were nucleoside analogues, and two were immune response modifiers. The nucleoside analogues, except for acyclovir and zidovudine, were all active *in vitro* against HBV in the 2.2.15 cell system [11]. Drugs were ranked based on their *in vitro* selective indices (SI) (Table 2). Acyclovir and zidovudine, which had no selectivity in 2.2.15 cells, had no antiviral effect in the woodchuck model of HBV infection. AraAMP, which had moderate antiviral activity *in vitro* had significant antiviral activity in woodchucks *in vivo* at the 15 mg/kg/day

**Table 2.** Comparative antiviral activity and toxicity of antiviral agents *in vitro* and *in vivo*

| Drug* | Rank | Selective index (2.2.15 cells)† | Dose (mg/kg/day) | Route | Treatment duration (days) | Toxicity‡ | Antiviral efficacy§ |
|---|---|---|---|---|---|---|---|
| (–)-FTC | 1 | 9054 | 10 | p.o. | 28 | – | +++ |
| Lamivudine | 2 | 8900 | 5 | p.o. | 28 | – | ++ |
| | | | 15 | p.o. | 28 | – | +++ |
| | | | 5 | p.o. | 84 | – | +++ |
| L-FMAU | 3 | 838 | 10 | p.o. | 84 | – | ++++ |
| 2'CDG | 4 | 126 | 1.5 | i.p. | 7 | ++++ | + |
| | | | 0.15 | i.p. | 7.17 | ++++ | Not tested |
| | | | 0.075 | i.p. | 28 | +++ | +++ |
| | | | 0.06 | p.o. | 14 | ++ | ++ |
| | | | 0.019 | p.o. | 28 | + | ++ |
| IFN-α | 5 | 76 | 5 MIU/kg/2 days | s.c. | 84 | – | + |
| Lobucavir | 6 | 50 | 20 | p.o. | 84 | + | ++++ |
| BW816U88 | 7 | 26 | 15 | i.p. | 84 | – | + |
| BW145U87 | 8 | 18 | 15 | i.p. | 84 | – | + |
| BW1592U89 | 8 | 18 | 15 | i.p. | 84 | – | + |
| D-FIAU | 9 | 9 | 0.3 | i.p. | 28 | – | +/– |
| | | | 1.5 | i.p. | 28 | – | ++ |
| | | | 1.5 | p.o. | 84 | ++++ | ++++ |
| araAMP | 10 | 5 | 15 | i.p. | 28 | – | ++ |
| Ribavirin | 10 | 5 | 40 | i.p. | 28 | + | + |
| D-FEAU | 11 | 2.6 | 2.0, 0.2 | i.p. | 84 | ++++ | +++ |
| Zidovudine | 12 | Negative | 15 | i.p. | 28 | – | – |
| Acyclovir | 12 | Negative | 40 | p.o. | 28 | – | – |

*Chemical formulae: FTC: cis-5-fluoro-1-[2-(hydroxymethyl)-1,3-oxathiolan-5-yl]cytosine; lamivudine (3TC): (–)-β-L-2′,3′-dideoxy-3′-thiacytidine; L-FMAU: 1-(2-fluoro-5-methyl-β-L-arabinofuranosyl)-uracil; 2'CDG: carbocyclic 2′-deoxyguanosine; IFN-α: rhuIFN-α B/D, recombinant human IFN-α B/D; lobucavir (BMS-180194): [IR-(1α, 2β, 3α)]-2-amino-9-[2,3-bis(hydroxymethyl)cyclobutyl]-1,9-dihydro-6H-purin-6-one; BW816U88: (±)-cis-4-(2-amino-6-(cyclopropylamino)-9H-purin-9-yl)-2-cyclopentene-1-methanol, a ddG prodrug; BW145U87: (2R,5S)-2-amino-6-(cyclopropy-lamino)-9-(tetrahydro-5-(hydroxymethyl)-2-furyl)-9H-purine, a ddG prodrug; BW1592U89: (1S,4R)-4-(2-amino-6-(cyclopropylamino)- 9H-purin-9-yl)-2-cyclopentene-1-methanol, a ddG prodrug; D-FIAU: 2′-deoxy-2′-fluoro-1-β-D-arabinofuranosyl-5-iodo-uracil; araAMP: adenine arabinoside 5′-monophosphate; ribavirin: 1-β-D-ribofuranosyl-1,2,4 triazole-3-carboxamide; D-FEAU: 2′-deoxy-2′-fluoro-1-β-D-arabinofuranosyl-5-ethyl-uracil; zidovudine (AZT): 3′-azido-3′-deoxythymidine; acyclovir: 9-(2-hydroxyethoxymethyl)guanine.
†The Selective Index (SI) is defined as the EC$_{90}$ (the concentration of drug at which 90% of HBV DNA production was inhibited) divided by the CC$_{50}$ (the concentration of drug at which cytotoxicity of 50% of 2.2.15 cells was observed).
‡2'CDG produced prompt multiorgan failure in a dose-dependent manner. Both FIAU and FEAU produced delayed toxicity not recognizable clini- cally or with biochemical tests until 7 weeks or more of antiviral drug therapy. With all three drugs, the actual mechanism(s) of toxicity are not known but with each there was evidence of multiorgan failure. Ribavirin toxicity was limited to reversible anaemia. Uniformly fatal responses were classified as (+++) or (++++), the latter being the most prompt. Clinically significant but reversible toxicity were identified as (+) or (++) responses.
§Antiviral activity was defined as (+) if there was at least a 10-fold reduction in serum WHV DNA at the end of the treatment period compared to controls; (++) and (+++) responses were defined as 2- and 3-log reductions in serum WHV DNA compared to controls; a (++++) response was defined as a greater than 3-log reduction of serum WHV DNA at the end of treatment compared to controls.
Abbreviations: p.o., per oral; i.p. intraperitoneal; s.c., subcutaneous.

dose [12]. Most nucleoside analogues with interme- diate antiviral activity *in vitro* against HBV had inter- mediate antiviral activity *in vivo* except for D-FIAU, which had potent antiviral activity in woodchucks but was highly toxic (see below). Lobucavir also had inter- mediate *in vitro* activity in the 2.2.15 cell system but at the dosage studied, was a highly potent antiviral

drug against WHV [13].
2'CDG had very potent antiviral activity in wood- chucks with chronic WHV infection, but was also remarkably toxic. Lamivudine, which had the second highest SI *in vitro*, was a potent antiviral drug in woodchucks and was without toxicity at doses of 5 or 15 mg/kg/day for 28 days.

Extended treatment of woodchucks with chronic WHV infections has delayed the development of HCC and significantly extended survival [14]. (–)-FTC, which had the highest *in vitro* selective index, was also a remarkably potent drug and was without toxicity. With most nucleosides tested, including (–)-FTC and lamivudine, withdrawal of drug treatment was followed by prompt return of serum WHV DNA to pretreatment levels, characteristically within 1 or 2 weeks after treatment ended. When D-FIAU was withdrawn after 4 weeks of treatment, return of serum WHV DNA to the pretreatment value was delayed for more than 12 weeks. A similar delay in WHV recrudescence of 13 weeks was observed following lobucavir withdrawal. The most potent of the nucleoside analogues so far tested is L-FMAU. After 12 weeks of treatment, serum WHV DNA was undetectable in all treated woodchucks and remained undetectable for more than 28 weeks after treatment ended in three of four chronic WHV carriers [15].

Interferon alpha (IFN-α) and thymosin alpha 1 (TA1) are immune response modifiers that were tested in woodchucks. The IFN-α used in woodchucks (rhuIFN-α B/D) did have significant antiviral activity *in vitro* (Table 2) and *in vivo* [16]. TA1 given at a dose of 900 µg/m$^2$ twice weekly by subcutaneous injection also produced a highly significant antiviral effect in chronic WHV carriers [17,18] but had no detectable *in vitro* activity (data not shown). As with the effective nucleosides, however, serum WHV DNA returned to near pretreatment levels following withdrawal of both IFN-α and TA1 within 12 weeks.

## TOXICITY OF ANTIVIRAL DRUGS

In addition to its use in assessment of antiviral efficacy, a potentially valuable use of the woodchuck is in the assessment of drug toxicity. The majority of antiviral drugs tested so far have been found to be without toxicity after 4 or 12 weeks of treatment. However, 2'CDG was highly toxic at a dose as low as 0.06 mg/kg/day, and D-FEAU [19] and D-FIAU [20] were toxic after extended treatment (Table 2). The closely related D-FMAU also has been shown to be toxic in woodchucks [15,18,21], while the L-FMAU isomer is not apparently toxic [15].

Toxicity of 2'CDG was observed within days after administration of the drug was initiated. The three pyrimidine drugs, D-FEAU, D-FIAU and D-FMAU, demonstrated a different pattern of toxicity. D-FEAU did not appear to be toxic either after 10 days or 4 weeks of treatment, but after 12 weeks of continued treatment at 0.2 mg/kg/day, the drug was definitely

toxic and treatment was associated with very high mortality. In a preliminary trial of D-FIAU, using doses of 0.3 and 1.5 mg/kg/day given intraperitoneally for 4 weeks, no significant toxicity was observed but signs of delayed toxicity were observed after 7 to 8 weeks of treatment [20]. A similar pattern of delayed toxicity was observed with D-FMAU [15].

A study using D-FIAU in HBV-infected patients conducted in 1993 was prematurely ended because of severe clinical toxicity [22]. Prior to the clinical trial, preclinical toxicological investigations of D-FIAU had been performed using conventional laboratory animal species with normal livers and the question was raised of whether the severe hepatotoxicity associated with D-FIAU treatment in patients with chronic HBV infection might have been related to their existing chronic hepatitis. A study was designed specifically to investigate the possibility that chronic viral infection might have influenced the toxicity in patients with chronic hepatitis associated with HBV infection using the woodchuck model [20]. The study involved four groups of woodchucks. One group was WHV-negative and received placebo. Woodchucks of the second group were also WHV-negative and received D-FIAU at a dose of 1.5 mg/kg/day. The third group of WHV-carrier woodchucks received placebo, and the fourth group of carriers received D-FIAU at the 1.5 mg/kg/day dose.

After 7 weeks of treatment, a reduction in mean body weight was observed in both D-FIAU-treated groups, compared to placebo-treated groups which gained weight. From 7 weeks onward, when food intake was first measured, there was a progressive reduction in food intake in the D-FIAU-treated groups compared to placebo groups.

D-FIAU treatment was associated with severe metabolic acidosis. After 8 weeks, serum bicarbonate levels began to fall gradually and then fell precipitously during the final days of life. The base deficit in the two D-FIAU-treated groups was significantly greater than that of the two groups not treated with D-FIAU. Acidosis was also associated with significant elevation in serum lactate, a finding also observed in human patients with D-FIAU toxicity [22]. Additional evidence of liver disease in the D-FIAU-treated groups compared with the placebo-treated animals included decreases in the serum fibrinogen concentration and increases in prothrombin time.

Pancreatitis and the occurrence of fatty liver were two of the most serious signs of toxicity in the human clinical trial [22]. The effects of D-FIAU on serum lipase activity and the extent of fatty liver was therefore of particular interest in the animal study.

Elevations in serum lipase activity occurred prior to death in several D-FIAU-treated animals but, at autopsy, none of these animals showed evidence of acute pancreatitis. There were signs of pancreatic acinar atrophy in the D-FIAU treated animals, but because food intake was not controlled, it was impossible to determine whether this effect was directly due to the drug or was secondary to anorexia.

The D-FIAU-treated animals developed fatty liver which was primarily microvesicular in type and, as such, was similar to that seen in humans [19]. Using an arbitrary scoring system to quantify the amount of steatosis present, it was found that significant amounts of fatty change were present only in the D-FIAU treated animals. Half of the D-FIAU-treated woodchucks died after 12 weeks or less. D-FIAU was stopped according to protocol after 12 weeks, and the remaining woodchucks in the treated groups all died within 4 weeks after treatment ended. Survival was not influenced by the presence or absence of chronic WHV infection, suggesting that the woodchuck was susceptible to D-FIAU toxicity – a situation similar to that seen in humans, but different to that observed in mice and rats [20].

Ironically, D-FIAU was found to be a very potent antiviral drug. At a dose of 1.5 mg/kg/day, the serum WHV DNA decreased to undetectable levels within 8 weeks. D-FIAU treatment also produced a significant decrease in the levels of hepatic WHV replicative intermediates and in the expression of WHc and WHs antigen in hepatic tissue.

Chu and Cheng have synthesized and tested the L-isomers of FEAU, FIAU, and FMAU, and have compared their cytotoxicity and anti-HBV activity *in vitro* to that of the D-isomers. All three L-isomers were remarkably less cytotoxic than the D-isomers, and L-FMAU was found to have very significant *in vitro* antiviral activity against HBV [23,24]. The pharmacokinetic [25] and pharmacodynamic [15] studies so far completed, and the absence of clinical toxicity in the woodchuck, suggests that L-FMAU is among the most important drug candidates available for development as therapy for chronic HBV infection.

## CONCLUSIONS

The woodchuck model has a valuable role to play in the investigation of the pathogenesis of hepadnaviral infections and hepatocarcinogenesis. It also has become valuable in the development of antiviral drugs, and may possibly be useful in evaluating new forms of immunotherapy both for efficacy and potential toxicity. In particular, the woodchucks seem

to be ideal for studying the impact of antiviral and immunotherapy on the outcome of hepadnavirus infection and on survival. The median life expectancy of the chronic WHV carrier woodchuck is 29 months and almost all develop HCC, providing an opportunity to determine the effects of new forms of therapeutic intervention in a relatively short period of time.

## ACKNOWLEDGEMENTS

This work was supported by Contracts NO1-AI-35164 (BCT) and NO1-AI-45179 (JLG) from the National Institute of Allergy and Infectious Diseases, National Institutes of Health, USA.

## REFERENCES

1. Tennant BC & Gerin JL. The woodchuck model of hepatitis B virus infection. In *The Liver: Biology and Pathobiology. 3rd edition* 1994; pp. 1455–1466. Edited by IM Arias, JL Boyer, N Fausto, WB Jakoby, DA Schachter & DA Shafritz. New York: Raven Press.
2. Summers J, Smolec JM & Snyder R. A virus similar to human hepatitis B virus associated with hepatitis and hepatoma in woodchucks. *Proceedings of the National Academy of Sciences, USA* 1978; 75:4533–4537.
3. Marion PL, Oshiro LS, Regnery DC, Scullard GH & Robinson WS. A virus in Beechey ground squirrels that is related to hepatitis B virus of humans. *Proceedings of the National Academy of Sciences, USA* 1980; 77:2941–2945.
4. Testut P, Renard C-A, Terradillos O, Vitvitski-Trepo L, Tekaia F, Degott C, Blake J, Boyer B & Buendia MA. A new hepadnavirus endemic in Arctic ground squirrels in Alaska. *Journal of Virology* 1996; in press.
5. Feitelson MA, Millman I, Halbherr T, Simmons H & Blumberg BS. A newly identified hepatitis B type virus in tree squirrels. *Proceedings of the National Academy of Sciences, USA* 1986; 83:2233–2237.
6. Feitelson MA, Millman I & Blumberg BS. Tree squirrel hepatitis B virus: antigenic and structural characterization. *Proceedings of the National Academy of Sciences, USA* 1986; 83:2994–2997.
7. Minuk GY, Shaffer EA, Hoar DI & Kelly J. Ground squirrel hepatitis virus (GSHV) infection and hepatocellular carcinoma in the Canadian Richardson ground squirrel (*Spermophilus richardsonii*). *Liver* 1986; 6:350–356.
8. Tennant BC, Mrosovsky N, McLean K, Cote PJ, Korba BE, Engle RE, Gerin JL, Wright J, Michener GR, Uhl E & King JM. Hepatocellular carcinoma in Richardson's ground squirrels (*Spermophilus richardsonii*): evidence for association with hepatitis B-like virus infection. *Hepatology* 1991; 13:1215–1221.
9. Mason WS, Seal G & Summers J. Virus of Pekin ducks with structural and biological relatedness to human hepatitis B virus. *Journal of Virology* 1980; 36:829–836.
10. Sprengel R, Kaleta EF & Will H. Isolation and characterization of a hepatitis B virus endemic in herons. *Journal of Virology* 1988; 62:3832–3839.
11. Korba BE & Gerin JL. Use of a standardized cell culture assay to assess activities of nucleoside analogs

against hepatitis B virus replication. *Antiviral Research* 1992; **19**:55–70.

12. Enriquez PM, Jung C, Josephson L & Tennant BC. Conjugation of adenine arabinoside 5′-monophosphate to arabinogalactan: synthesis, characterization, and antiviral activity. *Bioconjugate Chemistry* 1995; **6**: 195–202.

13. Tennant BC, Baldwin BH, Bellezza CA, Cote PJ, Korba BE & Gerin JL. Antiviral activity of BMS-180194 in the woodchuck model of hepatitis B virus infection. *36th Interscience Conference on Antimicrobial Agents and Chemotherapy*. New Orleans, Louisiana, USA, 15–18 September 1996; Abstract H22.

14. Peek SF, Tochkov IA, Erb HN, Schinazi RF, Korba BE, Cote PJ, Gerin JL & Tennant BC. 3′-thiacytidine (3TC) delays development of hepatocellular carcinoma (HCC) in woodchucks with experimentally induced chronic woodchuck hepatitis virus (WHV) infection. Preliminary results of a lifetime study. *Hepatology* 1997; **26**: 368A.

15. Peek SF, Jacob JR, Tochkov IA, Korba BE, Cote PJ, Gerin JL, Chu CK & Tennant BC. Substantial antiviral activity of 1-(2-fluoro-5-methyl-β-L-arabinofuranosyl) uracil (L-FMAU) in the woodchuck (*Marmota monax*) model of hepatitis B virus infection. *Hepatology* 1997; **26**:425a.

16. Gangemi JD, Korba BE, Tennant BC, Ueda H & Gilbert J. Antiviral and anti-proliferative activities of α interferons in experimental hepatitis B virus infections. *Antiviral Therapy* 1996; **1** (Supplement 4): 64–70.

17. Tennant BC, Korba BE, Baldwin BH, Goddard LA, Hornbuckle WE, Cote PJ & Gerin JL. Treatment of chronic woodchuck hepatitis virus infection with thymosin alpha-1 (TA1). *Antiviral Research* 1993; **20** (Supplement 1):163.

18. Gerin JL, Korba BE, Cote PJ & Tennant BC. A preliminary report of a controlled study of thymosin alpha-1 in the woodchuck model of hepadnavirus infection. In *Innovations in Antiviral Development and the Detection of Virus Infection*, 1992; pp. 121–123. Edited by TM Block, D Jungkind, RL Crowell, M Denison & LR Walsh. New York: Plenum Press.

19. Korba BE, Cote PJ, Tennant BC & Gerin JL. Woodchuck hepatitis virus infection as a model for the development of antiviral therapies against HBV. In *Viral Hepatitis and Liver Disease*, 1991; pp. 663–665. Edited by FB Hollinger, SM Lemon & H Margolis. Baltimore: Williams and Wilkins.

20. Tennant BC, Baldwin BH, Graham LA, Ascenzi MA, Hornbuckle WH, Rowland P, Tochkov IA, Yeager A, Erb H, Colacino J, Lopez C, Engelhardt J, Bowsher R, Richardson F, Lewis W, Cote P & Korba B. Antiviral activity and toxicity of fialuridine in the woodchuck model of hepatitis B virus infection. *Hepatology* 1998; (in press).

21. Fourel I, Hantz O, Watanabe KA, Jacquet C, Chomel B, Fox JJ & Trepo C. Inhibitory effects of 2′-fluorinated arabinosyl-pyrimidine nucleosides on woodchuck hepatitis virus replication in chronically infected woodchucks. *Antimicrobial Agents and Chemotherapy* 1990; **34**: 473–475.

22. McKenzie R, Fried MW, Sallie R, Conjeevaram H, Di Bisceglie AM, Park Y, Savarese B, Kleiner D, Tosokos M, Luciano C, Pruett T, Stotka JL, Straus S & Hoofnagle JH. Hepatic failure and lactic acidosis due to fialuridine (FIAU), an investigational nucleoside analogue for chronic hepatitis B. *New England Journal of Medicine* 1995; **333**:1099–1105.

23. Ma T, Pai SB, Zhu YL, Lin JS Shanmuganathan K, Du J, Wang C, Kim H, Newton MG, Cheng YC & Chu CK. Structure–activity relationships of 1-(2-deoxy-2-fluoro-β-L-arabinofuranosyl) pyrimidine nucleosides as anti-hepatitis B virus agents. *Journal of Medicinal Chemistry* 1996; **39**:2835–2843.

24. Pai SB, Liu S-H, Zhu Y-L, Chu CK & Cheng Y-C. Inhibition of hepatitis B virus by a novel L-nucleoside, 2-fluoro-5-methyl-β-L-arabinofuranosyl uracil. *Antimicrobial Agents and Chemotherapy* 1996; **40**: 380–386.

25. Witcher JW, Boudinot FD, Baldwin BH, Ascenzi MA, Tennant BC, Du JF & Chu CK. Pharmacokinetics of 1-(2-fluoro-5-methyl-β-L-arabinofuranosyl) uracil in woodchucks. *Antimicrobial Agents and Chemotherapy* 1997; **41**:2184–2187.

# 20 Antiviral therapy for chronic hepadnavirus infections

## William S Mason*, Tianlun Zhou, Fred Nunes, Lynn D Condreay, Samuel Litwin and Jesse Summers

## SUMMARY

Long-term antiviral therapy with lamivudine transiently suppresses viraemia in woodchucks chronically infected with woodchuck hepatitis virus (WHV). However, after 6 to 12 months, virus titres begin to return towards pre-treatment levels. This rebound is associated with the appearance of virus that is mutated in the active site of the viral reverse transcriptase. An attempt has therefore been made to increase the efficacy of lamivudine therapy by inducing an intrahepatic immune response to infection with a second virus, a replication defective adenovirus vector expressing β-galactosidase. The adenovirus efficiently infected the hepatocyte population of the liver; however, this superinfection did not induce clearance of WHV. In this manuscript, we review these experiments in the context of current knowledge about the biology of infection.

## INTRODUCTION

Hepatitis B virus (HBV) causes chronic infections of which the potential consequences, including active liver disease, cirrhosis, and hepatocellular carcinoma (HCC), are well known. The basis for disease activity is thought to be the cytotoxic lymphocyte (CTL) response to viral antigens that may be displayed on infected hepatocytes. Virtually 100% of the hepatocytes are presumed to be infected. However, CTL killing of hepatocytes may be primarily due to recognition of antigens expressed exclusively during virus replication: active liver injury generally abates in individuals in whom virus replication ceases, despite the fact that viral envelope proteins continue to be produced by hepatocytes, possibly from integrated, replication defective, viral DNA. Thus, the immediate goal of antiviral therapy is to shut down virus replication, not to eliminate all viral gene expression. In fact, blocking expression of viral envelope proteins which continues after replication has ceased is probably beyond the reach of current ideas about

antiviral therapies. Nonetheless, the pathogenic effect of envelope protein expression in carriers no longer producing appreciable amount of virus, while generally unknown, may have to be considered as a target for future therapeutic approaches, especially if inhibition of replication does not reduce the risk of HCC.

Two animal models are currently used to evaluate the efficacy of agents designed to inhibit virus replication, the domestic duck, congenitally infected with duck hepatitis B virus (DHBV), and the woodchuck, infected at birth with woodchuck hepatitis virus (WHV). The advantage of the duck model is that congenital infection, with virus replication very early in embryonic life [1], does not produce an immune response to viral antigens [2]. Thus, loss of virus during treatment with antiviral agents may be attributed to direct (inhibition of virus replication) and/or indirect effects (such as liver toxicity [3]) of the treatment. In woodchucks, chronic infection is normally created by infection at birth and is associated with an ongoing hepatitis. A disadvantage of this model is that virus replication may spontaneously shut down late in life, presumably as a consequence of the immune response to the infection [4].

One possible advantage of the woodchuck model is that there may be a higher rate of hepatocyte destruction, due to the immune response to viral antigens, which may augment the effects of inhibitors of virus replication. For instance, viral RNA is transcribed from episomal DNA (approximately 10–50 copies) present in the nucleus of infected hepatocytes. Hepatocytes have a very low proliferation rate in normal conditions (half-life $\geq 6$ months), which probably favours survival of this episomal DNA, unless it is adapted to segregate to daughter nuclei during mitosis. If it were not, enhanced hepatocyte division, in the presence of an inhibitor of viral DNA replication, would accelerate clearance of virus by leading to daughter cells which are free of viral DNAs. A second advantage of the woodchuck is that it should be possible to use this model to determine how

©1998 International Medical Press

to augment the host's immune response against the viral infection.

In this article, we review our experience from a preliminary, long-term study of lamivudine therapy in chronically infected woodchucks [4], with respect to effects on liver damage, fraction of infected hepatocytes, and outgrowth of drug resistant variants of WHV. Preliminary efforts to enhance the rate of WHV loss, by superinfection of the liver with an unrelated virus, are also reviewed, with particular reference to the bystander effects observed after 'superinfection' of the liver of HBV transgenic mice [5,6].

## THE HEPADNAVIRUS REPLICATION CYCLE

The replication cycle of HBV and the other hepadnaviruses is summarized in Figure 1 [7]. Most virion DNA (approximately 95%) has an open circular conformation, but a small fraction has a linear conformation. Infection begins with translocation of virion DNA to the nucleus and its conversion to a covalently closed circular DNA (cccDNA). Circular and linear DNAs are equally likely to participate in cccDNA formation [8,9]. The cccDNA is found in the cell nucleus [10,11], where it serves as the template for transcription of the viral mRNAs. However, sequences can be lost when linear viral DNA infects the cell, and the resultant cccDNA may not be competent to support a complete cycle of virus replication or subsequent round of infection.

For the mammalian hepadnaviruses, there are four distinct promoters in cccDNA, whereas DHBV has only three. It had been thought that none of the viral RNAs was normally spliced, but this idea has been challenged with the identification of a spliced DHBV transcript that is essential for virus replication [12]. Among the several viral RNAs, one of the largest (known as the pre-genome), is not just the mRNA for translation of viral core protein, the subunit of the viral nucleocapsid, but has two other functions. It is the mRNA for the viral reverse transcriptase (RT) as well as the template for reverse transcription. Synthesis of RT is limited compared with that of core protein because RT binds in cis to its own mRNA, at a sequence called epsilon (Fig. 1), and the complex is then packaged into viral nucleocapsids. Thus, the pregenomic mRNA is the only viral transcript needed for DNA synthesis [13]. In addition to the RT, core protein is also essential (J Summers, unpublished observations), possibly as reflected by the fact that viral DNA synthesis occurs entirely within immature viral nucleocapsids.

After completion of the (−)-strand of viral DNA (the reverse transcript) and partial synthesis of the (+)-strand (Fig. 1), nucleocapsids are either coated with viral envelope proteins by budding into the endoplasmic reticulum, and transported from the cell, or, if not enveloped, they may be transported to the nucleus. When nucleocapsids are transported to the nucleus, viral DNA is converted to a cccDNA conformation, as during the initiation of infection. In this intracellular pathway, the copy number of cccDNA is ultimately determined by a regulatory process that is controlled by viral proteins, in particular, the viral envelope proteins [14]. In general, the copy number of cccDNA appears to be amplified to, and maintained at, approximately 10 to 50 per productively infected cell [15,16].

cccDNA is highly important in devising strategies for therapy of chronic infections, since its elimination is the ultimate goal of therapy. Though one recent cell culture study has suggested that cccDNA is unstable in non-dividing primary hepatocytes, with a half-life of 3–5 days [17], in vivo studies have not yet led to a similar conclusion. Moreover, in another cell culture study, again employing primary hepatocyte cultures, treatment with inhibitors of viral DNA synthesis did not cause a detectable loss of cccDNA [18]. Thus, a reasonable conclusion is that cccDNA is quite stable, in vivo, in the absence of cell division. This implies that either the death or proliferation of infected cells, or a combination of both, may be essential steps in virus clearance.

These considerations imply that to cure chronic infections by treatment with an inhibitor of RT, it might be necessary to block new cccDNA formation for a sufficiently long time that all the cccDNA-containing cells either die or else lose cccDNA as they pass through the cell cycle. How long this might actually take would be dependent upon the rate of cell death and proliferation in the liver. Techniques such as bromodeoxyuridine (BUdR) labelling of nuclear DNA and immunostaining to detect proliferating cell nuclear antigen (PCNA) can be used as indicators of changes in cell cycling in vivo, but none of these techniques gives an adequate indication of actual proliferation rates. If the half-life for hepatocytes were normally 10 months (for example, rat hepatocytes appear to have a half-life of 6–12 months [19]), then the PCNA data predict that half-life is decreased to 3–30 days by chronic infection. However, the half-life for hepatocytes in normal liver is not precisely known for any species, and calculations of changes in the half-life may also be unreliable. Nonetheless, a completely different approach, involving measurements of changes in viraemia during initiation

# Figure 1. The replication cycle of hepatitis B virus and other hepadnaviruses

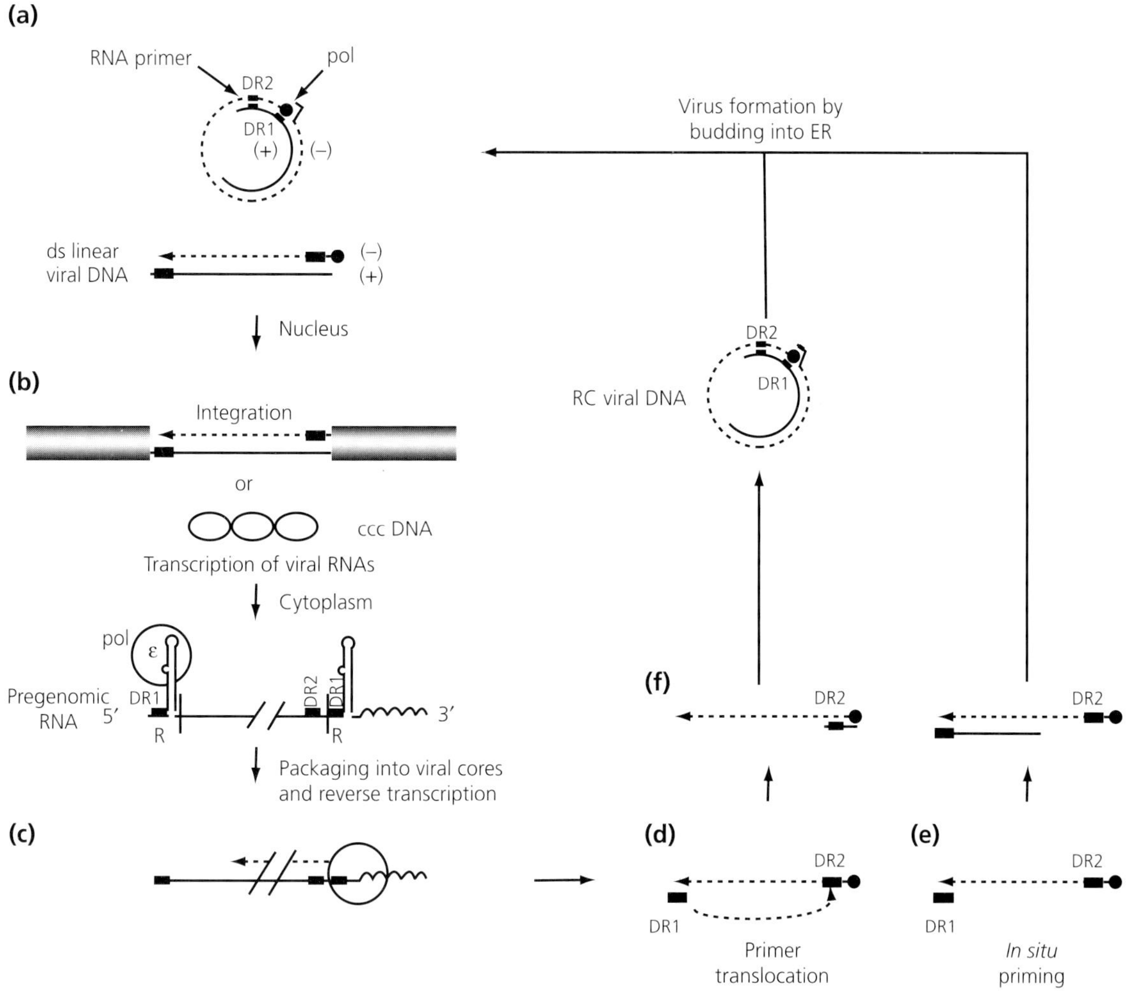

Virus, shown at the top left **(a)**, may contain either relaxed circular (RC) or linear DNA. The viral reverse transcriptase (pol) is covalently bound to the 5' end of the (–)-strand DNA, and an RNA is attached to the 5' end of the (+)-strand. The (+)-strand of RC DNA is always incomplete, but is finished during initiation of a new round of infection. In addition, during initiation, attached RNA and protein is removed. Both RC and linear DNAs may be converted to covalently closed circular DNA (cccDNA) [8,9] **(b)**, though conversion of linear DNA induces alterations around the ends that may interfere with production of replication-competent progeny virus. There is also suggestive evidence that linear DNA is a preferential substrate for integration into host DNA [27,28], an event which is presumed to be rare, but whose actual frequency is unknown. Among the RNAs transcribed from the cccDNA, one of the largest, a terminally redundant RNA known the pregenome, serves as mRNA for the nucleocapsid subunit and for the viral polymerase, a reverse transcriptase. The pol protein binds to the sequence known as epsilon at the 5' end of its own mRNA to initiate viral DNA synthesis [31,32]; at the same time, the complex is packaged into viral nucleocapsids, where the bulk of viral DNA synthesis occurs. Reverse transcription is primed from a tyrosine located in the N-terminal domain of pol [33,34]. After reverse transcription of a four-nucleotide sequence located in a bulge in the stem–loop structure of epsilon, the complex transfers to a sequence in a region known as DR1 in the 3' terminal redundancy-region of the pregenome, where the four-nucleotide sequence can anneal by base pairing **(c)**. Reverse transcription then continues to the 5' end of the RNA, which is degraded by a viral RNase-H activity of pol, except for a 17-base RNA extending from the CAP through the 5' copy of DR1 **(d-f)**. This RNA can either prime (+)-strand synthesis *in situ*, to generate linear DNA [35], or translocate to a sequence known as DR2, which is homologous to DR1, to generate circular DNA. As the (+)-strand nears completion, viral nucleocapsids undergo a maturation event which facilitates their packaging into viral envelopes at the endoplasmic reticulum for subsequent release as mature virus. The cores may also migrate to the nucleus to produce additional cccDNA, a process which appears to be blocked as long as sufficient viral envelope protein is produced.

and termination of lamivudine therapy in human carriers, suggested half-lives for chronically infected hepatocytes of as little as 2 weeks in some carriers [20].

To indicate the potential role of hepatocyte proliferation during antiviral therapy, we have calculated the fraction of infected cells that would remain after different intervals, using four different models for loss of infected hepatocytes. In each model, we assume that the antiviral drug will completely block new cccDNA synthesis and that the total number of hepatocytes stays constant. We also assume that there is no mechanism for eliminating cccDNA from cells that do not pass through mitosis. In model one, infected hepatocytes die at a constant rate and are replaced by proliferation of uninfected hepatocytes or hepatocyte progenitors. In the second model, infected hepatocytes die because of specific and non-specific killing, with the rate of non-specific killing being 10% of the rate of specific killing. Non-specific killing affects both infected and uninfected hepatocytes equally. Both uninfected and infected hepatocytes can divide to replace hepatocytes that have been destroyed, and cccDNA is lost during cell division; thus, the progeny of infected hepatocytes are virus-free. The third model is similar to the second, except that the immune response to infected hepatocytes produces secondary effects which lead to non-specific killing at an equal rate to specific killing. Infected cells still die at a higher rate than uninfected cells, since infected cells are also still subject to specific killing. Model four assumes an equal rate of killing of infected and uninfected hepatocytes. Such a model probably has no basis in the killing mediated by the immune response to viral antigens, but defines an upper limit to the rapidity of clearance if killing is, for example, due primarily to toxicity of the antiviral agent.

In Figure 2, we have plotted the loss of infected cells during antiviral therapy wth time measured in units of half-life. Thus, if the initial overall killing rate indicated a half-life of 30 days, a 99% reduction in the fraction of virus-infected hepatocytes would take about 200 days with model 1, 150 days with model 2, 120 days with model 3 and 90 days with model 4. Moreover, these models do not consider that a therapy may be ineffective in preventing new cccDNA formation, following cell division, from pre-existing, relatively mature viral DNA in nucleocapsids that are present in the cytoplasm of infected hepatocytes, or that cccDNA may actually survive through cell division. For instance, if there were 100 copies of cccDNA precursor at the start of therapy, and each daughter cell acquired 10 copies of cccDNA, infected hepatocytes could still have essentially normal amounts of cccDNA at the third generation. In other words, the appearance of substantial numbers of uninfected hepatocytes would only begin after three half-lives. Thus, a major challenge for antiviral therapy with viral DNA synthesis inhibitors, especially in carriers experiencing less overt disease activity, will be either to suppress virus replication for very long intervals or to shorten therapy times by

**Figure 2.** The role of cell death and cell proliferation in clearance of hepadnavirus infections

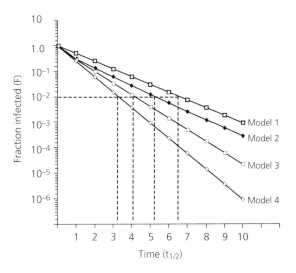

The models assume that all cells are infected at t=0 and that the total cell number, F (infected)+U (uninfected) stays constant. For this to be true, the length of the cell cycle must be short compared to the rate of cell killing. $t_{1/2}$ is the half-life of infected cells due to specific killing.

Model 1: infected cells die at a constant rate due to CTL killing and other factors associated with their infected state. There is no non-specific killing, and infected cells are replaced by division of uninfected cells. Then $dF/dt=-(\ln(2)/t_{1/2}\times F)$ and $F=\exp(-\ln(2)/t_{1/2}\times t)$, or if $t_{1/2}=1$, $F=\exp(-\ln(2)\times t)$.

Model 2: infected cells have a half-life of $t_{1/2}$ due to specific killing, and there is also a background turnover of cells due to cell death that applies to both infected and uninfected cell populations. This background turnover is unrelated to the immune response. In model 2, this background death rate is 10% of the rate of death of infected cells. Infected cells can be lost due to either death or cell division, which may occur in response to death of infected and uninfected cells. Thus, $dF/dt=-\ln(2)/t_{1/2}\times F-0.1\times\ln(2)/t_{1/2}\times F-F\times\ln(2)/t_{1/2}\times F-0.1\times F\times\ln(2)/t_{1/2}\times F-0.1\times F\times\ln(2)/t_{1/2}\times(1-F)=-1.2\times\ln(2)/t_{1/2}\times F-\ln(2)/t_{1/2}F^2$, where the expression sums the rate of loss of infected cells due to (i) specific killing of infected cells, $-\ln(2)/t_{1/2}\times F$, (ii) non-specific (background) killing of infected cells, $-0.1\times\ln(2)/t_{1/2}\times F$, (iii) regeneration due to specific killing of infected cells, $-F\times(\ln(2)/t_{1/2})\times F$, and (iv) regeneration due to non-specific killing of infected and uninfected cells, $-0.1\times F\times\ln(2)/t_{1/2}\times F-0.1\times F\times\ln(2)/t_{1/2}\times(1-F)$. If $t_{1/2}=1$, then $F=[1.2\times\exp(-1.2\times\ln(2)\times t)]/[2.2-\exp(-1.2\times\ln(2)\times t)]$.

Model 3: this model is similar to model 2, except that the background rate of killing is composed of two effects, the effect included above and an additional killing due to secondary effects of the immune response. If this rate of non-specific killing is as high as the rate due to specific killing alone, then in model 2 the factor 0.1 is replaced by 1. Then $F=[3\times\exp(-3\times\ln(2)\times t)]/[4-\exp(-3\times\ln(2)\times t)]$.

Model 4: this model is similar to model 2, except that infected and uninfected hepatocytes are assumed to be killed at the same rate (for example, as a result of drug toxicity). Thus, if $t_{1/2}=1$, $dF/dt=-(\ln(2))\times F-(\ln(2))\times F\times(F+(1-F))$, and $F=\exp(-2\times\ln(2)\times t)$. In plotting the different models, we assume that the overall rate of killing of infected cells at t=0 is the same. Thus, the half-life of infected cells due to specific killing in model 3 is twice the half-life in model 1. In model two, the half life of infected cells due to specific killing is 1.1 times the half-life in model 1. With model 4, all killing is non-specific.

inducing increased hepatocyte proliferation (for example, by immuno-therapy). A potential problem with the former approach, using only a single antiviral drug, is illustrated in Figure 3. Within a year, virus replication rebounded in all woodchucks treated with lamivudine, apparently as a consequence of the outgrowth of drug resistant virus ([4]; T Zhou and WS Mason, unpublished observations). Sequencing through the active site of the viral RT, in a region surrounding the YMDD motif, suggested that the ultimate failure of lamivudine therapy was due to WHV variants with mutations in the B domain of the RT, which maps just upstream of the YMDD motif [4]. The possible benefits of enhanced cell killing during therapy are illustrated by treatment with 2'carbodeoxyguanosine (2'CDG), which both inhibits viral DNA synthesis and causes an early burst of liver toxicity, as reflected by a very high BUdR-labelling index (10–20% after two weeks of 2'CDG administration). The fraction of infected hepatocytes was reduced to about 10% after 5 weeks of 2'CDG administration, while 6 weeks of administration of a non-toxic drug, which was also a good inhibitor of viral DNA synthesis, was essentially without effect [21].

## THE HOST IMMUNE RESPONSE AND CHRONIC HBV INFECTIONS

Because it is reasonably clear that the host immune response contributes to elevated hepatocyte destruction in carriers, it is a bit puzzling that this response does not lead to complete elimination of the virus, as it does during transient infection. To understand why this is so, it will ultimately be helpful to understand how the immune response can clear an infection, either by spontaneous activation in a chronic carrier or during transient infections. Consideration of the latter as a paradigm for therapy of chronic infections is also appropriate because virus clearance is often initiated only after a viraemia of many weeks duration and the infection of virtually the entire hepatocyte population [16,22]. That is, there is a long latent period before the immune system develops the qualitative or quantitative responses necessary for clearance.

A key to understanding how transient infections are cleared (but not the long delay) comes from the recent work of Guidotti and colleagues, who demonstrated that the cytokines, including tumour necrosis factor (TNF)-α, interferon (IFN)-α and IFN-γ, that are released by effector cells, can induce pathways leading to degradation of virus replication intermediates in HBV-transgenic mice [6,23]. Within a day after injection of activated CTLs specific for HBV surface antigen (HBsAg), viral DNA replication intermediates and viral proteins disappeared from the cytoplasm of hepatocytes. Viral mRNAs disappeared a few days later. The data also indicated that neither process depended upon hepatocyte killing, which appeared to involve a much lower percentage of hepatocytes than were actually expressing the virus. Thus, it is possible to make a simple three-step model to explain clearance

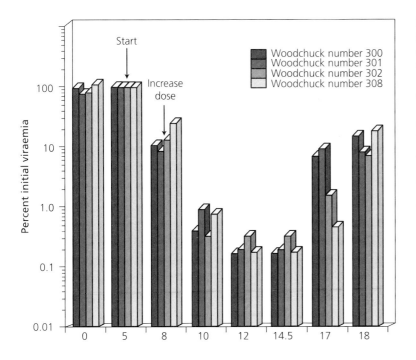

**Figure 3.** Effect of long term lamivudine therapy on virus titres in woodchucks chronically infected with WHV

Woodchucks were infected at birth and lamivudine administration was started at approximately 15 months of age. The initial dose of 40 mg/kg body weight was increased to 200 mg/kg at the indicated time. Virus titres were determined by Southern blot analysis and are summarized from a more detailed study published elsewhere [4]. The titre at the start of therapy in each woodchuck (approximately $10^9$ to $10^{10}$) was defined as 100%. The first sample was collected when the woodchucks were 10 months of age.

of transient infections: (1) Cytokines elaborated by infiltrating lymphocytes induce loss of viral replicative intermediates, including precursors to cccDNA, from infected hepatocytes; (2) greater than 50% of the infected hepatocytes are killed by viral antigen-specific CTLs; and (3) cccDNA is lost as surviving hepatocytes proliferate to maintain liver mass. An alternative model can also be derived from the work of Guidotti and colleagues [23]. Cytokines may also induce loss of cccDNA, thereby eliminating the infection without any need for cell killing and proliferation (steps 2 and 3).

It has not so far been possible to investigate whether or not cytokines can induce loss of cccDNA from hepatocytes, as HBV-transgenic mice do not make this DNA. Instead, viral mRNAs are produced in these mice from the viral transgene. However, other aspects of the mouse model apparently help explain how transient infections are resolved. Indeed, there is preliminary data to show that hepatocytes can recover from an infection, as would be predicted by the mouse experiments, though the role of hepatocyte proliferation in recovery is still unresolved [16]. Also, this [16] and another study [24] suggest that the actual recovery phase may not require the generation of neutralizing antibodies, which would be difficult to explain unless the immune response, as again predicted by the mouse studies, was able to stop infectious virus production within infected cells (for example, by intracellular degradation of replication intermediates).

Is spontaneous clearance of virus in chronic carriers mediated by the same mechanisms? In cases where clearance is associated with acute liver disease, the answer is probably yes. However, more than 50% of long-term carriers are virus-free, or produce virus at extremely low levels ($<10^6$ per ml of serum) [25]. It is not known if this shutdown of virus production is due to a transient increase in immune reactivity to viral antigens with an episode of acute liver disease. Interpretation of virus loss from long-term carriers is made more difficult by the observation that most remain HBsAg-seropositive, releasing large amounts of this viral antigen into the blood stream. Perhaps, if this HBsAg is produced from integrated DNA, it might function to inhibit new cccDNA synthesis [26] and/or provide superinfection resistance, which could contribute to loss of productively infected hepatocytes. This would make a contribution to the cessation of virus replication during a chronic infection which would not be a factor during transient infections. How important this factor might be is unknown. Recent evidence suggests that the linear forms of viral DNA are recombinagenic and that integration of viral DNA into host DNA may be a frequent event [8,9,27,28].

Unfortunately, the importance of transcription of integrated DNA in HBsAg production in nonviraemic carriers has not yet been systematically evaluated. It therefore remains speculative as to whether or not expression of HBsAg from integrated DNA does play, or even has the potential to play, a role in freeing hepatocytes of replicating virus. Thus, while transient infections provide a useful paradigm to design therapies for chronic infections, and even to understand the biology of such infections, their relevance to the latter is still uncertain.

In order to address the ability of cytokines to induce the clearance of viral proteins and DNAs from infected hepatocytes, we carried out a preliminary study to determine if the immune response to superinfection of the liver with another virus would lead to a loss of replicating WHV DNA. For this purpose, woodchucks were started on lamivudine therapy and after a week, superinfected with an adenovirus 5 vector expressing β-galactosidase [29]. In HBV transgenic mice, infection with this vector produces a bystander effect, in which cytokines elaborated during the immune response to the adenovirus induce loss of HBV proteins and replicating DNA during the first week post-infection [30]. In the woodchucks, liver biopsies were taken 3 and 30 days post-infection, with the idea that the lamivudine administration would prevent the return of any replicating DNAs that were destroyed by a bystander effect in the first few weeks following the adenovirus injection. Under these experimental conditions, no clear indication of a bystander effect was detected, despite evidence that 40 to 80% of the hepatocytes were superinfected. That is, we did not observe a drop in the amount of viral DNAs in the liver beyond the small amount that might be expected if superinfected hepatocytes were killed by adenovirus-specific CTLs. Whether this reflects a technical problem in our protocol, or a difference between the mouse and woodchuck responses to the adenovirus, is unknown. In this regard, it may be important that the work of Cavanaugh *et al.* [30] reveals that the cytokine-mediated bystander effect obtained with this adenovirus vector is much less vigorous than achieved by superinfection with murine cytomegalovirus, or lymphocytic choriomeningitis virus [6].

## CONCLUSIONS

It would appear that the most rapid elimination of infected hepatocytes during antiviral therapy with an inhibitor of viral DNA synthesis would occur if there was an interval where there was a high rate of hepatocyte turnover, in which infected hepatocytes were killed by CTLs, as well as by indirect effects of this specific response, and uninfected hepatocytes were killed by the indirect effects (Fig. 2). There is no conclusive evidence to suggest that hepadnavirus infection is intrinsically unstable in hepatocytes and it is possible that blocking viral DNA synthesis, in the absence of hepatocyte turnover, would be insufficient to clear the virus. However, the actual rate of hepatocyte death, both in infected and uninfected liver, remains a major uncertainty in evaluating various models for virus clearance. Another major uncertainty is whether or not the immune response can remove all episomal forms of viral DNA from non-dividing hepatocytes.

# ACKNOWLEDGEMENTS

This work was supported by USPHS grants AI-18641, CA-42542, CA-57425, CA-40737 and CA-06927 from the National Institutes of Health and by an appropriation from the Commonwealth of Pennsylvania.

# REFERENCES

1. Urban MK, O'Connell AP & London WT. Sequence of events in natural infection of Pekin duck embryos with duck hepatitis B virus. *Journal of Virology* 1985; **55**:16–22.
2. Halpern MS, Mason WS, Coates L, O'Connell AP & England JM. Humoral immune responsiveness in duck hepatitis B virus-infected ducks. *Journal of Virology* 1987; **61**:916–920.
3. Fourel I, Cullen JM, Saputelli J, Aldrich CE, Schaffer P, Averett DR, Pugh J & Mason WS. Evidence that hepatocyte turnover is required for rapid clearance of duck hepatitis B virus during antiviral therapy of chronically infected ducks. *Journal of Virology* 1994; **68**:8321–8330.
4. Mason WS, Cullen J, Moraleda G, Saputelli J, Aldrich CE, Miller DS, Tennant B, Frick L, Averett D, Condreay LD & Jilbert AR. Lamivudine therapy of WHV infected woodchucks. *Virology* 1998; **245**:18–32.
5. Cavanaugh VJ, Guidotti LG & Chisari FV. Inhibition of hepatitis B virus replication during adenovirus and cytomegalovirus infection with HBV transgenic mice. *Journal of Virology* 1998; **72**:2630–2637.
6. Guidotti LG, Borrow P, Hobbs MV, Matzke B, Gresser I, Oldstone MB & Chisari FV. Viral cross talk: Intracellular inactivation of the hepatitis B virus during an unrelated viral infection of the liver. *Proceedings of the National Academy of Sciences, USA* 1996; **93**:4589–4594.
7. Seeger C & Mason WS. Reverse transcription and amplification of the hepatitis B virus genome. In *DNA Replication in Eukaryotic Cells* 1996; pp. 815–831. Edited by M DePamphilis. New York: Cold Spring Harbor Laboratory Press.
8. Yang W, Mason WS & Summers J. Covalently closed circular viral DNA formed from two types of linear DNA in woodchuck hepatitis virus-infected liver. *Journal of Virology* 1996; **70**:4567–4575.
9. Yang W & Summers J. Illegitimate replication of linear hepadnavirus DNA through nonhomologous recombination. *Journal of Virology* 1995; **69**:4029–4036.
10. Miller RH & Robinson WS. Hepatitis B virus DNA forms in nuclear and cytoplasmic fractions of infected human liver. *Virology* 1984; **137**:390–399.
11. Newbold JE, Xin H, Tencza M, Sherman G, Dean J, Bowden S & Locarnini S. The covalently closed duplex form of the hepadnavirus genome exists in situ as a heterogeneous population of viral minichromosomes. *Journal of Virology* 1995; **69**:3350–3357.
12. Obert S, Zachmann BB, Deindl E, Tucker W, Bartenschlager R & Schaller H. A spliced hepadnavirus RNA that is essential for virus replication. *EMBO Journal* 1996; **15**:2565–2574.
13. Huang MJ & Summers J. Infection initiated by the RNA pregenome of a DNA virus. *Journal of Virology* 1991; **65**:5435–5439.
14. Lenhoff RJ & Summers J. Coordinate regulation of replication and virus assembly by the large envelope protein of an avian hepadnavirus. *Journal of Virology* 1994; **68**:4565–4571.
15. Jilbert AR, Burrell CJ, Gowans EJ & Rowland R. Histological aspects of in situ hybridization. Detection of poly (A) nucleotide sequences in mouse liver sections as a model system. *Histochemistry* 1986; **85**:505–514.
16. Kajino K, Jilbert AR, Saputelli J, Aldrich CE, Cullen J & Mason WS. Woodchuck hepatitis virus infections: Very rapid recovery after a prolonged viremia and infection of virtually every hepatocyte. *Journal of Virology* 1994; **68**:5792–5803.
17. Civitico GM & Locarnini SA. The half-life of duck hepatitis B virus supercoiled DNA in congenitally infected primary hepatocyte cultures. *Virology* 1994; **203**:81–89.
18. Moraleda G, Saputelli J, Aldrich CE, Averett D, Condreay L & Mason WS. Lack of effect of antiviral therapy in nondividing hepatocyte cultures on the closed circular DNA of woodchuck hepatitis virus. *Journal of Virology* 1997; **71**:9392–9399.
19. MacDonald RA. 'Lifespan' of liver cells. *Archives of Internal Medicine* 1960; **107**:335–343.
20. Nowak MA, Bonhoeffer S, Hill AM, Boehme R, Thomas HC & McDade H. Viral dynamics in hepatitis B virus infection. *Proceedings of the National Academy of Sciences, USA* 1996; **93**:4398–4402.
21. Fourel I, Cullen JM, Saputelli J, Aldrich CE, Schaffer P, Averett D, Pugh J & Mason WS. Evidence that hepatocyte turnover is required for rapid clearance of DHBV during antiviral therapy of chronically infected ducks. *Journal of Virology* 1994; **68**:8321–8330.
22. Jilbert AR, Wu TT, England JM, Hall PM, Carp NZ, O'Connell AP & Mason WS. Rapid resolution of duck hepatitis B virus infections occurs after massive hepatocellular involvement. *Journal of Virology* 1992; **66**:1377–1388.
23. Guidotti LG, Ishikawa T, Hobbs MV, Matzke B, Schreiber R & Chisari FV. Intracellular inactivation of the hepatitis B virus by cytotoxic T lymphocytes. *Immunity* 1996; **4**:25–36.
24. Ponzetto A, Cote PJ, Ford EC, Purcell RH & Gerin JL. Core antigen and antibody in woodchucks after infection with woodchuck hepatitis virus. *Journal of Virology* 1984; **52**:70–76.
25. Mason WS, Evans AA & London WT. Hepatitis B virus replication, liver disease, and hepatocellular carcinoma. *In Human Tumor Viruses* 1998; pp. 251–281. Edited by D McCance, Washington: ASM publications.
26. Summers J, Smith PM & Horwich AL. Hepadnavirus envelope proteins regulate covalently closed circular DNA amplification. *Journal of Virology* 1990; **64**:2819–2824.
27. Gong SS, Jensen AD & Rogler CE. Loss and acquisition of duck hepatitis B virus integrations in lineages of

LMH-D2 chicken hepatoma cells. *Journal of Virology* 1996; **70**:2000–2007.

28. Gong SS, Jensen AD, Wang H & Rogler CE. Duck hepatitis B virus integrations in LMH chicken hepatoma cells: identification and characterization of new episomally derived integrations. *Journal of Virology* 1995; **69**: 8102–8108.

29. Kozarsky KF & Wilson JM. Gene therapy: adenovirus vectors. *Current Opinion in Genetics and Development* 1993; **3**:499–503.

30. Cavanaugh VJ, Guidotti L & Chisari FV. Inhibition of Hepatitis B virus replication during adenovirus and cytomegalovirus infections with transgenic mice. *Journal of Virology* 1998; **72**:2630–2637.

31. Wang GH & Seeger C. Novel mechanism for reverse transcription in hepatitis B viruses. *Journal of Virology* 1993; **67**:6507–6512.

32. Wang G-H, Zoulim F, Leber EH & Seeger C. Role of RNA in enzymatic activity of the reverse transcriptase of hepatitis B viruses. *Journal of Virology* 1994; **68**:8437–8442.

33. Zoulim F & Seeger C. Reverse transcription in hepatitis B viruses is primed by a tyrosine residue of the polymerase. *Journal of Virology* 1994; **68**:6–13.

34. Weber M, Bronsema V, Bartos H, Bosserhoff A, Bartenschlager R & Schaller H. Hepadnavirus P protein utilizes a tyrosine residue in the TP domain to prime reverse transcription. *Journal of Virology* 1994; **68**:2994–2999.

35. Staprans S, Loeb DD & Ganem D. Mutations affecting hepadnavirus plus-strand DNA synthesis dissociate primer cleavage from translocation and reveal the origin of linear viral DNA. *Journal of Virology* 1991; **65**:1255–1262.

# 21 Maternal and foetal vaccination strategies for hepatitis B surface antigen in non-human primate models: evaluation of therapeutic modalities during pregnancy

Allison M Watts, John R Stanley, Michael H Shearer and Ronald C Kennedy*

## SUMMARY

Our laboratory is interested in developing new immunotherapeutic strategies directed toward preventing vertical transmission of hepatitis B virus (HBV). We are examining the safety and immunogenicity of candidate HBV vaccines administered during pregnancy in non-human primate models. Included among our interests are the induction and characterization of the immune response in vaccinated pregnant females, the placental transfer of specific antibodies from mother to foetus during the third trimester of pregnancy, the induction and characterization of the foetal immune response after direct active *in utero* immunization, and the effects of maternally derived antibodies and/or direct active *in utero* immunization on the ability of the infant to respond to subsequent vaccination. Previously, we have investigated the interspecies variability of the antibody response to HBV surface antigen (HBsAg) immunization and HBV infection by determination of the serological, molecular, and structural characteristics of the antibody variable regions that recognize an immunodominant protective group-specific *a* epitope on HBsAg. In this article, we discuss the advantages of the baboon as the non-human primate model of choice and describe preliminary studies that examine the humoral immune response of mother, foetus and infant to both maternal and foetal vaccinations during pregnancy through the characterization of antibody isotype and specificity for HBsAg.

## INTRODUCTION

In developing countries, vertical transmission of HBV may be one of the prevalent modes of transmission; the rate being more than 9% in Caucasian populations and 40 to 50% in Oriental populations [1]. Transmission of the virus from mother to offspring may occur via the birth canal or, less frequently, *in utero*. An estimated 40% of chronic infections results from vertical transmission of HBV to infants [2]. Chronic carriers of HBV are at risk of cirrhosis and primary hepatocellular carcinoma. It is currently recommended by the Centers for Disease Control and Prevention that neonates born to hepatitis B surface antigen (HBsAg)-positive mothers receive hepatitis B immunoglobulin (HBIg) within 12 hours of birth and HBsAg vaccination within 7 days of birth [3]; vertical transmission of HBV being prevented about 90% of the time by this combination of passive immunoglobulin and HBsAg vaccination of the infant.

Age of infection has a considerable impact upon the development of chronic hepatitis. An infection occurring during the first 2 or 3 months of life has an 80 to 85% chance of becoming chronic (as opposed to 2 to 10% in adult infections) [1]. Presumably, this is due to the immaturity of the neonatal immune system. The premature immune system contains defects in the complement pathway, phagocytosis, chemotaxis, and opsonic activity. In addition, the humoral immune response of the neonate is depressed as compared to the adult. Immunoglobulin synthesis in the foetus has been detected as early as 8 to 10 weeks gestation [4,5], however the serum of a term infant contains only about 10% of the adult level of IgM and very little IgA. IgM reaches adult levels around 1 to 2 years of age, while IgA does not reach adult levels until puberty.

The only immunoglobulin transferred transplacentally to the foetus is IgG. The Fc region of the IgG molecule is recognized by Fc-γ receptors on trophoblast cells of the placenta concentrated on the area of the syncytiotrophoblast that makes direct contact with the maternal circulation. The maternal IgG binds the receptor, undergoes receptor-mediated endocytosis, and is released in the foetal circulation through vesicle exocytosis [6,7]. The rate of transplacental IgG transport increases during gestation [8]. This maternally derived IgG is responsible for much of the neonatal immune protection. IgG levels in the foetus increase from around 17 weeks gestation to reach maternal levels at around 40 weeks gestation. Levels peak at birth and then begin to fall rapidly during the first three months of life. Consequently, the infant of 3 to 4 months is most susceptible to infection. Adult IgG levels are not reached until around 4 to 6 years of age [9,10]

The progress related to the study of maternal vaccination during pregnancy to protect the neonate from bacterial and viral infection has been slow. Slow progress is partly due to the lack of available vaccines for many serious neonatal infections and the poor understanding of the mechanisms involved in the transfer of immunity from the mother to the foetus. Much of the information on maternal vaccination during pregnancy has been obtained through the use of the tetanus toxoid vaccine. These studies consistently demonstrated improved maternal and neonatal survival [11–13]. Vaccination with tetanus toxoid has served as a model for the protection and benefit of both the mother and infant and is presently administered during pregnancy in many developing countries. With the advent and emerging development of new and improved vaccines against common neonatal pathogens, including, but not limited, to *Haemophilus influenzae* type b (Hib) and group B *Streptococcus* (GBS), interest in maternal vaccination concepts has been renewed.

Although transfer of maternal antibodies protects neonates against various pathogens, there are a number of immunological concerns about maternal vaccination strategies during pregnancy. The presence of maternal antibodies has often been shown to interfere with subsequent active immunization of the neonate [14–17]. Studies investigating the effects of maternally transferred antibodies on the immune response of the neonate in a murine rabies virus model revealed that the presence of maternal antibodies results in a decrease in specific B and T cell-mediated immune responses to later rabies virus vaccine antigen. Even when vaccinated at a time when protec-

tive levels of maternal antibody were no longer present, neonates did not develop a protective immune response to the vaccine antigen [18]. The mechanism that causes this decrease in immune responsiveness has not been thoroughly investigated. Maternal antibodies may interfere by reducing the antigenic load below a threshold required for immune response activation. The B-cell response could be affected by low levels of antibodies inhibiting activation of primary B-cell responses through immune complex formation [19], or by alteration of antigen presentation affecting the stimulation of T helper cells. Additional concerns relate to what effects maternal antibodies that express immunogenic variable (V) regions in the form of idiotypic determinants may have on the ability of the neonate to respond to later vaccination. Therefore, in the development of maternal vaccination strategies for prevention of neonatal infection, it is important to consider potential adverse effects that may result from foetal exposure to maternal antibody.

The immunological response of the foetus after direct exposure to antigen *in utero* has not been well characterized. The ability of the foetus to respond to antigenic stimulation has been questionable because of the immaturity of the foetal immune system. Studies have demonstrated a foetal IgM response to maternal immunization with tetanus toxoid [20] and as the result of congenital infections such as rubella, toxoplasma, cytomegalovirus (CMV), and human immunodeficiency virus (HIV) [21–23]. However, these IgM responses do not occur in all foetuses with congenitally acquired infection and may only occur in late gestation. Studies in foetal lambs demonstrated an ability of the foetuses to mount an immune response to certain antigens such as viruses and ovalbumin, although other antigens such as diphtheria toxoid and BCG could only induce a response after 40 days of post-natal life (reviewed in [24]). The notion that the foetus may be able to generate an immune response to a particular antigen is of interest as direct active immunization of the foetus *in utero* may allow protective levels of specific vaccine-induced antibodies to be present prior to, during, and soon after birth, providing protection to the developing foetus and neonate.

As with exposure to maternal antibody, one aspect of *in utero* exposure to antigen that has been considered is the induction of a state of immunological tolerance in the neonate. Tolerance induction of foetal and premature infant lymphocytes due to antigen exposure has become a paradigm for neonatal responsiveness. Studies by Owen in 1957 of neonatal cattle revealed that genetically non-identical twins sharing the same placenta *in utero*, and therefore exposed to each others blood cells, failed to reject allogenic grafts between each other as adults and were therefore tolerant [25]. Kuzu and colleagues also provided direct evidence of differences in tolerance susceptibility between foetal, neonatal, and adult CD8+ T cells by studying the effect of *in vivo* priming of cytotoxic lymphocytes by an influenza virus nucleoprotein peptide in various stages of development [26]. This study showed that whereas tolerance induction was easy to achieve during the foetal stage of development, it was not achieved in neonatal or adult mice [26]. *In utero* foetal vaccination has not been closely examined, partly because of this paradigm of neonatal tolerance, but also because of the lack of appropriate animal models that mimic the human maternal–foetal unit.

Ontogeny, reproductive physiology, placentation and immunology of an animal species must be taken into account when searching for a relevant animal model to use in studies of maternal and foetal immunization strategies. Although hominoid primates, including the chimpanzee, are the non-human primates most closely related to humans, these animals are considered endangered and threatened, and the cost for their use in biomedical research is prohibitive. Baboons are an Old World monkey species belonging to the taxonomic superfamily Cercopithecoidea, subfamily Papiinae. The baboon is a more feasible animal model and is excellent for use in such studies due to a high degree of immunological and reproductive physiological similarity to man. In addition, unlike rhesus monkeys, the baboon is not infected with herpes B virus, relieving animal handlers and their staff from any danger of infection by cross-species transmission.

Baboons and humans are similar in both humoral and cell-mediated aspects of the immune response. Studies using immunoelectrophoresis have shown that immunoglobulins express cross-reactive determinants [27–29]. The rhesus monkey has only three subclasses of immunoglobulins [30]. An additional similarity between baboons and humans is that baboon IgG is transferred transplacentally to the foetus, while IgM does not cross the placenta [31]. This suggests that the transfer of maternal antibodies and vaccine antigen across the placenta should be very similar for man and baboon, making the baboon a comparable model for maternal and foetal vaccination studies that should be relevant to the human situation.

The baboon breeds well year-round in captivity and, due to the reproductive nature of the female baboon, dates of conception and gestational age can be assigned as accurately as within ±2 days. The adult female baboon has an average menstrual cycle of 33 days and the state of ovarian activity can be easily identified by observation of the perianal sex skin which becomes turgescent for 8 to 10 days prior to ovulation and deturgescent approximately 3 days after ovulation. Pregnancy is indicated by failure to have bleeding and a dusty rose colour of the non-swollen perianal skin. Therefore, pregnancies can be accurately timed, allowing the immunological response to maternal or foetal vaccination to be further characterized by the gestational age of the foetus.

The baboon is the best readily available model for the study of human placental physiology since the developmental sequence and structure of the baboon placenta is similar to that of humans. *Macacca* spp. exhibit a double discoid placenta and differ from humans in the maternal–foetal unit. The maternal-foetal transfer of immunoglobulin and vaccine antigen in macaques may not be representative and similar to that of man. However, baboons and humans are similar in that they form a single discoid placenta classified as villous haemochorial [32]. Histological and electron microscopic examination of the baboon placenta have shown that it closely resembles the human placenta [33], and although the trophoblast of the baboon placenta does not invade into the myometrium as in the human placenta, the morphology of the chorionic villi, the functional unit of the placenta and the point of exchange between mother and the foetus, is equivalent.

In developing a non-human primate model to evaluate maternal and foetal HBV vaccination strategies, the identification and characterization of serological reagents for use in examining the structural basis of the specific antibody response to the vaccine antigen can prove invaluable. We have previously characterized anti-HBsAg (anti-HBs) responses generated in a variety of animal species, including primates, after HBsAg immunization [34–37]. These studies revealed that HBsAg immunization induced a dominant anti-HBs response recognizing a protective group *a* epitope across the species barrier [35,38]. Additionally, we have described the functional duality of anti-HBs V regions through epitope mapping and idiotype expression [38,39]. The immunodominance of the group *a* epitope and its protective role in preventing HBV infection represents a serological marker for examining the induction of anti-HBs responses and will aid us in discerning antibody responses in the infant that are either maternally derived or actively induced via direct antigen exposure. In this report, we discuss observations obtained from preliminary studies of both maternal and foetal vaccination of the baboon with

HBsAg. We have examined the immune response of mother, foetus and infant to this vaccine antigen through the characterization of antibody isotype and HBsAg specificity. These studies should provide information and insight into immunotherapeutic strategies that prevent vertical transmission of HBV from an infected mother to her infant.

## MATERIALS AND METHODS

### HBsAg

The recombinant HBsAg vaccine (Recombivax HB) was purchased from Merck and company and administered according to manufacturers instructions. Pregnant adult female baboons *(Papio anubis)* received 10 µg recombinant HBsAg in an alum adjuvant. Foetal baboons received 5 µg of the recombinant HBsAg in an alum adjuvant, the dose of Recombivax HB recommended for high-risk infants.

### Timed pregnancies

Mature baboon breeding harems were assembled to establish stable social groups and to document menstrual cycles. Female baboons were housed in gang cages in the social groups with a male and observed three times weekly for changes in the perianal sex skin to record menstrual cycles. The follicular phase of the baboon menstrual cycle is indicated by turgescence. Deturgescence is indicative of the luteal phase. Ovulation occurs two days prior to deturgescence. Failure to mense approximately 14 to 17 days post-deturgescence is the first sign of pregnancy. The day of conception for each female can be estimated within ±2 days. Approximately 30 days after conception the pregnant female was scanned by ultrasound to confirm pregnancy.

### Maternal vaccination

Pregnant baboons were vaccinated at approximately 30, 60 and 150 days gestation intramuscularly with 10 µg recombinant HBsAg in alum. Maternal blood samples were obtained from the cephalic vein just distal to the elbow prior to vaccination and at 90, 130 and 165 days gestation. Additional blood samples were obtained at 1, 7, 21, 60, 90 and 120 days post partum. All procedures were performed with Institutional Animal Care and Utilization Committee approval and in accordance with the Principles and Procedures of the NIH Guidelines for Care and Use of Laboratory Animals.

### Foetal blood sampling

In order to obtain levels of transplacentally transferred maternal antibody and to analyse the time in gestation when the foetal immune system develops the ability to respond to vaccination, we obtained foetal blood samples via percutaneous umbilical blood sampling (PUBS) at approximately 90, 135 and 165 days gestation. Maternal blood was drawn simultaneous to each foetal blood sampling. PUBS technique consists of a needle being guided by ultrasound through the anterior abdominal wall and uterine wall into the umbilical vein. Mothers were immobilized initially with ketamine (10 mg/kg) and xylazine (0.5 mg/kg) followed by anaesthesia to a surgical plane with halothane (1.5%) and nitrous oxide (40%). Less than 4 ml of foetal blood was removed from the foetus. In order to ensure that no maternal blood was contained, an APT test (to detect adult haemoglobin) was performed on all samples.

### Foetal vaccination

Foetuses were vaccinated *in utero* at approximately 90, 120 and 150 days gestation with 5 µg of Recombivax HB by intramuscular injection into the foetal thigh. Aspiration was performed prior to the vaccine injection to insure that the needle was intramuscular, not intravenous or intraamniotic. The schedule of the vaccination was chosen such that the foetus would be large enough to easily inject *in utero*, and the doses were given at intervals during the pregnancy such that development of a response during gestation could be detected. For foetal vaccination, mothers were immobilized as described above. The site of inoculation was located using Doppler ultrasound guidance. Under sterile conditions, a Teflon coated sonolucent 22 gauge needle was introduced through the anterior abdominal wall and uterus into the foetal thigh. Foetal heart rate was monitored intermittently during the procedure using Doppler ultrasound. Maternal electrocardiogram and blood pressure were also monitored during the procedure.

### Analysis of IgM/IgG levels

Levels of baboon IgM and IgG were determined by radial immunodiffusion (RID) employing commercial assays (The Binding Site Ltd). RID kits contained anti-human µ-chain and γ-chain monospecific antibody that cross reacted with baboon IgG and IgM, respectively, in an agarose gel. Three calibrator solutions containing the appropriate immunoglobulin at known low, medium, and high concentrations were loaded into wells on the agar plates, along with a positive control (all supplied in the RID kits) and the respective baboon serum samples. Following incubation, the diameter of the precipitin rings around the wells was determined in millimetres. The square of the diameter of the known immunoglobulin calibrators was plotted against their concentrations to generate a standard curve. Immunoglobulin concentration was determined in grams per litre. All serum samples were assayed in duplicate.

## Anti-HBs levels

A commercial solid-phase enzyme immunoassay (EIA) kit was used for the titration of antibodies to anti-HBs in baboon sera (AUSAB EIA, Abbott Laboratories). In this double sandwich EIA, HBsAg-coated beads are used to bind anti-HBs present in the serum and enzyme-labelled HBsAg serves as the indicator of binding. Anti-HBs titres were determined from individual binding curves in milli-international units per millilitre (mIU/ml) of sera according to the manufacturers instructions. These methods have been described in detail elsewhere [35]. Studies have demonstrated that anti-HBs titres greater than 8 mIU/ml are indicative of protective levels of antibodies in humans.

## RESULTS

To determine the level of maternal antibody induced in pregnant female baboons following HBsAg vaccination and to examine any immunoglobulin that had been placentally transferred to the foetus from the mother, we evaluated anti-HBs levels and quantitated IgM and IgG (Table 1). Maternal IgG half-life in the baboon infant was approximately 25 days and appears to be similar to that reported in humans. Of the three maternally vaccinated baboons, both total IgM and IgG levels in maternal serum slightly increased above baseline levels and these levels were sustained after birth. Serum IgM was not present in any foetal samples, however, foetal IgG levels increased with maternal levels, reaching maternal levels by the time approximating birth. IgG in infant serum of maternally vaccinated animals consistently fell back to baseline foetal levels by two months of age. These data suggest that maternal IgG is being transferred from mother to foetus while IgM is not. The rate in increase of foetal IgG levels increases with the time of gestation. This suggests an increase in the transfer of maternal IgG across the placenta in late gestation. The rate of IgG decay in baboon foetus seems to correlate with that of the human foetal IgG. Since no IgM was transferred,

**Table 1.** Antibody isotype and anti-HBs levels after maternal vaccination

### Mother/infant pair #1

| Sample | IgM (g/l) | IgG (g/l) | HBsAg reactivity (mIU/ml) |
|---|---|---|---|
| Baseline | 0.78 | 21.10 | 0 |
| Mother 130 days | 0.95 | 18.90 | 62 |
| Mother 165 days | 1.50 | 20.60 | 330 |
| Mother 24 h pp | 1.35 | 27.35 | 275 |
| Mother 7 days pp | 1.50 | 26.60 | 330 |
| Mother 21 days pp | 1.23 | 23.10 | 359 |
| Mother 60 days pp | 0.63 | 19.00 | 176 |
| Mother 120 days pp | 1.07 | 19.20 | 150 |
| Foetus 130 days | 0 | 8.00 | 169 |
| Foetus 165 days | 0 | 13.30 | 339 |
| Infant 24 h | 0 | 19.25 | 383 |
| Infant 7 days | 0.34 | 15.10 | 377 |
| Infant 21 days | 0.38 | 12.40 | 347 |
| Infant 60 days | 0.04 | 5.30 | 389 |
| Infant 120 days | 0.02 | 6.20 | 97 |

### Mother/infant pair #2

| Sample | IgM (g/l) | IgG (g/l) | HBsAg reactivity (mIU/ml) |
|---|---|---|---|
| Baseline | 0.93 | 18.20 | 0 |
| Mother 130 days | 0.98 | 19.35 | 99 |
| Mother 165 days | 0.88 | 14.23 | 388 |
| Mother 7 days pp | 1.26 | 16.60 | 334 |
| Mother 60 days pp | 0.81 | 18.47 | 289 |
| Mother 90 days pp | 0.88 | 17.80 | 163 |
| Mother 120 days pp | 0.81 | 13.80 | 118 |
| Foetus 130 days | 0 | 7.80 | 153 |
| Foetus 165 days | 0 | 13.70 | 350 |
| Infant 7 days | 0 | 16.00 | 344 |
| Infant 60 days | 0 | 7.10 | 277 |
| Infant 90 days | 0 | 4.10 | 130 |
| Infant 120 days | 0 | 4.40 | 158 |

### Mother/infant pair #3

| Sample | IgM (g/l) | IgG (g/l) | HBsAg reactivity (mIU/ml) |
|---|---|---|---|
| Baseline | 0.98 | 17.60 | 0 |
| Mother 130 days | 1.00 | 15.10 | 351 |
| Mother 165 days | 0.95 | 10.00 | 250 |
| Mother 24 h pp | 0.84 | 20.60 | 278 |
| Mother 7 days pp | 1.20 | 15.10 | 250 |
| Mother 21 days pp | 1.32 | 17.70 | 219 |
| Mother 60 days pp | 1.30 | 14.20 | 150 |
| Mother 90 days pp | 1.29 | 15.40 | 120 |
| Foetus 130 days | 0 | 9.85 | 173 |
| Foetus 165 days | 0 | 12.40 | 319 |
| Infant 24 h | 0 | 14.80 | 345 |
| Infant 7 days | 0.16 | 14.80 | 305 |
| Infant 21 days | 0.25 | 12.20 | 250 |
| Infant 60 days | 0.30 | 6.50 | 125 |
| Infant 90 days | 0.25 | 6.30 | 130 |

Abbreviation: p.p., post-partum.

the transplacental transfer of IgG and IgM in the baboon appears similar to the human. Baseline levels of IgM and IgG observed for the animals reveal variation between individuals. Both mother and foetus in animal pair #1 reached an increased level of total IgG after vaccination. Mothers from animal pairs #2 and #3 did not greatly increase in levels of total IgG following HBsAg vaccination, however, the foetuses and infants of these pairs did attain maternal IgG levels similar to levels seen in the infant in pair #1 (Table 1).

In examining anti-HBs reactivity of maternal serum, we observed high levels of reactivity for all animals. Studies have previously demonstrated that anti-HBs titres greater than 8 mIU/ml are indicative of protective levels of antibodies in humans. The peak levels of anti-HBs reactivity observed for mothers of animal pairs #1, #2, and #3 were 359 mIU/ml, 388 mIU/ml, and 351 mIU/ml, respectively. This indicates that vaccination with HBsAg did induce a specific anti-HBs humoral response in all three pregnant baboons. In addition, foetuses from these animal pairs reached similar titres of anti-HBs as their mothers. Therefore, vaccination with HBsAg is producing specific maternal antibody that is being efficiently transferred to the foetus. Since IgG was the only immunoglobulin isotype observed in foetal serum, maternally derived IgG appears responsible for the foetal anti-HBs response. Anti-HBs levels in foetal serum correlates with IgG levels in two of the three animal pairs. At the time of birth, two of the three infants contained their maximum anti-HBs titres. Anti-HBs levels began to fall after birth but were maintained at levels indicative of protective immunity for at least the follow-up time period that was observed.

In preliminary studies with one animal pair (pair #4) on foetal vaccination with HBsAg, we observed no greater increase in total IgM or IgG levels over time in maternal serum. The mother of this pair contained higher than average IgG levels when compared to the three maternally vaccinated mothers that remained consistent throughout the sampling. The foetus of this animal pair contained no detectable IgM. Foetal IgG levels increased during gestation, however remained lower than maternal levels (Table 2). No anti-HBs was detected in the maternal serum, whereas foetal anti-HBs levels reached levels similar to that seen with maternal vaccinations. This indicates that no HBsAg vaccine antigen was exposed to the maternal immune system after foetal vaccination. More importantly, this preliminary data suggests that the foetus is able to mount an IgG response to direct *in utero* vaccination. The foetal IgG anti-HBs did not appear to cross the

placenta and was not detected in the maternal serum. Further studies will examine the effects of maternal and foetal vaccination on the ability of the infant to respond to similar vaccination.

## DISCUSSION

The development of new and more immunogenic vaccines continues to lead to better protection of young children from viral and bacterial pathogens. Unfortunately, neonates and very young infants who are most vulnerable to serious infectious diseases are not protected by current vaccine regimens. Prematurity complicates approximately 10% of births in the USA. Since the greatest amount of transfer of maternal antibodies to the foetus transplacentally occurs late in gestation, premature infants receive lower levels of maternal antibody and may not be protected regardless of maternal levels of specific antibody. For the prematurely delivered infant, acceleration of transplacental immunoglobulin transfer from mother to foetus is invariably needed to prevent neonatal humoral immune deficiency. Vaccination of the mother during pregnancy can result in higher levels of specific protective antibodies which may be passively transferred to the foetus.

Of the three animal pairs that underwent maternal vaccination, all mothers produced high levels of HBsAg-specific antibody. The foetuses of these pairs possessed anti-HBs IgG levels that were elevated to maternal levels at around the time of birth and were maintained into infancy. The baboon efficiently trans-

Table 2. Antibody isotype and anti-HBs reactivity after foetal vaccination

**Mother-infant pair #4**

| Sample | IgM (g/l) | IgG (g/l) | HBsAg reactivity (mIU/ml) |
|---|---|---|---|
| Mother 135 days | 0.74 | 31.00 | 0 |
| Mother 165 days | 0.74 | 31.00 | 0 |
| Mother 24 h p.p. | 0.74 | 32.00 | 0 |
| Mother 7 days p.p | 1.03 | 31.00 | 0 |
| Mother 21 days p.p | 1.13 | 31.00 | 0 |
| Mother 60 days p.p | 0.91 | 25.20 | 0 |
| Foetus 135 days | 0 | 11.00 | 27 |
| Foetus 165 days | 0 | 20.40 | 40 |
| Infant 24 h | 0 | 23.00 | 287 |
| Infant 7 days | 0.10 | 13.70 | 366 |
| Infant 21 days | 0.22 | 7.00 | 260 |
| Infant 60 days | 0.38 | 13.90 | 234 |

Abbreviation: p.p., post-partum

ferred maternal antibody to the foetus at rates similar to that seen in humans. Because of the similar response of the adult baboon and humans to this vaccine regimen in rates of antibody increase and decline, isotype transfer limitations, and rate and level of passively transferred maternal antibody, the baboon has proven to be an ideal animal model for use in studies of maternal vaccination with recombinant HBsAg and the transfer of HBsAg-specific maternal antibody to the foetus.

Active immunization of the foetus *in utero* may be able to provide protection at birth when maternal antibody is not available, as with maternal immunoglobulin deficiencies and autoimmune diseases. Mothers with an immunoglobulin deficiency present a problem for the foetus exposed *in utero* to HBV. The foetus must be supplemented with an antibody repertoire that is complete and quantitatively accurate. In autoimmune mothers, antibodies may be transferred to the foetus and damage neonatal tissues. Myasthenia gravis, Graves' disease and immune thrombocytopenia purpura are some examples. In these scenarios, to prevent damage to the foetus, blocking the placental uptake, processing, or secretion of maternal antibodies is often desirable. However, this would leave the foetus and neonate devoid of immune protection early in life [40]. This presents a need for vaccination strategies that will activate the underdeveloped foetal immune system and generate protective antibody in the absence of transplacental transfer of maternal antibody.

Preliminary data obtained in our studies of foetal vaccination suggest that the baboon foetus is able to generate a specific IgG response to direct active immunization with HBsAg. The vaccinated foetus generated anti-HBs levels similar to maternally derived levels seen in the maternal vaccination studies. No anti-HBs reactivity was observed in the serum of the mother of the vaccinated foetus, suggesting that the foetal vaccination procedure did not result in the generation of a maternal immune response to the vaccine antigen and that no maternally derived antibody was responsible for the foetal anti-HBs response. The lack of IgG anti-HBs in this mother also indicates that transplacental transfer of immunoglobulin occurs in only one direction, from the mother to the foetus and not from the foetus to the mother. These observations shed new light on the feasibility of employing foetal vaccination strategies in immunodeficient and autoimmune mothers to protect the premature infant and neonate.

Safety is of great concern in the development of new vaccination strategies. The PUBS procedure is now being used extensively in human pregnancies for indications such as isoimmunization and intrauterine blood transfusions and for the diagnosis of foetal thrombocytopenia, congenital infections, and genetic disorders. In human pregnancies, PUBS has been performed routinely as early as 18 weeks gestation with foetal loss rates of 1–2% [41,42]. PUBS is much less invasive than a hysterotomy which involves the placement of foetal catheters. PUBS is associated with little increased risk of abortion or preterm delivery and no reported risk of maternal complications. Therefore, monitoring of the foetal immune response to vaccination using the PUBS procedure to obtain foetal blood samples makes the study of foetal vaccination safe and efficient.

The main difficulty in developing vaccines for protection of the neonate is providing vaccines that result in rapid and high immunogenicity in an immature immune system. Foetal immunization may result in tolerance or non-responsiveness to similar vaccination in infancy. In addition, exposure of the foetus to certain vaccine antigens may impede responses to different childhood vaccinations. Recent studies have shown that the HBsAg component of the quadrivalent $DTP_W$-HB vaccine does not interfere with the immune response to diphtheria, tetanus, and whole-cell *Bordetella pertussis* components of the vaccine in healthy infants [43]. The possibility of interference such as this must be examined for foetal vaccination protocols as well, since it is possible that the effectiveness of later childhood immunizations may be effected by previous *in utero* vaccination.

There exist several potential advantages to routine maternal or foetal vaccination during pregnancy. In addition to the benefit of improving both neonatal morbidity and mortality, there is a cost benefit of an efficacious vaccine that would boost neonatal antibody when compared to alternative strategies such as the use of high-titre human immunoglobulin administered intravenously after delivery. Also, maternal health programs already in place could be utilized to administer vaccines during pregnancy. The benefit would be to protect neonates from pathogenic organisms at a period in life when they are most susceptible, thus providing a time- and cost-effective method for preventing common neonatal diseases.

Our studies of maternal and foetal vaccination in the baboon are in preliminary stages. Future studies will be better able to evaluate the safety and immunogenicity of these methods of vaccination. It will also be important to address the possibility of adverse effects on future vaccination of infants with both similar and alternative vaccine antigens. The work in our laboratory on maternal and foetal vaccination strategies in a relevant non-human primate model will contribute much needed information on the foetal immune response and the effects of maternal and foetal vaccination that mimics the situation in humans.

## ACKNOWLEDGEMENTS

This work was supported in part by grants and contracts AI35156, RR12317 and AI07634 from the National Institutes of Health and a grant from the Oklahoma Center for the Advancement of Science and Technology.

## REFERENCES

1. Levine AJ. *Virology*. 1992; p. 189. New York: Scientific American Library.
2. Kane MA, Hadler SC, Margolis HS & Maynard JE. Routine prenatal screening for hepatitis B surface antigen. *Journal of the American Medical Association* 1988; **259**:408–409.
3. Update on adult immunization. Recommendations of the Immunization Practices Advisory Committee. *Morbidity and Mortality Weekly Report* 1991; **40** (RR12):1–94.
4. Gitlin D & Biasucci A. Development of γG, γA, γM, γ1C-β1a, C1 esterase inhibitor, ceruloplasmin, transferrin, hemopexin, haptoglobin, fibrinogen, plasminogen, α1-antitrypsin, orosomucoid, β-lipoprotein, β2-macroglobulin, and prealbumin in the human conceptus. *Journal of Clinical Investigation* 1969; **48**: 1433–1446.
5. Vakil M & Kearney JF. Functional characterization of monoclonal auto-anti-idiotypic antibodies isolated from the early B-cell repertoire of BALB/c mice. *European Journal of Immunology* 1986; **16**: 1151–1158.
6. Brown PJ & Johnson PM. Fcγ receptor activity of isolated human placental syncytiotrophoblast plasma membrane. *Immunology* 1981; **42**: 313–319.
7. Pearse BM. Coated vesicles from human placenta carry ferritin, transferrin, and immunoglobulin G. *Proceedings of the National. Academy of Sciences, USA* 1982; **79**:451–455.
8. Pitcher-Wilmott RW, Hindocha P & Wood CB. The placental transfer of IgG subclasses in human pregnancy. *Clinical and Experimental Immunology* 1980; **41**:303–308.
9. Allansmith M, McClellan BH, Butterworth M & Maloney JR. The development of immunoglobulin levels in man. *Journal of Pediatrics* 1968; **72**:276–290.
10. Buckley RH, Dees SC & O'Fallon WM. Serum immunoglobulins: I. Levels in normal children and in uncomplicated childhood allergy. *Pediatrics* 1968; **41**:600–611.
11. Schoenfeld FD, Tucker VM & Westbrook GR. Neonatal tetanus in New Guinea: effect of active immunization in pregnancy. *British Medical Journal* 1961; **2**:785–789.
12. Chen ST, Edsau G, Peel MM & Sinnathuray TA. Timing antenatal tetanus immunization for effective protection of the neonate. *Bulletin of the World Health Organization* 1983; **161**:159–165.
13. Rahman M, Chen LC, Chakraborty J, Yunus M, Chowdhury AI, Sarder AM, Bhatia S & Curlin GT. Use of tetanus toxoid for the prevention of neonatal tetanus: I. Reduction of neonatal mortality by immunization of non-pregnant and pregnant women in rural Bangladesh *Bulletin of the World Health Organization* 1982; **60**:261–267.
14. Albracht P, Ennis FA, Saltzman EJ & Krugman S. Persistence of maternal antibody in infants beyond 12 months: mechanism of measle vaccine failure. *Journal of Pediatrics* 1977; **91**:715–719.
15. Bangham CRM. Passively acquired antibodies to respiratory syncytial virus impair the secondary cytotoxic T-cell response in the neonatal mouse. *Immunology* 1986; **59**:37–41.
16. Francis MJ & Black L. Response of young pigs to foot-and-mount disease oil emulsion vaccination in the presence and absence of maternally derived neutralizing antibodies. *Research in Veterinary Science* 1986; **41**:33–39.
17. Harte PG & Playfair JHL. Failure of malaria vaccination in mice born to immune mothers. II. Induction of specific suppressor cells by maternal IgG. *Clinical and Experimental Immunology* 1983; **51**:157–164.
18. Xiang ZQ & Ertl HCJ. Transfer of maternal antibodies results in inhibition of specific immune responses in the offspring. *Virus Research* 1992; **24**:297–314.
19. Uhr JW & Moller G. Regulatory effect of antibody on the immune response. *Advances in Immunology* 1968; **8**:81–127.
20. Gill TJ, Repetti CF, Metlay LA, Rabin BS, Taylor FH, Thompson DS & Cortese AL. Transplacental immunization of the human fetus to tetanus by immunization of the mother. *Journal of Clinical Investigation* 1983; **72**:987–996.
21. Enders G. Serologic test combinations for safe detection of rubella infections. *Reviews in Infectious Disease* 1985; **7**:S113–S122.
22. Naot YD, Desmonts G & Remington JS. IgM enzyme-linked immunosorbent assay test for the diagnosis of congenital toxoplasma infection. *Journal of Pediatrics* 1981; **98**:32–36.
23. Griffiths PD, Stagno S & Pass RF. Congenital cytomegalovirus infection: diagnostic and prognostic significance of the detection of specific immunoglobulin M antibodies in cord serum. *Pediatrics* 1982; **69**:544–550.
24. Silverstein AM. *Development of Host Defense*. 1977. New York: Raven.
25. Owen RD. Erythrocyte antigenes and tolerance phenomena. *Proceedings of the Royal Society of London. Series B: Biological Sciences* 1957; **146**:8–18.
26. Kuzu H, Kuzu Y, Zaghuani H & Bona CA. *In vivo* priming effect during various stages of ontogeny of an influenza A virus nucleoprotein peptide. *European Journal of Immunology* 1993; **23**:1397–1400.
27. Attanasio R, Allan JS, Anderson SA, Chanh TC & Kennedy RC. Anti-idiotypic antibody response to monoclonal anti-CD4 in non-human primate species. *Journal of Immunology* 1991; **146**:507–514.
28. Kim KH, Park MK, Peeters C, Shearer MH, Kennedy RC & Nahm MH. Comparison of non-human primate antibodies against *Haemophilus influenzae* type b polysaccharide with human antibodies in oligoclonality and *in vivo* protective potency. *Infection and Immunity* 1994; **62**: 2037–2045.
29. Zaghouani H, Anderson SA, Sperber KE, Daian C, Kennedy RC, Mayer L & Bona CA. Induction of antibodies to the human immunodeficiency type 1 by

immunization of baboons with immunoglobulin molecules carrying the principal neutralizing determinant of the envelope protein. *Proceedings of the National Academy of Sciences, USA* 1995; **92:**631–635.

30. Martin LN. Chromatographic fractionation of rhesus monkey *(Macacca mulatta)* IgG subclasses using DEAE cellulose and protein A sepharose. *Journal of Immunological Methods* 1982; **50:**319–329.

31. Shearer MH, Lucas AH, Anderson PW, Carey KD, Jenson HB, Stanley JR & Kennedy RC. The baboon as a non-human primate model for assessing the effects of maternal immunization with *Haemophilus influenzae* type b polysaccharide vaccines. *Infection and Immunity* 1997; **65:**3267–3270.

32. Hendricx AG. *Embryology of the Baboon.* 1971. Chicago: University of Chicago Press.

33. Wynn RM, Panigel M & Maclennan AH. Fine structure of the placenta and fetal membranes of the baboon. *American Journal of Obstetrics and Gynecology* 1971; **109:**638–648.

34. Kennedy RC & Dreesman GR. Common idiotypic determinants associated with antibodies to hepatitis B surface antigen. *Journal of Immunology* 1983; **130:**385–389.

35. Kennedy RC, Ionescu-Matiu I, Sanchez Y & Dreesman GR. Detection of interspecies idiotypic cross-reactions associated with antibodies to hepatitis B surface antigen. *European Journal of Immunology* 1983; **13:**232–235.

36. Kennedy RC, Eichberg JW, Lanford RE & Dreesman GR. Anti-idiotypic antibody vaccine for type B viral hepatitis in chimpanzees. *Science* 1986; **232:**220–223.

37. Anderson SA, Ostberg LG, Ehrlich PH & Kennedy RC. Characterization of private and cross-reactive idiotypes associated with human antibodies to hepatitis B surface antigen. *International Immunology* 1992; **4:**135–145.

38. Kennedy RC, Shearer MH, Chanh TC, Jenson HB & Stanley JR. Molecular and structural characterization of antibodies to hepatitis B surface antigen: developing a non-human primate model to evaluate maternal therapeutic vaccination strategies during pregnancy. *Antiviral Therapy* 1996; **1** (Supplement 4):76–83.

39. Lohman KL, Kieber-Emmons T & Kennedy RC. Molecular characterization and structural modeling of immunoglobulin variable regions specific for hepatitis B virus surface antigen. *Molecular Immunology* 1993; **30:**1295–1306.

40. Landor M. Maternal-fetal transfer of immunoglobulins. *Annals of Allergy, Asthma and Immunology* 1995; **74:** 279–283.

41. Daffos F, Capella-Pavlovsky M & Forestier F. Fetal blood sampling during pregnancy with the use of a needle guided by ultrasound: a study of 606 consecutive cases. *American Journal of Obstetrics and Gynecology* 1985; **153:**655.

42. Ludomirsky A. *Sixth International Conference on Cordocentesis.* Philadelphia, Pennsylvania, USA, 1991; Abstract.

43. Diez-Delgado J, Dal-Re R, Llorente M, Gonzalez A & Lopez J. Hepatitis B component does not interfere with the immune response to diphtheria, tetanus and whole-cell *Bordetells pertussis* components of a quadrivalent (DTP$_W$-HB) vaccine: a controlled trial in healthy infants. *Vaccine* 1997; **12:**1418–1422.

# 22 Antiviral and anti-proliferative activities of α interferons in experimental hepatitis B virus infections

J David Gangemi*, Brent E Korba, Bud C Tennant, John L Gerin, Paul J Cote, Hiroyuki Ueda and Gilbert Jay

## SUMMARY

Interferon α (IFN-α) has been the drug of choice for the treatment of chronic hepatitis B virus (HBV) infections for the past 20 years, yet little more is known about the mechanism(s) of action (antiviral and immunomodulatory) of this cytokine today than in 1975 when some of the first clinical trials were performed. Much of this can be attributed to the limitation in experimental models with which to dissect the direct and indirect activities of IFN on (i) cytotoxic T lymphocyte (CTL) development and activation; (ii) viraemia and histopathology; and (iii) antibody production and seroconversion. In addition, even in those animal models that are currently used to study viral pathogenesis (such as woodchuck, duck and transgenic mice), human IFN-α is biologically inactive and the comparable animal IFN is either not available or too expensive to use in long-term therapy studies. Clearly, a cross-species active human IFN could resolve some of these difficulties. In contrast to the α IFNs currently approved for clinical use in man (IFN-α 2a and 2b), experimental hybrids, consisting of two IFN-α subtypes (for example A/D and B/D), are active in a variety of animal species including woodchucks, mice and ducks. These hybrids provide a unique opportunity to study the direct and indirect mechanism(s) of IFN action alone or in combination with other drugs in experimental animal models of HBV disease. This chapter reviews the results of studies in which a hybrid IFN (IFN-α B/D) was used to assess (i) direct antiviral activity in hepatocyte cultures; (ii) the antiviral and immunomodulatory effects in chronically infected woodchucks; and (iii) the antiproliferative activity in mice with HBV-induced hepatocellular carcinoma (HCC). The activity of IFN-α B/D used in combination with the nucleoside analogue lamivudine is also presented.

## INTRODUCTION

### IFN-α in HBV infections

The IFN-α family has at least 20 subtypes, some of which are more closely related than others [1,2]. The biological activities of these subtypes are similar, but may be distinguished when evaluated in cells of different lineage. For example, infection of peripheral blood leukocytes (PBLs) with some RNA viruses may result in the release of a predominant IFN-α subtype, α-2, which is highly effective in enhancing the antiviral activity of PBLs. While this IFN-α subtype is effective for viruses infecting these cells, it is not the most effective subtype for use against viruses infecting other cell types (such as hepatocytes) [3,4]. Thus, the virus type (RNA or DNA), the site of infection and cell type infected may determine the subtype of IFN-α that is most effective in treatment. Likewise, these same factors will determine the subtype that will be released from infected cells.

Infection with some viruses results in the induction of multiple subtypes of IFN-α. While the biological roles of α subtypes are uncertain, some could play auxiliary roles in immune stimulation and/or in triggering the release of other cytokines [5]. Both α and γ interferons have been found in sera and in culture fluids from the PBLs of individuals with acute and chronic hepatitis [6,7]; however, HBV-infected cells respond

---

poorly to the direct antiviral effects of IFN [8,9]. α IFNs can act in either a positive or negative regulatory fashion in both acute and chronic disease. For example, they may enhance CTL activity and thereby exacerbate inflammatory responses, or they may inhibit the induction of CTLs and reduce hepatocyte injury [10,11]. It is uncertain which α subtypes are induced during acute and chronic infection. Moreover, the subtypes that are most effective in inhibiting HBV replication or modulating CTL activity are not known. Thus, it is quite possible that subtypes of IFN-α, other than those now being used, could enhance the current response rate (20–30%) [12,13].

## IFN-α hybrids

The α IFN family is unique in that it contains a number of biologically active subtypes. Because of this subtype heterogeneity [2], one approach to developing a more effective α IFN involves genetic tailoring or engineering of chimeric molecules that capture the best qualities of two or more subtypes. For example, IFN-α B has potent antiviral activity, but is produced in rather limited amounts following infection. This subtype can be combined with other subtypes such as α-D, which has potent anti-proliferative and anti-tumour properties, to make a highly active chimeric molecule which has better antiviral and antiproliferative activities than either parent. Such a chimera has been produced and developed by investigators at Novartis in Basel, Switzerland [14].

To produce the IFN-α B/D hybrid, it was necessary to splice both the α-B and α-D genes and select for a molecule that, in this case, had parts of the α-D gene inserted into the α-B gene. DNA splicing resulted in a molecule with amino acids 61–92 from α-D inserted into the α-B chain [14]. This substitution resulted in a molecular conformation that was different from either parent (α-B or α-D) and which resulted in cross-species activity. IFN-α B/D is biologically active in a number of experimental animal species [15] and in a variety of experimental virus infection models [16]. Other human IFN-α hybrids, such as A/D, have similar biological profiles [1]. Why these human IFN hybrids are biologically active in other species is unclear; however, their ability to bind to conserved regions of the type 1 IFN receptor may play a key role in their cross-species activity [14].

## Combination therapy

The standard treatment of a chronic hepatitis B e antigen (HBeAg)-positive, HBV DNA-positive patient is 10 MU of IFN-α three times a week for 16 weeks. Nonetheless, the overall therapeutic effect, as measured by disappearance of HbeAg, is estimated to be at best 20–30%. Improvement is possible by better selection of the patient, modification in the treatment schedule, or combination therapy [17,18]. In the selection of possible candidates for combination therapy, the second generation nucleoside analogues with activity against HBV are promising [17]. In this regard Korba [19] has shown that combinations of lamivudine and IFN-α B/D are more effective than either drug alone in inhibiting virus replication in a human hepatocyte cell line. The fact that each of these drugs affects different viral targets results in their combined efficacy. This observation has provided a rationale for additional combination studies in experimental animal models in which the antiviral and immunomodulating effects of IFN can be evaluated together with the chain terminating activity of selected nucleoside analogues.

## METHODS

### Antiviral assays

The 2.2.15 hepatoblastoma cell line, which produces HBV from integrated viral DNA, was used. Confluent cultures of these productively infected cells were maintained in 96-well flat-bottomed tissue culture plates in RPMI 1640 medium with 2% fetal bovine serum and were treated with nine consecutive daily doses of test compounds as previously described [20]. Virus replication was measured by assaying HBV DNA in supernatants or replicative intermediates in cells. Virion DNA levels were measured using the blot hybridization method described previously [20]. A total of eight individual cultures, on two plates, were used for each of six serial, threefold dilutions of each drug or drug combination.

For the combination treatments, antiviral agents were mixed at ratios to approximately match their 90% effective concentrations ($EC_{90}$). Thus, two drugs with equal potency would be mixed at a 1:1 molar ratio. Serial dilutions were then made of the drug mixtures, maintaining the same ratio for all dilutions. The $EC_{90}$ values were determined by linear regression analysis and analysis of synergism was performed using the COMBOSTAT program (Combostat) [19]. Lamivudine [(−)-β-L-2′,3′-dideoxy-3′-thiacytidine; 3TC] was obtained from R Schinazi (Emory University, Atlanta, Georgia, USA) and lyophilized recombinant human IFN-α B/D (32 MIU/0.4 mg) was obtained from H-K Hochkeppel (Novartis, Basel, Switzerland).

## Woodchuck hepatitis

Six 10-month-old woodchucks that had been experimentally infected with woodchuck hepatitis virus (WHV) at 3 days of age and had become chronic WHV carriers [21] were treated every other day for 12 weeks with IFN-α B/D at a dose of 5 MIU/kg administered subcutaneously. Saline-treated and untreated groups of chronic WHV carriers of identical age served as controls.

Serum WHV DNA was measured by blot hybridization and WHV DNA replicative intermediates were measured in hepatic biopsies obtained before, during and after treatment. Both liver biopsies and serum biochemical analyses were taken before, during and after treatment to assess organ function.

## Transgenic mice

HBx transgenic mice were derived by microinjection of a 1.15 kb HBV subtype *adr* DNA fragment, which spans nucleotide positions 707–1856 in the viral genome, into single cell embryos derived from outbred CD1 mice [22]. This segment of DNA contains not only the entire coding region of the HBx gene, but also the transcriptional enhancer, the principal RNA start sites and the polyadenylation site. Mice from the CL1 transgenic line were used in this study. Immunohistochemical staining of liver sections from young transgenic mice with antibody directed against the HBx protein revealed selective expression only in cells that form altered foci. The expression of HBx in this subset of cells appeared to reflect the need for specific transcriptional factors required for the activation of viral regulatory elements. These factors were present only in cells at a specific differentiation state.

**Table 1.** IFN treatment of 2.2.15 cells: suppression of HBV replication

| Treatment* | HBV DNA (pg/ml)† | | | |
|---|---|---|---|---|
| | Day 0 | Day 3 | Day 6 | Day 9 |
| None | 37 | 90 | 69 | 74 |
| Ara-A (50 μM) | 112 | 6 | 0 | 0 |
| Lymphoblastoid IFN | 69 | 85 | 53 | 44 |
| rIFN-α A | 73 | 76 | 75 | 91 |
| rIFN-β | 70 | 80 | 68 | 56 |
| rIFN-γ | 63 | 70 | 75 | 81 |
| rIFN-α B/D | 89 | 69 | 8 | 2 |

*IFN (1000 IU/ml) was added daily for 9 days and viral DNA in culture medium was assayed on day 10.

†1 pg/ml represents approximately $3 \times 10^5$ virions.

Accumulation of the HBx protein was limited to the cytoplasm.

## Immunohistochemical staining for HBx

Sections of paraffin-embedded liver were mounted on saline-coated slides, dewaxed, rehydrated and treated with 0.1% trypsin for 30 min at 30°C. Sections were incubated overnight at 4°C with the appropriate antibody. All immunostained sections were combined with diaminobenzidine substrate using the avidin–biotin horseradish peroxidase system (Vector Laboratories).

## RESULTS

### Suppression of HBV replication in human hepatocytes

The antiviral activity of IFN-α B/D was compared with other IFNs considered for use in the treatment of chronic HBV infection. Antiviral activity was measured in the HBV-producing human hepatoblastoma cell line 2.2.15, with the nucleoside analogue adenosine arabinoside (Ara-A), as an internal standard. As illustrated in Tables 1 and 3, Ara-A suppressed the release of virus 3 days after addition to the culture system whereas IFN-α B/D was effective by day 6 following addition. In contrast, neither of the parental subtypes (α-B or α-D), lymphoblastoid, α-2a, α-2b, β or γ IFNs were active. Similar results were observed when the levels of HBV replicative intermediates were examined following IFN treatment (Table 3). It is also interesting to note that the only other active IFN was another recombinant human IFN-α hybrid, IFN-α A/D (Table 2). Why only hybrid forms of IFN-α are capable of eliciting an anti-HBV response in 2.2.15 cells is unclear. Future studies that focus on the nature of the type 1 receptor interactions and the transmembrane signalling events that result from binding may shed some light on this phenomenon.

Although IFN-α B/D is able to suppress HBV replication in human hepatoblastoma cells, it should be noted that relatively high concentrations (300–1000 IU/ml) are required. This rather poor response to exogenous IFN is typical of cells infected with HBV. Because of this, we initiated combination therapies in which IFN-α was administered together with nucleoside analogues. As illustrated in Table 4, combinations with one promising nucleoside analogue, lamivudine, were synergistic. The synergy observed resulted in a significant increase in the selectivity

**Table 2.** IFN-α B/D and A/D hybrids in 2.2.15 cells: effects on HBV replicative intermediates

| Treatment* | HBV DNA (pg/mg cell DNA)† | | |
| --- | --- | --- | --- |
| | Integrated | Episomal | RI‡ |
| None | 1.0 | 2.5 | 77 |
| Ara-A | 1.3 | 1.1 | 1 |
| rIFN-α | | | |
| B/D | 1.3 | 1.7 | 6 |
| B | 1.2 | 2.2 | 22 |
| D | 1.0 | 2.3 | 68 |
| A/D | ND | 2.3 | 6 |
| A | ND | 2.4 | 67 |
| D | ND | 2.1 | 81 |

*IFN (1000 IU/ml) was added daily for 9 days; Ara-A was used at 30 µM.
†Analysis of intercellular HBV DNA was performed 24 h after the 9th day of treatment. The levels of episomal 3.2 kb HBV genomes and HBV DNA replicative intermediates (RI) were determined from total cell DNA extracts as described by Korba & Gerin [12]. One pg/mg cell DNA represents approximately 3–5 genomic copies. ND, not determined.

**Table 3.** Summary of IFN activities in 2.2.15 cells

| Treatment* | Inhibition† | |
| --- | --- | --- |
| | RI | Virus |
| Ara-A | +++ | +++ |
| rIFN-α B/D | ++ | ++ |
| rIFN-α A/D | ++ | ++ |
| rIFN-α B | – | – |
| rIFN-α D | – | – |
| rIFN-α 2a | – | – |
| rIFN-α 2b | – | – |
| Lymphoblastoid IFN | – | – |

*IFN was added daily (1000 IU/ml) for 9 days.
†Inhibition was scored as follows: +++, 100% inhibition; ++, > 80% inhibition; –, < 4.2% inhibition.

index of IFN alone. This effect was maximized when the 3000:1 ratio (units IFN:µM lamivudine) was evaluated.

## Therapy of chronic woodchuck hepatitis

Although IFN-α B/D is able to suppress HBV replication in hepatocytes through direct interaction with these cells, the immune system is needed to eliminate virus from chronically infected livers. In order that we might examine the immunomodulatory effects of IFN therapy, woodchucks were chronically infected with WHV and then treated with IFN-α B/D. As illustrated in Figures 1 and 2, the levels of WHV in serum and liver were significantly reduced after 12 weeks of therapy. This effect was, however, transient and virus titres returned to pretreatment levels 12 weeks after therapy was discontinued. While it is likely that the initial virus reduction (that observed during the first 2 weeks of treatment) results from a direct antiviral effect, the

reduction that continues over the next 10 weeks of treatment is thought to result from immune destruction of virus-infected hepatocytes. Support for this hypothesis comes from the observed elevated serum enzyme levels and the development of an intense inflammatory response late in the course of treatment. Unfortunately, we were not able to obtain natural woodchuck IFN-α to see whether treatment with this IFN would result in a similar antiviral response. Likewise, other human IFNs such as IFN-α 2a did not induce an antiviral response in woodchuck hepatocytes and, therefore, were not evaluated. It should be noted that in Chapter 18 of this book, Morrey, Korba and Sidwell present the results of their study in which HBV transgenic mice treated with IFN-α B/D reveal a similar reduction in viraemia and rebound effect following the removal of IFN.

## Lamivudine and IFN-α in the woodchuck model

The lamivudine/IFN combination studies used five groups of chronic carrier animals. Two groups of animals were given either daily oral doses of lamivudine (three animals; 1 mg/kg) or subcutaneous doses of IFN

**Table 4.** Anti-HBV activity of IFN-α B/D plus lamivudine combinations

| Treatment* | $CC_{50}$ (IU/ml) | $EC_{90}$ (IU/ml) | SI ($CC_{50}/EC_{90}$) | COMBOSTAT analysis (at $EC_{90}$) |
| --- | --- | --- | --- | --- |
| IFN-α B/D | 60000±3400 | 989±71 | 60 | – |
| IFN-α B/D plus lamivudine (3000:1) | 68000±4000 | 146±15 | 466 | Synergism |
| IFN-α B/D plus lamivudine (10000:1) | 55900±4000 | 409±45 | 135 | Synergism |

*Fresh drug was added to each well containing 2.2.15 cells every day for 9 days. In IFN-α/lamivudine combinations, either 3000 or 10000 IU/ml of IFN-α was present for each 1.0 µM lamivudine (3000:1 or 10000:1 ratios, respectively). See Methods for full description of assay. The $EC_{90}$ of lamivudine used alone and as a single antiviral agent was 0.241 µM in this assay. When used in combination with IFN, the lamivudine $EC_{90}$ levels dropped to 0.045 µM and 0.041 µM, respectively, for the 3000:1 and 10000:1 ratios.

**Figure 1.** IFN-α B/D suppression of WHV DNA in the sera of chronically infected animals

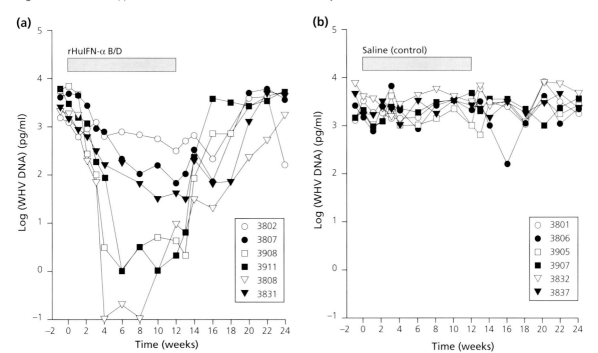

Woodchucks were infected as described in Methods and then treated every other day with 5×10⁶ U/kg of IFN subcutaneously for 3 months. DNA was measured using blot hybridization.

**Figure 2.** IFN-α B/D suppression of WHV DNA in the livers of chronically infected animals

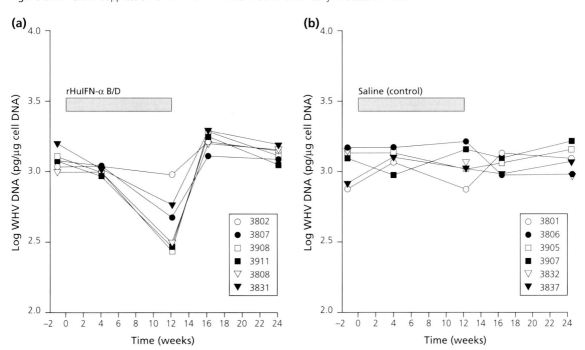

Woodchucks were infected as described in Methods and then treated every other day with 5×10⁶ U/kg of IFN subcutaneously for 3 months. Liver biopsies were taken at selected times and the cells were evaluated for the presence of replicative intermediates.

every 48 hours (six animals; 100000 IU/kg) for 24 weeks. A control group of six untreated animals was included. Two different combination treatment protocols were used. The concentrations and dosing schedules of lamivudine and IFN in the two combination groups were the same as in the monotherapy groups.

The two combination protocols were designed to compare the relative effectiveness of a regimen in which both drugs were given simultaneously or in a staggered fashion. In the simultaneous protocol, both drugs were given together for 24 weeks. In the staggered protocol, lamivudine was given initially for 12 weeks, followed by treatment with both drugs for an additional 12 weeks. At the end of the first 24 week period, lamivudine was discontinued and IFN alone was administered for a final 12 week period. The logic behind the 'staggered' protocol is that patients with high levels of HBV replication and low levels of active liver disease markers do not respond well to IFN therapy. Thus, this protocol was designed to lower HBV replication prior to the initiation of IFN therapy in the hope of better mimicking the levels of virus replication in a 'typical responder profile' and, thereby, increasing the likelihood of successful antiviral response to IFN. It should be noted that simply reducing viraemia and virus replication is not necessarily a complete parallel to the status of HBV in such patients, which most likely involves a complex interaction of virus with the host immune system.

The levels of lamivudine and IFN used in the combination study were approximately fivefold and 10-fold lower, respectively, than doses used in monotherapy studies. The IFN dose used is approximately equivalent to that used to treat chronic HBV infection ($7–10\times10^6$ IU), and the dose of lamivudine is approximately fourfold lower than the metabolic dose equivalent of the dose used in human clinical trials (100 mg). These drug doses were chosen to permit the discrimination of enhanced antiviral effects due to the combination treatments.

Both groups of animals treated with a combination of lamivudine and IFN showed reductions in viraemia that were significantly more pronounced than those observed in either of the monotherapy groups (Table 5). However, in both groups of animals treated with the combination therapies, viraemia returned to pretreatment levels following removal of therapy, essentially as rapidly as in the monotherapy groups. In the group of animals receiving the staggered lamivudine–IFN regimen, the decline in viraemia during treatment was accelerated once IFN therapy was added at week 12. Viraemia continued to decline under the influence of IFN alone following the removal of lamivudine. Although it took longer for viraemia to decline in the staggered combination treatment regimen than with the simultaneous combination therapy, viraemia was sustained at a more reduced level and for a substantially longer period by the staggered regimen. These observations indicate that the reduction in viraemia induced by lamivudine prior to the administration of IFN therapy may have partially mimicked the virus status in the 'IFN responder profile'.

An estimation of the 'expected' reductions in viraemia for the lamivudine/IFN combination treatments at the end of the two treatment protocols is shown in Table 5. Both lamivudine/IFN combination therapies produced antiviral effects significantly greater than that predicted from the monotherapies.

The levels of WHV DNA replication intermediates (WHV RI) in the liver tissues of animals in this study were well correlated with the levels of viraemia (data not shown). No changes in the levels of WHV RI were observed in the untreated group of animals. None of the treatments induced significant changes in the levels of 3.2 kb episomal WHV monomeric genomes or in the levels of WHV RNA or in WHsAg serum levels.

No obvious treatment-related clinical (for example, body weight loss), haematological, or serological indications of toxicity, including hepatic toxicity [for example, ALT, succinate dehydrogenase], were observed during either the treatment or post-treatment follow-up periods in any of the animals in either the treatment or the control groups.

In summary, combination therapy reduces hepadnavirus replication more effectively than monotherapy both in cell culture and in chronically infected woodchucks. In this regard, the predictivity of the 2.2.15 cell culture system for antiviral effectiveness *in vivo* has been verified [19].

**Table 5.** Fold reduction in viraemia at end of treatment period

| Treatment | Expected (±SD)* | Observed (±SD)* |
|---|---|---|
| Lamivudine (1 mg/kg) | | 37±75 |
| IFN ($10^5$ IU/kg) | | 1155±332 |
| Lamivudine plus IFN (simultaneous dosing) | 174000±76000 | 419000±179000 ($P=0.02$)† |
| Lamivudine plus IFN (staggered dosing) | 174000±76000 | 2600000±676000 ($P=0.001$) |

*Expected reductions in viraemia were estimated by Bliss Independence [$Z=X+Y(1-X)$] [26] using the average of all possible combinations of data from each individual animal treated with the monotherapies.
†Significance value calculated by Student's two-tailed $t$-test, with corrections for small population size.

## Anti-proliferative activity in HBx transgenic mice

The association between HCC and HBV infection is well known; however, the mechanism by which tumours develop as a result of infection is unclear. One HBV gene, HBx, has attracted much interest in this regard since the transcriptional trans-activator protein encoded by this gene has been shown to induce progressive neoplastic changes in the livers of transgenic mice [22,23]. Since one mechanism by which interferon is known to exert an anti-proliferative effect is through the regulation of viral oncogene expression [12], we wanted to learn what, if any, effect IFN-α has on tumour induction and hepatocyte proliferation in the HBx transgenic mouse. These mice develop progressive neoplastic changes in the liver and malignancies develop through a progression from vacuolated cells with increased glycogen storage, through adenomas and eventually on to carcinomas which arise from a background of adenoma cells [22]. In each stage of this malignancy, histochemical staining of tumour cells confirms the expression of cytoplasmic HBx. Moreover, sequential sections of tumours, stained with anti-p53 antibody, reveal the accumulation of this tumour suppressor protein in the cytoplasm; whereas, in normal cells of the same liver, p53 accumulates in the nucleus. Similar to observations with other viral oncoproteins, HBx complexes with p53 in the cytosol and prevents p53 migration to the nucleus [23].

HBx transgenic mice (4–6 months of age) were treated with IFN-α B/D at an early stage of tumour development (Group I) or at a later stage (Group II) when adenomas and/or carcinomas had developed.

**Table 6**. Anti-neoplastic activity of IFN-α B/D: effects in HBx transgenic mice

| Group | IFN | HBx expression | Liver pathology |
|---|---|---|---|
| I (4–6 months)* | No | +++ | Micro-foci around blood vessels |
| | Yes | – | Normal histology |
| II (18–20 months)† | No | +++ | Adenomas/carcinomas |
| | Yes | – | Apoptosis/tumour regression |

*Group I mice were 4–6 months of age. Littermates were HBx-positive with microfocal liver lesions. Treated mice received $1 \times 10^6$ IU of IFN-α B/D intraperitoneally every other day for 4 months.
†Group II mice were 18–20 months of age. Littermates were HBx-positive with adenomas or carcinomas in all of the animals examined. Treated mice received $1 \times 10^6$ IU of IFN-α B/D intraperitoneally every other day for 4 months.

Treatment of both groups resulted in a dramatic reduction in the expression of HBx, and a change in the pattern of p53 accumulation and tumour growth (Table 6). As previously mentioned, there is an unusually high accumulation of HBx and p53 in the cytoplasm of tumour cells from untreated animals. Following interferon treatment, HBx and p53 are no longer observed in the cytosol and p53 appears in the nucleus. The appearance of p53 in the nucleus of tumour cells precedes the apoptotic death of these cells (Table 6). Thus, it appears that when HBx is produced it complexes with p53 and prevents migration of this tumour suppressor protein to the nucleus. Cells lacking nuclear p53 do not possess normal regulatory signals for cell division and neoplastic changes develop. IFN-α appears to prevent the uncontrolled proliferation of hepatocytes by suppressing the expression of HBx.

## DISCUSSION

The human recombinant IFN-α hybrids, IFN-α B/D and A/D, are effective in inhibiting HBV replication in a human hepatocyte cell line, whereas other interferons are not. This observation suggests that the receptor binding dynamics of chimeric forms of IFN-α differ from those of other interferons. Such binding differences could result in unique transmembrane signals which escape inactivation by HBV-coded proteins [8,24]. Moreover, these observations indicate that the antiviral responses reported in clinical studies evaluating treatment with IFN-α-2a, IFN-α-2b and lymphoblastoid interferons may be due to activation of the immune system rather than to direct antiviral effects.

Since IFN-α B/D is effective in reducing virus loads in an experimental WHV model of HBV chronicity, it may now be possible to delineate the immune mechanisms which play a role in IFN induced clearance of virus. Moreover, the enhanced therapeutic indices observed when lamivudine was combined with IFN-α B/D suggests that this combination may be useful for those individuals who do not respond to IFN therapy. In addition, it will be interesting to see whether this synergy can eliminate virus from chronically infected hepatocytes and/or prevent the emergence of lamivudine-resistant variants. The data presented from therapy of chronically infected woodchucks indicates that combination therapy is more effective than monotherapy; nonetheless, a rebound effect was observed after removal of both drugs. Thus, elimination of virus from infected hepatocytes did not occur. Most importantly, however, is the fact that combination therapy reduces the concentrations of both drugs and thus the long-term toxicity which often follows therapy with either interferon or lamivudine.

Both RNA and DNA tumour viruses code for oncoproteins that interfere with cell regulation. These oncoproteins are ideal targets for antiviral therapy; yet, most attempts to control their expression have failed. We have recently reported that IFN-α B/D is able to suppress the expression of both E6 and E7 oncoproteins of human papillomaviruses [25]. This inhibition restored the biological activity of both p53 and Rb tumour suppressor proteins and suppressed clonal proliferation of human papillomavirus 16 (HPV-16)-transfected human keratinocytes. Similar observations were made following treatment of HBx mice and suggest that IFN-α may be quite effective in regulating expression of the HBx oncogene. This raises the obvious questions regarding the potential of IFN therapy early in the course of HBV disease to prevent HBx expression and possibly eliminate or slow progression from chronic disease to HCC. Likewise, future clinical trials should re-evaluate interferon therapy of HCC with the possibility of combining the antiviral, immunomodulating and anti-proliferative properties of this cytokine with other anti-neoplastic agents.

In conclusion, we have demonstrated that a novel human IFN hybrid (IFN-α B/D) is highly active in a variety of experimental animal models of HBV disease. This cross-species activity makes this IFN a valuable tool with which to probe the antiviral and immunomodulating properties of IFN in treatment of chronic disease. Likewise, this IFN allows for the *in vivo* evaluation of drug combinations and the identification of synergistic modalities.

# REFERENCES

1. Pestka S. The human interferons – from protein purification and sequence to cloning and expression in bacteria: before, between, and beyond. *Archives of Biochemistry and Biophysics* 1983; **22**:1–37.
2. Zoon KC. Human interferons: structure and function. In *Interferon 9*, 1987; pp. 1–12. Edited by I Gresser. New York: Academic Press.
3. Dianzani F & Capobianchi MR. Mechanism of induction of alpha interferon. In *The Interferon System: A Current Review to 1987*, 1987; pp. 21–30. Edited by S Baron, F Dianzani, GJ Stanton & WR Fleischman Jr. Austin: University of Texas Medical Branch.
4. Dianzani F. Interferon treatments: how to use an endogenous system as a therapeutic agent. *Journal of Interferon Research* 1992; **12**:109–118.
5. De Maeyer E & De Maeyer-Guignard J. Interferon effects on cellular and humoral immunity. In *The Interferon System: A Current Review to 1987*, 1987; pp. 21–30. Edited by S Baron, F Dianzani, GJ Stanton & WR Fleischman Jr. Austin: University of Texas Medical Branch.
6. Chu CM, Sheen IS, Yeh CT, Hsieh SY, Tsai SL & Liaw YF. Serum levels of interferon-alpha and -gamma in acute and chronic hepatitis B virus infection. *Digestive Diseases and Sciences* 1995; **40**:2107–2112.
7. Vingerhoets J, Michielsen P, Vanham G, Bosmans E, Paulij W, Ramon A, Pelckmans P, Kestens L & Leroux-Roels G. HBV-specific lymphoproliferative and cytokine responses in patients with chronic hepatitis B. *Journal of Hepatology* 1998; **28**:8–16.
8. Tolentino P, Dianzani F, Zucca M & Giacchino R. Decreased interferon response by lymphocytes from children with chronic hepatitis. *Journal of Infectious Diseases* 1975; **132**:459–463.
9. Ikeda T, Lever AML & Thomas HC. Evidence for a deficiency of interferon production in patients with chronic hepatitis B virus infection acquired in adult life. *Hepatology* 1986; **6**:962–965.
10. Rehermann B, Lau D, Hoofnagle JH & Chisari FV. Cytotoxic T lymphocyte responsiveness after resolution of chronic hepatitis B virus infection. *Journal of Clinical Investigation* 1996; **97**:1655–1665.
11. Isono E, Yamauchi K, Haruta I, Kamogawa Y & Hayashi N. Effect of alpha-interferon on hepatitis B virus-specific cytotoxic T cells. *Journal of Gastroenterology and Hepatology* 1995; **10**:24–29.
12. Estrov Z, Kurzrock R & Taltaz M. Interferon in viral diseases. In *Interferon Basic Principles and Clinical Applications*, 1993; pp. 38–52. Austin: RG Lands.
13. Lau DT, Everhart J, Kleiner DE, Park Y, Vergalla J, Schmid P & Hoofnagle JH. Long-term follow-up of patients with chronic hepatitis B treated with interferon alfa. *Gastroenterology* 1997; **113**:1660–1667.
14. Meister A, Uze G, Mogenson K, Gresser I, Tovey MG, Grutter M & Meyer F. Biological activities and receptor binding of two human recombinant interferons and their hybrids. *Journal of General Virology* 1986; **67**: 1633–1643.
15. Horisberger MA & De Staritzky KA. A recombinant human interferon-alpha B/D hybrid with a broad host range. *Journal of General Virology* 1987; **68**: 945–948.
16. Gangemi JD, Lazdins J, Dietrich FM, Matter A, Poncioni B & Hochkeppel HK. Antiviral activity of a novel recombinant human interferon-alpha B/D hybrid. *Journal of Interferon Research* 1989; **9**:227–237.
17. De Man RA, Heijtink RA, Niesters HG & Schalm SW. New developments in antiviral therapy for chronic hepatitis B infection. *Scandinavian Journal of Gastroenterology* 1995; **212**:100–104.
18. Van Thiel DH, Fridlander L, Kania RJ, Molloy PJ, Hassanein T & Faruki H. A preliminary experience with GM-CSF plus interferon in patients with HBV and HCV resistant to interferon therapy. *Journal of Viral Hepatitis* 1997; **1**:101–106.
19. Korba BE. *In vitro* evaluation of combination therapies against hepatitis B virus replication. *Antiviral Research* 1996; **29**:49–51.
20. Korba BE & Gerin JL. Use of a standardized cell culture system to evaluate nucleoside analogues for activity against hepatitis B virus replication. *Antiviral Research* 1992; **19**:55–70.
21. Chen HS, Kaneko S, Girones R, Anderson RW, Hornbuckle WE, Tennant BC, Cote PJ, Gerin JL, Purcell RH & Miller RH. The woodchuck hepatitis virus X gene is important in the establishment of virus infection in woodchucks. *Journal of Virology* 1993; **67**:1218–1226.

22. Kim CM, Koike K, Saito I, Miyamura T & Jay G. The HBx gene of hepatitis B virus induces liver cancer in transgenic mice. *Nature* 1991; **351**:317–320.

23. Ueda H, Ullrich SJ, Gangemi JD, Kappel C, Ngo L, Feitleson MA & Jay G. Functional inactivation but not structural mutation of p53 causes liver cancer. *Nature Genetics* 1995; **9**:41–47.

24. McNair AN & Kerr IM. Viral inhibition of the interferon system. *Pharmacological Therapies* 1992; **56**:79–95.

25. Johnson J & Gangemi JD. Control of tumor suppressor and oncoprotein expression in HPV-16 immortalized human cells by recombinant interferon α (rIFN-α) *96th General Meeting of the American Society for Microbiology*, 19–23 May 1996, New Orleans, USA. Abstract.

26. Pritchard MN & Shipman C Jr. Analysis of combinations of antiviral drugs and design of effective multidrug therapies. *Antiviral Therapy* 1996; **1**:9–20.

# Section V

## ANTIVIRAL TARGETS
## FOR HEPATITIS C

# 23

# Molecular virology of hepatitis C virus: an update with respect to potential antiviral targets

Keril J Blight, Alexander A Kolykhalov, Karen E Reed, Eugene V Agapov and Charles M Rice*

## INTRODUCTION

Despite the decreased incidence of post-transfusion hepatitis caused by hepatitis C virus (HCV), this chronic viral infection remains a major human health concern affecting about 3% of the population worldwide [1]. Chronic HCV infection is strongly associated with progressive liver pathology, including cirrhosis and the development of hepatocellular carcinoma. Chronic hepatitis C virus infection is treated with interferon α (IFN-α) alone, or in combination with ribavirin; however a significant fraction of patients either fail to respond or relapse after cessation of therapy [2]. Thus, there is an obvious need to develop effective therapeutic strategies to improve the clinical treatment of HCV-associated hepatitis. Over the past 9 years there has been a great deal of progress in our understanding of HCV genome structure and expression. These advances have already begun to reveal a number of viral functions which may provide attractive targets for the development of new and more effective anti-HCV therapies. In this report, we briefly summarize what is currently known in this area, highlighting potential targets including HCV-encoded enzymatic activities, conserved *cis* RNA elements, and protein–protein interactions likely to be required for viral replication.

## HCV classification, genome organization and translation

HCV has been grouped with the classical flaviviruses (such as yellow fever virus) and pestiviruses (such as bovine viral diarrhoea virus) in the family *Flaviviridae*. All members of this family are small, enveloped viruses containing a positive-sense, single-stranded RNA genome with a single, long open reading frame (ORF). In the case of HCV, the genome RNA is ~9.6 kb in length, and the ORF is flanked by 5′ and 3′ non-translated regions (NTRs) (Fig. 1). The highly conserved 5′ NTR is 341–344 bases in length. Multiple stem–loop structures in this region contribute to an internal ribosome entry site (IRES), mediating cap-independent translation of viral RNA [3–6]. The high degree of conservation in this RNA element and its function in translation of the polyprotein makes it an attractive target for nucleic acid-based antiviral approaches. For instance, several groups have described inhibition of HCV translation by antisense oligonucleotides complementary to sequences within or overlapping the 5′ NTR [7–11]. Although the mechanisms of inhibition by antisense oligonucleotides are not clearly understood, RNase H-dependent cleavage of target RNAs hybridized to oligonucleotides appears to be responsible for some of the antisense inhibition observed for HCV; however, RNase H-independent mechanisms have also been implicated [8]. Furthermore, ribozymes designed to cleave conserved sequences within the 5′ NTR were expressed from recombinant adenovirus vectors and shown to efficiently eliminate HCV RNA from infected human hepatocytes [12].

IRES-mediated translation of the HCV ORF leads to the production of a polyprotein of more than 3000 amino acid residues with the structural proteins located in the N-terminal portion followed by the non-structural (NS) proteins in the remainder. The HCV polyprotein is proteolytically processed into at least ten individual proteins (Fig. 1). The gene order in the polyprotein is: NH$_2$-C–E1–E2–p7–NS2–NS3–NS4A–NS4B–NS5A–NS5B-COOH. Processing in the structural–NS2 region (at the C/E1, E1/E2, E2/p7 and p7/NS2 sites) is catalysed by a host signal peptidase, located in the lumen of the endoplasmic reticulum (ER) [13–19]. On the other hand, cleavages within the NS region of the polyprotein are mediated by two over-

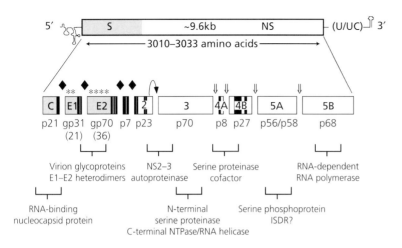

**Figure 1.** HCV genome structure, polyprotein processing and protein features

The viral genome is depicted in the upper part of the diagram, with the structural (S) and non-structural (NS) protein coding regions, the 5′ and 3′ NTRs, and the putative 3′ secondary structure. Boxes below the genome represent proteins generated by the proteolytic processing cascade. Putative S proteins are indicated by shaded boxes and the NS proteins by open boxes. Contiguous stretches of uncharged amino acids are shown by black bars. Asterisks denote proteins with N-linked glycans, but do not necessarily indicate the position or number of sites utilized. Cleavage sites for host signalase (◆), the NS2-3 proteinase (curved arrow), and the NS3-4A serine protease (⇓) are also marked. Roles of the HCV proteins in the virus replication cycle are listed below. See text for additional protein properties and interactions with cellular factors.

lapping HCV-encoded proteases that have different catalytic mechanisms and cleavage site specificities (see below). The NS2 protein coupled with the N-terminal one-third of NS3 form an autoproteinase responsible for *cis* (intramolecular) cleavage at the 2/3 site [20,21]. The remaining four cleavages (3/4A, 4A/4B, 4B/5A and 5A/5B) are mediated by the N-terminal serine protease domain of NS3 complexed with NS4A [22–25].

## Structural proteins

C, E1 and E2 are thought to be the structural components of the HCV virion. C is a highly conserved basic protein, believed to associate with genome RNA to form the nucleocapsid. The C protein has RNA-binding [18,26] and multimerization [27,28] properties, consistent with this hypothesis. The 21 kDa C protein is ER-membrane associated [13,18,29–34], but smaller forms have been observed. These smaller forms are transported into the nucleus, owing to the presence of clusters of basic amino acids which act as nuclear localization signals, coupled with the absence of C-terminal domains responsible for association of C with the ER membrane [29,33,35–37]. The generality and biological relevance of the smaller forms of C and localization of C in the nucleus are still unclear. The C protein has been shown to inhibit hepatitis B virus [38] and human immunodeficiency virus [39] replication, modulate transcription/translation of several cellular genes [31,40–42] and cooperate in Ras-mediated transformation of rat embryo fibroblasts [43]. The latter observation is in contrast to a recent report which

showed that C was unable to transform rat embryo fibroblasts in conjunction with the H-*ras* oncogene; however, transformed phenotypes were exhibited after C expression in the Rat-1 cell line [44]. Furthermore, C can specifically suppress apoptotic cell death in artificial systems [45] and interact with the cytoplasmic tail of the lymphotoxin-β receptor [46,47] implicating a possible immunomodulatory function.

The E1 and E2 proteins are heavily modified by Asn-linked glycosylation with apparent molecular masses of approximately 31 kDa and 70 kDa, respectively [13,48–56]. They contain hydrophobic domains in their C-terminal regions which presumably act as membrane anchors giving the proteins a type I membrane topology [57]. Although E1 has been shown to associate through its C terminus with the C protein [58], other studies have focused on the interaction between E1 and E2. E1 and E2 associate slowly to form heterodimers stabilized by non-covalent interactions [59,60], and although a direct analysis of the infectious HCV virion has not been performed, the E1–E2 heterodimers are thought to represent the functional subunits embedded in the lipid envelope of the HCV virus particle. Folding and heterodimer formation occur in association with the ER chaperone calnexin [60], and evidence suggests that this interaction plays a role in the productive folding of the HCV glycoproteins [61]. Assembled glycoprotein complexes appear to be retained in the ER with no evidence of translocation to the Golgi [62]. Recently, at least one signal for ER retention of the E1–E2 heterodimers was found to reside in the C-terminal transmembrane domain of E2. This domain has also been implicated in E1–E2 complex formation [63]. Intracellular 'virus-like' particles have been visualized by electron microscopy following expression of the full-length HCV ORF in hepatoma cell lines [64,65] or the structural region in insect cells using a recombinant baculovirus [66]. Thus far, secretion of unmodified HCV glycoproteins or 'virus-like' particles has not been observed in any of these reports; as a consequence virus maturation and release have not been amenable to study.

To date, nothing is known about the function of the small, hydrophobic polypeptide, p7, which is cleaved inefficiently from the C terminus of E2 [15–17,19]. Whether p7 is a component of the HCV virion or a non-structural protein remains to be ascertained. However, in pestiviruses, p7 and E2–p7 do not appear to be major components of the virion [67].

## Non-structural proteins

NS2 is a hydrophobic 23 kDa integral membrane protein [68], which, together with the N-terminal one-third of NS3 (polyprotein residues ~900–1207), forms a zinc-stimulated protease responsible for autocatalytic cleavage at the 2/3 site [20,21]. Site-directed mutagenesis studies have identified His-952 and Cys-993 as important residues for enzymatic activity [20,21]. Based on these studies and comparative modelling with other viral cysteine proteases, the NS2-3 protease has been proposed to be a cysteine protease [69] rather than a metalloprotease [21]. Additionally, cleavage at the 2/3 junction is dramatically inhibited by mutations that are likely to disrupt the local conformation of the 2/3 cleavage site. For instance, Pro substitutions at the P1 or P1′ position, deletion of both amino acids at P1 and P1′, or simultaneous substitution of multiple Ala residues all inhibit cleavage [70,71]. The hydrophobicity of NS2 and the autocatalytic nature of 2/3 cleavage pose a challenge for purification of an active NS2-3 protease. This in turn may hinder the design of effective antivirals to this autoprotease. Nevertheless, an *in vitro* assay has been developed which allows the NS2-3 protease to be activated post-translationally [72]. Moreover, this assay has been used to identify several protease inhibitors capable of inactivating the NS2-3 protease.

NS3, a 70 kDa protein, has been subject to intensive study because it is a multifunctional molecule with a serine proteinase catalytic domain residing in the N-terminal 181 residues and an RNA nucleoside triphosphatase (NTPase)/helicase domain in the C-terminal

two-thirds. The NS3 serine protease directs both a *cis* cleavage at the 3/4A junction, as well as *trans* (intermolecular) cleavages at three downstream sites (4A/4B, 4B/5A, and 5A/5B) [22,24,73,74]. The residues His-1083, Asp-1107 and Ser-1165 in NS3 form the catalytic triad of the protease, and N-terminal sequence analysis has defined the cleavage sites in which the residues flanking these sites are highly conserved and conform to the sequence Cys (Thr)⇓Ser (Ala) [75–77]. While a Cys residue is present at all P1 positions of the *trans*-cleavage sites, a Thr residue is found at the P1 position of the 3/4A *cis*-cleavage site. Substitutions at the P1 position tend to have the most detrimental effects on cleavage. In contrast, site-directed mutagenesis revealed that substitutions at the P1′ site are well tolerated and the conserved acidic Asp or Glu residue found upstream at the P6 position is not essential [78–81]. Generally, mutations abolishing cleavage at one site do not affect processing at the other serine proteinase-dependent sites.

The NS3 serine protease domain and the 54-residue NS4A protein form a stable complex which is a prerequisite for cleavage at the 3/4A and 4B/5A sites and enhances processing at the 4A/4B and 5A/5B sites [22–25]. A central hydrophobic region in NS4A and the N-terminal portion of NS3 have been shown to be important for NS3-4A complex formation and for NS4A cofactor-stimulated proteolytic activity [25,82–89]. A highly active NS3 serine protease domain, which can be stimulated by synthetic NS4A cofactor peptide, has now been purified from *Escherichia coli* [83,88,90–93]. These advances have led to the structure determination of the protease complex (see below) and have facilitated a growing number of biochemical studies.

The elucidation of the three-dimensional crystal structure of the NS3 protease domain [94] and of the proteinase domain complexed with a synthetic NS4A cofactor peptide [95] confirmed that this enzyme (~20 kDa) adopts a chymotrypsin-like fold. The serine protease consists of two principal subdomains each forming a β barrel, with both subdomains contributing residues to the active site of the enzyme and the substrate-binding groove [94,95]. Unlike other chymotrypsin family proteases, the substrate binding groove of the HCV serine protease is relatively flat and featureless, and consequently it is anticipated that the design of highly specific low molecular weight inhibitors will prove challenging [95]. Consistent with earlier mutagenesis studies, the NS4A cofactor peptide forms an integral part of the serine proteinase structure [95]. The N-terminal domain folds into eight β strands, including one contributed directly by the NS4A cofactor peptide. The contact surface between the NS4A peptide and the N-terminal residues of NS3 was found to be extensive and may represent an alternative site for pharmacological intervention. A zinc atom is found in the C-terminal subdomain and is tetrahedrally coordinated by Cys-1123, Cys-1125, Cys-1171, and indirectly by His-1175 via a water molecule [94,95]. Although individual mutations of any of the metal-coordinating Cys residues to Ala greatly reduced the proteolytic activity [21,96], the distance of the zinc-binding site from the catalytic centre [94,95] and additional biochemical evidence [97] support a structural rather than a catalytic function for zinc. Hence, the zinc-binding site presents yet another option for drug development.

Some NS3 serine protease inhibitors have begun to emerge. These include competitive peptide inhibitors mimicking the 5A/5B cleavage site [91], as well as some low molecular weight compounds [98–100]. Gene therapy approaches targeting the NS3 protein are also being explored. For example, tight-binding oligonucleotide ligands (aptamers) have been shown to efficiently inhibit the NS3 proteolytic activity *in vitro*. Moreover, two aptamers were also effective inhibitors of the helicase activity of NS3 [101]. Macromolecular ligands of the NS3 protease domain such as minimized variable domain antibody fragments [102,103] and variants of the human pancreatic secretory trypsin inhibitor [102] have been applied and shown to competitively inhibit the protease activity.

The C-terminal domain of HCV NS3 contains an Asp–Glu–Cys–His (DECH) motif at positions 1315–1318 of the polyprotein which identifies it as a member of the DEXH subfamily of DEAD box helicases. Similar to other members of this helicase family, NS3 also contains a Gly–X–Gly–Lys motif at positions 1233–1237 and a cluster of basic residues at positions 1486–1493. Purified NS3 expressed in *E. coli* exhibits RNA-stimulated NTPase [104–109] and RNA helicase [104,106–108,110,111] activities. The purified enzyme was shown to bind RNA substrates with a minimal RNA-binding region of between 7 and 20 nucleotides [104] and to unwind RNA:RNA, RNA:DNA and DNA:DNA duplexes in a 3′ to 5′ direction [104,105,111]. Deletion mapping showed that the functional domain of the NTPase/helicase resides between residues 1209 and 1608 [112]. In addition, the importance of the conserved motifs for each activity have started to be defined by site-directed mutagenesis experiments. As an example, within the DECH motif a Cys to Ser mutation disrupted both the helicase and

NTPase functions [113], while His to Ala either reduced or abolished the helicase activity leaving a functional NTPase [106,113].

The initial crystallization of the NS3 RNA helicase domain was conducted in the absence of nucleic acid, revealing a structure with distinct NTPase and RNA binding domains [114]. However, the recent X-ray crystal structure of the NS3 helicase (amino acids 1215–1652 of the polyprotein) complexed with a single-stranded DNA oligonucleotide revealed three distinct structural domains as well as the nucleic acid- and ATP-binding sites [115]. The oligonucleotide contacted relatively few residues in a groove between the first two domains and the third. The conserved residues line an interdomain between the first two domains, both of which adopt an adenylate kinase-like fold. Hence, further structural and biochemical analysis will not only aid in the determination of the mechanism of nucleic acid unwinding and translocation, but will hopefully uncover attractive targets for ongoing drug design.

Despite the fact that NS3 encodes three enzymatic activities, there is no evidence to suggest that the N- and C-terminal domains are separated by proteolysis. Recent observations from Morgenstern [116] have shown that the protease, NTPase and helicase activities could be modulated by the addition of polynucleotides to the assay system, suggesting that interdomain communication may modulate the various NS3 catalytic activities. Hence, the diverse function of NS3 in the viral replication cycle and the availability of the structural details of both domains makes this protein a very attractive target for the development of antiviral therapies.

Besides the enzymatic activities of NS3 there may be additional functions for this protein. For instance, the N-terminal half of NS3 has been reported to transform NIH 3T3 mouse fibroblasts and induce tumours in nude mice [117]. This may be related to the observation that NS3 specifically interacts with the catalytic subunit of PKA (cAMP-dependent protein kinase) [118,119]. However, the relevance of these observations to viral pathogenesis has not been investigated.

The NS proteins NS4B (27 kDa) and NS5A (56 kDa) have not been assigned functions. However, the NS5A protein is post-translationally phosphorylated on multiple Ser residues [120,121] and a minor fraction of Thr residues [121]. Site-directed mutagenesis and deletion mapping experiments have identified three Ser residues in the central region of NS5A as potential phosphorylation sites, along with additional residues in the C-terminal region of NS5A [122]. In addition, interaction of amino acids 2135–2139 of NS5A with NS4A stimulates hyperphosphorylation of NS5A, resulting in a 58 kDa form [123]. To date, the kinase(s) responsible for NS5A phosphorylation has not been identified, although the addition of phosphate groups in the absence of other HCV-encoded proteins [121–123] suggests the associated Ser/Thr kinase may be of cellular origin. Protein phosphorylation regulates many protein–protein and protein–nucleic acid interactions important for biological processes; if NS5A phosphorylation is essential in the virus replication cycle, then identification of the responsible kinase may uncover yet another potential target for therapeutic intervention.

Apart from the possible role in replication, NS5A has been proposed to modulate the host interferon-stimulated antiviral response. This suggestion was initially based on observations that the degree of variation within the central region of NS5A (amino acids 2209–2248), termed the interferon-sensitivity-determining region (ISDR), appeared to correlate with the sensitivity of HCV genotype 1b viruses to interferon treatment [124,125]. Recently, NS5A was reported to directly interact with the interferon-stimulated protein kinase, PKR [126]. Evidence suggests the ISDR may be necessary for this interaction with PKR and the subsequent repression of PKR phosphorylation [126]. Hence, disrupting the interaction between PKR and NS5A may provide an avenue to increase the effectiveness of IFN-α therapy. Alternatively, considering that PKR is important for cell growth regulation, repression of PKR by a viral protein such as NS5A could be an important factor in the development of hepatocellular carcinoma.

The 68 kDa protein, NS5B, has been shown to possess an RNA-dependent RNA polymerase (RDRP) activity, and this activity presents another target for antiviral drug development. Purified NS5B expressed in *E. coli* [127,128] and from recombinant baculoviruses in insect cells [129,130] has been shown to exhibit primer-dependent RDRP activity capable of copying *in vitro* transcribed full-length HCV genomic RNA, which possibly indicates a high degree of enzyme processivity [130]. However, the NS5B protein was able to bind to and act on other RNA templates without any specificity [127–130]. RNA-dependent RNA polymerization by NS5B has been proposed to occur by a copy-back mechanism, in which the 3′ nucleotide of the template is used to prime synthesis of the complementary strand. Consistent with this hypothesis was the observation that synthesis from homopolymeric templates, incapable of intramolecular base pairing, or templates with a blocked 3′-hydroxyl group, was dependent on the addition of complementary DNA or RNA oligonucleotides. Besides the RDRP activity, recombinant baculovirus-produced NS5B exhibited a terminal transferase (TNTase) activity in which a non-templated base was added to the 3′ terminus of the input RNA [129]. However, the observations that the TNTase activity was: (i) not found in NS5B purified from *E. coli* [127,128]; (ii) present in control baculovirus extracts [130]; and (iii) not linked to the NS5B RDRP activity [130], suggest that this activity may not be intrinsic to NS5B.

## Conservative sequences at the 3′ terminus of the HCV genome

The 3′ NTR consists of three elements: (i) a short sequence (~28–42 nucleotides) after the termination codon that is poorly conserved among different genotypes; (ii) a homopolymeric poly(U) tract and a polypyrimidine stretch consisting of mainly U with interspersed C nucleotides; and (iii) a highly conserved 98 base sequence, also designated the X tail [131–134]. The function(s) of the 3′ NTR remain to be determined. Enzymatic and chemical probing techniques revealed that the 3′-terminal 46 bases form a stable stem–loop structure, SL I [135]. All base changes identified thus far appear within SL I; however, these base changes are compensatory, resulting in the preservation of SL I. On the other hand, the 5′ invariant 52 nucleotides of this sequence appear to be less ordered and exist in multiple conformations [135,136]. Conservation at the sequence and structural level suggests that this 98 base element may have functional importance in the viral replication cycle. For other RNA viruses, such sequences/structures often modulate translation, are involved in the initiation of minus-strand and plus-strand RNA synthesis and act as signals for selective packaging of viral RNA. These processes are likely to be mediated by interaction with viral and/or cellular factors, or RNA elements. To date, interactions between HCV-encoded proteins and the 98 base sequence have not been reported. In fact, only one cellular protein has been shown to interact with this element. Two independent studies described an interaction between the 98 bases and polypyrimidine tract binding protein (PTB) [136,137]. Site-directed mutagenesis mapped the PTB-binding domain within the invariant 52 bases [136]. Similarly, deletion mapping identified a more precise binding site, comprising 19 nucleotides in the invariant sequence and seven bases of the poly (U/UC) tract known as the transitional region [137]. The role of PTB in the viral replication cycle has yet to be determined. However, the identification of compounds able to block interaction of this element with its cognate host and/or viral factors may prove useful in controlling chronic HCV infections. In addition, the sequence conservation within this element makes it an attractive target for nucleic-acid-based antiviral approaches, such as antisense oligonucleotides and ribozymes, as discussed previously for the 5′ NTR.

## Infectious HCV cDNA clones and replication in cell culture

Genetic studies of HCV replication have been hampered by the lack of an infectious full-length cDNA clone for HCV. Recently, two reports described the preparation of infectious HCV RNA transcribed from cloned cDNA [138,139]. Both groups assembled full-length cDNA clones reflecting the consensus sequence for the H77 genotype 1a isolate of HCV, and viral replication was initiated following injection of HCV RNA transcribed *in vitro* directly into the liver of naive chimpanzees. Briefly, in the report from our laboratory [138], transfection of two chimpanzees was conducted, and alanine aminotransferase (ALT), a serum marker of liver damage, and circulating HCV RNA levels were monitored. The ALT levels fluctuated and then increased before peaking by week 13. Viraemia was detected in both animals as early as week 1 which gradually increased to $6–8\times10^6$ genome equivalents/ml by week 13, the onset of seroconversion. In addition, histological changes in liver biopsies indicative of HCV infection, such as portal inflammation and focal necrosis, were observed. These experiments provided the formal proof that HCV alone is the causative agent of disease, and defined the elements necessary for functional HCV genomic RNA. For instance, no additional 5′ and 3′ sequences were required for infectivity, and 3′ poly(U/UC) tracts of variable length were tolerated. Such clonal infections of chimpanzees can be used to facilitate studies on HCV evolution, pathogenesis and the host immune response, that are relevant to understanding the factors that determine viral clearance versus chronic infection.

Several studies have examined the ability of HCV to replicate in cell culture following infection with virus-containing inoculum or transfection with HCV RNA transcribed from cloned cDNA. Thus far, only low levels of HCV replication have been observed, and the reported systems are not readily applicable for antiviral screening or evaluation. Cell cultures which apparently support low levels of HCV replication after infection include hepatocyte cell lines [140–143], B lymphocytes [144–146], T lymphocytes [140,145, 147–150], Vero cells [151] and porcine kidney and testis cell lines [142]. Two groups have reported HCV replication after transfection of hepatoma cell lines with RNA transcribed *in vitro* [64,152]. Surprisingly, a requirement for the 3′ terminal 98 base sequence was not found, and these results need to be confirmed in view of the highly conserved nature of this RNA element [153]. The availability of functional cDNA clones where RNA infectivity has been confirmed in the chimpanzee model should greatly facilitate identification of permissive cell lines and optimal conditions for HCV replication. In addition, homogeneous virus stocks from transfected chimpanzees can be used for infection studies.

## Antiviral intervention

Since the molecular cloning of HCV in 1989, conserved RNA elements, protein products, and enzymatic activities – all elements likely to be essential for HCV replication – have begun to be defined. A number of attractive targets for antiviral intervention have been identified for HCV, including the virus-specific enzymatic activities NS2-3 protease, NS3 serine protease, NS3 NTPase/helicase and the RDRP activity of NS5B. Protein–protein interactions, such as those necessary for virion and RNA replicase assembly also present possible targets for therapeutic intervention. Finally, conserved RNA elements (for example IRES and 3′ NTR), which probably function via interaction with host and viral components, should also be considered in designing strategies to inhibit HCV replication. In the coming years our understanding of the mechanisms by which HCV proteins and RNA elements function will grow; with this expanded knowledge additional targets will undoubtedly emerge. This is important because multiple targets and combination therapy may be necessary for effective control of HCV replication, given the high error rate inherent in RNA virus replication, the existing HCV diversity and the likely emergence of resistant variants. The recent availability of infectious cDNA clones for HCV may facilitate the development of more efficient and standardized *in vitro* culture systems and alternative animal models, thus promoting, basic studies on HCV replication and pathogenesis, as well as antiviral drug screening and evaluation.

## ACKNOWLEDGEMENTS

Work in our laboratory on HCV was supported in part by grants CA57973 and AI40034 from the Public Health Service.

# REFERENCES

1. World Health Organization. Hepatitis C: global prevalence. *Weekly Epidemiological Record* 1997; **72**: 341–344.

2. Reichard O, Schvarcz R & Weiland O. Therapy of hepatitis C: alpha interferon and ribavirin. *Hepatology* 1997; **26**:108S–111S.

3. Honda M, Brown EA & Lemon SM. Stability of a stem–loop involving the initiator AUG controls the efficiency of internal initiation of translation on hepatitis C virus RNA. *RNA* 1996; **2**:955–968.

4. Honda M, Ping L-H, Rijnbrand RCA, Amphlett E, Clarke B, Rowlands D & Lemon SM. Structural requirements for initiation of translation by internal ribosome entry within genome-length hepatitis C virus RNA. *Virology* 1996; **222**:31–42.

5. Wang C, Le S-Y, Ali N & Siddiqui A. An RNA pseudo-knot is an essential structural element of the internal ribosome entry site located within the hepatitis C virus 5' noncoding region. *RNA* 1995; **1**:526–537.

6. Wang C & Siddiqui A. Structure and function of the hepatitis C virus internal ribosome entry site. *Current Topics in Microbiology and Immunology* 1995; **203**: 99–115.

7. Alt M, Renz R, Hofschneider PH, Paumgartner G & Caselmann WH. Specific inhibition of hepatitis C viral gene expression by antisense phosphorothioate oligodeoxynucleotides. *Hepatology* 1995; **22**:707–717.

8. Hanecak R, Brown-Driver V, Fox MC, Azad RF, Furusako S, Nozaki C, Ford C, Sasmor H & Anderson KP. Antisense oligonucleotide inhibition of hepatitis C virus gene expression in transformed hepatocytes. *Journal of Virology* 1996; **70**:5203–5212.

9. Mizutani T, Kato N, Hirota M, Sugiyama K, Murakami A & Shimotohno K. Inhibition of hepatitis C virus replication by antisense oligonucleotide in culture cells. *Biochemical and Biophysical Research Communications* 1995; **212**:906–911.

10. Seki M & Honda Y. Phosphorothioate antisense oligodeoxynucleotides capable of inhibiting hepatitis C virus gene expression: in vitro translation assay. *Journal of Biochemistry* 1995; **118**:1199–1204.

11. Wakita T & Wands JR. Specific inhibition of hepatitis C virus expression by antisense oligodeoxynucleotides. *Journal of Biological Chemistry* 1994; **269**:14205–14210.

12. Lieber A, He C, Polyak SJ, Gretch DR, Barr D & Kay MA. Elimination of hepatitis C virus RNA in infected human hepatocytes by adenovirus-mediated expression of ribozymes. *Journal of Virology* 1996; **70**:8782–8791.

13. Hijikata M, Kato N, Ootsuyama Y, Nakagawa M & Shimotohno K. Gene mapping of the putative structural region of the hepatitis C virus genome by in vitro processing analysis. *Proceedings of the National Academy of Sciences, USA* 1991; **88**:5547–5551.

14. Hüssy P, Langen H, Mous J & Jacobsen H. Hepatitis C virus core protein: carboxy-terminal boundaries of two processed species suggest cleavage by a signal peptide peptidase. *Virology* 1996; **224**:93–104.

15. Lin C, Lindenbach BD, Prágai B, McCourt DW & Rice CM. Processing of the hepatitis C virus E2–NS2 region: identification of p7 and two distinct E2–specific products with different C termini. *Journal of Virology* 1994; **68**:5063–5073.

16. Mizushima H, Hijikata M, Tanji Y, Kimura K & Shimotohno K. Analysis of N-terminal processing of hepatitis C virus nonstructural protein 2. *Journal of Virology* 1994; **68**:2731–2734.

17. Mizushima H, Hijikata H, Asabe S-I, Hirota M, Kimura K & Shimotohno K. Two hepatitis C virus glycoprotein E2 products with different C termini. *Journal of Virology* 1994; **68**:6215–6222.

18. Santolini E, Migliaccio G & La Monica N. Biosynthesis and biochemical properties of the hepatitis C virus core protein. *Journal of Virology* 1994; **68**:3631–3641.

19. Selby MJ, Glazer E, Masiarz F & Houghton M. Complex processing and protein:protein interactions in the E2:NS2 region of HCV. *Virology* 1994; **204**:114–122.

20. Grakoui A, McCourt DW, Wychowski C, Feinstone SM & Rice CM. A second hepatitis C virus-encoded proteinase. *Proceedings of the National Academy of Sciences, USA* 1993; **90**:10583–10587.

21. Hijikata M, Mizushima H, Akagi T, Mori S, Kakiuchi N, Kato N, Tanaka T, Kimura K & Shimotohno K. Two distinct proteinase activities required for the processing of a putative nonstructural precursor protein of hepatitis C virus. *Journal of Virology* 1993; **67**:4665–4675.

22. Bartenschlager R, Ahlborn-Laake L, Mous J & Jacobsen H. Kinetic and structural analyses of hepatitis C virus polyprotein processing. *Journal of Virology* 1994; **68**:5045–5055.

23. Failla C, Tomei L & DeFrancesco R. Both NS3 and NS4A are required for proteolytic processing of hepatitis C virus nonstructural proteins. *Journal of Virology* 1994; **68**:3753–3760.

24. Lin C, Pr‡gai B, Grakoui A, Xu J & Rice CM. Hepatitis C virus NS3 serine proteinase: trans-cleavage and processing kinetics. *Journal of Virology* 1994; **68**:8147–8157.

25. Tanji Y, Hijikata M, Satoh S, Kaneko T & Shimotohno K. Hepatitis C virus-encoded nonstructural protein NS4A has versatile functions in viral protein processing. *Journal of Virology* 1995; **69**:1575–1581.

26. Hwang SB, Lo S-Y, Ou J-H & Lai MMC. Detection of cellular proteins and viral core protein interacting with the 5' untranslated region of hepatitis C virus RNA. *Journal of Biomedical Sciences* 1995; **2**:227–236.

27. Matsumoto M, Hwang SB, Jeng K-S, Zhu N & Lai MMC. Homotypic interaction and multimerization of hepatitis C virus core protein. *Virology* 1996; **218**: 43–51.

28. Nolandt O, Kern V, Muller H, Pfaff E, Theilmann L, Welker R & Krausslich HG. Analysis of hepatitis C virus core protein interaction domains. *Journal of General Virology* 1997; **78**:1331–1340.

29. Chang SC, Yen J-H, Kang H-Y, Jang M-H & Chang M-F. Nuclear localization signals in the core protein of hepatitis C virus. *Biochemical and Biophysical Research Communications* 1994; **205**:1284–1290.

30. Harada S, Watanabe Y, Takeuchi K, Suzuki T, Katayama T, Takebe Y, Saito I & Miyamura T. Expression of processed core protein of hepatitis C virus in mammalian cells. *Journal of Virology* 1991; **65**:3015–3021.

31. Kim DW, Suzuki R, Harada T, Saito I & Miyamura T. Trans-suppression of gene expression by hepatitis C viral core protein. *Japanese Journal of Medical Science and Biology* 1994; **47**:211–220.

32. Moradpour D, Englert C, Wakita T & Wands JR. Characterization of cell lines allowing tightly regulated expression of hepatitis C virus core protein. *Virology* 1996; **222**:51–63.

33. Ravaggi A, Natoli G, Primi D, Albertini A, Levrero M

& Cariani E. Intracellular localization of full-length and truncated hepatitis C virus core protein expressed in mammalian cells. *Journal of Hepatology* 1994; **20**:833–836.

34. Suzuki T, Sato M, Chieda S, Shoji I, Harada T, Yamakawa Y, Watabe S, Matsuura Y & Miyamura T. In vivo and in vitro trans-cleavage activity of hepatitis C virus serine proteinase expressed by recombinant baculoviruses. *Journal of General Virology* 1995; **76**:3021–3029.

35. Lo S-Y, Selby M, Tong M & Ou J-H. Comparative studies of the core gene products of two different hepatitis C virus isolates: two alternative forms determined by a single amino acid substitution. *Virology* 1994; **199**:124–131.

36. Lo S, Masiarz F, Hwang SB, Lai MMC & Ou J. Differential subcellular localization of hepatitis C virus core gene products. *Virology* 1995; **213**:455–461.

37. Suzuki R, Matsuura Y, Suzuki T, Ando A, Chiba J, Harada S, Saito I & Miyamura T. Nuclear localization of the truncated hepatitis C virus core protein with its hydrophobic C terminus deleted. *Journal of General Virology* 1995; **76**:53–61.

38. Shih CM, Lo SJ, Miyamura T, Chen SY & Lee YH. Suppression of hepatitis B virus expression and replication by hepatitis C virus core protein in HuH-7 cells. *Journal of Virology* 1993; **67**:5823–5832.

39. Srinivas RV, Ray RB, Meyer K & Ray R. Hepatitis C virus core protein inhibits human immunodeficiency virus type 1 replication. *Virus Research* 1996; **45**:87–92.

40. Ray RB, Lagging LM, Meyer K, Steele R & Ray R. Transcriptional regulation of cellular and viral promoters by the hepatitis C virus core protein. *Virus Research* 1995; **37**:209–220.

41. Ray RB, Steele R, Meyer K & Ray R. Transcriptional repression of p53 promoter by hepatitis C virus core protein. *Journal of Biological Chemistry* 1997; **272**: 10983–10986.

42. Ray RB, Steele R, Meyer K & Ray R. Hepatitis C virus core protein represses p21WAF1/Cip1/Sid1 promoter activity. *Gene* 1998; **208**:331–336.

43. Ray RB, Lagging LM, Meyer K & Ray R. Hepatitis C virus core protein cooperates with ras and transforms primary rat embryo fibroblasts to tumorigenic phenotype. *Journal of Virology* 1996; **70**: 4438–4443.

44. Chang J, Yang S, Cho Y, Hwang SB, Hahn YS & Sung YC. Hepatitis C virus core from two different genotypes has an oncogenic potential but is not sufficient for transforming primary rat embryo fibroblasts in cooperation with the H-ras oncogene. *Journal of Virology* 1998; **72**:3060–3065.

45. Ray RB, Meyer K & Ray R. Suppression of apoptotic cell death by hepatitis C virus core protein. *Virology* 1996; **226**:176–182.

46. Chen C, You L, Hwang L & Lee Y. Direct interaction of hepatitis C virus core protein with the cellular lymphotoxin-β receptor modulates the signal pathway of the lymphotoxin-β receptor. *Journal of Virology* 1997; **71**:9417–9426.

47. Matsumoto M, Hsieh T, Zhu N, VanArsdale T, Hwang SB, Jeng K, Gorbalenya AE, Lo S, Ou J, Ware CF & Lai MMC. Hepatitis C virus core protein interacts with the cytoplasmic tail of lymphotoxin-β receptor. *Journal of Virology* 1997; **71**:1301–1309.

48. Grakoui A, Wychowski C, Lin C, Feinstone SM & Rice CM. Expression and identification of hepatitis C virus polyprotein cleavage products. *Journal of Virology* 1993; **67**:1385–1395.

49. Hsu HH, Donets M, Greenberg HB & Feinstone SM. Characterization of hepatitis C virus structural proteins with a recombinant baculovirus expression system. *Hepatology* 1993; **17**:763–771.

50. Kohara M, Tsukiyama-Kohara K, Maki N, Asano K, Yamaguchi K, Miki K, Tanaka S, Hattori N, Matsuura Y, Saito I, Miyamura T & Nomoto A. Expression and characterization of glycoprotein gp35 of hepatitis C virus using recombinant vaccinia virus. *Journal of General Virology* 1992; **73**:2313–2318.

51. Koike K, Moriya K, Ishibashi K, Matsuura Y, Suzuki T, Saito I, Iino S, Kurokawa K & Miyamura T. Expression of hepatitis C virus envelope proteins in transgenic mice. *Journal of General Virology* 1995; **76**:3031–3038.

52. Lanford RE, Notvall L, Chavez D, White R, Frenzel G, Simonsen C & Kim J. Analysis of hepatitis C virus capsid, E1, and E2/NS1 proteins expressed in insect cells. *Virology* 1993; **197**:225–235.

53. Matsuura Y, Harada S, Suzuki R, Watanabe Y, Inoue Y, Saito I & Miyamura T. Expression of processed envelope protein of hepatitis C virus in mammalian and insect cells. *Journal of Virology* 1992; **66**:1425–1431.

54. Matsuura Y, Suzuki T, Suzuki R, Sato M, Aizaki H, Saito I & Miyamura T. Processing of E1 and E2 glycoproteins of hepatitis C virus expressed in mammalian and insect cells. *Virology* 1994; **205**:141–150.

55. Ryu W-S, Choi D-Y, Yang J-Y, Kim C-H, Kwon Y-S, So H-S & Cho JM. Characterization of the putative E2 envelope glycoprotein of hepatitis C virus expressed in stably transformed Chinese hamster ovary cells. *Molecules & Cells* 1995; **5**:563–568.

56. Spaete RR, Alexander D, Rugroden ME, Choo Q-L, Berger K, Crawford K, Kuo C, Leng S, Lee C, Ralston R, Thudium K, Tung JW, Kuo G & Houghton M. Characterization of the hepatitis C virus E2/NS1 gene product expressed in mammalian cells. *Virology* 1992; **188**:819–830.

57. Rice CM. *Flaviviridae*: The viruses and their replication. In *Fields Virology* 3rd edn, vol. 1 1996; pp. 931–960. Edited by BN Fields, DM Knipe & PM Howley. Philadelphia: Lippincott-Raven Publishers.

58. Lo S, Selby MJ & Ou J. Interaction between hepatitis C virus core protein and E1 envelope protein. *Journal of Virology* 1996; **70**:5177–5182.

59. Dubuisson J, Hsu HH, Cheung RC, Greenberg H, Russell DR & Rice CM. Formation and intracellular localization of hepatitis C virus envelope glycoprotein complexes expressed by recombinant vaccinia and Sindbis viruses. *Journal of Virology* 1994; **68**: 6147–6160.

60. Dubuisson J & Rice CM. Hepatitis C virus glycoprotein folding: disulfide bond formation and association with calnexin. *Journal of Virology* 1996; **70**:778–786.

61. Choukhi A, Ung S, Wychowski C & Dubuisson J. Involvement of endoplasmic reticulum chaperones in the folding of hepatitis C virus glycoproteins. *Journal of Virology* 1998; **72**:3851–3858.

62. Deleersnyder V, Pillez A, Wychowski C, Blight K, Xu J, Hahn YS, Rice CM & Dubuisson J. Formation of native hepatitis C virus glycoprotein complexes. *Journal of Virology* 1997; **71**:697–704.

63. Cocquerel L, Meunier J, Pillez A, Wychowski C & Dubuisson J. A retention signal necessary and sufficient for endoplasmic reticulum localization maps to the transmembrane domain of hepatitis C virus glycoprotein E2. *Journal of Virology* 1998; **72**:2183–2191.

64. Dash S, Halim A, Tsuji H, Hiramatsu N & Gerber MA. Transfection of HepG2 cells with infectious hepatitis C virus genome. *American Journal of Pathology* 1997;

151:363–373.

65. Mizuno M, Yamada G, Tanaka T, Shimotohno K, Takatani M & Tsuji T. Virion-like structures in Hela G cells transfected with the full-length sequence of the hepatitis C virus genome. *Gastroenterology* 1995; 109:1933–1940.

66. Baumert TF, Ito S, Wong DT & Liang JT. Hepatitis C virus structural proteins assemble into viruslike particles in insect cells. *Journal of Virology* 1998; 72:3827–3836.

67. Elbers K, Tautz N, Becher P, Stoll D, Rumenapf T & Thiel HJ. Processing in the pestivirus E2–NS2 region: identification of proteins p7 and E2p7. *Journal of Virology* 1996; 70:4131–4135.

68. Santolini E, Pacini L, Fipaldini C, Migliaccio G & Monica N. The NS2 protein of hepatitis C virus is a transmembrane polypeptide. *Journal of Virology* 1995; 69:7461–7471.

69. Gorbalenya AE & Snijder EJ. Viral cysteine proteinases. *Perspectives in Drug Discovery and Design* 1996; 6:64–86.

70. Hirowatari Y, Hijikata M, Tanji Y, Nyunoya H, Mizushima H, Kimura K, Tanaka T, Kato N & Shimotohno K. Two proteinase activities in HCV polypeptide expressed in insect cells using baculovirus vector. *Archives of Virology* 1993; 133:349–356.

71. Reed KE, Grakoui A & Rice CM. The hepatitis C virus NS2–3 autoproteinase: cleavage site mutagenesis and requirements for bimolecular cleavage. *Journal of Virology* 1995; 69:4127–4136.

72. Pieroni L, Santolini E, Fipaldini C, Pacini L, Migliaccio G & La Monica N. In vitro study of the NS2–3 protease of hepatitis C virus. *Journal of Virology* 1997; 71:6373–6380.

73. Tanji Y, Hijikata M, Hirowatari Y & Shimotohno K. Identification of the domain required for trans-cleavage activity of hepatitis C viral serine proteinase. *Gene* 1994; 145:215–219.

74. Tomei L, Failla C, Santolini E, DeFrancesco R & La Monica N. NS3 is a serine protease required for processing of hepatitis C virus polyprotein. *Journal of Virology* 1993; 67:4017–4026.

75. Eckart MR, Selby M, Masiarz F, Lee C, Berger K, Crawford K, Kuo C, Kuo G, Houghton M & Choo Q-L. The hepatitis C virus encodes a serine protease involved in processing of the putative nonstructural proteins from the viral polyprotein precursor. *Biochemical and Biophysical Research Communications* 1993; 192:399–406.

76. Grakoui A, McCourt DW, Wychowski C, Feinstone SM & Rice CM. Characterization of the hepatitis C virus-encoded serine proteinase: determination of proteinase-dependent polyprotein cleavage sites. *Journal of Virology* 1993; 67:2832–2843.

77. Pizzi E, Tramontano A, Tomei L, La Monica N, Failla C, Sardana M, Wood T & DeFrancesco R. Molecular-model of the specificity pocket of the hepatitis C virus protease: implications for substrate recognition. *Proceedings of the National Academy of Sciences, USA* 1994; 91:888–892.

78. Bartenschlager R, Ahlborn-Laake L, Yasargil K, Mous J & Jacobsen H. Substrate determinants for cleavage in cis and in trans by the hepatitis C virus NS3 proteinase. *Journal of Virology* 1995; 69:198–205.

79. Kolykhalov AA, Agapov EV & Rice CM. Specificity of the hepatitis C virus serine proteinase: effects of substitutions at the 3/4A, 4A/4B, 4B/5A, and 5A/5B cleavage sites on polyprotein processing. *Journal of Virology* 1994; 68:7525–7533.

80. Leinbach SS, Bhat RA, Xia S-M, Hum W-T, Stauffer B, Davis AR, Hung PP & Mizutani S. Substrate specificity

of the NS3 serine proteinase of hepatitis C virus as determined by mutagenesis at the NS3/NS4A junction. *Virology* 1994; 204:163–169.

81. Tanji Y, Hijikata M, Hirowatari Y & Shimotohno K. Hepatitis C virus polyprotein processing: kinetics and mutagenic analysis of serine proteinase-dependent cleavage. *Journal of Virology* 1994; 68:8418–8422.

82. Bartenschlager R, Lohmann V, Wilkinson T & Koch JO. Complex formation between the NS3 serine-type proteinase of the hepatitis C virus and NS4A and its importance for polyprotein maturation. *Journal of Virology* 1995; 69:7519–7528.

83. Butkiewicz NJ, Wendel M, Zhang RM, Jubin R, Pichardo J, Smith EB, Hart AM, Ingram R, Durkin J, Mui PW, Murray RG, Ramanathan L & Dasmahapatra B. Enhancement of hepatitis C virus NS3 proteinase activity by association with NS4A-specific synthetic peptides: identification of sequence and critical residues of NS4A for the cofactor activity. *Virology* 1996; 225:328–338.

84. Failla C, Tomei L & DeFrancesco R. An amino-terminal domain of the hepatitis C virus NS3 protease is essential for interaction with NS4A. *Journal of Virology* 1995; 69:1769–1777.

85. Koch JO, Lohmann V, Herian U & Bartenschlager R. In vitro studies on the activation of the hepatitis C virus NS3 proteinase by the NS4A cofactor. *Virology* 1996; 221:54–66.

86. Lin C, Thomson JA & Rice CM. A central region in the hepatitis C virus NS4A protein allows formation of an active NS3–NS4A serine proteinase complex in vivo and in vitro. *Journal of Virology* 1995; 69:4373–4380.

87. Satoh S, Tanji Y, Hijikata M, Kimura K & Shimotohno K. The N-terminal region of hepatitis C virus nonstructural protein 3 (NS3) is essential for stable complex formation with NS4A. *Journal of Virology* 1995; 69:4255–4260.

88. Shimizu Y, Yamaji K, Masuho Y, Yokota T, Inoue H, Sudo K, Satoh S & Shimotohno K. Identification of the sequence on NS4A required for enhanced cleavage of the NS5A/5B site by hepatitis C virus NS3 protease. *Journal of Virology* 1996; 70:127–132.

89. Tomei L, Failla C, Vitale RL, Bianchi E & DeFrancesco R. A central hydrophobic domain of the hepatitis C virus NS4A protein is necessary and sufficient for the activation of the NS3 protease. *Journal of General Virology* 1996; 77:1065–1070.

90. Kakiuchi N, Komoda Y, Hijikata M & Shimotohno K. Cleavage activity of hepatitis C virus serine proteinase. *Journal of Biochemistry* 1997; 122:749–755.

91. Landro JA, Raybuck SA, Luong YPC, O'Malley ET, Harbeson SL, Morgenstern KA, Rao G & Livingston DJ. Mechanistic role of an NS4A peptide cofactor with the truncated NS3 protease of hepatitis C virus: elucidation of the NS4A stimulatory effect via kinetic analysis and inhibitor mapping. *Biochemistry* 1997; 36:9340–9348.

92. Steinkuhler C, Urbani A, Tomei L, Biasiol G, Sardana M, Bianchi E, Pessi A & DeFrancesco R. Activity of purified hepatitis C virus protease NS3 on peptide substrates. *Journal of Virology* 1996; 70:6694–6700.

93. Urbani A, Bianchi E, Narjes F, Tramontano A, De Francesco R, Steinkuhler C & Pessi A. Substrate specificity of the hepatitis C virus serine protease NS3. *Journal of Biological Chemistry* 1997; 272:9204–9209.

94. Love RA, Parge H, Wickersham JA, Hostomsky Z, Habuka N, Moomaw EW, Adachi T & Hostomska Z. The crystal structure of hepatitis C virus NS3 proteinase reveals a trypsin-like fold and a structural zinc binding

site. *Cell* 1996; **87**:331–342.

95. Kim JL, Morgenstern KA, Lin C, Fox T, Dwyer MD, Landro JA, Chambers SP, Markland W, Lepre CA, O'Malley ET, Harbeson SL, Rice CM, Murcko MA, Caron PR & Thomson JA. Crystal structure of the hepatitis C virus NS3 protease domain complexed with a synthetic NS4A cofactor peptide. *Cell* 1996; **87**: 343–355.

96. Stempniak M, Hostomska Z, Nodes BR & Hostomsky Z. The NS3 proteinase domain of hepatitis C virus is a zinc-containing enzyme. *Journal of Virology* 1997; **71**:2881–2886.

97. DeFrancesco R, Urbani A, Nardi MC, Tomei L, Steinkuhler C & Tramontano A. A zinc binding site in viral serine proteinases. *Biochemistry* 1996; **35**:13282–13287.

98. Chu M, Mierzwa R, Truumees I, King A, Patel M, Berrie R, Hart A, Butkiewicz N, Dasmahapatra B, Chan TM & Puar MS. Structure of Sch 68631: a new hepatitis C virus proteinase inhibitor from *Streptomyces* sp. *Tetrahedron Letters* 1996; **37**:7229–7232.

99. Kakiuchi N, Komoda Y, Komoda K, Takeshita N, Okada S, Tani T & Shimotohno K. Non-peptide inhibitors of HCV serine proteinase. *FEBS Letters* 1998; **421**:217–220.

100. Sudo K, Matsumoto Y, Matsushima M, Fujiwara M, Konno K, Shimotohno K, Shigeta S & Yokota T. Novel hepatitis C virus protease inhibitors: thiazolidine derivatives. *Biochemical and Biophysical Research Communications* 1997; **238**:643–647.

101. Kumar PKR, Machida K, Urvil PT, Kakiuchi N, Vishnuvardhan D, Shimotohno K, Taira K & Nishikawa S. Isolation of RNA aptamers specific to the NS3 protein of hepatitis C virus from a pool of completely random RNA. *Virology* 1997; **237**: 270–282.

102. Dimasi N, Martin F, Volpari C, Brunetti M, Biasiol G, Altamura S, Cortese R, De Francesco R, Steinkuhler C & Sollazzo M. Characterization of engineered hepatitis C virus NS3 protease inhibitors affinity selected from human pancreatic secretory trypsin inhibitor and minibody repertoires. *Journal of Virology* 1997; **71**:7461–7469.

103. Martin F, Volpari C, Steinkuhler C, Dimasi N, Brunetti M, Biasiol G, Altamura S, Cortese R, De Francesco R & Sollazzo M. Affinity selection of a camelized VH domain antibody inhibitor of hepatitis C virus NS3 protease. *Protein Engineering* 1997; **10**:607–614.

104. Gwack T, Kim DW, Hang JH & Choe J. Characterization of RNA binding activity and RNA helicase activity of the hepatitis C virus NS3 protein. *Biochemical and Biophysical Research Communications* 1996; **225**:654–659.

105. Gwack Y, Kim DW, Han JH & Choe J. DNA helicase activity of the hepatitis C virus nonstructural protein 3. *European Journal of Biochemistry* 1997; **250**:47–54.

106. Heilek GM & Peterson MG. A point mutation abolishes the helicase but not the nucleoside triphosphatase activity of hepatitis C virus NS3 protein. *Journal of Virology* 1997; **71**:6264–6266.

107. Jin L & Peterson DL. Expression, isolation, and characterization of the hepatitis C virus ATPase/RNA helicase. *Archives of Biochemistry and Biophysics* 1995; **323**:47–53.

108. Preugschat F, Averett DR, Clarke BE & Porter DJT. A steady-state and pre-steady-state kinetic analysis of the NTPase activity associated with the hepatitis C virus NS3 helicase domain. *Journal of Biological Chemistry*

1996; **271**:24449–24457.

109. Suzich JA, Tamura JK, Palmer-Hill F, Warrener P, Grakoui A, Rice CM, Feinstone SM & Collett MS. Hepatitis C virus NS3 protein polynucleotide-stimulated nucleoside triphosphatase and comparison with the related pestivirus and flavivirus enzymes. *Journal of Virology* 1993; **67**:6152–6158.

110. Kim DW, Gwack Y, Han JH & Choe J. C-terminal domain of the hepatitis C virus NS3 protein contains an RNA helicase activity. *Biochemical and Biophysical Research Communications* 1995; **215**:160–166.

111. Tai C-L, Chi W-K, Chen D-S & Hwang L-H. The helicase activity associated with hepatitis C virus nonstructural protein 3 (NS3). *Journal of Virology* 1996; **70**:8477–8484.

112. Kim DW, Gwack Y, Han JH & Choe J. Towards defining a minimal functional domain for NTPase and RNA helicase activities of the hepatitis C virus NS3 protein. *Virus Research* 1997; **49**:17–25.

113. Kim DW, Kim J, Gwack Y, Han JH & Choe J. Mutational analysis of the hepatitis C virus RNA helicase. *Journal of Virology* 1997; **71**:9400–9409.

114. Yao N, Hesson T, Cable M, Hong Z, Kwong AD, Le HV & Weber PC. Structure of the hepatitis C virus RNA helicase domain. *Nature Structural Biology* 1997; **4**:463–467.

115. Kim JL, Morgenstern KA, Griffith JP, Dwyer MD, Thomson JA, Murcko MA, Lin C & Caron PR. Hepatitis C virus NS3 RNA helicase domain with a bound oligonucleotide: the crystal structure provides insights into the mode of unwinding. *Structure* 1998; **6**:89–100.

116. Morgenstern KA, Landro JA, Hsiao K, Lin C, Gu Y, Su MS & Thomson JA. Polynucleotide modulation of the protease, nucleoside triphosphatase, and helicase activities of a hepatitis C virus NS3–NS4A complex isolated from transfected COS cells. *Journal of Virology* 1997; **71**:3767–3775.

117. Sakamuro D, Furukawa T & Takegami T. Hepatitis C virus nonstructural protein NS3 transforms NIH 3T3 cells. *Journal of Virology* 1995; **69**:3893–3896.

118. Borowski P, Heiland M, Oehlmann K, Becker B, Kornetzky L, Feucht H & Laufs R. Non-structural protein 3 of hepatitis C virus inhibits phosphorylation mediated by cAMP-dependent protein kinase. *European Journal of Biochemistry* 1996; **237**:611–618.

119. Borowski P, Oehlmann K, Heiland M & Laufs R. Nonstructural protein 3 of hepatitis C virus blocks the distribution of the free catalytic subunit of cyclic AMP-dependent protein kinase. *Journal of Virology* 1997; **71**:2838–2843.

120. Kaneko T, Tanji Y, Satoh S, Hijikata M, Asabe S, Kimura K & Shimotohno K. Production of two phosphoproteins from the NS5A region of the hepatitis C viral genome. *Biochemical and Biophysical Research Communications* 1994; **205**:320–326.

121. Reed KE, Xu J & Rice CM. Phosphorylation of the hepatitis C virus NS5A protein in vitro and in vivo: properties of the NS5A-associated kinase. *Journal of Virology* 1997; **71**:7187–7197.

122. Tanji Y, Kaneko T, Satoh S & Shimotohno K. Phosphorylation of hepatitis C virus-encoded nonstructural protein NS5A. *Journal of Virology* 1995; **69**: 3980–3986.

123. Asabe S-I, Tanji Y, Satoh S, Kaneko T, Kimura K & Shimotohno K. The N-terminal region of hepatitis C virus-encoded NS5A is important for NS4A-dependent phosphorylation. *Journal of Virology* 1997; **71**:790–796.

124. Enomoto N, Sakuma I, Asahina Y, Kurosaki M, Murakami T, Yamamoto C, Izumi N, Marumo F & Sato C. Comparison of full-length sequences of interferon-sensitive and resistant hepatitis C virus 1b. *Journal of Clinical Investigation* 1995; **96**:224–230.

125. Enomoto N, Sakuma I, Asahina Y, Kurosaki M, Murakami T, Yamamoto C, Ogura Y, Izumi N, Marumo F & Sato C. Mutations in the nonstructural protein 5A gene and response to interferon in patients with chronic hepatitis C virus 1b infection. *New England Journal of Medicine* 1996; **334**:77–81.

126. Gale JM, Korth MJ, Tang NM, Tan S-L, Hopkins DA, Dever TE, Polyak SJ, Gretch DR & Katze MG. Evidence that hepatitis C virus resistance to interferon is mediated through repression of the PKR protein kinase by the nonstructural 5A protein. *Virology* 1997; **230**:217–227.

127. Al RH, Xie Y, Wang Y, Staercke CD, van Beers EH & Hagedorn CH. Expression of recombinant hepatitis C virus NS5B. *Nucleic Acids Symposium Series* 1997; **36**:197–199.

128. Yuan Z-H, Kumar U, Thomas HC, Wen Y-M & Monjardino J. Expression, purification, and partial characterization of HCV RNA polymerase. *Biochemical and Biophysical Research Communications* 1997; **232**:231–235.

129. Behrens SE, Tomei L & DeFrancesco R. Identification and properties of the RNA-dependent RNA polymerase of hepatitis C virus. *EMBO Journal* 1996; **15**:12–22.

130. Lohmann V, Körner F, Herian U & Bartenschlager R. Biochemical properties of hepatitis C virus NS5B RNA-dependent RNA polymerase and identification of amino acid sequence motifs essential for enzymatic activity. *Journal of Virology* 1997; **71**:8416–8428.

131. Kolykhalov AA, Feinstone SM & Rice CM. Identification of a highly conserved sequence element at the 3′ terminus of hepatitis C virus genome RNA. *Journal of Virology* 1996; **70**:3363–3371.

132. Tanaka T, Kato N, Cho M-J & Shimotohno K. A novel sequence found at the 3′ terminus of hepatitis C virus genome. *Biochemical and Biophysical Research Communications* 1995; **215**:744–749.

133. Tanaka T, Kato N, Cho M-J, Sugiyama K & Shimotohno K. Structure of the 3′ terminus of the hepatitis C virus genome. *Journal of Virology* 1996; **70**:3307–3312.

134. Yamada N, Tanihara K, Takada A, Yorihuzi T, Tsutsumi M, Shimomura H, Tsuji T & Date T. Genetic organization and diversity of the 3′ noncoding region of the hepatitis C virus genome. *Virology* 1996; **223**:255–261.

135. Blight KJ & Rice CM. Secondary structure determination of the conserved 98–base sequence at the 3′ terminus of hepatitis C virus genome RNA. *Journal of Virology* 1997; **71**:7345–7352.

136. Ito T & Lai MMC. Determination of the secondary structure of and cellular protein binding to the 3′-untranslated region of the hepatitis C virus RNA genome. *Journal of Virology* 1997; **71**:8698–8706.

137. Tsuchihara K, Tanaka T, Hijikata M, Kuge S, Toyoda H, Nomoto A, Yamamoto N & Shimotohno K. Specific interaction of polypyrimidine tract-binding protein with the extreme 3′-terminal structure of the hepatitis C virus genome, the 3′X. *Journal of Virology* 1997; **71**:6720–6726.

138. Kolykhalov AA, Agapov EV, Blight KJ, Mihalik K, Feinstone SM & Rice CM. Transmission of hepatitis C by intrahepatic inoculation with transcribed RNA. *Science* 1997; **277**:570–574.

139. Yanagi M, Purcell RH, Emerson SU & Bukh J. Transcripts from a single full-length cDNA clone of hepatitis C virus are infectious when directly transfected into the liver of a chimpanzee. *Proceedings of the National Academy of Sciences, USA* 1997; **94**:8738–8743.

140. Ikeda M, Kato N, Mizutani T, Sugiyama K, Tanaka K & Shimotohno K. Analysis of the cell tropism of HCV by using in vitro HCV-infected human lymphocytes and hepatocytes. *Journal of Hepatology* 1997; **27**: 445–454.

141. Kato N, Ikeda M, Mizutani T, Sugiyama K, Noguchi M, Hirohashi S & Shimotohno K. Replication of hepatitis C virus in cultured non-neoplastic human hepatocytes. *Japanese Journal of Cancer Research* 1996; **87**:787–792.

142. Seipp S, Mueller HM, Pfaff E, Stremmel W, Theilmann L & Goeser T. Establishment of persistent hepatitis C virus infection and replication in vitro. *Journal of General Virology* 1997; **78**:2467–2476.

143. Tagawa M, Kato N, Yokosuka O, Ishikawa T, Ohto M & Omata M. Infection of human hepatocyte cell lines with hepatitis C virus *in vitro*. *Journal of Gastroenterology and Hepatology* 1995; **10**:523–527.

144. Bertolini L, Iacovacci S, Ponzetto A, Gorini G, Battaglia M & Carloni G. The human bone-marrow-derived B-cell line CE, susceptible to hepatitis C virus infection. *Research in Virology* 1993; **144**: 281–285.

145. Nakajima N, Hijikata M, Yoshikura H & Shimizu YK. Characterization of long-term cultures of hepatitis C virus. *Journal of Virology* 1996; **70**:3325–3329.

146. Valli MB, Bertolini L, Iacovacci S, Ponzetto A & Carloni G. Detection of a 5′ UTR variation in the HCV genome after long-term in vitro infection. *Research in Virology* 1995; **146**:285–288.

147. Kato N, Nakazawa T, Mizutani T & Shimotohno K. Susceptibility of human T-lymphotropic virus type I infected cell line MT-2 to hepatitis C virus infection. *Biochemical and Biophysical Research Communications* 1995; **206**:863–869.

148. Mizutani T, Kato N, Saito S, Ikeda M, Sugiyama K & Shimotohno K. Characterization of hepatitis C virus replication in cloned cells obtained from a human T-cell leukemia virus type 1–infected cell line, MT-2. *Journal of Virology* 1996; **70**:7219–7223.

149. Mizutani T, Kato N, Ikeda M, Sugiyama K & Shimotohno K. Long-term human T-cell culture system supporting hepatitis C virus replication. *Biochemical and Biophysical Research Communications* 1996; **227**:822–826.

150. Shimizu YK, Iwamoto A, Hijikata M, Purcell RH & Yoshikura H. Evidence for in vitro replication of hepatitis C virus genome in a human T-cell line. *Proceedings of the National Academy of Sciences, USA* 1992; **89**:5477–5481.

151. Valli MB, Carloni G, Manzin A, Nasorri F, Ponzetto A & Clementi M. Hepatitis C virus infection of a Vero cell clone displaying efficient virus-cell binding. *Research in Virology* 1997; **148**:181–186.

152. Yoo BJ, Selby M, Choe J, Suh BS, Choi SH, Joh JS, Nuovo GJ, Lee H-S, Houghton M & Han JH. Transfection of a differentiated human hepatoma cell line (Huh7) with in vitro-transcribed hepatitis C virus (HCV) RNA and establishment of a long-term culture persistently infected with HCV. *Journal of Virology* 1995; **69**:32–38.

153. Lai MMC. An infectious hepatitis C virus RNA at last. *Hepatology* 1998; **27**:299–302.

# 24 Targets for inhibition of hepatitis C virus replication

## Margaret Littlejohn, Stephen Locarnini and Angeline Bartholomeusz*

## INTRODUCTION

Hepatitis C virus (HCV) is the major cause of what was previously termed non-A non-B hepatitis. The major site of viral replication is the liver and the half life of virus in serum is approximately 4 hours [1]. Chronic infection with HCV is a worldwide health problem, and approximately 1% of the world's population are infected with the virus. HCV infection can result in an asymptomatic carrier state, acute hepatitis, chronic active hepatitis, cirrhosis and hepatocellular carcinoma [2]. In a recent study of the natural history of hepatitis C, the median estimated time from infection to the progression of cirrhosis was 30 years [3].

HCV was the first virus to be identified using molecular techniques [4] and considerable progress has been made since characterising this virus in 1989. This chapter focuses on the recent advances in understanding how the virus replicates. These advances will aid in the design of new antiviral agents that may specifically reduce the spread of this virus in the community as well as treat existing chronic carriers. Studies into HCV replication and pathogenesis have been impeded by the inability to either grow the virus in cell culture or to produce an infectious clone. However, two independent clones which were infectious for chimpanzees have recently been developed [5,6]. In addition, HCV RNA from a clone containing full-length cDNA has been transfected into HepG2 cells to produce virus-like particles [7]. These pivotal experiments will now enable researchers to address questions on how HCV replicates at the cellular and molecular level.

Hepatitis C virus contains a positive-strand RNA genome and is a member of the family *Flaviviridae* [8]. The genomic RNA encodes a single polyprotein of 3,010 amino acids [4]. Two non-coding regions at the 5′ and 3′ termini contain 341 and approximately 230 nucleotides, respectively [9–11]. The RNA encodes a polyprotein in which the structural core (C) and envelope proteins (E1, E2 and p7) at the N-terminal

end are followed by the non-structural proteins NS2, NS3, NS4A, NS4B, NS5A and NS5B. These proteins have been identified by the cleavage of the HCV polyprotein in recombinant expression systems [12–15]. The processing of the structural proteins is mediated by a host signal peptidase [16]. The non-structural protease NS2/3 cleaves the junction between NS2 and NS3 [17] and the remaining non-structural proteins are cleaved by the NS3-4A protease complex [18]. The X-ray crystal structure of this NS3 protease with and without NS4A has been determined [19,20]. The elucidation of the crystal structure may aid advances in the design of molecules that may specifically inhibit protein processing and thus viral replication.

There are two untranslated regions at the 5′ and 3′ termini that are important for translation and the transcription of RNA. The proposed RNA secondary structure of the 5′ untranslated region of the genomic RNA of HCV is similar to that proposed for pestiviruses [9] and it contains an internal ribosome entry site (IRES) for the initiation of translation [21,22]. The 3′ untranslated region of the genomic RNA contains a stretch of polyuridine (poly U) ribonucleotides, followed by a region of 98 to 100 nucleotides [10,11,23,24]. This region is highly conserved and contains important signals for the initiation of RNA synthesis; it may also have a role in RNA stability or packaging of the RNA into viral core particles. The 3′ untranslated region of the negative-sense RNA contains RNA initiation signals for the synthesis of genomic sense RNA.

The proteins encoded by viral non-structural genes are necessary for genomic RNA replication. The NS3 protein has helicase activity and NS5B has polymerase activity [25–27], both proteins are relatively hydrophilic. In addition to these factors, it is likely that NS2, NS4A, NS4B and NS5A are involved in RNA replication and the membrane asso-

Positive-sense RNA template

RNA replication complex

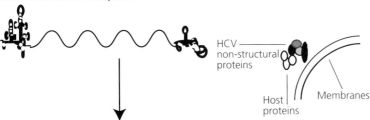

**Figure 1.** Synthesis of negative-sense RNA from a positive-sense RNA template

There is an initial interaction between proteins involved in RNA synthesis and between these proteins and cell membranes. This is followed by recognition and binding of the RNA template by the replication complex, the unwinding of the complex RNA secondary structures by an RNA helicase, elongation of newly synthesized RNA and the dissociation of the polymerase complex from the RNA.

Binding of the replication complex; priming and initiation

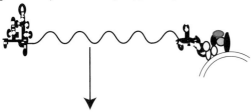

Unwinding of RNA secondary structures

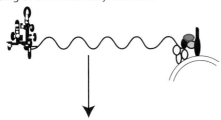

Elongation of newly synthesized RNA

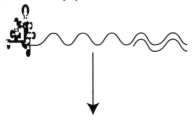

Termination and release of the replication complex from RNA

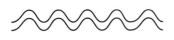

ciation of the RNA replication complex. It is known that RNA replication complexes of flaviviruses are associated with the membranes of the smooth endoplasmic reticulum [28].

The process of viral RNA replication for a positive-strand virus is complex. The genomic RNA must serve as a template for RNA synthesis and the direct production of non-structural proteins involved in RNA replication. Viral RNA synthesis involves several

steps and is outlined in Figure 1. The first step involves interactions between proteins involved in RNA synthesis and the association of these proteins with cellular membranes. The second step involves recognition of the RNA template by the replication complex, followed by priming and initiation. During the third step, the RNA helicase unwinds the proposed complex RNA secondary structures in the single-stranded RNA or the double-stranded replicative form (RF) of the

RNA template. The fourth step involves elongation of newly synthesized RNA; single-stranded RNA-binding proteins may bind to the nascent RNA strand. During the final step, the full-length genomic RNA (or double-stranded RNA) is released and dissociates the replication complex.

HCV RNA synthesis will probably involve most of these features. Some of these processes and the proteins involved have already been investigated. For example, the helicase and the NTPase activity of NS3 [25,29], the polymerase and nucleotidyl transferase activity of NS5B [26], and the binding of host proteins to the 3' untranslated RNA [24]. These virus-specific processes may be ideal targets for antiviral agents. However, the replication strategy of HCV will need to be determined in order to understand how these proteins interact and synthesize RNA. The flavivirus RNA replication strategy may be used as a model for HCV RNA synthesis.

## Flavivirus RNA replication strategy

Several RNA replicative intermediates have been investigated for flaviviruses and a replication strategy developed. *In vitro* polymerase assays using infected cell lysates have been established for a number of flaviviruses to investigate the RNA replication strategy [30–33]. In these experiments, RNA synthesis was detected by the incorporation of [$\alpha$-$^{32}$P]GTP into full-length genomic RNA, the double-stranded RF RNA, and the partially single-stranded replicative intermediate (RI). The genomic positive-sense strand is tran-

scribed into negative-sense RNA in flaviviruses [33]. The negative-sense RNA may exist as a single- or double-stranded RNA molecule [30,31]. Chu and Westaway have proposed that the negative strand of the RF molecule is used for the asymmetric and preferential synthesis of positive-sense genomic RNA (Fig. 2; [30]). Bartholomeusz and Wright have shown that the RF RNA can be used as a template in RNA synthesis [33]. When heterologous RF RNA templates were used in this assay, the RF RNA was converted to an RI, and the RI was subsequently converted into RF RNA.

## Growth of HCV in cell culture

Recent studies have shown virus-like particles after infection of hepatoma cells by HCV and the successful reinfection of naive cells [7,34–36]. In one such study, HCV propagation was observed for 50 days in a serum-free medium with stimulation of the low-density lipoprotein (LDL) receptor expression by lovastatin [35]. The LDL receptor may be involved in the uptake of HCV. Iacovacci *et al.* have detected virus-like particles and the presence of RNAse-resistant double-stranded RNA in HCV-infected human foetal hepatocytes [36]. Dash *et al.* have detected virus-like particles in HepG2 cells after transfection with HCV RNA [7]. The detection of virus-like particles in cell culture suggests this system may be used in the future to screen for potential antiviral agents. However, optimization of conditions in these cell culture systems will be required in order to differentiate real antiviral effects from variable virus growth conditions. The viral titres

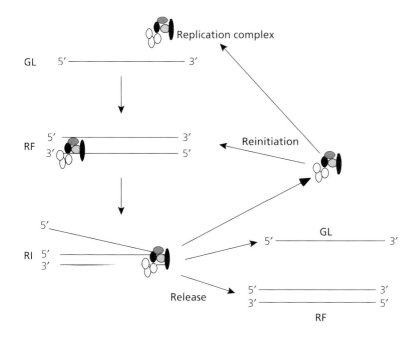

**Figure 2.** Model for the replication of flavivirus RNA, based on [30]

Genomic positive-sense RNA (GL) is translated into the proteins required for RNA replication and used as a template for the synthesis of negative-sense RNA. The negative-sense RNA may exist as part of a double-stranded RF molecule. The RF is used as a recycling template for the asymmetric synthesis of positive-strand RNA. The RF is converted to the RI, containing the newly synthesized strand as well as the RF template. The full-length genomic strand is released, allowing the RF and the replication complex to be reused.

in cell culture systems appear to be low, and reproducibility may be difficult to achieve. The benefits of growing HCV in cell culture systems include: (i) studies of all elements of authentic viral replication occurring during the complete viral replication cycle; (ii) the establishment of high-throughput screening to develop antiviral agents; (iii) toxicity studies of these agents in a cell culture system where the dual effects of viral infection and drug toxicity can be measured; and (iv) confirmation of the inhibitory activity of a compound found to be active in *in vitro*-based assays targeted to one step in the replication cycle.

## Targets for antiviral agents

Until recently, assays for testing antiviral compounds that inhibit the growth of HCV in cell culture have not been possible. The initial inability to grow the virus in cell culture has led to the development of *in vitro* assays designed for specific targets and large scale *in vitro* screening of compounds. The importance of combination therapies to multiple enzyme targets has been demonstrated in the clinical setting with HIV [37]. In the case of HCV, the current antiviral targets include protein synthesis, protein processing, the initiation of RNA transcription, the RNA helicase activity for unwinding double-stranded RNA regions and polymerase elongation activity. These targets are discussed in more detail below.

### Synthesis and processing of the non-structural proteins involved in viral RNA replication

Protein synthesis is initiated at the IRES within the 5′ untranslated region. The RNA within this region has a high degree of secondary structure which forms a pseudoknot containing a number of potential initiation (AUG) codons [9,21]. The synthesis of RNA and the confirmation of the initiating AUG has been investigated by many groups [22,38,39]. Antisense oligonucleotides and hammerhead ribozymes directed towards the IRES inhibit protein synthesis *in vitro* [40–43]. The complementary sequence to the 5′ untranslated region corresponds to the 3′ untranslated region of the negative-sense RNA. The secondary structure and sequence of this region of the RNA may have various constrains for the efficient translation and the transcription of positive-sense RNA.

The processing of HCV non-structural proteins is mediated by two virally encoded enzymes, NS2/3 and NS3 [12,13,18]. The NS2/3 protease is responsible for the *cis* cleavage between NS2 and NS3 [13,17]. The majority of NS2 and the N-terminal region of NS3 are required for this catalytic activity [44]. The region of NS3 involved in the NS2/3 protease activity overlaps with the serine protease domain of NS3; however, the NS2/3 proteolytic activity is distinct from the serine protease activity.

NS4A is a cofactor for NS3-mediated cleavage of NS3/4A and NS4B/5A and increases the efficiency of cleavage between NS5A/5B and NS4A/4B [45–50]. The interaction between NS4A and NS3 may be important in RNA replication, as the N-terminal residues of NS4A may form a transmembrane helix that can serve as an membrane anchor to tether NS3 and the RNA replication complex to membranes [46,47,51,52]. Interestingly, NS4A stimulates the phosphorylation of NS5A [53]. A number of pharmaceutical companies have developed high-throughput assays to screen for potential HCV protease inhibitors. The X-ray crystal structure of NS3 protease domain, with and without NS4A, may aid in the design and modification of inhibitors that can specifically inhibit HCV protease activity. The interaction between NS3 and NS4A or the zinc binding domain may serve as ideal targets for protease inhibitors, especially as the substrate-binding groove was described by Kim *et al.* to be relatively featureless [19]. There have been two published reports of HCV protease inhibitors. The first is based on an RNA aptamer of 120 base pairs, which was found to block the cleavage of the substrate (NS5A/5B) with a $K_i$ of 3 $\mu$M [54]. The second report found two potential inhibitors that were selected from two distinct libraries using phage display technology [55]. One of these protein-based inhibitors had a $K_i$ of 360 nM.

### Unwinding of HCV RNA by NS3

The NS3 helicase and NTPase activity of HCV is also present in flaviviruses and pestiviruses [25,29,56–61]. HCV can unwind 3′/3′ substrates, but not 5′/5′ substrates, suggesting that the HCV helicase is similar to the majority of RNA helicases, which can unwind only in a 3′ to 5′ direction [25]. The HCV helicase can unwind DNA–RNA and DNA–DNA substrates as well as RNA–RNA hybrids [25]. Recently the structure of the HCV helicase domain with and without a single-stranded oligonucleotide has been reported [62,63].

The helicase contains three domains; the oligonucleotide binds within a cleft that separates domain 3 from domains 1 and 2. In a model of the proposed HCV helicase, the binding of ATP results in the interaction of domains 1 and 2 and translocation of the single-stranded polynucleotide in a 5′ to 3′ direction, with respect to domains 1 and 3. Hydrolysis of ATP results in the reopening of the cleft and a net translocation of the enzyme in a 3′ to 5′ direction along the double-stranded polynucleotide [64]. Elucidation of the crystal structure of NS3 may aid the design and modification of antiviral agents targeted to various sites of the helicase, including the NTP-binding site, binding sites for the single- and double-stranded RNA or DNA, and regions of interaction between the domains, which may restrict the translocation of the molecule relative to the polynucleotide substrate. In addition, the interaction between NS3 and NS5B or the protease domain of NS3 may also be specific targets for the design of antiviral agents.

The bifunctional helicase/protease activities of NS3 may have a role in regulating viral replication. In a study using a clone containing both domains, it was found that poly U inhibited helicase activity, while it stimulated the protease and NTPase activity of NS3 [65]. HCV contains a poly U tract within the 3′ untranslated region. Morgenstern *et al.* have proposed that the binding of NS3 to the poly U region may localize NS5A/5B processing to the 3′ untranslated region, directing the assembly of the RNA replication complex and the initiation of minus-strand synthesis [65]. The publication of a study showing that an RNA aptamer inhibited both protease and helicase activity suggests that the dual functions of NS3 may be a ideal target [54].

## Elongation of HCV RNA by NS5B alone

Several groups have developed HCV polymerase assays containing recombinant NS5B, for which elongation activity was demonstrated [26,27,66]. Two groups expressed various NS5B gene constructs in baculovirus expression systems [26,27], and both found polymerase elongation activity associated with NS5B. Terminal transferase activity was identified by both groups by the detection of labelled RNA which was the same size as the input RNA. However, Lohmann *et al.* subsequently found this terminal transferase activity resulted from a cellular contaminant [27].

Using full-length HCV RNA as a template and a fully denaturing system to analyse the products, both groups detected a major species of ~20 kilobases (kb), as well as several smaller species [26,27]. Treatment with RNase to digest single-stranded RNA resulted in digestion of input RNA and a major product of ~10kb. Smaller RNA products disappeared when the input RNA was purified by denaturing polyacrylamide gel electrophoresis, and were presumed to be synthesized from primers present in the input RNA [27]. It was therefore concluded that complementary strands of RNA, covalently joined at one end by a stretch of single-stranded RNA, were the major RNA species synthesized in these assays. It was presumed these products represented the full-length HCV genome primed by a 'copy-back' mechanism. The authors proposed that priming of the negative-sense RNA occurs when NS5B binds to an RNA secondary structure at the 3′ terminus of the genomic RNA.

In these assays containing purified NS5B, no template specificity has been reported, as non-viral RNA could be used as a template. Lohmann *et al.* suggested that template specificity was not required, because HCV RNA synthesis would be compartmentalized within the cell [27]. NS5B alone was found by both groups to be sufficient for RNA synthesis, both groups postulating that the other non-structural proteins may aid in processivity, specificity, or other enhancement of the polymerase activity.

## Elongation of HCV RNA by NS5B in association with the other non-structural proteins

We have developed an assay using cloned HCV non-structural proteins [67]. The non-structural proteins (NS2–NS5) were translated using rabbit reticulocyte lysates and used in polymerase assays. Reaction mixtures contained either purified bovine diarrhoea virus (BVDV) RNA or HCV RNA transcripts from the non-coding region, uninfected cell extract and [α-$^{32}$P]GTP. A product migrating in a similar position to RI was detected in the test samples, which contained all the components of the reaction mix. When fully denatured in a formamide sample buffer, this RNA product was found to migrate at a similar position to the full-length genomic RNA. No product has been detected in the control samples, which contain the test assay mixture minus one component (that is, no template RNA, no uninfected cell extract, or no translated HCV protein).

In assays containing all the HCV non-structural proteins and host cell factors, either BVDV RNA or the 3′ negative-sense RNA could be used as a template, whereas the non-specific RNA (the 5′ untranslated region) was not used as a template. This suggests that the other non-structural proteins may be involved in template specificity. It is also unlikely that incorporation of radiolabel into the RNA products resulted from terminal nucleotidyl transferase activity, because the non-specific template was not radiolabelled. Either Vero or HepG2 cell lysates could be used as the source of cellular host factors for RNA replication, indicating the RNA replication is not dependent on liver-specific cell lines.

In the assay described above, BVDV RNA could be

used as a template, which indicates that BVDV and HCV may contain similar secondary structures. It has previously been shown that RNA from one flavivirus could be used as a template by the replication complex of another flavivirus in RNA-dependent RNA polymerase assays [33]. In an experiment using BVDV RNA as a template, a product migrating slightly slower than BVDV RF was detected. This RNA may have a different secondary structure or it may be a higher molecular weight species. This result suggests that the RNA template may be released from the replication complex; however, the efficiency of this process *in vitro* requires further investigation. RNA products have previously been detected that are twice the size of the template RNA in *vitro* assays for poliovirus, flaviviruses and HCV (A. Bartholomeusz, unpublished results; [26,68]).

## Synthesis of HCV RNA using HCV-infected human liver cell extracts and detection of HCV RNA replicative intermediates

We are carrying out preliminary assays in this laboratory to analyse HCV RNA replication using authentic HCV RNA replication complexes within cell extracts prepared from HCV-infected human liver [67]. Crude cell extracts were prepared by homogenizing uninfected and HCV-infected human liver tissue and removing the nuclei by low speed centrifugation. These cell extracts were stored at –70°C and used in assays containing a reaction mixture that included [α-$^{32}$P]GTP. No additional RNA template was added to the assay as authentic HCV replication complexes, including the RNA template from infected liver cells, were used. In these preliminary experiments, we detected radiolabelled products migrating in a similar positions to full-length genomic RNA and double-stranded RNA. These RNA products were not detected in the uninfected liver.

It has not been determined whether the 3′ terminus of the negative strand is duplexed with the complementary positive-sense strand; in addition, the role of the double-stranded RNA molecule in the transcription of HCV genomic RNA has not been clarified. In one report, Blight *et al.* were unable to detect double-stranded RNA in HCV-infected livers [69], although this may be due to lack of sensitivity of the detection method used. HCV has recently been shown to replicate in cell culture, and Iacovacci *et al.* have detected the presence of RNase-resistant double-stranded RNA in HCV-infected human foetal hepatocytes [36]. We have detected double-stranded RNA molecules in chronically infected BVDV-infected liver using RNase digestion, followed by PCR and hybridiza-

tion to increase the sensitivity of detection (M. Littlejohn and A. Bartholomeusz, unpublished results).

## Future directions for HCV RNA replication studies

Further work is required to determine how authentic negative-sense HCV RNA is primed and synthesized. To date, no group has investigated the synthesis of genomic positive-sense HCV RNA from a negative-sense (single- or double-stranded) RNA template, or the effects of interactions between individual non-structural proteins on the specificity and activity of the polymerase protein. NS5B has polymerase elongation activity, as clearly demonstrated by the groups of Lohmann and Behrens [26,27].

An important question that needs to be addressed is how NS3 helicase and NS5 polymerase activities interact. NS3 may be linked to membranes via NS4A. Morgenstern *et al.* have suggested that poly U, which is present within the 3′ non-coding region, may serve to stimulate the protease activity of NS3 [65]. In turn, the polymerase protein NS5B is cleaved from NS5A. All of these proteins may form part of a replication complex. However, the questions of how HCV RNA synthesis is initiated (especially the initiation of positive-sense RNA from the negative-sense RNA template, where there is no equivalent poly U), and whether the other non-structural proteins alter the specificity or the polymerase elongation activity of NS5B have yet to be answered. NS3 and NS5 interact in other flaviviruses [70] and other helicase and polymerase proteins of positive-strand RNA viruses interact [71,72]. Current studies are attempting to dissect the functions of some of the individual replication proteins, although more work on how they all interact is required.

## The future of antivirals directed against HCV

Interferon alone, or in combination with ribavirin, is the only current treatment for hepatitis C infection [73]. These treatments have a disappointingly low initial response rate and high relapse rate. The factors that contribute to the persistence of an RNA virus are poorly understood. New antiviral agents directed towards HCV that prevent viral replication and persistence are required. The two viral targets that have been extensively studied are the initiation of protein synthesis from the IRES and the protease activity of NS3. Antiviral agents directed against these two targets have now been reported. These include antisense oligonucleotides, ribozymes that cleave the HCV RNA, and RNA aptamers and small protein molecules that inhibit protease activity [40–43]. Compounds directed towards helicase, polymerase and RNA synthesis have yet to be reported. There are only limited numbers of published reports of antiviral compounds directed against RNA-dependent polymerases from positive-strand RNA viruses. A number of different classes of polymerase inhibitors have been tested against flaviviruses, including enzyme-binding compounds, template/primer-binding compounds, substrate analogues and modified nucleosides [74]. However, recent developments in understanding these molecules, and the establishment of *in vitro* screening assays, have suggested that new approaches to antiviral drugs that inhibit these activities may soon be available.

Combination therapy will be essential to treat HCV infection and prevent resistance to any one specific agent. The HCV RNA polymerase has a high error rate, as reflected by the number of quasispecies detected within one individual at any given time [75], and the high turnover of virus (HCV has a serum half life of approximately 4 hours [1]). These observations suggest there is the potential for rapid development of resistance. A number of different drugs directed against essential components of viral replication will therefore be required.

# REFERENCES

1. Fukumoto T, Berg T, Ku Y, Bechstein WO, Knoop M, Lemmens HP, Lobeck H, Hopf U & Neuhaus P. Viral dynamics of hepatitis C early after orthotopic liver transplantation: evidence for rapid turnover of serum virions. *Hepatology* 1996; **24**:1351–1354.

2. Hoofnagle JH. Hepatitis C: The clinical spectrum of disease. *Hepatology* 1997; **26** (Supplement 1):15S–20S.

3. Poynard T, Bedossa P & Opolon P. Natural history of liver fibrosis progression in patients with chronic hepatitis C. The OBSVIRC, METAVIR, CLINIVIR and DOSVIRC Groups. *Lancet* 1997; **349**:825–832.

4. Choo Q-L, Kuo G, Weiner A, Overby LR, Bradley DW & Houghton M. Isolation of a cDNA clone derived from a blood-borne non-A, non-B viral hepatitis genome. *Science* 1989; **244**:359–362.

5. Kolykhalov AA, Agapov EV, Blight KJ, Mihalik K, Feinstone SM & Rice CM. Transmission of hepatitis C by intrahepatic inoculation with transcribed RNA. *Science* 1997; **277**:570–574.

6. Yanagi M, Purcell RH, Emerson SU & Bukh J. Transcripts from a single full-length cDNA clone of hepatitis C virus are infectious when directly transfected into the liver of a chimpanzee. *Proceedings of the National Academy of Sciences, USA* 1997; **94**: 8738–8743.

7. Dash S, Halim AB, Tsuji T, Hiramatsu N & Gerber MA. Transfection of HepG2 cells with infectious hepatitis C virus genome. *American Journal of Pathology* 1997; **151**:363–373.

8. Houghton R. Hepatitis C viruses. In *Virology*, vol. 1 1996; pp. 1035–1058. Edited by BN Fields, DM Knipe,

PM Howley, Chanock RM, Melnick JL, Monath TP, Roizman B & Straus SE. Philadelphia: Lippincott-Raven.

9. Brown EA, Zhang H, Ping LH & Lemon SM. Secondary structure of the 5′ nontranslated regions of hepatitis C virus and pestivirus genomic RNAs. *Nucleic Acids Research* 1992; **20**:5041–5045.

10. Tanaka T, Kato N, Cho M-J, Sugiyama K & Shimotohno K. Structure of the 3′ terminus of the hepatitis C virus genome. *Journal of Virology* 1996; **70**:3307–3312.

11. Kolykhalov AA, Feinstone SM & Rice CM. Identification of a highly conserved sequence element at the 3′ terminus of hepatitis C virus genome RNA. *Journal of Virology* 1996; **70**:3363–3371.

12. Grakoui A, Wychowski C, Lin C, Feinstone SM & Rice CM. Expression and identification of hepatitis C virus polyprotein cleavage products. *Journal of Virology* 1993; **67**:1385–1395.

13. Hijikata M, Mizushima H, Tanji Y, Komoda Y, Hirowatari Y, Akagi T, Kato N, Kimuran K & Shimotohno K. Proteolytic processing and membrane association of putative nonstructural proteins of hepatitis C virus. *Proceedings of the National Academy of Sciences USA* 1993; **90**:10773–10777.

14. Tomei L, Failla C, Santolini E, De Francesco R & La Monica N. NS3 is a serine protease required for processing of hepatitis C virus polyprotein. *Journal of Virology* 1993; **67**:4017–4026.

15. Lin C, Lindenbach D, Pragai M, McCourt DW & Rice CM. Processing in the hepatitis C virus E2-NS2 region: identification of p7 and two distinct E2-specific products with different C termini. *Journal of Virology* 1994; **68**:5063–5073.

16. Hijikata M, Kato N, Ootsuyama Y & Nakagawa M. Gene mapping of the putative structural region of the hepatitis C virus genome by *in vitro* processing analysis. *Proceedings of the National Academy of Sciences, USA* 1993; **88**:5547–5551.

17. Grakoui A, McCourt DW, Wychowski C, Feinstone SM & Rice CM. A second hepatitis C virus-encoded proteinase. *Proceedings of the National Academy of Sciences, USA* 1993; **90**:10583–10587.

18. Grakoui A, McCourt DW, Wychowski C, Feinstone SM & Rice CM. Characterization of the hepatitis C virus-encoded serine proteinase: determination of proteinase-dependent polyprotein cleavage sites. *Journal of Virology* 1993; **67**:2832–2843.

19. Kim JL, Morgenstern KA, Lin C, Fox T, Dwyer MD, Landro JA, Chambers SP, Markland W, Lepre CA, O'Malley ET, Harbeson SL, Rice CM, Murcko MA, Caron PR & Thomson JA. Crystal structure of the hepatitis C virus NS3 protease domain complexed with a synthetic NS4A cofactor peptide. *Cell* 1996; **87**:343–355.

20. Love RA, Parge HE, Wickersham JA, Hostomsky Z, Habuka N, Moomaw EW, Adachi T & Hostomska Z. The crystal structure of hepatitis C virus NS3 proteinase reveals a trypsin-like fold and a structural zinc binding site. *Cell* 1996; **87**:331–342.

21. Honda M, Brown EA & Lemon SM. Stability of a stem-loop involving the initiator AUG controls the efficiency of internal initiation of translation on hepatitis C virus RNA. *RNA* 1996; **2**:955–968.

22. Honda M, Ping LH, Rijnbrand RC, Amplett E, Clarke B, Rowlands D & Lemon SM. Structural requirements for initiation of translation by internal ribosome entry within genome-length hepatitis C virus RNA. *Virology*

1996; **222**:31–42.

23. Yamada N, Tanihara K, Takada A, Yorihuzi T, Tsutsumi M, Shimomura H, Tsuji T & Date T. Genetic organization and diversity of the 3′ noncoding region of the hepatitis C virus genome. *Virology* 1996; **223**:255–261.

24. Ito T & Lai MM. Determination of the secondary structure of and cellular protein binding to the 3′-untranslated region of the hepatitis C virus RNA genome. *Journal of Virology* 1997; **71**:8698–8706

25. Tai CL, Chi WK, Chen, DS & Hwang LH. The helicase activity associated with hepatitis C virus nonstructural protein 3 (NS3). *Journal of Virology* 1996; **70**:8477–8484.

26. Behrens SE, Tomei L & de Francesco R. Identification and properties of the RNA-dependent RNA polymerase of hepatitis C virus. *EMBO Journal* 1996; **15**:12–22.

27. Lohmann V, Korner F, Herian U & Bartenschlager R. Biochemical properties of hepatitis C virus NS5B RNA-dependent RNA polymerase and identification of amino acid sequence motifs essential for enzymatic activity. *Journal of Virology* 1997; **71**:8416–8428.

28. Chu PWG & Westaway EG. Molecular and ultrastructural analysis of heavy membrane fractions associated with the replication of Kunjin virus RNA. *Archives of Virology* 1992; **125**:177–191.

29. Suzich JA, Tamura JK, Palmer-Hill F, Warrener P, Grakoui A, Rice CM, Feinstone SM & Collett MS. Hepatitis C virus NS3 protein polynucleotide-stimulated nucleoside triphosphate and comparison with the related pestivirus and flavivirus enzymes. *Journal of Virology* 1993; **67**:1720–1726.

30. Chu PW & Westaway EG. Replication stratey of Kunjin virus: evidence for recycling role of replicative form RNA as template in semiconservative and asymmetric replication. *Virology* 1985; **140**:68–79.

31. Chu PW & Westaway EG. Characterization of Kunjin virus RNA-dependent RNA polymerase: reinitiation of synthesis *in vitro*. *Virology* 1987; **157**:330–337.

32. Grun JB & Brinton MA. Dissociation of NS5 from cell fractions containing West Nile virus-specific polymerase activity. *Journal of Virology* 1987; **61**:3641–3644.

33. Bartholomeusz AI & Wright PJ. Synthesis of dengue virus RNA *in vitro*: evidence for initiation and involvement of proteins NS3 and NS5. *Archives of Virology* 1993; **128**:111–121.

34. Yoo BJ, Selby MJ, Choe J, Suh BS, Choi SH, Joh JS, Nuovo GJ, Lee H-S, Houghton, M & Han JH. Transfection of a differentiated human hepatoma cell line (Huh7) with *in vitro*-transcribed hepatitis C virus (HCV) RNA and establishment of a long-term culture persistently infected with HCV. *Journal of Virology* 1995; **69**:32–38.

35. Seipp S, Mueller HM, Pfaff E, Stremmel W, Theilmann L, Goeser, T. Establishment of persistent hepatitis C virus infection and replication *in vitro*. *Journal of General Virology* 1997; **78**:2467–2476.

36. Iacovacci S, Manzin A, Barca S, Sargiacomo M, Serafino A, Valli MB, Macioce G, Hassan HJ, Ponzetto A, Clementi M, Peschle C & Carloni G. Molecular characterization and dynamics of hepatitis C virus replication in human fetal hepatocytes infected *in vitro*. *Hepatology* 1997; **26**:1328–1337.

37. Corey L & Holmes KK. Therapy for human immunodeficiency virus infection - what have we learned? *New England Journal of Medicine* 1996; **335**:1142–1144.

38. Reynolds JE, Kaminski A, Carroll AR, Clarke BE, Rowlands DJ & Jackson RJ. Internal initiation of translation of hepatitis C virus RNA: the ribosome entry site is at the authentic initiation codon. *RNA* 1996; **2**:867–878.

39. Rijnbrand RC, Abbink TE, Haasnoot PC, Spaan WJ & Bredenbeek PJ. The influence of AUG codons in the hepatitis C virus 5′ nontranslated region on translation and mapping of the translation initiation window. *Virology* 1996; **226**:47–56.

40. Vidalin O, Major ME, Rayner B, Imbach JL, Trepo C & Inchauspe G. *In vitro* inhibition of hepatitis C virus gene expression by chemically modified antisense oligodeoxynucleotides. *Antimicrobial Agents and Chemotherapy* 1996; **40**:2337–2344.

41. Lima WF, Brown-Driver V, Fox M, Hanecak R & Bruice TW. Combinatorial screening and rational optimization for hybridization to folded hepatitis C virus RNA of oligonucleotides with biological antisense activity. *Journal of Biological Chemistry* 1997; **272**: 626–638.

42. Sakamoto N, Wu CH & Wu GY. Intracellular cleavage of hepatitis C virus RNA and inhibition of viral protein translation by hammerhead ribozymes. *Journal of Clinical Investigation* 1996; **98**:2720–2728.

43. Hanecak R, Brown-Driver V, Fox MC, Azad RF, Furusako S, Nozaki C, Ford C, Sasmor H & Anderson KP. Antisense oligonucleotide inhibition of hepatitis C virus gene expression in transformed hepatocytes. *Journal of Virology* 1996; **70**:5203–5212.

44. Reed KE, Grakoui A & Rice CM. Hepatitis C virus-encoded NS2-3 protease: cleavage-site mutagenesis and requirements for bimolecular cleavage. *Journal of Virology* 1995; **69**:4127–4136.

45. Bartenschlager R, Ahlborn-Laake L, Mous J & Jacobsen H. Kinetic and structural analyses of hepatitis C virus polyprotein processing. *Journal of Virology* 1994; **68**:5045–5055.

46. Bartenschlager R, Lohmann V, Wilkinson T & Koch JO. Complex formation between the NS3 serine-type proteinase of the hepatitis C virus and NS4A and its importance for polyprotein maturation. *Journal of Virology* 1995; **69**:7519–7528.

47. Faila C, Tomei L & de Francesco R. Both NS3 and NS4A are required for proteolytic processing of hepatitis C virus nonstructural proteins. *Journal of Virology* 1994; **68**:3753–3760.

48. Faila C, Tomei L & de Francesco R. An amino-terminal domain of the hepatitis C virus NS3 protease is essential for interaction with NS4A. *Journal of Virology* 1995; **69**:1769–1777.

49. Lin C, Thomson JA & Rice CM. A central region in the hepatitis C virus NS4A protein allows formation of an active NS3-NS4A serine proteinase complex *in vivo* and *in vitro*. *Journal of Virology* 1995; **69**:4373–4380.

50. Koch JO, Lohmann V, Herian U & Bartenschlager R. *In vitro* studies on the activation of the hepatitis C virus NS3 proteinase by the NS4A cofactor. *Virology* 1996; **221**:54–66.

51. Tanji Y, Hijikata M, Satoh S, Kaneko T & Shimotohno K. Hepatitis C virus-encoded nonstructural protein NS4A has versatile functions in viral protein processing. *Journal of Virology* 1995; **69**:1575–1581.

52. Santolini E, Pacini L, Fipaldini C, Migliaccio G & La Monica N. The NS2 protein of hepatitis C virus is a transmembrane polypeptide. *Journal of Virology* 1995; **69**:7461–7471.

53. Tanji Y, Kaneko T, Satoh S & Shimotohno K. Phosphorylation of hepatitis C virus-encoded nonstructural protein NS5A. *Journal of Virology* 1995;

**69:**3980–3986.

54. Kumar PK, Machida K, Urvil PT, Kakiuchi N, Vishnuvardhan D, Shimotohno K, Taira K & Nishikawa S. Isolation of RNA aptamers specific to the NS3 protein of hepatitis C virus from a pool of completely random RNA. *Virology* 1997; **237:** 270–282.

55. Dimasi N, Martin F, Volpari C, Brunetti M, Biasiol G, Altamura S, Cortese R, De Francesco R, Steinkuhler C & Sollazzo M. Characterization of engineered hepatitis C virus NS3 protease inhibitors affinity selected from human pancreatic secretory trypsin inhibitor and minibody repertoires. *Journal of Virology* 1997; **71:** 7461–7469.

56. Takegami T, Sakamuro D & Furukawa T. Japanese encephalitis virus nonstructural protein NS3 has RNA binding and ATPase activities. *Virus Genes* 1994; **9:**105–112.

57. Preugschat F, Averett DR, Clarke BE & Porter JT. A steady-state and pre-steady-state kinetic analysis of the NTPase activity associated with the hepatitis C virus NS3 helicase domain. *Journal of Biological Chemistry* 1996; **271:**24449–24457.

58. Gwack Y, Kim DW, Han JH & Choe J. Characterization of RNA binding activity and RNA helicase activity of the hepatitis C virus NS3 protein. *Biochemical and Biophysical Research Communications* 1996; **225:**654–659.

59. Warrener P & Collett MS. Pestivirus NS3 (p80) protein possesses RNA helicase activity. *Journal of Virology* 1995; **69:**1720–1726.

60. Warrener P, Tamura JK & Collett MS. RNA-stimulated NTPase activity associated with Yellow Fever virus NS3 protein expressed in bacteria. *Journal of Virology* 1993; **67:**989–996.

61. Tamura JK, Warrener P & Collett MS. RNA-stimulated NTPase activity associated with the p80 protein of the pestivirus Bovine Viral Diarrhea Virus. *Virology* 1993; **193:**1–10.

62. Yao N, Hesson T, Cable M, Hong Z, Kwong AD, Le HV & Weber PC. Structure of the hepatitis C virus RNA helicase domain. *Nature Structural Biology* 1997; **4:**463–467.

63. Kim JL, Morgenstern KA, Griffith JP, Dwyer MD, Thomson JA, Murcko MA, Lin C & Caron PR. Hepatitis C virus NS3 RNA helicase domain with a bound oligonucleotide: the crystal structure provides insights into the mode of unwinding. *Structure* 1998; **6:**89–100.

64. Kim JL & Caron PR. Crystal structure of hepatitis C virus NS3 RNA helicase reveals a possible enzyme mechanism and suggests multiple potential drug binding sites. *International Antiviral News* 1998; **6:**26–28.

65. Morgenstern KA, Landro JA, Hsiaw K, Lin C, Gu Y, Su

MSS & Thomson JA. Polynucleotide modulation of the protease, nucleoside triphosphatase, and helicase activities of a hepatitis C virus NS3-NS4A complex isolated from transfected COS cells. *Journal of Virology* 1997; **71:**3767-3775.

66. Yuan ZH, Kumar U, Thomas HC, Wen YM & Monjardino J. Expression, purification, and partial characterization of HCV RNA polymerase. *Biochemical and Biophysical Research Communications* 1997; **232:**231–235.

67. Bartholomeusz AI, Guo KJ, Edwards PC & Locarnini SA. Hepatitis C virus (HCV) RNA polymerase assay using cloned HCV non-structural proteins. *Antiviral Therapy* 1996; **1:**18–24.

68. Tuschall DM, Hiebert E & Flanegan JB. Poliovirus RNA dependent RNA polymerase synthesizes full-length copies of poliovirion RNA, cellular mRNA, and several plant RNAs *in vitro*. *Journal of Virology* 1982; **44:**209–216.

69. Blight K Trowbridge R & Gowans EJ. Absence of double-stranded replicative forms of HCV RNA in liver tissue from chronically infected patients. *Journal of Viral Hepatitis* 1996; **3:**29–36.

70. Kapoor M, Zhang L, Ramachandra M, Kusukawa J, Ebner KE & Padmanabhan R. Association between NS3 and NS5 proteins of dengue virus type 2 in the putative RNA replicase is linked to differential phosphorylation of NS5. *Journal of Biological Chemistry* 1995; **270:**19100–19106.

71. Kao CC, Quadt R, Hershberger RP & Ahlquist P. Brome Mosaic Virus RNA replication proteins 1a and 2a form a complex *in vitro*. *Journal of Virology* 1992; **66:**6322–6329.

72. Kao CC & Ahlquist P. Identification of the domains required for direct interaction of the helicase-like and polymerase-like RNA replication proteins of Brome Mosaic Virus. *Journal of Virology* 1992; **66:** 7293–7302.

73. Poynard T, Leroy V, Cohard M, Thevenot T, Mathurin P, Opolon P & Zarski JP. Meta-analysis of interferon randomized trials in the treatment of viral hepatitis C: effects of dose and duration. *Hepatology* 1996; **24:**778–789

74. Bartholomeusz A, Tomlinson E, Wright PJ, Birch C, Locarnini S, Weigold H, Marcuccio S & Holan G. Use of a flavivirus RNA-dependent RNA polymerase assay to investigate the antiviral activity of selected compounds. *Antiviral Research* 1994; **24:**341–350.

75. Martell M, Esteban JI, Quer J, Genesca J, Weiner A, Esteban R, Guardia J & Gomez J. Hepatitis C virus (HCV) circulates as a population of different but closely related genomes: quasispecies nature of HCV genome distribution. *Journal of Virology* 1992; **66:** 3225–3229.

# 25 Helicase, a target for novel inhibitors of hepatitis C virus

## Nanhua Yao and Patricia C Weber*

## SUMMARY

Virally encoded enzymes of hepatitis C virus (HCV) were identified from its genome sequence. This allows application of drug discovery strategies that rely on inhibition of enzymes unique to HCV. Discovery of high affinity inhibitors is facilitated by knowledge of the target enzyme's three-dimensional structure. For development of inhibitors of the HCV helicase, which belongs to a class of enzymes for which little structural information is available, the impact of structural information on the drug discovery process is greater than for targets belonging to well-characterized classes of enzymes. Here the structure of the HCV helicase is described. Regions required for enzymatic activity, which are also the preferred sites of drug interaction, are highlighted.

## INTRODUCTION

The HCV genome encodes at least four enzymatic activities within the non-structural (NS) region [1,2]. NS2 is a metalloprotease responsible for cleavage at the NS2–NS3 junction [3,4]. The gene product of NS5B is an RNA-dependent RNA polymerase required for viral replication [5]. The 631 residue NS3 protein is a bifunctional enzyme. The N-terminal domain is a serine protease which cleaves the non-structural polyprotein into NS3, NS4A, NS4B, NS5A and NS5B proteins [6,7]. An RNA helicase activity resides in the C-terminal 450 residues of NS3 [8,9]. The helicase removes double-stranded segments of RNA to form a single-stranded molecule, which is required during translation and transcription.

Inhibitors of HCV enzymes are being developed for use as anti-HCV agents. Treatment of viral infections with inhibitors specific for virally encoded enzymes has proven successful for treatment of human immunodeficiency virus (HIV) infections. Currently, both HIV protease and reverse transcriptase inhibitors are available.

## STRUCTURAL STUDIES OF THE NS3 PROTEASE DOMAIN

The NS3 protease belongs to a well-characterized and extensively studied class of enzymes [10,11]. The wealth of knowledge about the serine protease mechanism broadly impacts discovery of NS3 serine protease inhibitors. Available information aids in the development of assays to screen for inhibitors and assists in the interpretation of observed inhibition data. In addition, structural studies of serine proteases both in complex with substrates and inhibitors can be exploited in inhibitor design.

Crystallographic studies of the NS3 serine protease domain revealed that it is structurally similar to previously characterized proteases [12,13]. The molecular fold consists of two β-barrels and resembles that of the chymotrypsin class of serine proteases. The catalytic residues, Ser-139, His-57 and Asp-81, participate in a hydrogen bond network which is a signature of serine proteases. The catalytic triad spans the β-barrels, as does the proposed substrate binding site [12,13].

## STRUCTURAL STUDIES OF RNA POLYMERASES

Less is known about the mechanism and inhibition of RNA-dependent RNA polymerases. The structure of the poliovirus RNA polymerase was recently determined [14] and may guide design of inhibitors of the HCV enzyme. In addition, structures of related DNA-dependent RNA and DNA polymerases are available [14]. Comparison of the structures to find conserved features may provide additional insights useful for drug design.

## STRUCTURAL AND ENZYMATIC STUDIES OF HELICASES

Unlike serine proteases and polymerases, structural information on helicases has become available only recently. Within the last year, the structures of DNA

**Figure 1.** Ribbon representation of the HCV RNA helicase domain of NS3

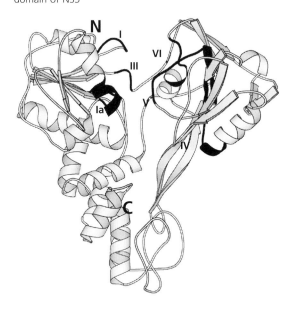

The molecule folds into three domains with a deep groove separating the first and third domains from the second. In this view, the first and third domains are on the left; the N and C termini correspond to NS3 residues 187 and 629, respectively. The black sections of the ribbon indicate amino acid motifs (numbered) conserved among superfamily II helicases.

helicases from *Bacillus stearothermophilus* and *Escherichia coli* have been reported [15,16]. Both molecules fold into two structurally similar domains exhibiting canonical βαβ folds. Each domain possesses a large insertion which folds into an α-helical subdomain. A similar fold within the NTP binding site is one of several structural features shared by the DNA helicases and the HCV RNA helicase domain [17], whose structure was recently reported [18].

Enzymatic characterization of the helicase reaction provides some insights into possible means for inhibition of these enzymes [19,20]. Helicases recognize double-stranded nucleic acids and unwind the DNA or RNA duplexes during genomic replication. Helicase activity requires NTP hydrolysis. The NTP binding site and regions that bind the nucleic acid substrate are common helicase features that provide possible sites for inhibitor interaction [18,21,22]. In addition to questions about substrate recognition, a major unanswered puzzle about the helicase mechanism relates to how NTPase hydrolysis is coupled to unwinding. If features of the coupling machinery are structurally distinct from the NTP and nucleic acid binding sites, a molecule capable of uncoupling NTP hydrolysis and RNA binding might also effectively inhibit the helicase.

**Figure 2.** Comparison of NTPase domains and NTP binding residues

**(a)**

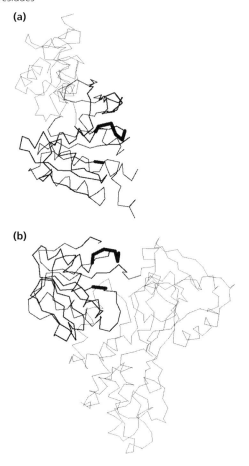

**(b)**

**(c)**

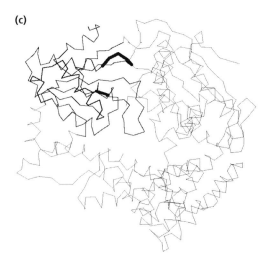

Bold lines highlight Walker motifs A and B which directly ligate NTP. Darker lines indicate the NTPase domains, and lighter lines show the remainder of the protein. (a) *E. coli* RecA [Protein Database (PDB) entry: 1REA]; (b) HCV RNA helicase (PDB entry: 1HE1); (c) *E. coli* Rep helicase [16] (PDB entry: 1UAA).

Structural studies of the HCV helicase were undertaken to apply structure-based approaches for inhibitor design and development. In addition, features of the NTP and RNA binding sites were expected to aid design of inhibitor screening strategies. The overall structure of the HCV helicase domain has been determined [18]. Here we describe in more detail features of the structure important for its activity that may also serve as sites for inhibitor binding.

## OVERALL STRUCTURE OF THE HCV RNA HELICASE

The HCV helicase is folded into three, nearly equal-sized domains (Fig. 1). The first and second domains possess similar βαβ architectures where α-helices pack about a central β-sheet. The third domain is composed of α-helices. The first and third domains are closely packed, while a deep groove separates the first and third domains from the second.

## Conserved amino acids

Sequence comparisons have been used to group helicases into three superfamilies [23,24]. The HCV helicase is a member of superfamily II (SFII) which includes the initiation factor eIF-4A, and other viral helicases from bovine viral diarrhoea pestivirus, plum pox potyvirus and vaccinia virus. Seven conserved

sequences have been identified in SFII helicases [23,24]. Figure 1 shows the location of conserved sequences in the three-dimensional structure of the HCV RNA helicase. Many conserved amino acids are located near the interface that separates the second domain from the first and third [18]. Clustering of conserved sequences near the interdomain interface identifies this channel as a mechanistically important feature of the structure.

## NTP binding site

All helicases contain conserved amino acids associated with NTP binding [18,23,24]. These include Walker motif A, which binds the terminal phosphate groups of the NTP cofactor, and Walker motif B, responsible for chelating the Mg$^{2+}$ ion of the Mg–NTP complex. As shown in Figure 1, sequences important for binding NTPs are localized in the first helicase domain. The residues exhibit an overall folding pattern observed in other NTP binding sites (Fig. 2).

## Residues important for NTPase activity

While sequence homology with other NTPases identified functional roles for Walker motifs A and B, the roles of other conserved sequence motifs were less well defined by comparison of amino acid sequences. Instead, structural and genetic studies were conducted

**Figure 3.** Stereoscopic views of residues Asp290–Glu291–Cys292–His293, Thr322–Ala323–Thr324 and Gln460–Arg461–Arg462–Gly463–Arg464–Thr465–Gly466–Arg467 of SFII motifs II, III and IV, respectively

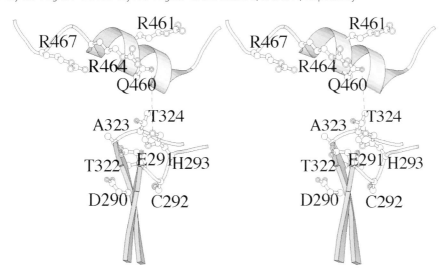

The structure of the non-liganded form of the RNA helicase was determined [18]. In the absence of NTP and nucleic acids, a complex hydrogen bond network interconnects the side chain of His293 of the DECH box with side chains of Thr322, Thr324, Arg461, Arg464 and Gln460. Arg467 is also oriented toward the NTPase domain. Single circles denote carbon atoms, double circles nitrogen, triple circles oxygen and four circles sulphur.

**Figure 4.** Relative domain rotations in the HCV RNA helicase

**(a)**

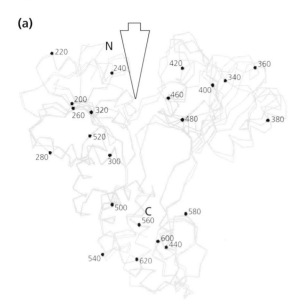

**(b)**

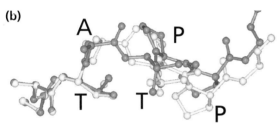

**(c)**

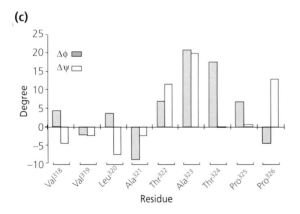

(a) Superposition of the first and third domains of each monomer in the crystallographic asymmetric unit reveals a relative rotation of the second domain. (b) Conformational changes in residues Val318– Val319–Leu320– Ala321–Thr322–Ala323–Thr324–Pro325–Pro326, a portion of the 'switch region' involved in coupling NTP hydrolysis to unwinding, are shown in detail; in (a), an arrow indicates the location of these residues in the structure. Every 20th residue, and the N and C termini, are labelled. (c) Changes in the backbone conformational angles φ and ψ for this region are shown as shaded and white bars, respectively. The changes in backbone torsional angles are nearly twice the standard deviation for all residues in the protein.

to determine the function of other conserved residues. For example, a role for motif IV residues in NTPase activity was suggested by the structure [18] and established by site-directed mutagenesis studies [25]. Single substitutions of histidine for glutamine at residue 460 and lysine for arginine at residue 467 abolishes ATPase and helicase activities. Poly(U)-dependent ATPase activity and helicase activity are also lost when alanine replaces arginine at residue 464. In the three-dimensional structure, these residues are oriented toward the NTPase domain and are involved in an interdomain hydrogen bond network (Fig. 3).

Arg461 is also conserved within motif IV. Mutation of this residue to alanine slightly alters ATPase and helicase activities [25]. In contrast to Gln460, Arg464 and Arg467, the Arg461 side chain is oriented away from the NTP binding domain (Fig. 3). However, in this non-liganded form of the protein, it remains within hydrogen bond distance of Gln460.

## Structural flexibility

Comparison of the two helicase molecules in the crystallographic asymmetric unit reveals that the second domain can pivot relative to the remainder of the structure (Fig. 4). Overall, the second domain rotates about 4° about an axis approximately collinear with residues 481–485. Because of the location of these residues near the bottom of the interdomain cleft, rotation of the second domain results in larger movements near the 'top' of the cleft than near the strands interconnecting the domains.

Structural comparisons suggested that the conserved Thr322–Ala323–Thr324 sequence was part of the 'switch region' responsible for transmission of conformational changes accompanying NTP hydrolysis [18]. Consistent with this hypothesis, molecules with Thr322 changed to alanine exhibited a 50% reduction in helicase activity while retaining wild-type ATPase activity [25].

## THE HELICASE 'ACTIVE SITE'

The structure of the HCV RNA helicase revealed that amino acids conserved among helicases lined either side of the deep groove separating the second domain from the first and third. Site-directed mutagenesis studies confirmed that this region contains residues required for NTP hydrolysis and RNA unwinding. The interdomain cleft then constitutes part of the helicase active site. Consequently, molecules binding to this region with high affinity would be expected to inhibit helicase activity.

# REFERENCES

1. Clarke B. Molecular virology of hepatitis C virus. *Journal of General Virology* 1997; **78**:2397–2410.

2. Pozzetto B, Bourlet T, Grattard F & Bonnevial L. Structure, genomic organization, replication and variability of hepatitis C virus. *Nephrology Dialysis Transplantation* 1996; **11**:2–5.

3. Grakoui A, McCourt DW, Wychowski C, Feinstone SM & Rice CM. A second hepatitis C virus-encoded proteinase. *Proceedings of the National Academy of Sciences, USA* 1993; **90**:10583–10587.

4. Hijikata M, Mizushima H, Akagi T, Mori S, Kakiuchi N, Kato N, Tanaka T, Kimura K & Shimotohno K. Two distinct proteinase activities required for the processing of a putative non-structural precursor protein of hepatitis C virus. *Journal of Virology* 1993; **67**:4665–4675.

5. Behrens S-E, Tomei L & De Francesco R. Identification and properties of the RNA-dependent RNA polymerase of hepatitis C virus. *EMBO Journal* 1996; **15**:12–22.

6. Grakoui A, McCourt DW, Wychowski C, Feistone SM & Rice CM. Characterization of the hepatitis C virus-encoded serine proteinase: determination of proteinase-dependent polyprotein cleavage sites. *Journal of Virology* 1993; **67**:2832–2843.

7. Bartenschlager R, Ahlborn-Laake L, Mous J & Jacobsen H. Nonstructural protein 3 of the hepatitis C virus encodes a serine-type proteinase required for cleavage at the NS3/4 and NS4/5 junctions. *Journal of Virology* 1993; **67**:3835–3844.

8. Jin L & Peterson DL. Expression, isolation, and characterization of the hepatitis C virus ATPase/RNA helicase. *Archives of Biochemistry and Biophysics* 1995; **323**:47–53.

9. Kim DW, Gwack Y, Han JH & Choe C. C-terminal domain of the hepatitis C virus NS3 protein contains an RNA helicase activity. *Biochemical and Biophysical Research Communications* 1995; **215**:160–166.

10. Edwards PD & Bernstein PR. Synthetic inhibitors of elastase. *Medicinal Research Reviews* 1994; **14**:127–194.

11. Babe LM & Craik CS. Viral proteases: evolution of diverse structural motifs to optimize functions. *Cell* 1997; **91**:427–430.

12. Love RA, Parge HE, Wickersham JA, Hostomsky Z, Habuka N, Moomaw EW, Adachi T & Hostomska Z. The crystal structure of hepatitis C virus NS3 proteinase reveals a trypsin-like fold and a structural zinc binding site. *Cell* 1996; **87**:331–342.

13. Kim JL, Morgenstern KA, Lin C, Fox T, Dwyer MD, Landro JA, Chambers SP, Markland W, Lepre CA, O'Malley ET, Harbeson SL, Rice CM, Murcko MA, Caron PR & Thomson JA. Crystal structure of the hepatitis C virus NS3 protease domain complexed with a synthetic NS4A cofactor peptide. *Cell* 1996; **87**:343–355.

14. Hansen JL, Long AM & Schultz SC. Structure of the RNA-dependent RNA polymerase of poliovirus. *Structure* 1997; **5**:1109–1122.

15. Subramanya HS, Bird LE, Brannigan JA & Wigley DB. Crystal structure of a DExx box DNA helicase. *Nature* 1996; **384**:379–383.

16. Korolov S, Hsieh J, Gauss GH, Lohman TM & Waksman G. Major domain swiveling revealed by the crystal structures of complexes of *E. coli* Rep helicase bound to single-stranded DNA and ADP. *Cell* 1997; **90**:635–637.

17. Yao N, Hesson T, Cable M, Hong Z, Kwong AD, Le HV & Weber PC. Structure of the hepatitis C virus RNA helicase domain. *Nature Structural Biology* 1997; **4**:463–467.

18. Korolev S, Yao N, Lohman TM, Weber PC & Waksman G. Comparisons between the structures of HCV and Rep helicases reveal structural similarities between SF1 and SF2 superfamilies of helicases. *Protein Science* 1998; **7**:1–6.

19. Lohman TM & Bjornson KP. Mechanisms of helicase-catalyzed DNA unwinding. *Annual Review of Biochemistry* 1996; **65**:169–214.

20. Preugschat F, Averett DR, Clarke BE & Porter DJT. A steady-state and pre-steady-state kinetic analysis of the NTPase activity associated with the hepatitis C virus NS3 helicase domain. *Journal of Biological Chemistry* 1996; **271**:24449–24457.

21. Gross CH & Shuman S. Vaccinia virus RNA helicase: nucleic acid specificity in duplex unwinding. *Journal of Virology* 1996; **70**:2615–2619.

22. Walker JE, Saraste M, Runswick MJ & Gay NJ. Distantly related sequences in the α- and β-subunits of ATP synthetase, myosin, kinases and other ATP-requiring enzymes and a common nucleotide binding fold. *EMBO Journal* 1982; **1**:945–951.

23. Gorbalenya AE & Koonin EV. Helicases: amino acid sequence comparisons and structure–function relationships. *Current Opinions in Structural Biology* 1993; **3**:419–429.

24. Kadare G & Haenni A-L. Virus-encoded RNA helicase. *Journal of Virology* 1997; **71**:2583–2590.

25. Kim DW, Kim J, Gwack Y, Han J & Choe J. Mutational analysis of the hepatitis C virus RNA helicase. *Journal of Virology* 1997; **71**:9400–9404.

# 26

# The hepatitis C virus NS3 proteinase: structure and function of a zinc-containing serine proteinase

Raffaele De Francesco*, Antonello Pessi and Christian Steinkühler

## INTRODUCTION

Hepatitis C virus (HCV) is now recognized as the leading cause of blood-borne and community-acquired non-A, non-B viral hepatitis. The number of people infected with this virus has been estimated to be in excess of 1% of the world's population. Infection with HCV is typically followed by a mild onset of the disease and is often asymptomatic. Acute liver illness is reported to occur in only around 20% of infected individuals. In most cases, however, HCV establishes a persistent infection that results in chronic active hepatitis and eventually leads to cirrhosis of the liver and possibly to hepatocellular carcinoma [1].

Presently, there is no vaccine available to prevent HCV infection. In addition, current therapies for HCV-associated chronic hepatitis are costly and seldom efficacious: treatment with interferon α provides long-term therapeutic benefit to only about 25% of treated patients [2]. Thus, there is an urgent need to develop novel therapeutic strategies.

As is the case for other proven antiviral agents, virally encoded enzymes that are essential for replication are the targets of choice for an anti-HCV therapy [3]. The search for such targets has been severely hampered by the lack of a reliable system to grow HCV in cell culture and by the lack of small animal models to study infection. In spite of this limitation, molecular cloning of the viral genome combined with the powerful tools of recombinant DNA technology has ultimately led to the identification of several viral enzymatic functions that are believed to be essential for viral replication [4,5].

Among the proteins considered to be part of the viral replication machinery, non-structural protein 3 (NS3) has been the focus of much attention and

intensive research in several pharmaceutical and biotechnology companies, as well as in many academic groups. HCV NS3 protein is a multifunctional enzyme: the N-terminal third contains a serine proteinase domain essential for the proteolytic processing of most of the non-structural region of the viral polyprotein. The remainder of the protein contains an RNA/DNA helicase and a polynucleotide-stimulated NTPase. In the past few years, several unique and unexpected properties of the NS3 serine proteinase have emerged that make the discovery of small molecule inhibitors of this enzyme a very exciting, but very challenging task.

## NS3 serine proteinase and polyprotein processing

HCV represents a novel genus of the family *Flaviviridae* [6]. Investigation of the molecular biology underlying the replication cycle of this virus was thus facilitated by the homology of the HCV genome structure to that of flavi- and pestiviruses, the two other genera of the family *Flaviviridae*. HCV has a single-stranded RNA genome of approximately 9.6 kb with positive polarity containing a single open reading frame (ORF). This ORF encodes a polyprotein of 3010–3033 amino acids that is processed into at least 10 mature viral proteins (Fig. 1). Both cellular signal peptidases and two virally encoded proteolytic enzymes are involved in this maturation process. Whereas the structural HCV proteins arise through the action of cellular proteinases, viral enzymes are required for the processing of the non-structural region. The NS2–NS3 junction is cleaved by a zinc-dependent autoproteinase associated with NS2 and the N-terminal region of the NS3 protein [7,8]. A

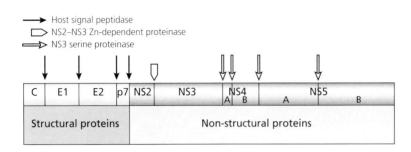

Figure 1. Scheme of the HCV polyprotein organization and processing

See text for details.

serine proteinase domain is contained within the N-terminal 180 amino acids of NS3; the enzymatic activity associated with this domain is responsible for the proteolytic processing of the downstream region of the viral polyprotein. Thus, the NS3 serine proteinase mediates proteolysis at the NS3–NS4A, NS4A–NS4B, NS4B–NS5A and NS5A–NS5B cleavage sites [8–14]. Differences exist in the mechanism by which NS3 effects these cleavages: processing at the NS3–NS4A junction has been shown to occur exclusively in *cis*, that is within the same polyprotein molecule. Conversely, the remaining cleavage sites were found to be also processed in *trans* when exogenous NS3 was added to polyprotein derivatives containing the target cleavage sites [10,11,15,16].

Based on studies carried out with yellow fever virus, a member of the flavivirus genus [17], it is believed that inactivation of the serine proteinase activity associated with NS3 would be deleterious for HCV replication. The NS3 serine proteinase of HCV has thus become one of the major targets for the discovery of novel anti-HCV drugs.

## NS4A cofactor

Although the 180 residue NS3 proteinase domain possesses intrinsic proteolytic activity, NS4A has been shown to be an essential cofactor for efficient NS3-dependent processing of the HCV polyprotein [15,18–20]. Interaction of NS3 with the NS4A cofactor was demonstrated to be an absolute requirement for the cleavage of the NS3–NS4A, NS4A–4B and NS4B–NS5A junctions. Cleavage at the NS5A–NS5B site was observed in the absence of the NS4A protein, although the presence of the cofactor greatly increased the efficiency of NS3-dependent proteolysis at this site. These observations suggested that a direct molecular interaction between NS3 and NS4A might take place. Several studies have subsequently shown that, in cells expressing the HCV

polyprotein, NS3 in fact exists as a detergent-stable complex with NS4A [21–25]. In addition to modulating its serine proteinase activity, NS4A targets the NS3 protein to the membranes of the endoplasmic reticulum (ER) and significantly increases the metabolic stability of NS3 in the cytoplasm of cultured cells [20]. The region of NS3 involved in the interaction with the NS4A cofactor has been mapped by deletion mutagenesis to the N-terminal extremity of the proteinase [22,24,26]. The 22 N-terminal amino acids of NS3 were thus found to be indispensable both for NS3–NS4A complex formation and for the modulation of the proteolytic activity by NS4A. Consistently, the same region did not appear to be required for the NS4A-independent residual serine proteinase activity of NS3 measured on the NS5A–NS5B site.

NS4A is a protein of 54 amino acids and is predicted to be membrane-bound. Analysis of hydropathy plots and secondary structure prediction highlight the presence of three distinct regions within NS4A. The first region encompasses residues 1–20, is highly hydrophobic and is predicted to form a trans-membrane α-helix [27]. This domain possibly has the function of anchoring the NS3–NS4A complex onto the ER membrane. The second region, residues 21–34, is also hydrophobic and it is predicted to fold in an extended β-strand conformation [28]. This central region of NS4A is required and sufficient for the NS3 serine proteinase cofactor activity [23,26,28,29]. Synthetic peptides with the amino acid sequence of this region have been found to bind to the NS3 enzyme with a 1:1 stoichiometry and to activate its proteolytic activity *in vitro* [23,26,28–32]. The third region of NS4A, corresponding to the 20 C-terminal residues, is more hydrophilic and its function is not yet known.

Deletion experiments have shown that the helicase and proteinase domains of NS3 can work independently of each other, with the separate polypeptide

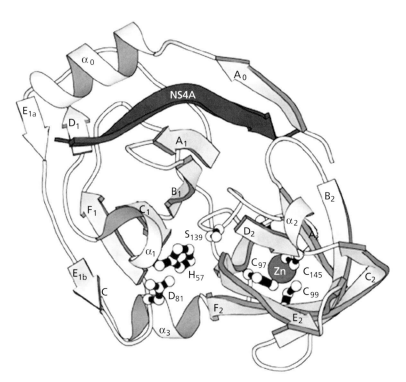

**Figure 2.** Schematic representation of the three-dimensional structure of the HCV NS3 proteinase domain complexed with an NS4A-derived peptide

The side chains of the amino acids of the catalytic triad (His-57, Asp-81, Ser-139) and of the amino acids involved in metal coordination (Cys-97, Cys-99 and Cys-145) are shown. The side chain of the fourth zinc ligand, His-149, is hidden by strand β-D2. The strand contributed by NS4A is shown in dark grey. The coordinates used to generate the picture are deposited in the Protein Data Base (PDB entry: 1JXP) and refer to the HCV genotype 1b NS3–NS4A complex [46].

chains expressing the respective activities [14,15,19,22,33–38]. This has led many researchers to adopt a minimalist approach, focusing on the characterization of a system composed of the isolated recombinant 20 kDa NS3 proteinase domain and a synthetic peptide as an NS4A cofactor mimic. Purification of the truncated enzyme using several different heterologous expression systems has been reported [30,31,39–43] and the effort has ultimately resulted in the solution of the crystal structure of the NS3 proteinase domain in the absence [44] and presence of the cofactor peptide [45,46].

Analysis of the X-ray structure of the NS3 N-terminal domain complexed with NS4A-derived peptides [45,46] revealed that the NS3 serine proteinase adopts a canonical chymotrypsin-like fold, consisting of two nearly symmetrical β-barrel domains, with the residues of the catalytic triad located at the interface between the two domains (Fig. 2). The C-terminal domain (residues 94–180) contains a conventional six-stranded β-barrel and ends with a structurally conserved C-terminal helix. Conversely, the N-terminal domain (NS3 residues 1–93 and NS4A residues 21–34) contains eight β-strands: as described below, one of the two additional strands is contributed by the extreme N terminus of the proteinase ($A_0$) and the other by the NS4A peptide. The NS4A cofactor assumes an extended structure and forms a β-strand that intercalates in an anti-parallel fashion between the two β-strands $A_0$ and $A_1$ in the N-terminal barrel of the enzyme (Fig. 2). The region of the NS3 protein that interacts with the NS4A peptide adopts a β–α–β fold, with an α-helix ($α_0$) packing in a perpendicular fashion against the N-terminal portion of the NS4A peptide. The 22 N-terminal residues of NS3, which were implicated by deletion mapping in the stabilization of the NS3–NS4A complex, encompass strand $A_0$ and helix $α_0$. Consistent with deletion mapping results, these two structural elements form a sort of molecular clamp that locks the NS4A cofactor onto the NS3 proteinase domain. Strand $A_0$ and helix $α_0$ have no counterparts in other structurally characterized serine proteinases: this is in line with the earlier finding that deletion of the corresponding region of NS3 resulted in an enzyme that retains the basal, NS4A-independent proteolytic activity.

Overall, about 2400 $Å^2$ of surface area is buried by the interaction between the enzyme and the cofactor [45]. In agreement with the large buried surface area, the NS3–NS4A complex has been shown to be very stable in the cytoplasm of cultured cells expressing the HCV polyprotein: Bartenschlager *et al.* [25] have shown that the complex, once formed in the cytoplasm of cells transfected with HCV cDNA, does not dissociate for up to 5 hours. For these reasons, NS4A has been suggested to be an integral structural component of the proteinase [45].

In the crystal structure without NS4A, the C-terminal β-barrel of the NS3 proteinase domain adopts substantially the same fold observed in the complex. Conversely, the N-terminal domain of the protein assumes a significantly different conformation: the N-terminal 30 amino acids of NS3 extend away from the protein core and interact with hydrophobic surface patches of neighbouring molecules in the crystallographic asymmetric unit [44]. In solution, the N-terminal region of NS3 is probably disordered when not engaged in the interaction with NS4A, thus providing an explanation for the enhanced metabolic stability of the NS3–NS4A complex with respect to the uncomplexed enzyme [20].

## Mechanisms of NS4A activation

Complex formation with NS4A causes the NS3 proteinase to undergo several conformational changes. As described above, the most obvious changes impact the N-terminal region of the NS3 proteinase. Along with the rearrangement of the N-terminal part of the molecule, a less obvious but crucial conformational change takes place at the proteinase active site upon cofactor binding. In all known serine proteinases, the enzyme catalytic residues are arranged in a so-called catalytic triad [47]. Ser-139, His-57 and Asp-81 form the catalytic triad of the HCV NS3 proteinase. In the NS3–NS4A complex structure, the side chain of Asp-81 is hydrogen bonded to the His-57 imidazole. In this way the imidazole ring of His-57 is polarized and can act as a general base to extract a proton from the enzyme nucleophile, the hydroxyl group of Ser-139. In the structure of the uncomplexed NS3 proteinase, the carboxyl group of Asp-81 points away from His-57 and forms a hydrogen bond with the guanidinium moiety of Arg-155. Similarly, the imidazole ring of His-57 is too far away from Ser-139 to effectively assist the deprotonation of the serine hydroxyl group.

In summary, the conformational reorganization of the NS3 proteinase N-terminal domain induced by NS4A binding ultimately results in the proper alignment of the enzyme active site residues, thus making efficient catalysis possible. It is worth noting, however, that relatively minor readjustments would be sufficient to correctly position the side chain of Asp-81 and His-57, even in the absence of the cofactor, suggesting that in this case also, a classic catalytic triad configuration could probably exist during catalysis [44]. This hypothesis would be consistent with the observation that uncomplexed NS3 retains intrinsic proteinase activity and that complex formation with NS4A does not alter the $pK_a$ value of His-57, as determined by activity titration and NMR [48,49].

## NS3 serine proteinase contains a structural zinc

The presence of a metal-binding site within the serine proteinase domain of HCV NS3 was first predicted on the basis of a three-dimensional model of the protein [50]. Analysis of the alignment of the NS3 amino acid sequence of different HCV isolates with the NS3 region of the related GB viruses has highlighted three Cys and one His residues that are strictly conserved in the serine proteinase domain. In the homology model of the HCV NS3 proteinase domain originally proposed by Failla *et al.* [50], these conserved residues were located on the side of the molecule opposite from the active site and clustered in space. This observation led to the hypothesis that these residues could serve as ligands of a tetradentate metal-binding site [51]. This prediction was confirmed experimentally by the finding that the purified NS3 proteinase domain contains stoichiometric amounts of zinc [51,52] and ultimately by the solution of the enzyme three-dimensional structure (Fig. 2). Since the metal-binding site is remote from the active site, zinc is very unlikely to have a role in catalysis and is thought to have a structural function. Nevertheless, zinc is essential for enzyme activity. Thus, zinc addition was shown to enhance the proteinase activity of an *in vitro*-translated NS3 protein in cell-free experiments [52]. Furthermore, zinc addition was required for the production of soluble NS3 proteinase in *Escherichia coli* [51]. The assignment of the metal ligands has ultimately been confirmed by X-ray crystallography: the zinc ion was shown to be tetrahedrally coordinated by Cys-97, Cys-99 and Cys-145 and, through a bridging water molecule, by His-149 [44–46]. The residues coordinating the metal ion are located on a long loop connecting the two domains of NS3 (Cys-97 and Cys-99) and in a hairpin–loop situated in the second domain (Cys-145 and His-149). Since the residues of the catalytic triad are positioned at the interface between the N-terminal and the C-terminal domain, the relative orientation of the two β-barrels is expected to affect, indirectly, the enzymatic activity. Interestingly, picornavirus 2A proteinases contain two sequence motifs, Cys-X-Cys and Cys-X-His, that are located in a region which is topologically equivalent to the one containing the metal-binding site of HCV NS3 proteinase. Picornavirus 2A proteinase has also been found to contain a tightly bound zinc ion that is required for the formation of an active enzyme and is an essential component of the native structure [53]. The structural conservation of a metal-binding site between HCV NS3 and picornavirus 2A is striking from an evolutionary point of view, since picornavirus 2A proteinases also adopt a chymotrypsin-like fold, but are cysteine, not serine proteinases. The metal-binding site is thus even more conserved than the catalytic site. Similar metal-binding motifs have not been found in any other cellular or viral serine proteinases.

## Substrate specificity of NS3 serine proteinase

The locations of the sites cleaved by the NS3 proteinase within the HCV polyprotein were obtained by N-terminal sequencing of the mature NS4A, NS4B, NS5A and NS5B proteins [9,54]. Based on a comparative analysis of the sequences flanking the cleaved peptide bonds (Fig. 3), it has been possible to derive the following consensus sequence for the NS3-dependent cleavage site (P6 to P1'): Asp/GluXaa$_4$-Cys/Thr-Ser/Ala (we follow the nomenclature of Schechter and Berger [55] in designating the cleavage sites as P6-P5-P4-P3-P2-P1...P1'-P2'-P3'-P4'-, with the scissile bond between P1 and P1' and the C terminus of the substrate on the prime side). It is interesting to note that cleavage occurs after a Cys residue in all *trans* cleavage sites, whereas the intramolecular site between NS3 and NS4A is unique in this respect, having a Thr residue at the P1 position. When incorporated into peptide substrates, this residue has been shown to decrease cleavage efficiency by almost two orders of magnitude [56], suggesting that factors other than maximized cleavage efficiency led to the selection of a suboptimal residue at the P1 position of the NS3–NS4A junction. The other features common to all of the cleavage sites are a conserved negatively charged residue at the P6 position, and a Ser or Ala residue at the P1' position. Site-directed mutagenesis experiments using polyprotein substrates have identified P1 as the major determinant of substrate specificity, at least in the case of the *trans* cleavage sites [57–60]. In apparent contrast with this finding, the P1 position of the NS3–NS4A *cis* cleavage site has turned out to be very insensitive to amino acid substitutions, leading to the suggestion that intramolecular cleavage at the NS3–NS4A site is governed primarily by polyprotein folding and not by its sequence [57,59–61]. Both the consensus P1' and P6 positions have been found to be very tolerant to substitutions [57,60]. In particular, the acidic residue conserved at the P6 position of all cleavage sites was shown not to be essential for polyprotein processing. It was noticed,

**Figure 3**. HCV NS3 serine proteinase-dependent cleavage sites

**NS3–NS4A**

| | |
|---|---|
| 1a(Hcv-1) | CMSA**D**LEVV**T**-**S**TWVLVGGVL |
| 1b(Hcv-Bk) | CMSA**D**LEVV**T**-**S**TWVLVGGVL |
| 2a(Hcv-J6) | CMQA**D**LEVM**T**-**S**TWVLAGGVL |
| 2b(Hcv-J8) | CMQA**D**LEIM**T**-**S**SWVLAGGVL |
| 3a(Hcv-Nzl1) | CMSA**D**LEVT**T**-**S**TWVLLGGVL |

**NS4A–NS4B**

| | |
|---|---|
| 1a(Hcv-1) | YREF**D**EMEE**C**-**S**QHLPYIEQG |
| 1b(Hcv-Bk) | YQEF**D**EMEE**C**-**A**SHLPYIEQG |
| 2a(Hcv-J6) | YEAF**D**EMEE**C**-**A**SRAALIEEG |
| 2b(Hcv-J8) | YEAF**D**EMEE**C**-**A**SKAALIEEG |
| 3a(Hcv-Nzl1) | YQQY**D**EMEE**C**-**S**QAAPYIEQA |

**NS4B–NS5A**

| | |
|---|---|
| 1a(Hcv-1) | WISS**E**CTTP**C**-**S**GSWLRDIWD |
| 1b(Hcv-Bk) | WINE**D**CSTP**C**-**S**GSWLRDVWD |
| 2a(Hcv-J6) | WITE**D**CPIP**C**-**S**GSWLRDVWD |
| 2b(Hcv-J8) | WITE**D**CPVP**C**-**S**GSWLQDIWD |
| 3a(Hcv-Nzl1) | WINE**D**YPSP**C**-**S**DDWLRTIWD |

**NS5A–NS5B**

| | |
|---|---|
| 1a(Hcv-1) | EANA**E**DVVC**C**-**S**MSYSWTGAL |
| 1b(Hcv-Bk) | EEAS**E**DVVC**C**-**S**MSYTWTGAL |
| 2a(Hcv-J6) | SEED**D**SVVC**C**-**S**MSYSWTGAL |
| 2b(Hcv-J8) | SDQE**D**SVIC**C**-**S**MSYSWTGAL |
| 3a(Hcv-Nzl1) | DSEE**Q**SVVC**C**-**S**MSYSWTGAL |

The amino acids surrounding NS3–NS4A, NS4A–NS4B, NS4B–NS5A and NS5A–NS5B are aligned for the most common HCV genotypes: 1a, 1b, 2a, 2b and 3a. The P6, P1 and P1' positions are shown in bold type.

however, that additional acidic residues are present in the P regions of all cleavage sites (Fig. 3), suggesting that they might substitute for a mutated P6 residue [60]. It has indeed been found that, while substitution of the P6 Asp is well tolerated, simultaneous mutagenesis of both acidic residues present in the P region of the NS5A–NS5B junction abolishes cleavage [58].

In contrast to host serine proteinases such as trypsin or chymotrypsin, the HCV enzyme cannot cleave small peptide substrates. For efficient *in vitro* activity on synthetic substrates, purified NS3 proteinase requires at least decamer peptide substrates spanning P6–P4' [31]. P6–P4' decamer substrates corresponding to the three *trans* cleavage sites were hydrolysed by the NS3 proteinase with the same order as the corresponding junctions in the context of the polyprotein (NS5A–NS5B>NS4A–NS4B>NS4B–NS5A). This was taken as evidence for primary structure being a major determinant for *trans* cleavage efficiency [31,48]. Alanine-scanning experiments performed on peptide substrates based either on the NS4A–NS4B [56] or NS5A–NS5B [62] cleavage confirmed that the

P1 and, to a lesser extent, the P6, P3 and P4′ residues contribute to substrate recognition by the NS3 proteinase.

P1 substitutions in the context of an NS4A–NS4B-based substrate gave the following order of decreasing cleavage efficiency: Cys>hCys>Alg>Abu>Thr>NVal> Val (hCys, homocysteine; Alg, allylglycine; Abu, α-aminobutyric acid; Nval, norvaline). Ser, Ala, Gly or Leu at the P1 position yielded uncleavable substrates [56]. Using a decapeptide substrate based on the NS5A/5B sequence, Landro *et al.* [48] revealed a similar order for the influence of P1 on substrate binding: Cys>Abu>Cys(SMe)>Thr>Ala [Cys(SMe), S-methylcysteine], while Zhang *et al.* [62], using a longer substrate, found Cys>hCys>Cys(SMe)> Cys(SEt)~Met>Ala>Ser>Thr~(D)Cys [Cys(SEt), S-ethylcysteine]. The preference displayed by the NS3 serine proteinase for cleavage after a Cys residue can be rationalized on the basis of the structure of the enzyme P1 specificity pocket. The X-ray structure has revealed a specificity pocket that is shallow and hydrophobic, being closed at the bottom by the aromatic ring of Phe-154. The side chains of Ala-157 and Leu-135 constitute the sides of the P1-binding pocket [44–46,54]. The side chain of Cys in the substrate P1 position has been suggested to engage in a favourable sulphhydryl–aromatic interaction with the electron-rich π clouds on the ring system of Phe-154.

The requirement for long peptide substrates and the apparent lack of strong specific interactions with distal subsites can also be readily explained by the structural features of the enzyme substrate-binding site.

Apart from the P1 pocket, the surface of the enzyme involved in substrate recognition is wide, shallow and almost completely solvent-exposed. All major loops connecting the β-strands, which in other serine proteinases contact the P2, P3 and P4 moieties of substrates, are absent in NS3 [44–46]. Two positively charged residues, Arg-161 and Lys-165, have been shown to engage in interactions with the conserved negatively charged residue in the P6 position of the NS3 substrate [44]. As has emerged from molecular modelling studies [44,48], substrates appear to be stabilized in the enzyme active site by at least three types of interactions: (i) the interaction between the P1 Cys side chain and the Phe ring at the bottom of the P1-binding site; (ii) main-chain hydrogen bonding interactions between the enzyme on one side and the substrate P2–P5 region, and possibly the P′ region on the other side; and (iii) the ionic interaction provided by the complementary charges of the side chains of the substrate P6 amino acid with the side chains of Arg-161 and Lys-165. This unique substrate recognition mechanism thus appears to require an interaction that extends over several peptide bonds and provides an explanation of why the binding of small peptide substrates to the NS3 proteinase active site is very inefficient.

## Inhibitors of the NS3 proteinase

### Non-peptide inhibitors

Since the elucidation of the pivotal role of the NS3 proteinase in HCV polyprotein processing, a considerable effort has been devoted towards the development of expression systems, purification protocols and *in vitro* activity assays for this enzyme. Preliminary *in vitro* inhibition studies have shown that NS3 is only modestly inactivated by classical serine proteinase inhibitors such as chloromethylketones or PMSF [16,30,40–42,63–65]. Many of the assay systems that have been developed [16,30,31,39,40–43,62,63, 65–76] are presently used to screen for selective NS3 proteinase inhibitors that could be used as leads for the development of therapeutic agents. First reports on the identification of such compounds have appeared in the literature.

Chu *et al.* [77] reported the isolation of a phenan-threnequinone from a fermentation culture broth of *Streptomyces* sp. This natural product inhibited proteinase activity in an *in vitro* translation assay. The mechanism of inhibition by this compounds was not elucidated.

Several small molecule non-peptide inhibitors, active in the micromolar range, were identified in an HPLC-based screening assay using an NS3–NS4A complex, expressed in *E. coli* as a maltose binding protein, and peptide substrates based on the sequence of the NS5A–NS5B cleavage site [78–80]. The reported compounds belong to different structural classes, and include thiazolidine derivatives [78], 2,4,6-trihydroxy,3-nitro-benzamide derivatives [79] and halogenated benzanilides [80]. All of these compounds were found to inhibit the proteinase in a non-competitive manner, thus suggesting that they do not bind to the enzyme active site. In addition, compounds of the first two classes [78–79] show poor selectivity when tested against a panel of unrelated serine proteinases. The significance of these findings with respect to drug design and development remains to be established.

### Peptide inhibitors

Landro *et al.* [48] have reported the development of two different classes of competitive inhibitors of the

HCV NS3 serine proteinase, both derived from the sequence of the NS5A–NS5B substrate. The first class lacks P′ residues and binds to the enzyme in a way that is independent of the presence of the NS4A cofactor. A representative of this class of inhibitors is the hexapeptide aldehyde with the sequence Glu-Asp-Val-Val-Abu-Val-CHO. This compound inhibits the NS3 serine proteinase activity with a $K_i$ of around 50 μM, both in the presence and absence of the NS4A cofactor. Inhibitors belonging to the second class extend into the P′ region and display a large increase in NS3-binding affinity when NS4A is bound to the enzyme. These NS4A-dependent inhibitors contain cyclic amino acids as replacements for the P1′ naturally occurring serine residue and extend in the prime region. Thus, substitution of bulky cyclic aromatics [Tic (tetrahydroisoquinoline-3-carboxylic acid)] or smaller cyclic alkyls [Pro or Pip (pipecolinic acid)] in the context of a substrate decapeptide yielded peptides that were no longer cleaved, but retained a high binding affinity for the enzyme active site. The decapeptide Glu-Asp-Val-Val-Leu-Cys-Tic-Nle-Ser-Tyr was shown to be a competitive inhibitor of the NS3 proteinase with a $K_i$ of 340 nM in the presence of NS4A and 28 μM in the absence of the cofactor. Deletion of up to three prime residues of this decapeptide (P4′-P2′) resulted in a 40-fold decrease in affinity for the NS3–NS4A complex, but only a fourfold decrease in affinity for the free NS3 proteinase. Conversely, the progressive deletion of amino acids from the P side of the molecule led to roughly the same loss of affinity for both complexed and uncomplexed NS3 proteinase. Overall, this study suggests that, while the interaction of the enzyme with the P side of the substrate is contributing most of the inhibitor binding energy, the formation of auxiliary P′ subsites is promoted directly or indirectly by the NS4A cofactor [48].

Another unique and unexpected feature of the NS3 serine proteinase was pointed out in the recent work of Steinkühler et al. [81]. These authors found that the N-terminal cleavage products of substrate peptides corresponding to the NS4A–NS4B, NS4B–NS5A and NS5A–NS5B cleavage sites are rather potent competitive inhibitors of the NS3 proteinase. Conversely, no inhibition is observed with the N-terminal cleavage product of the intramolecular NS3–NS4A junction. The $K_i$ values found for hexamer P6–P1 products are in the micromolar range (NS4A 0.6 μM; NS5A 1.4 μM; NS4B 180 μM). Remarkably, the enzyme displays an affinity for the products that is up to one order of magnitude higher than for the corresponding substrates. The P1 α-carboxylate function appears to play a crucial role in determining the potency of the P

side hexamer inhibitors. In the case of the hexapeptide sequence derived from the NS4A product, amidation of the P1 α-carboxylate or its substitution with an alcohol caused a decrease in potency of more than two orders of magnitude [82]. Inspection of the structure of the active site of the NS3 proteinase, site-directed mutagenesis experiments and the pH dependence of the observed product inhibition have suggested that the side chain of Lys-136 may be selectively contributing to the stabilization of the bound product inhibitor, possibly by establishing an ionic interaction with the P1 α-carboxylate negative charge (Fig. 4).

Other possible interactions between the product inhibitor and the active site of the NS3 proteinase are shown in Figure 4: the oxygen atoms of the carboxylic acid of the product inhibitor may engage in hydrogen bond formation with the backbone amido groups of residues Ser-139 and Gly-137 (the NS3 serine proteinase oxyanion hole) and with the $N^{\epsilon 2}$ of the catalytic His-57.

The question as to whether product inhibition of the NS3 proteinase has any physiological relevance is, at the moment, unresolved. In this regard, however, it is interesting to note that in the intramolecular NS3–NS4A cleavage site, a suboptimum Thr residue is absolutely conserved in the substrate P1 position. The cleavage product obtained from a peptide with the sequence of this cleavage site does not inhibit the enzyme to any significant extent. It could be argued that a suboptimum P1 position at the NS3–NS4A site is evolutionarily advantageous in order to prevent

**Figure 4.** Schematic representation of the product inhibitor bound to the active site of the NS3 serine proteinase (Gly-137–Ser-139)

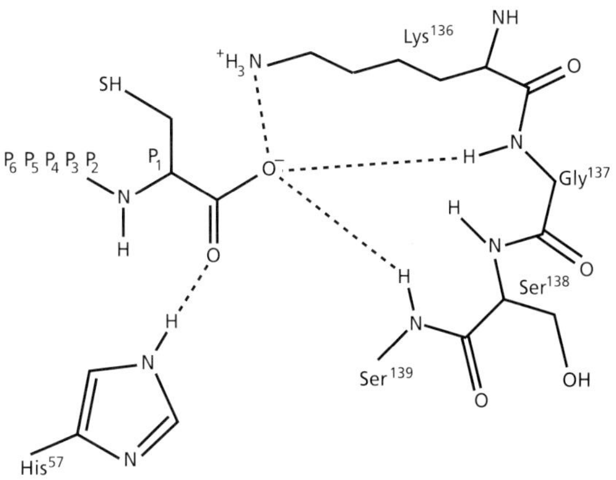

The P1 α-carboxylate is accepting hydrogen bonds from the $N^{\epsilon 2}$ of the catalytic His-57, and the amido groups of Gly-137 and Ser-139. An ionic interaction is established between the negatively charged P1 α-carboxylate and the positively charged side chain of Lys-136.

premature inhibition of the NS3 serine proteinase by the first intramolecular cleavage product.

The phenomenon of product inhibition of the NS3 proteinase was exploited to develop hexapeptide inhibitors active in the low nanomolar range. Using the sequence of the best peptide inhibitors derived from cleavage of the natural substrates as a starting point, a series of product analogues was synthesized with the goal of defining the structure–activity relationship of the product inhibitors. It was concluded that: (i) the main contribution to the binding energy derives from the P1 amino acid, through both its side chain and its free carboxylate; (ii) as in the case of the substrate, the side chain providing optimum occupancy of the P1-binding pocket of the enzyme is Cys, followed in decreasing order of potency by Abu, Cys(SMe), Val and Ser; significantly, deletion of the P1 residue leads to a >1000-fold loss in inhibitory potency; (iii) deletion of the acidic amino acid in the P6 position leads to a >10-fold drop in inhibitory potency; however, achiral diacids with a $C_4$ or $C_5$ carbon chain (such as succinic or glutaric acid) are good substitutes for the Glu or Asp normally found in this position; (iv) a negative charge in the P5 position is not strictly necessary for high inhibitory potency; amino acids with an aromatic side chain such as Tyr and Fno (4-nitrophenylalanine) are as effective as the acidic residues in this position; furthermore, amino acids with D-chirality were tolerated or even advantageous at this position; (v) the P4 position revealed a sharp preference for bulky hydrophobic amino acids, with either aromatic or aliphatic side chains; (vi) Glu, Leu or Val proved to be optimum in the P3 position, suggesting a dual mode of interaction by the side chain of the amino acid at this position and the enzyme; (vii) similarly, both negatively charged and hydrophobic amino acids are tolerated at the P2 position, whereas positively charged and conformationally constrained residues are not accepted.

By sequential optimization of the P5–P2 positions, the peptide Ac-Asp-(D)Gla-Leu-Ile-Cha-Cys-OH (Gla, γ-carboxyglutamic acid) was synthesized by Ingallinella et al. [82] and shown to inhibit the NS3 serine proteinase with an $IC_{50}$ of 1.5 nM. This is the most potent active site-directed inhibitor of the NS3 serine proteinase thus far reported and should serve as a useful lead for the development of anti-HCV compounds.

## CONCLUSIONS

Almost a decade has now elapsed since the molecular cloning of the HCV genome. Despite the inability to propagate this virus in the laboratory, we have witnessed an explosion of novel information regarding the structure and function of virally encoded proteins that are believed to be fundamental for the replication of HCV in the infected liver. The NS3 viral protein contains a proteinase that is likely to be necessary for the production of new infectious viruses and therefore represents a key target for therapeutic intervention. The structure of this important enzyme has now been solved at the atomic level, revealing several unique features of the enzyme that might provide opportunities to design new potent and specific antiviral drugs that block the HCV proteinase and disrupt the HCV replication cycle. The unique features of the NS3 proteinase suggest at least three ways of achieving inhibition of the enzyme. The first, most obvious way, is that of designing compounds that bind to the enzyme at the active site. The requirement of extended interactions spanning at least 10 residues in the substrate, the need for a Cys as optimum P1 residue and the absence of P2, P3 and P4 binding loops make the development of potent and selective NS3 proteinase active site inhibitors a very difficult task. In this respect, the recent publication of hexapeptide inhibitors of the enzyme, active in the low nanomolar range, should serve as the basis for the future development of peptidomimetic drugs. A second theoretical way to inhibit the proteinase action is by interference with the activation of the enzyme by its NS4A cofactor. However, the interaction between the NS3 protein and the cofactor is a very intimate one: the N terminus of NS3 literally wraps around the cofactor, providing a complex whose half-life presumably exceeds the time-span necessary for the proteinase to complete a full round of polyprotein processing. Since the formation of NS3–NS4A is presumably cotranslational, the window of intervention to block this interaction may, in practical terms, be too narrow. Finally, it should be pointed out that because of the absolute conservation of this site among HCV, GB viruses and picornaviruses, in spite of the high sequence variability of the viral RNA genomes, the zinc-binding site of HCV NS3 might provide a very attractive target for antiviral therapy.

## REFERENCES

1. Houghton M. Hepatitis C viruses. In *Fields' Virology*, 3rd edn, pp. 1035–1058; 1996. Edited by BN Fields, DM Knipe & PM Howley. Philadelphia: Lippincott-Raven.
2. Fried MW & Hofnagle JH. Therapy of hepatitis C. *Seminars in Liver Disease* 1995; **15**:82–91.
3. Blair CS, Haydon GH & Hayes PC. Current perspectives on the treatment and prevention of hepatitis C infection. *Expert Opinion in Investigational Drugs* 1996; **5**:1657–1671.

4. Bartenschlager R. Molecular targets in inhibition of hepatitis C virus replication. *Antiviral Chemistry and Chemotherapy* 1997; **8**:281–301.

5. Neddermann P, Tomei L, Steinkühler C, Gallinari P, Tramontano A & De Francesco R. The nonstructural proteins of the hepatitis C virus: structure and functions. *Biological Chemistry* 1997; **378**:469–476.

6. Francki RIB, Fauquet CM, Knudson DL & Brown F. Classification and nomenclature of viruses: fifth report of the International Committee on Taxonomy of Viruses. *Archives of Virology* 1991; **2** (Supplement):223–233.

7. Grakoui A, McCourt DW, Wychowski C, Feinstone SM & Rice CM. A second hepatitis C virus-encoded proteinase. *Proceedings of the National Academy of Sciences, USA* 1993; **90**:10583–10587.

8. Hijikata M, Mizushima H, Akagi T, Mori S, Kakiuchi N, Kato N, Tanaka T, Kimura K & Shimotohno K. Two distinct proteinase activities required for the processing of a putative nonstructural precursor protein of hepatitis C virus. *Journal of Virology* 1993; **67**:4665–4675.

9. Grakoui A, McCourt DW, Wychowski C, Feinstone SM & Rice C. Characterization of the hepatitis C virus-encoded serine proteinase: determination of proteinase-dependent polyprotein cleavage sites. *Journal of Virology* 1993; **67**:2832–2843.

10. Tomei L, Failla C, Santolini E, De Francesco R & La Monica N. NS3 is a serine proteinase required for processing of hepatitis C virus polyprotein. *Journal of Virology* 1993; **67**:4017–4026.

11. Bartenschlager R, Ahlborn-Laake L, Mous J & Jacobsen H. Nonstructural protein 3 of the hepatitis C virus encodes a serine-type proteinase required for cleavage at the NS3/4 and NS4/5 junctions. *Journal of Virology* 1993; **67**:3835–3844.

12. Eckart MR, Selby M, Masiarz F, Lee C, Berger K, Crawford K, Kuo G, Houghton M & Choo QL. The hepatitis C virus encodes a serine proteinase involved in processing of the putative nonstructural proteins from the viral polyprotein precursor. *Biochemical and Biophysical Research Communications* 1993; **192**:399–406.

13. D'Souza EDA, O'Sullivan E, Amphlett EM, Rowlands DJ, Sangar DV & Clarke BE. Analysis of NS3-mediated processing of the hepatitis C virus non-structural region *in vitro*. *Journal of General Virology* 1994; **75**:3469–3476.

14. Manabe S, Fuke I, Tanishita O, Kaji C, Gomi Y, Yoshida S, Mori C, Takamizawa A, Yosida I & Okayama H. Production of nonstructural proteins of hepatitis C virus requires a putative viral proteinase encoded by NS3. *Virology* 1994; **198**:636–644.

15. Lin C, Pragai BM, Grakoui A, Xu J & Rice CM. Hepatitis C virus NS3 serine proteinase: *trans*-cleavage requirements and processing kinetics. *Journal of Virology* 1994; **68**:8147–8157.

16. Lin C & Rice CM. The hepatitis C virus NS3 proteinase and NS4A cofactor: establishment of a cell-free trans-processing assay. *Proceedings of the National Academy of Sciences, USA* 1995; **92**:7622–7626.

17. Chambers TJ, Weir RC, Grakoui A, McCourt DW, Bazan JF, Fletterick RJ & Rice CM. Evidence that the N-terminal domain of nonstructural protein NS3 from yellow fever virus is a serine proteinase responsible for site-specific cleavages in the viral polyprotein. *Proceedings of the National Academy of Sciences, USA* 1990; **87**:8898–8902.

18. Failla C, Tomei L & De Francesco R. Both NS3 and NS4A are required for proteolytic processing of hepatitis C virus nonstructural proteins. *Journal of Virology* 1994; **68**:3753–3760.

19. Bartenschlager R, Ahlborn Laake L, Mous J & Jacobsen H. Kinetic and structural analyses of hepatitis C virus polyprotein processing. *Journal of Virology* 1994; **68**:5045–5055.

20. Tanji Y, Hijikata M, Satoh S, Kaneko T & Shimotohno K. Hepatitis C virus-encoded nonstructural protein NS4A has versatile functions in viral protein processing. *Journal of Virology* 1995; **69**:1575–1581.

21. Hijikata M, Mizushima H, Tanji Y, Komoda Y, Hirowatari Y, Akagi T, Kato N, Kimura K & Shimotohno K. Proteolytic processing and membrane association of putative nonstructural proteins of hepatitis C virus. *Proceedings of the National Academy of Sciences, USA* 1993; **90**:10733–10737.

22. Failla C, Tomei L & De Francesco R. An amino-terminal domain of the hepatitis C virus NS3 proteinase is essential for interaction with NS4A. *Journal of Virology* 1995; **69**:1769–1777.

23. Lin C, Thomson JA & Rice CM. A central region in the hepatitis C virus NS4A protein allows formation of an active NS3-NS4A serine proteinase complex *in vivo* and *in vitro*. *Journal of Virology* 1995; **69**:4373–4380.

24. Satoh S, Tanji Y, Hijikata M, Kimura K & Shimotohno K. The N-terminal region of hepatitis C virus nonstructural protein 3 (NS3) is essential for stable complex formation with NS4A. *Journal of Virology* 1995; **69**:4255–4260.

25. Bartenschlager R, Lohman V, Wilkinson T & Koch JO. Complex formation between the NS3 serine-type proteinase of the hepatitis C virus and NS4A and its importance for polyprotein maturation. *Journal of Virology* 1995; **69**:7519–7528.

26. Koch JO, Lohmann V, Herian U & Bartenschlager R. *In vitro* studies on the activation of the hepatitis C virus NS3 proteinase by the NS4A cofactor. *Virology* 1996; **221**:54–66.

27. Rost B, Casadio R, Fariselli P & Sander C. Transmembrane helices predicted at 95% accuracy. *Protein Science* 1995; **4**:521–533.

28. Tomei L, Failla C, Vitale RL, Bianchi E & De Francesco R. A central hydrophobic domain of the hepatitis C virus NS4A protein is necessary and sufficient for the activation of the NS3 proteinase. *Journal of General Virology* 1996; **77**:1065–1070.

29. Shimizu Y, Yamaji K, Masuho Y, Yokota T, Inoue H, Sudo K, Satoh S & Shimotohno K. Identification of the sequence of NS4A required for enhanced cleavage of the NS5A/5B site by hepatitis C virus NS3 proteinase. *Journal of Virology* 1996; **70**:127–132.

30. Steinkühler C, Tomei L & De Francesco R. *In vitro* activity of hepatitis C virus proteinase NS3 purified from recombinant baculovirus-infected Sf9 cells. *Journal of Biological Chemistry* 1996; **271**:6367–6373.

31. Steinkühler C, Urbani A, Tomei L, Biasiol G, Sardana M, Bianchi E, Pessi A & De Francesco R. Activity of purified hepatitis C virus proteinase NS3 on peptide substrates. *Journal of Virology* 1996; **70**:6694–6700.

32. Bianchi E, Urbani A, Biasiol G, Brunetti M, Pessi A, De Francesco R & Steinkühler C. Complex formation between the hepatitis C virus serine proteinase and a synthetic NS4A cofactor peptide. *Biochemistry* 1997; **36**:7890–7897.

33. Tanji Y, Hijikata M, Hirowatari Y & Shimotohno K. Identification of the domain required for trans-cleavage activity of hepatitis C viral serine proteinase. *Gene* 1994; **145**:215–219.

34. Han DS, Hahm B, Rho HM & Jang SK. Identification of the serine proteinase domain in NS3 of the hepatitis C virus. *Journal of General Virology* 1995; **76**:985–993.

35. Kim DW, Gwack Y, Han JH & Choe J. C-terminal domain of the hepatitis C virus NS3 protein contains an RNA helicase activity. *Biochemical and Biophysical Research Communications* 1995; **215**:160–166.

36. Jin L & Peterson DL. Expression, isolation, and characterization of the hepatitis C virus ATPase/RNA helicase. *Archives of Biochemistry and Biophysics* 1995; **323**:47–53.

37. Yao N, Hesson T, Cable M, Hong Z, Kwong AD, Le HV & Weber PC. Structure of the hepatitis C virus RNA helicase domain. *Nature Structural Biology* 1997; **4**:463–467.

38. Kim JL, Morgenstern KA, Griffith JP, Dwyer MD, Thomson JA, Murcko MA, Lin C & Caron PR. Hepatitis C virus NS3 RNA helicase domain with a bound oligonucleotide: the crystal structure provides insight into the mode of unwinding. *Structure* 1998; **6**:89–100.

39. Suzuki T, Sato M, Chieda S, Shoji I, Harada T, Yamakawa Y, Watabe S, Matsuura Y & Miyamura T. In vivo and in vitro trans-cleavage activity of hepatitis C virus serine proteinase expressed by recombinant baculoviruses. *Journal of General Virology* 1995; **76**:3021–3029.

40. Shoji I, Suzuki T, Chieda S, Sato M, Harada T, Chiba T, Matsuura Y & Miyamura T. Proteolytic activity of NS3 serine proteinase of hepatitis C virus efficiently expressed in *Escherichia coli*. *Hepatology* 1995; **22**:1648–1655.

41. Mori A, Yamada K, Kimura J, Koide T, Yuasa S, Yamada E & Miyamura T. Enzymatic characterization of purified NS3 serine proteinase of hepatitis C virus expressed in Escherichia coli. *FEBS Letters* 1996; **378**:37–42.

42. Markland W, Petrillo RA, Fitzgibbon M, Fox T, McCarrick R, McQuaid T, Fulghum JR, Chen W, Fleming MA, Thomson JA & Chambers SP. Purification and characterization of the NS3 serine proteinase domain of hepatitis C virus expressed in *Saccharomyces cerevisiae*. *Journal of General Virology* 1997; **78**:39–43.

43. Vishnuvardan D, Kakiuchi N, Urvil PT, Shimotohno K, Kumar PKR & Nishikawa S. Expression of highly active recombinant NS3 proteinase domain of hepatitis C virus in E. coli. *FEBS Letters* 1997; **402**:209–212.

44. Love RA, Parge HE, Wickersham JA, Hostomsky Z, Habuka N, Moomaw EW, Adachi T & Homstomska Z. The crystal structure of hepatitis C virus NS3 proteinase reveals a trypsin-like fold and a structural zinc binding site. *Cell* 1996; **87**:331–342.

45. Kim JL, Morgenstern KA, Lin C, Fox T, Dwyer MD, Landro JA, Chambers SP, Markland W, Lepre CA, O'Malley ET, Harbeson SL, Rice CM, Murcko MA, Caron PR & Thomson JA. Crystal structure of the hepatitis virus NS3 proteinase domain complexed with a synthetic NS4A cofactor peptide. *Cell* 1996; **87**:343–355.

46. Yan Y, Li Y, Munshi S, Sardana V, Cole J, Sardana M, Steinkühler C, Tomei L, De Francesco R, Kuo L & Chen Z. Complex of NS3 proteinase and NS4A peptide of BK strain hepatitis C virus: a 2.2 Å resolution structure in a hexagonal crystal form. *Protein Science* 1998; **7**:837–847.

47. Lesk AM & Fordham WD. Conservation and variability in the structure of serine proteinases of the chymotrypsin family. *Journal of Molecular Biology* 1996; **258**:501–537.

48. Landro JA, Raybuck SA, Luong YPC, O'Malley ET, Harbeson SL, Morgenstern KA, Rao G & Livingston DJ. Mechanistic role of an NS4A peptide cofactor with the truncated NS3 proteinase of hepatitis C virus: elucidation of the NS4A stimulatory effect via kinetic analysis and inhibitor mapping. *Biochemistry* 1997; **36**:9340–9348.

49. Urbani A, Bazzo R, Nardi MC, Cicero DO, De Francesco R, Steinkühler C & Barbato G. The metal binding site of the hepatitis C virus NS3 protease. A spectroscopic study. *Journal of Biological Chemistry* 1988;**273**:18760-18769.

50. Failla C, Pizzi E, De Francesco R & Tramontano A. Redesigning the substrate specificity of the hepatitis C virus proteinase. *Folding and Design* 1996; **1**:35–42.

51. De Francesco R, Urbani A, Nardi MC, Tomei L, Steinkühler C & Tramontano A. A zinc binding site in viral serine proteinases. *Biochemistry* 1996; **35**:13282–13287.

52. Stempniak M, Hostomska Z, Nodes BR & Hostomsky ZO. The NS3 proteinase domain of hepatitis C virus is a zinc-containing enzyme. *Journal of Virology* 1997; **71**:2881–2886.

53. Voss T, Meyer R & Sommergruber WO. Spectroscopic characterization of rhinoviral proteinase 2A: Zn is essential for structural integrity. *Protein Science* 1995; **4**:2526–2531.

54. Pizzi E, Tramontano A, Tomei L, La Monica N, Failla C, Sardana M, Wood T & De Francesco R. Molecular model of the specificity pocket of the hepatitis C virus proteinase: implications for substrate recognition. *Proceedings of the National Academy of Sciences, USA* 1994; **91**:888–892.

55. Schechter I & Berger A. On the size of the active site in proteinases. I. Papain. *Biochemical and Biophysical Research Communications* 1967; **27**:157–162.

56. Urbani A, Bianchi E, Narjes F, Tramontano A, De Francesco R, Steinkühler C & Pessi A. Substrate specificity of the hepatitis C virus serine proteinase NS3. *Journal of Biological Chemistry* 1997; **272**: 9204–9209.

57. Kolykhalov AA, Agapov EV & Rice CM. Specificity of the hepatitis C virus NS3 serine proteinase: effects of substitutions at the 3/4A, 4A/4B, 4B/5A, and 5A/5B cleavage sites on polyprotein processing. *Journal of Virology* 1994; **68**:7525–7533.

58. Komoda Y, Hijikata M, Sato S, Asabe SI, Kimura K & Shimotohno K. Substrate requirements of hepatitis C virus serine proteinase for intermolecular polypeptide cleavage in *Escherichia coli*. *Journal of Virology* 1994; **68**:7351–7357.

59. Tanji Y, Hijikata M, Hirowatari Y & Shimotohno K. Hepatitis C virus polyprotein processing: kinetics and mutagenic analysis of serine proteinase-dependent cleavage. *Journal of Virology* 1994; **86**:8418–8422.

60. Bartenschlager R, Ahlborn-Laake L, Yasargil K, Mous J & Jacobsen H. Substrate determinants for cleavage in cis and in trans by the hepatitis C virus NS3 proteinase. *Journal of Virology* 1995; **69**:198–205.

61. Leinbach SS, Bhat RA, Xia SM, Hum WT, Stauffer B, Davis A, Hung PP & Mizutani S. Substrate specificity of the NS3 serine proteinase of hepatitis C virus as determined by mutagenesis at the NS3/NS4A junction. *Virology* 1994; **204**:163–169.

62. Zhang R, Durkin J, Windsor WT, McNemar C, Ramanathan L & Le HV. Probing the substrate specificity of hepatitis C virus NS3 serine proteinase by using synthetic peptides. *Journal of Virology* 1997; **71**:6208–6213.

63. Bouffard P, Bartenschlager R, Ahlborn-Laake L, Mous J, Roberts N & Jacobsen H. An *in vitro* assay for hepatitis C virus NS3 serine proteinase. *Virology* 1995; **209**:52–59.

64. Hahm B, Han DS, Back SH, Song OK, Cho MJ, Kim CJ, Shimotohno K & Jang SK. NS3-4A of hepatitis C virus is a chymotrypsin-like proteinase. *Journal of Virology* 1995; **69**:2534–2539.

65. Sudo K, Inoue H, Shimizu Y, Yamaji K, Konno K, Shigeta S, Kaneko T, Yokota T & Shimotohno K. Establishment of an in vitro assay system for screening hepatitis C virus proteinase inhibitors using high performance liquid chromatography. *Antiviral Research* 1996; **32**:9–18.

66. Kakiuchi N, Hijikata M, Komoda Y, Tanji Y, Hirowatari Y & Shimotohno K. Bacterial expression and analysis of cleavage activity of HCV serine proteinase using recombinant and synthetic substrate. *Biochemical and Biophysical Research Communications* 1995; **210:** 1059–1065.

67. D'Souza EDA, Grace K, Sangar DV, Rowlands DJ & Clarke BE. *In vitro* cleavage of hepatitis C virus polyprotein substrates by purified recombinant NS3 proteinase. *Journal of General Virology* 1995; **76**:1729–1736.

68. Overton H, McMillan D, Gillespie F & Mills J. Recombinant baculovirus-expressed NS3 proteinase of hepatitis C virus shows activity in cell-based and *in vitro* assay. *Journal of General Virology* 1995; **76**:3009–3019.

69. Hamarake R, Wang HGH, Butcher JA, Bifano M, Clark G, Hernandez D, Zhang D, Racela J, Standring D & Colonno R. Establishment of an in vitro assay to characterize hepatitis C virus NS3-4A proteinase *trans*-processing activity. *Intervirology* 1996; **39**:249–258.

70. Bianchi E, Steinkühler C, Taliani M, Urbani A, De Francesco R & Pessi A. Synthetic depsipeptide substrates for the assay of human hepatitis C virus proteinase. *Analytical Biochemistry* 1996; **23**:239–244.

71. Taliani M, Bianchi E, Narjes F, Fossatelli M, Urbani A, Steinkühler C, De Francesco R & Pessi A. A continuous assay of hepatitis C virus proteinase based on resonance energy transfer depsipeptide substrates. *Analytical Biochemistry* 1996; **240**:60–67.

72. Lipovsek Sali D, Ingram R, Wendel M, Gupta D, McNemar C, Tsarbopoulos A, Chen JW, Hong Z, Chase R, Risano C, Zhang R, Yao N, Kwong AD, Ramanathan L, Le HV & Weber PC. Serine proteinase of hepatitis C virus expressed in insect cells as the NS3/4A complex. *Biochemistry* 1998; **37**:3392–3401.

73. Kakiuchi N, Komoda Y, Hijikata M & Shimotono K. Cleavage activity of hepatitis C virus serine proteinase. *Journal of Biochemistry* 1997; **122**:749–755.

74. Wilkinson TCI, Bunyard PR, Quirk K & Wilkinson C. Characterisation of an HCV NS3/NS4A proteinase fusion protein expressed in *E. coli* using synthetic peptide substrates. *Biochemical Society Transactions* 1997; **25**:90.

75. Hirowatari Y, Hijikata M & Shimotono K. A novel method for analysis of viral proteinase activity encoded by hepatitis C virus in cultured cells. *Analytical Biochemistry* 1995; **225**:113–120.

76. Song O-k, Cho OH, Hahm B & Jang SK. Development of an *in vivo* assay system suitable for screening inhibitors of hepatitis C viral proteinase. *Molecules and Cells* 1996; **6**:183–189.

77. Chu M, Mierzwa R, Truumees I, King A, Patel M, Berrie R, Hart A, Butkiewicz N, DasMahapatra B, Chan TM & Puar MS. Structure of Sch 68631: a new hepatitis C virus proteinase inhibitor from *Streptomyces* sp. *Tetrahedron Letters* 1996; **37**: 7229–7232.

78. Sudo K, Matsumoto Y, Matsushima M, Fujiwara M, Konno K, Shimotohno K, Shigeta S & Yokota T. Novel hepatitis C virus proteinase inhibitors: thiazolidine derivatives. *Biochemical and Biophysical Research Communications* 1997; **238**:643–647.

79. Sudo K, Matsumoto Y, Matsushima M, Konno K, Shimotohno K, Shigeta S & Yokota T. Novel hepatitis C virus proteinase inhibitors: 2,4,6-trihydroxy,3-nitro-benzamide derivatives. *Antiviral Chemistry and Chemotherapy* 1997; **8**:541–544.

80. Kakiuchi N, Komoda Y, Komoda K, Takeshita N, Okada S, Tani T & Shimotono K. Non-peptide inhibitors of HCV serine proteinase. *FEBS Letters* 1998; **421**:217–220.

81. Steinkühler C, Biasiol G, Brunetti M, Urbani A, Koch U, Cortese R, Pessi A & De Francesco R. Product inhibition of the hepatitis C virus NS3 protease. *Biochemistry* 1998; **37**:8899–8905.

82. Ingalinella S, Altamura S, Bianchi E, Taliani M, Ingenito R, Cortese R, De Francesco R, Steinkühler C & Pessi A. Potent peptide inhibitors of human hepatitis C virus NS3 protease are obtained by optimising the cleavage products. *Biochemistry* 1998; **37**:8906–8914.

# 27 Conformational changes in hepatitis C virus NS3 proteinase during NS4A complexation: correlation with enhanced cleavage and implications for inhibitor design

Robert A Love, Hans E Parge, John A Wickersham, Zdenek Hostomsky, Noriyuki Habuka, Ellen W Moomaw, Tsuyoshi Adachi, Steve Margosiak, Eleanor Dagostino and Zuzana Hostomska*

## SUMMARY

Hepatitis C virus (HCV) NS3 proteinase activity is required for the release of HCV non-structural proteins and is thus a potential antiviral target. The proteinase must complex with another protein, NS4A, located downstream of NS3 on the polyprotein, for efficient processing. Comparison of the proteinase three-dimensional structure before and after NS4A binding can help to elucidate the mechanism of NS4A-dependent enzyme activation. We solved the crystal structure of NS3 proteinase of the HCV BK isolate (residues 1–189), and the crystal structure of this proteinase complexed with a central region of HCV BK NS4A (residues 21–34). The core region of the enzyme (residues 30–178) without NS4A (designated NS3P) or with bound NS4A (NS3P/4A) is folded into a trypsin-like conformation. However, the loop that connects catalytic residues His-57 and Asp-81 shifts away from the NS4A binding site in NS3P/4A relative to NS3P, sterically accommodating the peptide. His-57 and Asp-81 move closer to Ser-139 in NS3P/4A, and their side chains adopt more 'traditional' (trypsin-like) orientations, consistent with the enhancement of NS3P's weak residual activity upon NS4A binding. The N terminus (residues 1–30), while extended in NS3P, is folded into an α-helix and β-strand that partially cover bound NS4A in the NS3P/4A complex.

Our modelling of peptide substrates shows that a new binding surface is formed from both the refolded N terminus and NS4A, potentially affecting substrate residues immediately downstream (P′ side) of the cleavage site. However, the binding surface for P-side substrate residues (including the P1 specificity pocket) changes little after NS4A complexation. These modelling results agree with recent experiments exploring cleavage before and after NS4A complexation. Based on our two structures, we propose a sequence of conformational changes that could occur during NS4A binding, and present a model for the NS3/NS4 polyprotein just prior to the intramolecular *cis* cleavage, in order to conceptualize these early stages of HCV replication.

## INTRODUCTION

HCV, a member of the family *Flaviviridae*, is the major agent of parenterally transmitted non-A, non-B hepatitis. Most HCV infections become chronic and often lead to liver cirrhosis and hepatocellular carcinoma. It is estimated that there are hundreds of millions of carriers worldwide. Given the absence of any preventative vaccination, there is an urgent need for effective treatment. Recent studies have focused on gaining detailed structural and functional infor-

---

mation about essential HCV replication components. HCV has a positive single-stranded RNA genome of about 9400 nucleotides encoding a polyprotein precursor of about 3020 amino acid residues. Non-structural (NS) proteins are released by the action of two virus-encoded proteinases: NS2-3 and NS3. NS2-3 performs a single cut to release the N terminus of NS3. The N-terminal one-third of NS3 contains a proteinase (NS3P) that yields all remaining NS proteins: NS4A, NS4B, NS5A and NS5B. NS3P is thus a potential antiviral target, and is the focus of this report. NS3P is activated after forming a heterodimer with the protein NS4A, located immediately downstream of NS3 on the polyprotein. It has been shown that a central hydrophobic region of NS4A is sufficient for complex formation and proteolytic activation of NS3P. The NS3/NS4A site is cleaved first in a rapid intramolecular event (in *cis*), followed by intermolecular cleavages (in *trans*) at NS5A/NS5B, NS4A/NS4B and NS4B/NS5A. The consensus sequence at HCV *trans* cleavage sites involves Cys–Ser at the P1–P1′ positions and an acidic residue at P6. Recent reviews provide further details of this system [1–3].

Here we describe the crystal structure of NS3 proteinase from the HCV BK isolate (residues 1–189) alongside the crystal structure of the proteinase complexed with a central region of HCV BK NS4A (residues 21–34). They are designated NS3P and NS3P/4A, respectively. NS3P was solved by MIRAS methods (multiple isomorphous replacement) from R32 crystals and refined at 2.4Å [4]. NS3P/4A was solved by MIRAS methods from P3$_1$21 crystals and refined at 2.8 Å. (X-ray structures for NS3P/4A have been reported by two other groups [5,6] using different crystal forms.) Comparison of the NS3P three-dimensional structure before and after NS4A complexation can give clues to the mechanism of NS4A-dependent enzyme activation. The expected binding mode of peptide substrates can be modelled into both, and the results correlated with experimental cleavage patterns. This modelling also lays ground for a discussion of inhibitor design.

## CONFORMATION OF THE CORE REGION WITH AND WITHOUT NS4A

A direct comparison between the two enzyme conformations is shown in Figure 1. The core region of the enzyme (residues 30–178) with or without NS4A is folded into a trypsin-like motif, with essentially the same secondary structure, zinc site and general location of catalytic triad His-57/Asp-81/Ser-139. The

largest difference between the two cores involves the D1–E1 double-stranded β-loop (residues 62–72), which is shifted away (up to 10 Å) from the NS4A-binding site in NS3P/4A relative to NS3P; this sterically accommodates NS4A residues 21–25. The D1–E1 loop of NS3P/4A is packed against both the N-terminal α-helix and NS4A, resulting in more restraint on residues located (sequentially) between catalytic His-57 and Asp-81. In NS3P/4A, His-57 and Asp-81 move closer to Ser-139, and their side chains adopt more 'traditional' trypsin-like orientations than in NS3P. The observation that the catalytic triad is only approximately formed in NS3P, then optimized in NS3P/4A, is consistent with the residual enzymatic activity of NS3P being enhanced after NS4A binding, particularly through the cleavage rate as measured by $k_{cat}$ [7–9].

Another consequence of the D1–E1 shift is that Trp-85 becomes significantly more buried in NS3P/4A than in NS3P, the indole ring being covered by the D1–E1 loop. This is consistent with fluorescence studies suggesting that at least one tryptophan of NS3P acquires a more hydrophobic environment upon NS4A complexation [10].

Despite changes in the D1–E1 loop and N terminus (see below), features of the enzyme surface complementing NS4A residues 27–33 in NS3P/4A exist essentially unchanged from the NS3P structure, including the orientation of groups that hydrogen-bond to NS4A. Thus, about half of the enzyme's NS4A-binding site is 'preformed' in the NS3P structure. This subsite may be crucial for the initial recognition of NS4A (residues 27–33) during polyprotein folding.

## CONFORMATION OF THE N TERMINUS WITH AND WITHOUT NS4A

The largest overall difference between the NS3P and NS3P/4A crystal structures involves the N terminus (residues 1–30). In NS3P, this is extended and interacts with neighbouring molecules in the crystal lattice, whereas in NS3P/4A it is folded into an α-helix (residues 13–22) and β-strand (residues 2–10) that partially cover the NS4A peptide (Fig. 1). In the NS3P crystal, a central patch on each enzyme is contacted by two N-terminal strands originating from different neighbouring molecules; the position of these strands closely mimics NS4A residues 29–32 and enzyme residues 2–6 from the NS3P/4A structure (Fig. 2). Specifically, side chains of neighbouring NS3P residues Cys-16 and Ile-18 interact with the central patch in a manner that sterically mimics NS4A Ile-29

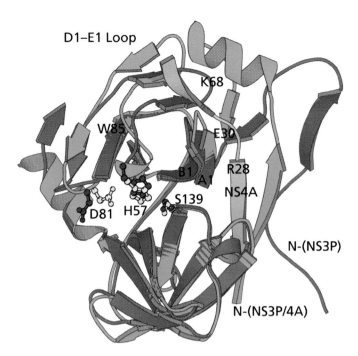

**Figure 1.** Superposition of the two NS3P proteinase crystal structures

The two NS3P structures are shown without NS4A (magenta ribbon, red side chains) and with bound NS4A peptide (green ribbon, yellow side chains and blue NS4A). Side chains for the catalytic triad are Asp-81, His-57 and Ser-139 (labelled D81, H57 and S139). Side chains of Asp-81 and His-57 rearrange substantially after NS4A complexation (from red to yellow), adopting more traditional trypsin-like positions. The overall fold within the core region is very similar between structures, but the N terminus (residues 1–30) is extended in NS3P (magenta strand on right), whereas it is folded in NS3P/4A (green strand/helix); Glu-30 (E30) defines the 'hinge' about which the N terminus displays structural variation. Another large conformational change involves a shift of the D1–E1 loop (top left), which permits complete binding of the NS4A peptide. NS4A Arg-28 (R28), along with enzyme Arg-92 (not shown), may play a role in correctly orienting part of the N terminus by salt-bridging to Glu-30; these interactions also appear to disrupt a Glu-30 to Lys-68 (K68) salt bridge in NS3P and thus allow movement of the D1–E1 loop during complexation.

and Leu-31 of NS3P/4A. Alongside this, neighbouring NS3P residues 2–6 interact with the patch almost exactly, as does the intramolecular segment 2–6 in NS3P/4A. The fact that the NS3P patch employed during intermolecular strand exchange includes the enzyme's 'preformed' NS4A binding site (NS4A residues 27–33) further suggests that this subsite might serve as the key recognition locus for NS4A.

It is not known whether the NS3P N-terminal conformation or exchange represents a situation that could exist outside of crystallization conditions. Some spectroscopic experiments with purified protein have suggested that, in certain solutions, the N terminus of NS3P has secondary structure closer to that in NS3P/4A [10]. In any case, the N terminus must undergo a substantial tertiary rearrangement during complexation, since it partially covers NS4A in NS3P/4A.

## CONCERTED REARRANGEMENTS DURING NS4A COMPLEXATION

The amino acid Glu-30 defines a 'hinge', or origin of conformational variation, for the N terminus as it emerges from the core of the enzyme (Fig. 1). In the NS3P structure, Glu-30 is salt-bridged to Lys-68 on the D1–E1 loop. But in NS3P/4A, the Glu-30 side chain rotates 180° away from the D1–E1 loop, and interacts with Arg-92 as well as NS4A residue Arg-

28. These two new salt bridges thus appear to be responsible for reorientation of Glu-30 and, consequently, of several residues sequentially preceding Glu-30. One scenario for NS4A peptide complexation could be as follows: NS4A residues 27–33 would first bind to NS3P at the 'preformed' NS4A subsite, and Glu-30 would flip, due to favourable interactions with NS4A Arg-28 and NS3P Arg-92. This would effectively lock the 'base' of the N terminus (approximately residues 27–30) into its 'correct' orientation. The D1–E1 loop could shift after being released from the Glu-30/Lys-68 salt bridge, thus creating a new complementary binding surface for the remainder of NS4A (residues 21–26). Finally, the bulk of the N terminus would fold, adopting secondary/tertiary structure driven partly by interactions with the solvent-exposed side of bound NS4A and with the enzyme's surface. Such a kinetic scheme of cooperative rearrangement is consistent with the slow association rates observed for the binding of NS3P and NS4A [10].

An important functional role for Arg-28 of NS4A has been suggested by experiments in which non-positive amino acid substitutions at position 28 in an NS4A peptide greatly reduce its ability to enhance NS3P activity, although the altered peptide still binds to NS3P competitively with native peptide [7]. Applying the hypothesis above, one would expect this mutant NS4A peptide to bind partially at the

**Figure 2.** Molecular packing in the NS3P crystal, showing N-terminal strand exchange among the three molecules of the asymmetric unit

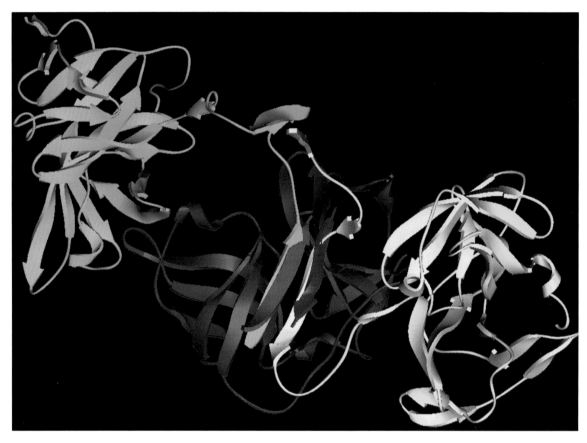

Two neighbouring molecules (green and yellow) each contribute a different portion of their N terminus (residues 2–6 and 16–20) to bind at a central patch of the third molecule (blue). If the NS3P/4A complex is aligned to the blue molecule, and only NS4A residues 27–33 (red ribbon) and enzyme residues 2–6 (purple ribbon) of NS3P/4A are displayed, then these segments are seen to overlap with the NS3P exchanged strands (yellow and green). The exchanged NS3P strands thus mimic internal components of the NS3P/4A structure. This is possible because of nearly identical enzyme surfaces on NS3P and NS3P/4A at the strand-exchange region, along with the ability of NS3P side chains 16–18 to mimic those of NS4A 29–31.

'preformed' site on NS3P, via NS4A residues 28–33. But without a positive charge at NS4A-28, the enzyme's Glu-30 could not be reoriented, nor could the Glu-30/Lys-68 salt link (restraining the D1–E1 loop) be disrupted to provide a site for NS4A residues 21–27. Therefore, concerted enzyme movements necessary for complete NS4A binding, complete N-terminal folding, and ultimately catalytic triad rearrangement, would not occur. The appearance would be competitive binding by the mutant NS4A peptide without a capacity to induce the fully active enzyme configuration.

## MODELLING OF PEPTIDE SUBSTRATES

To explore further the conformational consequences of NS4A binding, we modelled four decapeptide substrates spanning P6 to P4' into the active site of NS3P and NS3P/4A; these peptides contained the endogenous NS3P cleavage sites on the viral polyprotein. Positioning of the substrates was based on the known configuration of peptidic inhibitors bound to trypsin-like proteases [11]. Each peptide was modelled as a transition state adduct with the enzyme and then energetically minimized. An example is shown in Figure 3 for the NS4B/NS5A cleavage site.

When the enzyme–substrate interface for each modelled peptide is compared between NS3P and NS3P/4A, it is clear that substrate residues on the P side of a cleavage site (P1 to P6) will encounter no significant differences. Before and after NS4A binding, the S1 pocket accommodates the P1 cysteine with the same steric complementarity, and β-sheet hydrogen bonds exist between substrate and enzyme from P1 to

**Figure 3.** Model of a bound decapeptide substrate (P6 to P4′) containing the NS4B/NS5A cleavage site

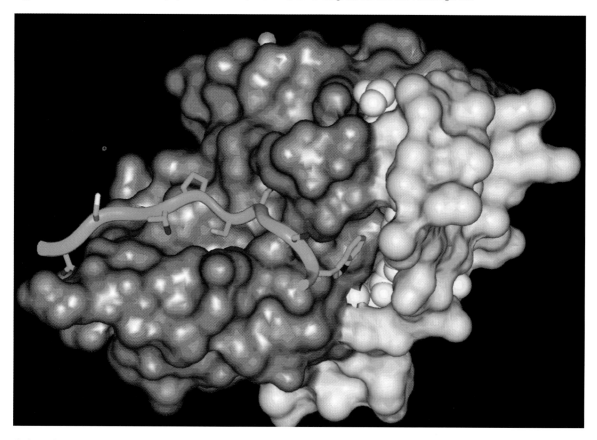

The bound decapeptide displayed with the molecular surface of NS3P/4A in magenta, except for N-terminal residues 2–30, whose surface is shown in blue. NS4A residues 21–34 are shown in yellow. There is a hydrophobic pocket on the P′ side of the substrate-binding surface which can readily accommodate a large side chain, such as this P4′ tryptophan of the NS4B/NS5A substrate. The pocket does not exist before binding of NS4A and refolding of the enzyme's N terminus. Since tryptophan is found at P4′ only in the NS4B/NS5A cleavage site, the favourable interaction depicted may explain the observation that binding affinity for this site is more enhanced by NS4A complexation than for other sites.

P6. However, substrate residues on the P′ side (P1′ to at least P4′ or P5′) will encounter large changes, since a new surface is formed from both the N terminus and NS4A in NS3P/4A; there is also minor repositioning of an enzyme loop between strands A1 and B1. Generally these observations agree with experiments investigating the importance of P′ amino acids in HCV substrates [8,9].

Cleavage at the NS4B/NS5A site, either within the polyprotein context or as a decapeptide, is highly dependent upon activation by NS4A, with cleavage efficiency being enhanced via improved $k_{cat}$ and $K_M$ [8]. Relative to other cleavages, NS4B/NS5A involves the greatest change in $K_M$ after NS4A complexation, thus its binding affinity is the most enhanced. From our model of NS4B/NS5A in NS3P/4A (Fig. 3), we find that the P4′ tryptophan indole could readily insert into a hydrophobic pocket formed by the enzyme's N terminus and bound NS4A. This tryptophan is the

largest hydrophobic side chain found at P4′ among the cleavage sites (the closest is the more polar tyrosine of NS5A/NS5B). Thus, this potential interaction may partially explain the greatly enhanced affinity of NS4B/NS5A decapeptides toward NS3P/4A relative to NS3P.

## MODEL OF THE NS3/NS4A FOLD BEFORE *CIS* CLEAVAGE

Modelling of the decapeptide NS3/NS4A cleavage site into NS3P/4A led us to broader structure–function considerations. For example, just prior to the *cis* cleavage event, NS3 and NS4 (plus NS5) exist as a single polypeptide chain, with some substrate specificity probably contributed by the folding of NS4A residues 1–20 as well as the binding of the central NS4A region (residues 21–34). The presence of folding-related contributions is suggested by the fact

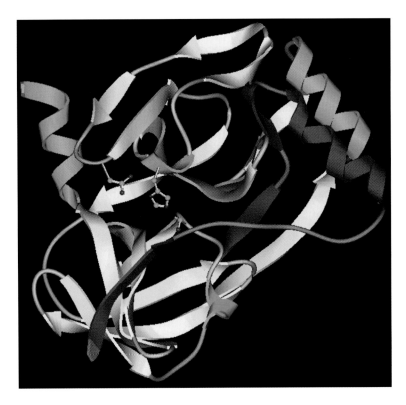

**Figure 4.** Proposed model for NS3P following NS4A complexation but prior to *cis* cleavage at NS3/NS4A

This model is based on the crystal structure of NS3P plus NS4A (residues 21–34), but hypothetically extends the NS4A peptide backward from residue 21 to form an α-helix for residues 8–20 (violet coil), and then further back to join the NS3/NS4A cleavage sequence (modelled independently) at the enzyme's active site. After *cis* cleavage by the catalytic serine, the NS4A hydrophobic helix would be free to swing away and associate with membranes. The enzyme's N-terminal α-helix (green coil on right), presenting a solvent-exposed non-polar surface, might assist in anchoring the otherwise highly charged NS3 complex to a membrane.

that NS3/NS4A has the least favourable P1 residue (threonine), and its cleavage is the least sensitive to mutation at P1 [11]. The first 20 residues of NS4A are extremely hydrophobic and have been proposed to form an α-helix which eventually inserts into a membrane [12]. Since the structure of bound NS4A residues 21–34 is experimentally known (from NS3P/4A), and we have a possible configuration for NS4A residues 1–4 (based on the NS3/NS4A decapeptide model), it is tempting to connect these two segments by constructing a model for NS4A residues 5–20 as they might exist just prior to the *cis* cleavage event. Therefore, we built a hypothetical conformation for NS4A, in which residues 8–20 form an α-helix that packs tightly against the enzyme and lies parallel to the enzyme's N-terminal α-helix (Fig. 4). Cleavage at NS3/NS4A would free the NS4A helix to swing away from the enzyme (pivoting perhaps at residues 20–21) and associate with a membrane. The nearby enzyme α-helix, being hydrophobic yet surprisingly solvent-exposed in the NS3P/4A structure, might improve the overall anchoring of the enzyme close to a membrane. The entire process of NS3-folding/NS4A-binding/*cis* cleavage/membrane association may represent a viral control mechanism that has evolved to ensure simultaneous protease activation and membrane localization of NS3.

## IMPLICATIONS FOR DRUG DESIGN

The exercise of modelling various substrates into the HCV NS3 proteinase reveals the challenges that this enzyme presents for inhibitor design. There is a lack of deep pockets or strong interactions (except possibly a P6 salt bridge) along the enzyme–substrate interface; this is partly because of the shortness of certain loops connecting the central β-strands when compared to other trypsin-like proteases [4,5]. Several experiments support the notion that ground-state binding of substrate is accomplished through multiple interactions, while the P1–S1 contact is the primary determinant of successful hydrolysis [13–15]. The specificity pocket S1 is shallow and relatively non-polar, but is quite selective for cysteine at P1 in most cleavages; the precise basis of this selectively (direct interaction of P1 sulphhydryl and Phe-154 versus a purely steric fit) has yet to be firmly established. These aspects might argue for design of relatively large inhibitors that can form numerous interactions; however, such an approach typically encounters problems of cellular entry and drug stability. But clearly, the development of peptidic inhibitors is a rational starting point for the identification of critical recognition elements.

HCV NS3P is unusual as a serine protease, given its poor response to low concentrations of standard (small molecule) protease inhibitors which target the nucleophile. Target sites on the enzyme other than the cleavage site, such as the NS4A site or the structural zinc site, seem unlikely candidates for enzyme inhibition. NS4A binding is a rapid, cotranslational event that involves intricate intramolecular folding and an effectively high local concentration of NS4A due to the single polyprotein construction. The structural zinc, presumably added during initial enzyme folding, remains tightly bound, and the site itself offers no obvious features that would ensure specific recognition by metal-chelating inhibitors. Nevertheless, these alternative sites should not be excluded from consideration. Ultimately, a combination of approaches, such as variations on a peptidic inhibitor theme, along with carefully chosen small molecule library screening, will be needed to identify the most promising drug type and the most promising enzyme target site. A few reports have recently appeared involving inhibition of NS3P by small compounds [16,17] and peptidic molecules [9,18].

## CONCLUSIONS

By comparing the X-ray structures of NS3P and NS3P/4A, we observe a structural basis for the enhanced substrate turnover and affinity that follow complexation of HCV NS3P with NS4A. There is improved anchoring/orientation of the enzyme's catalytic triad, and increased surface area for substrate interaction on the P′ side of the cleavage site. Modelling of the peptide cleavage sites into these structures has allowed us to define key components of recognition that can be exploited during inhibitor design on the P side, or P′ side, or both. We have also postulated a sequence of structural rearrangements that could occur during NS4A complexation, and have presented a hypothetical configuration for bound NS4A prior to the *cis* cleavage event; both hypotheses may suggest strategies for interfering with early stages of HCV polyprotein processing.

## REFERENCES

1. Houghton M. Hepatitis C viruses. In *Fields Virology*, 3rd edn 1996; pp. 1035–1058. Edited by BN Fields, DM Knipe & PM Howley. New York: Raven Press.
2. Rice CM. *Flaviviridae*: the viruses and their replication. In *Fields Virology*, 3rd edn 1996; pp. 931–960. Edited by BN Fields, DM Knipe & PM Howley. New York: Raven Press.
3. Bartenschlager R. Molecular targets in inhibition of hepatitis C virus replication. *Antiviral Chemistry and Chemotherapy* 1997; **8**:281–301.
4. Love R, Parge HE, Wickersham JA, Hostomsky Z, Habuka N, Moomaw EW, Adachi T & Hostomska Z. The crystal structure of hepatitis C virus NS3 proteinase reveals a trypsin-like fold and a structural zinc binding site. *Cell* 1996; **87**:331–342.
5. Kim JL, Morgenstern KA, Lin C, Fox T, Dwyer MD, Landro JA, Chambers SP, Markland W, Lepre CA, O'Malley ET, Harbeson SL, Rice CM, Murcko MA, Caron PR & Thompson JA. Crystal structure of the hepatitis C virus NS3 protease domain complexed with a synthetic NS4A cofactor peptide. *Cell* 1996; **87**:343–355.
6. Chen Z, Yan Y, Munshi S, Li Y, Sardana V, Blue J, Johns B, Cole J, Steinkueler C, Tomei L & DeFrancesco R. Crystal structure of hepatitis C virus (HCV) NS3 protease–NS4A(21–34) complex. *American Crystallographic Association Annual Meeting*, July 19–25 1997, St Louis, Missouri, USA; Abstract P77.
7. Shimizu Y, Yamaji K, Masuho Y, Yokota T, Inoue H, Sudo K, Satoh S & Shimotohno K. Identification of the sequence on NS4A required for enhanced cleavage of the NS5A/5B site by hepatitis C virus NS3 protease. *Journal of Virology* 1996; **70**:127–132.
8. Steinkuhler C, Urbani A, Tomei L, Biasiol G, Sardana M, Bianchi E, Pessi A & DeFrancesco R. Activity of purified hepatitis C virus protease NS3 on peptide substrates. *Journal of Virology* 1996; **70**: 6694–6700.
9. Landro JA, Raybuck SA, Luong YP, O'Malley ET, Harbeson SL, Morgenstern KA, Rao G & Livingston DJ. Mechanistic role of an NS4A peptide cofactor with the truncated NS3 protease of hepatitis C virus: elucidation of the NS4A stimulatory effect via kinetic analysis and inhibitor mapping. *Biochemistry* 1997; **36**:9340–9348.
10. Bianchi E, Urbani A, Biasiol G, Brunetti M, Pessi A, De Francesco R & Steinkuhler C. Complex formation between the hepatitis C virus serine protease and a synthetic NS4A cofactor peptide. *Biochemistry* 1997; **36**:7890–7897.
11. Read RJ & James MNG. Introduction to the protein inhibitors: X-ray crystallography. In *Proteinase Inhibitors* 1986; pp. 301–336. Edited by AJ Barret & G Salvesen. Amsterdam, New York, Oxford: Elsevier Science.
12. Tanji Y, Hijikata M, Satoh S, Kaneko T & Shimotohno K. Hepatitis C virus-encoded nonstructural protein NS4A has versatile functions in viral protein processing. *Journal of Virology* 1995; **69**:1575–1581.
13. Urbani A, Bianchi E, Narjes F, Tramontano A, DeFrancesco R, Steinkuhler C & Pessi A. Substrate specificity of the hepatitis C virus serine protease NS3. *Journal of Biological Chemistry* 1997; **272**:9204–9209.
14. Koch JO & Bartenschlager R. Determinants of substrate specificity in the NS3 serine proteinase of the hepatitis C virus. *Virology* 1997; **237**:78–88.
15. Zhang R, Durkin J, Windsor WT, McNemar C, Ramanathan L & Hung L. Probing the substrate specificity of hepatitis C virus NS3 serine protease by using synthetic peptides. *Journal of Virology* 1997; **71**: 6208–6213.
16. Chu M, Mierzwa R, Truumees I, King A, Patel M, Berrie R, Hart A, Butkiewicz N, DasMahapatra B, Chan TM & Puar MS. Structure of Sch 68631: a new hepatitis C virus proteinase inhibitor from *Streptomyces* sp. *Tetrahedron Letters* 1996; **37**: 7229–7232.

17. Sudo K, Matsumoto Y, Matsushima M, Fujiwara M, Konno K, Shimotohno K, Shigeta S & Yokota T. Novel hepatitis C virus protease inhibitors: thiazolidine derivatives. *Biochemical and Biophyscial Research Communications* 1997; **238:**643–647.

18. Martin F, Volpari C, Steinkuhler C, Dimasi N, Brunetti M, Biasiol G, Altamura S, Cortese R, DeFrancesco R & Sollazzo M. Affinity selection of a camelized $V_H$ domain antibody inhibitor of hepatitis C virus NS3 protease. *Protein Engineering* 1997; **10:**607–614.

# 28

# Hepatitis C virus non-structural region 5A protein is a potent transcriptional activator

Naoya Kato*, Keng-Hsin Lan,
Suzane Kioko Ono-Nita, Hideo Yoshida,
Yasushi Shiratori and Masao Omata

## SUMMARY

Hepatitis C virus (HCV) non-structural region 5A (NS5A) protein is a serine phosphoprotein containing a nuclear localization signal sequence. However, the function of the NS5A protein is still unknown. Here we report that the NS5A protein, without its 146 N-terminal amino acids and fused to the DNA-binding domain (DNA-BD) of GAL4, a yeast transcriptional activator, strongly activates transcription in yeast and human hepatoma cells. Analysis of various NS5A protein deletion mutants revealed that the transcriptional activation domain resides in the central region of the NS5A protein, between amino acids 2135 and 2331. This region contains two acidic regions and one proline-rich region which appear to be consensus motifs for transcriptional activation. Transcriptional activation by the HCV NS5A protein may play a role in viral replication and hepatocarcinogenesis.

## INTRODUCTION

HCV is a positive-stranded RNA virus with an approximately 10 kb genome and is distantly related to the flaviviruses and the pestiviruses of the family *Flaviviridae* [1,2]. Using the assay method of reverse transcription followed by PCR (RT–PCR), HCV RNA is frequently detected in the serum of patients with non-A, non-B hepatitis. RT–PCR analysis of HCV RNA shows that the majority of anti-HCV-positive patients with chronic liver disease are HCV carriers [3]. The HCV genome contains a large open reading frame (ORF) encoding a polyprotein precursor of 3010–3033 amino acids and untranslated regions (UTR) at the 5′ and 3′ ends of the genome. The putative organization of the HCV genome includes the 5′ UTR, three structural proteins, seven non-structural (NS) proteins, and the 3′ UTR, in order from the 5′

end [4]. One of the NS proteins, NS5A, is a serine phosphoprotein with two isoforms, p56 and p58 (the hyperphosphorylated form of p56) [5]. Clinically, a close association was demonstrated between mutations in the NS5A gene of HCV-1b and the response to interferon α (IFN-α) in patients with chronic active hepatitis [6,7]. Recently, the NS5A protein was shown to bind to the IFN-induced antiviral protein, PKR (double-stranded RNA-dependent protein kinase), and inhibit its kinase activity [8]. However, the function of the NS5A protein is still not fully understood. The NS5A protein was found to possess a nuclear localization-like signal sequence and to be localized in the nuclear periplasmic membrane fraction, so it seems that it may have some function related to transcription or translation [9].

In this study we have shown that N-terminally deleted HCV NS5A protein fused with the DNA-BD of GAL4 strongly activates transcription in yeast and mammalian cells (Huh7 human hepatoma cells) [10]. In addition, the transcriptional activation domain of the NS5A protein was analysed using deletion mutants.

## MATERIALS AND METHODS

### Construction of pGBT9-NS5A plasmids

HCV RNA was extracted from the sera of patients with chronic HCV type 1b infection using SepaGene-RV (Sankyo Junyaku Company). HCV genotyping was performed using PCR with type-specific primers [11]. The nucleotide sequences of the synthetic primers used in the RT-nested PCR are listed in Table 1. Part of the HCV NS5A region was amplified by reverse transcription followed by semi-nested PCR using primers F10 and R9 in the first PCR and primers

**Table 1.** PCR oligonucleotide primers used to construct the pGBT9–NS5A and pM–NS5A plasmids

| Primer | Sequence (5′ to 3′) | Position |
|---|---|---|
| Sense primer | | |
| FK | CTCTCCAGCCTTACCATCAC | 6171–6190 |
| F5 | cgcggaTCCGCTCCGGCTCGTGGCTAAAGGA | 6246–6265 |
| F10 | TGGATGGAGTGCGGTTGCACAGGTA | 6703–6727 |
| F11 | cgcggatcCCGGCGTGCAGACCTCTCCT | 6732–6751 |
| F14 | cgcggatccACAAGGTGGTGGTCCTAGACT | 7072–7092 |
| F15 | cgcggatccGGACGGTTGTCCTGACAGAGTC | 7321–7342 |
| F16 | cgcggatccCTTCAGCTAGCCAGTTGTCTG | 6913–6951 |
| F18 | cgcggatcCGGGTGGGGGGATTTCCACTA | 6612–6631 |
| F19 | cgcggatcCCATGTCAAAAACGGTTCCATGA | 6441–6462 |
| F20 | cgcggatCCCCGAATTCTTCACGGAAT | 6683–6702 |
| Antisense primer | | |
| RK | TCCTTGAGCACTGCCCGGTA | 7795–7776 |
| R5 | cgcggatccGCAGCAGACGATGTCGTCGC | 7586–7567 |
| R9 | cgcggatccCCTCTTTCTCCGTGGAGGTGG | 7322–7302 |
| R13 | cgcggatccATTCTCTGACTCCACACGGGTGA | 7073–7051 |
| R17 | cgcggatccAGAGTGGCCAAGGAGGGGG | 6932–6913 |

Nucleotides complementary to the HCV genome are shown in capitals. *Bam*HI sites are underlined. Nucleotide positions are given relative to the position in the prototype HCV type 1b, HCV-J [37].

F11 and R9 in the second PCR. RT–PCR was performed as previously described [12]. Amplified products were digested with *Bam*HI and then cloned into the *Bam*HI site of pGBT9 (Clontech Laboratories), a yeast expression vector, to generate a fusion protein of NS5A and GAL4 DNA-BD. Cloned plasmids were purified using the Qiagen plasmid kit (Qiagen). Nucleotide sequencing of the cloned plasmids, pGBT9-NS5A/UK1 and pGBT9-NS5A/UK2 from different patients with chronic HCV type 1b, was performed using an autosequencer (PE Applied Biosystems) and the dye-termination method as described previously [13]. Then, the amino acid sequences of the NS5A/UK1 and NS5A/UK2 segments were compared using the computer software package Genetyx-Mac (Software Development Company).

## Transformation of yeast with pGBT9-NS5A and β-galactosidase assay

Experiments with yeast and mammalian cells were performed using the TransAct assay kit (Clontech). The yeast reporter strain used was Y187 (genotype: MAT^a, ura3-52, his3-200, ade2-101, *trp*1-901, *leu*2-3, 112, *gal*4D, met–, *gal*80D, *URA3::GAL1*$_{UAS}$-GAL1$_{TATA}$-*lacZ*) containing an integrated *lacZ* reporter construct which was regulated by the wild-type GAL1 promoter (Clontech). Yeast cells were

made competent for transformation by treatment with lithium acetate as described previously [14]. pCL1 (Clontech), a yeast expression plasmid encoding the full-length wild-type GAL4, was used as a positive control, and pGBT9-HA (Clontech), a yeast expression plasmid encoding a GAL4 DNA-BD/haemagglutinin epitope fusion protein, was used as a weak-positive control. Competent cells were transformed with pGBT9, pCL1, pGBT9-HA, pGBT9-NS5A/UK1 or pGBT9-NS5A/UK2. β-Galactosidase activity was determined using o-nitrophenyl β-D-galactopyranoside as the substrate as previously described [15]. Assays were performed in triplicate.

## Construction of pM-NS5A plasmids

HCV RNA was extracted as outlined above from the serum of a male patient aged 53 years with HCV type 1b chronic active hepatitis. The full-length NS5A region was amplified by the long RT-nested PCR method using the LA RT–PCR kit (Takara Shuzo Company) with primers FK and RK for the first PCR and primers F5 and R5 for the second PCR. The amplified product was digested with *Bam*HI and cloned into the *Bam*HI site of pM (Clontech), a mammalian expression vector, to generate a GAL4 DNA-BD/NS5A hybrid protein under the control of an SV40 promoter. Subsequent PCRs using pM-

NS5A/F5-R5 (full-length NS5A-cloned pM) as the template were performed using primers of various NS5A regions to prepare various deletion mutants (Table 1). PCR products were digested with *Bam*HI and then cloned into the *Bam*HI site of pM. Nucleotide sequences of these plasmids were determined using an autosequencer.

## Transfection of pM-NS5A into Huh7 cells

Huh7 cells (Human Science Research Resource Bank, Osaka, Japan) were grown in RPMI 1640 supplemented with 0.5% fetal bovine serum (FBS) and 10 % lactalbumin at 37°C in a 5% $CO_2$ atmosphere [16]. Approximately $1\times10^6$ Huh7 cells were plated onto 6 cm tissue culture plates (Iwaki Glass Co, Chiba, Japan) 24 h before transfection. Transfection of plasmids into Huh7 cells was performed using Lipofectamine (Gibco BRL). The efficiency of transfection was checked by cotransfection of the β-galactosidase expression plasmid pCMVβ (Clontech) with a series of pM-NS5A plasmids and pG5CAT (Clontech), a chloramphenicol acetyltransferase (CAT) reporter plasmid possessing five GAL4 binding sites and an adenovirus E1b minimum promoter upstream from the CAT gene. Briefly, transfection was carried out by adding to each tissue culture plate 3 ml Opti-MEM I reduced serum medium (Gibco BRL) containing 2.5 μg pM-NS5A, 2.5 μg pG5CAT, 1 μg pCMVβ, and 24 μl lipofectamine. pM3-VP16 (Clontech), a mammalian expression plasmid encoding the herpes simplex virus protein VP16 fused with GAL4 DNA-BD, was used as a positive control. After 16 h, 3 ml RPMI 1640 supplemented with 1% FBS and 20% lactalbumin was added to each dish. After 24 h, the medium was replaced with regular medium.

## CAT assay

Cells were harvested 48 h after transfection. CAT assays were carried out as described previously except that 1-deoxy [dichloroacetyl-1-$^{14}$C] chloramphenicol

**Table 2.** β-galactosidase activities of the pGBT9 plasmids

| Plasmid | β-Galactosidase activity units (mean±SD) |
| --- | --- |
| pGBT9 | 0.1±0.05 |
| pGBT9-HA | 0.2±0.03 |
| pCL | 338±59 |
| pGBT9-NS5A/UK1 | 18±3 |
| pGBT9-NS5A/UK2 | 5±1 |

(Amersham International) was used as the substrate [15]. Assays were performed in triplicate. Autoradiography was performed and CAT activity was quantified using a BAS2000 image analyser (Fuji Photo Film Company) and normalized for transfection efficiency based on β-galactosidase activity.

## RESULTS

### β-Galactosidase assay of pGBT9-NS5A

pGBT9-NS5A/UK1 and pGBT9-NS5A/UK2 transformants exhibited marked β-galactosidase activity when assayed in liquid culture. β-Galactosidase units were calculated as described previously [17]. Data are shown in Table 2. The activities of pGBT9-NS5A/UK1 and pGBT9-NS5A/UK2 transformants were 90- and 25-fold higher, respectively, than the activity of the pGBT9-HA transformant, the weak positive control. Amino acid sequence analysis showed that the sequence identity between the NS5A/UK1 segment and the NS5A/UK2 segment was 85% (168 amino acid residues were identical out of 197 amino acids; Fig. 1).

### CAT assay of pM-NS5A

The N-terminal (146 amino acids) deletion mutants of the HCV NS5A protein fused with GAL4 DNA-BD (pM-NS5A/F20-R5) showed strong transcriptional activation, but the plasmid expressing the full-length

**Figure 1.** Amino acid sequences of the NS5A/UK1 segment and NS5A/UK2 segment

Numbers represent the amino acid position of the prototype HCV type 1b, HCV-J [37]. Two acidic regions are underlined, a proline-rich region is double-underlined.

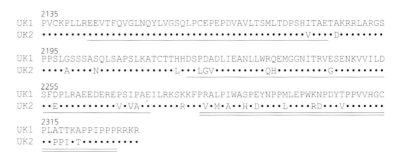

HCV NS5A protein (pM-NS5A/F5-R5) showed no transcriptional activation (Fig. 2).

Of the N-terminal deletion mutants, pM-NS5A/F19-R5 (amino acid residues 2038–2419) and F18-R5 (residues 2095–2419) showed weak or no transcriptional activation, but the longer deletion mutants, F20-R5 (residues 2119–2419) and F11-R5 (residues 2135–2419) showed strong transcriptional activation, the even longer deletion mutants, F16-R5 (residues 2202–2419), F14-R5 (residues 2249–2419) and F15-R5 (residues 2332–2419) showed weak or no transcriptional activation. The C-terminal (88 amino acids) deletion mutants showed a pattern similar to that obtained with the N-terminal deletion mutants. That is, of these C-terminal deletion mutants, pM-NS5A/F5-R9 (residues 1973–2331), F19-R9 (residues 2038–2331) and F18-R9 (residues 2095–2331) showed little or no activity, but F20-R9 (residues 2119–2331) and F11-R9 (residues 2135–2331) activated transcription strongly, and F16-R9 (residues 2202–2331) and F14-R9 (residues 2249–2331) showed weak or no transcriptional activation. The longer deletion mutants, pM-NS5A/F11-R13 (residues 2135–2248) still showed distinct transcriptional activation, while F11-R17 (residues 2135–2201), the N-terminal part of F11-R13, and F16-R13 (residues 2202–2248), the C-terminal part of F11-R13, showed weak or no transcriptional activation. Expression of the fusion proteins was examined by Western blot using soluble protein cell extracts and a monoclonal antibody against the GAL4 DNA-BD (Clontech) following standard Western blotting procedures (Kato and Lan, data not shown) [18].

Analysis of the NS5A protein deletion mutants revealed that the transcriptional activation domain may exist within the F11-R9 segment of the HCV NS5A protein (residues 2135–2331), because other deletion mutants (pM-NS5A/F16-R9, F14-R9, F11-R13, F16-R13, and F11-R17) which have longer deletions showed weak or no transcriptional activa-

Figure 2. Identification of the HCV NS5A segment responsible for transcriptional activation

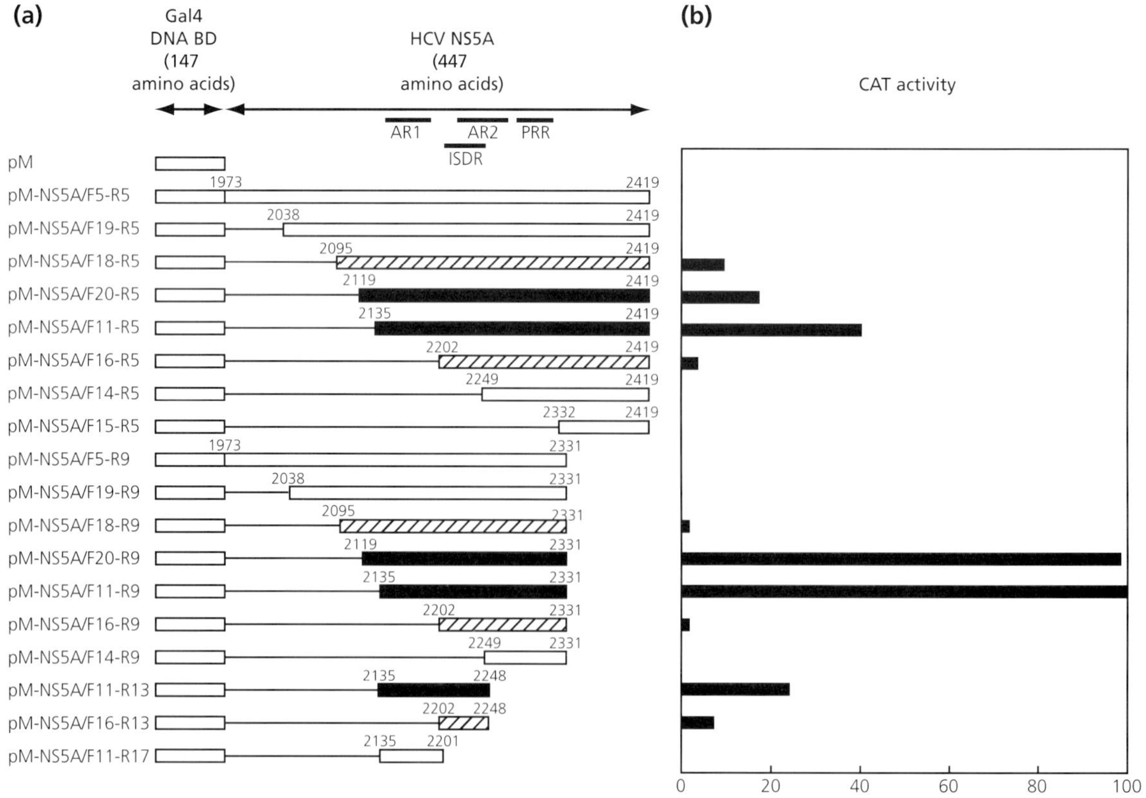

(a) Bars represent the segments of the HCV NS5A protein which are present. Solid bars, hatched bars and open bars indicate the HCV NS5A protein mutants that activate transcription strongly, poorly or not at all, respectively. Numbers indicate the amino acid position in the prototype HCV type 1b, HCV-J [37]. AR1, acidic region 1; AR2, acidic region 2; PRR, proline-rich region; ISDR, interferon sensitivity determining region. (b) CAT activity was normalized by taking the highest activity (pM-NS5A/F11-R9) as 100. Results are expressed as the mean of three experiments by solid bar.

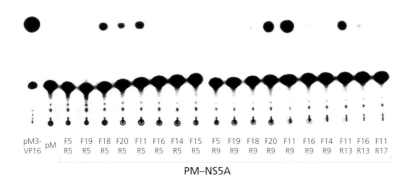

**Figure 3.** Representative CAT assay of transcriptional activation by pM-NS5A

pM3-VP16 was used as the positive control; VP16 is a herpes virus protein which is a strong transcriptional activator. pM is a wild-type plasmid used as the negative control.

| pM3-VP16 | pM | F5 R5 | F19 R5 | F18 R5 | F20 R5 | F11 R5 | F16 R5 | F14 R5 | F15 R5 | F5 R9 | F19 R9 | F18 R9 | F20 R9 | F11 R9 | F16 R9 | F14 R9 | F11 R13 | F16 R13 | F11 R17 |

PM–NS5A

```
2135          2145          2155          2165          2175          2185
+      +--                           -    -              -          -   +++   +
PACRPLLRDE VTFQVGLNQY PVGSQLPCEP EPDVTVITSM LTDPSHITAE AAKRRLARGS

2195          2205          2215          2225          2235          2245
                     +       -  -     -  -        +    -          +   - - -    -
PPSLASSSAS QLSAPSLKAT CTTWHDSPDA DLIEANLLWR QEMGGNITRV ESENEVVVLD

2255          2265          2275          2285          2295          2305
  -    +  ---   -+-      -  ++ ++  •    •   • +•      •• •••    +  •   ••
SFEPLRAEED EREVSVAAEI LRKTRRFPAA MPVWARPDYN PPLLESWKNP XYVPPVVHGC

2315          2325
•  •• • •• •••++++
PLPPTRAPPI PPPRRKR
```

**Figure 4.** Amino acid sequence of the F11-R9 segment of the HCV NS5A protein

Numbers represent the amino acid position in the prototype HCV type 1b, HCV-J [37]. Positively charged residues (R and K) are marked '+' and negatively charged residues (D and E) are marked '–'. The two acidic regions are underlined and the proline-rich region (PRR) is double-underlined. Proline residues in the PRR are indicated by dots.

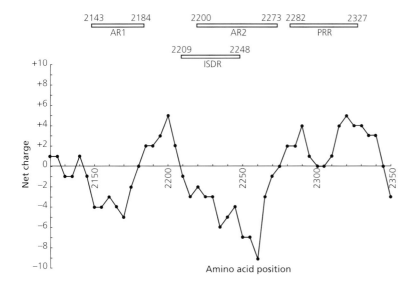

**Figure 5.** Purported functional regions and charge distribution within the F11-R9 segment of the HCV NS5A protein

Shown is the net charge of 30 sequential amino acids measured at five amino acid intervals. Numbers indicate the amino acid position in the prototype HCV type 1b, HCV-J [37]. AR1, acidic region 1; AR2, acidic region 2; PRR, proline-rich region; ISDR, interferon sensitivity determining region.

tion. A representative CAT assay result is shown in Figure 3. The nucleotide sequence of the F11-R9 segment was confirmed bidirectionally and then deduced into amino acids (Fig. 4). The net charge of 30 sequential amino acids was measured at five amino acid intervals (see Fig. 5 for charge distribution within the NS5A/F11-R9 segment). Analysis of the amino acid sequence of the F11-R9 segment revealed that the purported transcriptional activation domain contained two acidic regions (AR1 and AR2) and one proline-rich region (PRR). The HCV NS5A/F11-R9 segment showed no similarity with previously reported amino acid sequences as analysed using the Genetyx-Mac/CD computer software package.

## DISCUSSION

The NS5A protein is a serine phosphoprotein with two isoforms, p56 and p58. The p58 isoform is a hyper-phosphorylated form of p56, and its presence depends on the presence of NS4A protein [5]. The NS5A protein possesses a nuclear localization-like signal sequence and is present in the nuclear periplasmic membrane fraction, which indicates that it may have some function related to transcription or translation [9]; however, its exact function is still unknown. We found that when deleted of its 146 N-terminal amino acids, the NS5A protein acted as a strong transcriptional activator. Analysis of various NS5A deletion mutants shows that the transcriptional activation domain should lie within the F11-R9 segment (197 amino acids, from residues 2135–2331) of the HCV NS5A protein. This segment contains two acidic regions, AR1 and AR2, and one proline-rich region, PRR. AR1 consists of 42 amino acids (from residues 2143 to 2184 of the HCV NS5A region) with seven acidic residues (Glu or Asp) (17%), and AR2 consists of 54 amino acids (from residues 2220–2273) with 16 acidic residues (Glu or Asp) (30%). PRR consists of 46 amino acids (from residues 2282–2327) with 16 proline residues (35%). These acidic and proline-rich domains in addition to a glutamine-rich domain are considered consensus motifs of a transcriptional activation domain [19–21]. As examples, an acidic domain exists in GAL4 and GCN4 of yeast and VP16 of herpes simplex virus [22–24]. A proline-rich domain exists in CTF/NF-1, Jun, AP-2 and Oct-2 [25]. Although the actual contribution to transcriptional activation of the AR1, AR2 and PRR domains is as yet unknown, their contribution seems to be co-operative because mutants with more extensive deletions showed weak or no transcriptional activation. AR1 and AR2 seem to be essential for transcriptional activation, and although PRR seems not to be essential for transcriptional activation it seems to enhance it, since the pM-NS5A/F11-R13 mutant, lacking the PRR of the pM-NS5A/F11-R9 mutant, showed distinct transcriptional activation.

The full-length HCV NS5A protein fused with GAL4 DNA-BD did not activate transcription. The 146 N-terminal amino acids may mask the function of transcriptional activation. It may be that the 146 N-terminal amino acids are a regulatory region. For example, HCV NS4A protein (p4) was found to bind to the N-terminal region of the NS5A protein, and the NS5A protein is hyperphosphorylated at serine residues in an NS4A-dependent manner [26]. Therefore, it is possible that the NS4A protein functions as a regulatory factor. A similar phenomenon has been demonstrated for hMTF-1, a heavy metal-responsive transcription regulator in humans. Full-length hMTF-1 shows only weak transcriptional activation in the absence of heavy metals. The N-terminal part of hMTF-1 is a regulatory domain for metal induction. Therefore, hMTF-1 with the N-terminal region deleted shows transcriptional activation when fused to the GAL4 DNA-BD [27].

Although we have shown that HCV NS5A protein is a potent transcriptional activator, its actual function is still not known. HCV is a causative agent of hepatocellular carcinoma (HCC), which occurs all over the world, although the mechanism for HCC is still unknown [28–30]. It is possible that the NS5A protein plays a role in hepatocarcinogenesis, since many other viral proteins that play a role in carcinogenesis often function as transcriptional activators. Actually, retroviral oncogenes such as *myc*, *fos*, *jun*, *myb*, *rel*, *maf* and *ets* are all DNA-binding transcriptional activators. The human T cell leukaemia virus type 1 oncogene *tax* (transcriptional activator coded in the X-region) is also a transcriptional activator but it has no DNA-binding ability [31]. In fact, DNA virus oncogenes such as adenovirus early region 1A (E1A), simian virus 40 (SV40) large T antigen, and papillomavirus E6/E7 are transcriptional activators that have no DNA-binding ability [32–34]. Recently it was shown that NIH 3T3 mouse fibroblasts could be transformed with HCV NS3 cDNA and were then tumorigenic in nude mice [35]. Transformation of cells with the NS5A protein should be investigated with respect to oncogenic activity.

In a recent study, the amino acid residues 2209 to 2248 (IFN sensitivity determining region; ISDR) of the HCV-1b NS5A protein were implicated in responsiveness to IFN-$\alpha$ therapy in patients with chronic active hepatitis and the levels of serum HCV RNA [6,7]. The NS5A F11-R9 segment (amino acids 2135–2419) contains the ISDR (amino acids 2209–2248). Thus, it may be that the NS5A protein affects the response to IFN and viral replication through the function of transcriptional activation by regulating the transcription of certain cellular factors that have antiviral functions or play a role in replication. Mutations in this region affected transcription in yeast (Table 1 and Fig. 1) and in Huh7 cells (Kato and Lan, unpublished observations). Sequence analysis of many strains of HCV revealed that there is a high degree of interstrain as well as intrastrain non-homology, which suggests that different strains with different capacities for transcriptional activation may be a reason for the clinical differences between patients infected with different strains of HCV [36].

The results of this study clearly show that the HCV NS5A protein is a potent transcriptional activator. However, its DNA-binding ability, cellular target and the relationship between its activity and state of phosphorylation are still not known. Further investigations are necessary to elucidate the functions of this protein.

# REFERENCES

1. Choo Q-L, Kuo G, Weiner AJ, Overby LR, Bradley DW & Houghton M. Isolation of a cDNA clone derived from a blood-borne non-A, non-B viral hepatitis genome. *Science* 1989; **244**:359–362.
2. Miller RH & Purcell RH. Hepatitis C virus shares amino acid sequence similarity with pestiviruses and flaviviruses as well as members of two plant virus supergroups. *Proceedings of the National Academy of Sciences, USA* 1990; **87**:2057–2061.
3. Kato N, Yokosuka O, Omata M, Hosoda K & Ohto M. Detection of hepatitis C virus ribonucleic acid in the serum by amplification with polymerase chain reaction. *Journal of Clinical Investigation* 1990; **86**:1764–1767.
4. Choo Q-L, Richman KH, Han JH, Berger K, Lee C, Dong C, Gallegos C, Coito D, Medina-Selby R, Barr PJ, Weiner AJ, Bradley DW, Kuo G & Houghton M. Genetic organization and diversity of the hepatitis C virus. *Proceedings of the National Academy of Sciences, USA* 1991; **88**:2451–2455.
5. Kaneko T, Tanji Y, Satoh S, Hijikata M, Asabe S, Kimura K & Shimotohno K. Production of two phosphoproteins from the NS5A region of the hepatitis C virus genome. *Biophysical and Biochemical Research Communications* 1994; **205**:320–326.
6. Enomoto N, Sakuma I, Asahina Y, Kurosaki M, Murakami T, Yamamoto C, Izumi N, Marumo F & Sato C. Comparison of full-length sequences of interferon-sensitive and resistant hepatitis C virus 1b: Sensitivity to interferon is conferred by amino acid substitutions in the NS5A region. *Journal of Clinical Investigation* 1995; **96**:224–230.
7. Enomoto N, Sakuma I, Asahina Y, Kurosaki M, Murakami T, Yamamoto C, Ogura Y, Izumi N, Marumo F & Sato C. Mutations in the nonstructural protein 5A gene and response to interferon in patients with chronic hepatitis C virus 1b infection. *New England Journal of Medicine* 1996; **334**:77–81.
8. Gale MJ Jr, Korth MJ, Tang NM, Tan S-L, Hopkins DA, Dever TE, Polyak SJ, Gretch DR & Katze MG. Evidence that hepatitis C virus resistant to interferon is mediated through repression of the PKR protein kinase by the nonstructural 5A protein. *Virology* 1997; **230**:217–227.
9. Tanji Y, Kaneko T, Satoh S & Shimotohno K. Phosphorylation of hepatitis C virus-encoded nonstructural protein NS5A. *Journal of Virology* 1995; **69**:3980–3986.
10. Kato N, Lan K-H, Ono-Nita SK, Shiratori Y & Omata M. Hepatitis C virus nonstructural region 5A protein is a potent transcriptional activator. *Journal of Virology* 1997; **71**:8856–8859.
11. Okamoto H, Sugiyama Y, Okada S, Kurai K, Akahane Y, Sugai Y, Tanaka T, Sato K, Tsuda F, Miyakawa Y & Mayumi M. Typing hepatitis C virus by polymerase chain reaction with type-specific primers: application to clinical surveys and tracing infectious sources. *Journal of General Virology* 1992; **73**:673–679.
12. Kato N, Yokosuka O, Hosoda K, Ito Y, Ohto M & Omata M. Detection of hepatitis C virus RNA in acute non-A, non-B hepatitis as an early diagnostic tool. *Biochemical and Biophysical Research Communications* 1993; **192**:800–807.
13. Togo G, Toda N, Kanai F, Kato N, Shiratori Y, Kishi K, Imazeki F, Makuuchi M & Omata M. A transforming growth factor b type II receptor gene mutation common in sporadic cecum cancer with microsatellite instability. *Cancer Research* 1996; **56**:5620–5623.
14. Becker DM & Guarente L. High-efficiency transformation of yeast by electroporation. In *Methods in Enzymology*, vol. 194, Guide to yeast genetics and molecular biology 1991; pp. 182–187. Edited by Guthrie C & Fink GR. San Diego: Academic Press.
15. Sambrook J, Fritsch EF & Maniatis T. Expression of cloned genes in cultured mammalian cells. In *Molecular Cloning, A Laboratory Manual*. 2nd edn 1989; pp. 16.1–16.81. Edited by Nolan C Plainview: Cold Spring Harbor Laboratory Press.
16. Nakabayashi H, Taketa K, Miyano K, Yamane T & Sato J. Growth of human hepatoma cell lines with differentiated functions in chemically defined medium. *Cancer Research* 1982; **42**:3858–3863.
17. Miller JH. *Experiments in molecular genetics*. 1972. Cold Spring Harbor: Cold Spring Harbor Laboratory Press.
18. Sambrook J, Fritsch EF & Maniatis T. Detection and analysis of proteins expressed from cloned genes. *In Molecular Cloning, A Laboratory Manual*. 2nd edn 1989; pp 18.1–18.88. Edited by Nolan C Plainview: Cold Spring Harbor Laboratory Press.
19. Courey AJ & Tjian R. Analysis of Sp1 *in vivo* reveals multiple transcriptional domains, including a novel glutamine-rich activation motif. *Cell* 1988; **55**:887–898.
20. Ma J & Ptashne M. A new class of yeast transcriptional activators. *Cell* 1987; **51**:113–119.
21. Mermod N, O'Neill EA, Kelly TJ & Tjian R. The proline-rich transcriptional activator of CTF/NF-1 is distinct from the replication and DNA binding domain. *Cell* 1989; **58**:741–753.
22. Campbell ME, Palfreyman JW & Preston CM. Identification of herpes simplex virus DNA sequences which encode a trans-acting polypeptide responsible for stimulation of immediate early transcription. *Journal of Molecular Biology* 1984; **180**:1–19.
23. Hope IA & Struhl K. Functional dissection of a eukaryotic transcriptional activator protein, GCN4 of yeast. *Cell* 1986; **46**:885–894.
24. Ma J & Ptashne M. Deletion analysis of GAL4 defines two transcriptional activating segments. *Cell* 1987; **48**:847–853.
25. Mitchell PJ & Tjian R. Transcriptional regulation in mammalian cells by sequence-specific DNA binding proteins. *Science* 1989; **245**:371–378.
26. Asabe S, Tanji Y, Satoh S, Kaneko T, Kimura K & Shimotohno K. The N-terminal region of hepatitis C virus-encoded NS5A is important for NS4A-dependent

phosphorylation. *Journal of Virology* 1997; **71**:790–796.

27. Radtke F, Georgiev O, Muller H-P, Brugnera E & Schaffner W. Functional domains of the heavy metal-responsive transcription regulator MTF-1. *Nucleic Acids Research* 1995; **23**:2277–2286.

28. Kuo G, Choo Q-L, Alter HJ, Gitnick GL, Redeker AG, Purcell RH, Miyamura T, Dienstag JL, Alter MJ, Stevens CE, Tegtmeier GE, Bonino F, Colombo M, Lee AS, Kuo C, Berger K, Shuster JR, Overby LR, Bradley DW & Houghton M. An assay for circulating antibodies to a major etiologic virus of human non-A, non-B hepatitis. *Science* 1989; **344**:362–364.

29. Okuda K. Hepatocellular carcinoma: Recent progress. *Hepatology* 1992; **15**:948–963.

30. Saito I, Miyamura T, Ohbayashi A, Harada H, Katayama T, Kikuchi S, Watanabe Y, Koi S, Onji M, Ohta Y, Choo Q-L, Houghton M & Kuo G. Hepatitis C virus infection is associated with the development of hepatocellular carcinoma. *Proceedings of the National Academy of Sciences, USA* 1990; **87**:6547–6549.

31. Seiki M, Inoue J, Takeda T & Yoshida M. Direct evidence that p40x of human T-cell leukemia virus type I is a trans-acting transcriptional activator. *EMBO Journal* 1986; **5**:561–565.

32. Berk AJ. Adenovirus promoters and E1A transactivation. *Annual Review of Genetics* 1986; **20**:45–79.

33. Manfredi JJ & Prives C. The transforming activity of simian virus 40 large tumor antigen. *Biochemica et Biophysica Acta* 1994; **1198**:65–83.

34. Schwarz E, Freese UK, Gissmann L, Mayer W, Roggenbuck A, Stremlau B & zur Hausen H. Structure and transcription of human papillomavirus sequences in cervical carcinoma cells. *Nature* 1985; **314**: 111–114.

35. Sakamuro D, Furukawa T & Takegami T. Hepatitis C virus nonstructural protein NS3 transforms NIH 3T3 cells. *Journal of Virology* 1995; **69**:3893–3896.

36. Kato N, Shiratori Y & Omata M. Hepatitis C virus genotypes: molecular basis and clinical significance. In *Progress in Liver Diseases*, vol. XIV 1996; pp. 223–244. Edited by Boyer JL & Ockner RK. Philadelphia: WB Saunders Company.

37. Kato N, Hijikata M, Ootsuyama Y, Nakagawa N, Ohkoshi S, Sugimura T & Shimotohno K. Molecular cloning of the human hepatitis C virus genome from Japanese patients with non-A, non-B hepatitis. *Proceedings of the National Academy of Sciences, USA* 1990; **87**:9524–9528.

# 29 Protein processing of hepatitis C virus and investigation of the effects of viral proteins on cell proliferation

Shinya Satoh, Masami Hirota, Michiharu Inudoh, Nobuyuki Kato, Makoto Hijikata and Kunitada Shimotohno*

## INTRODUCTION

Hepatitis C virus (HCV), has a positive sense, single-stranded RNA genome of about 9.4 kb, and is the major cause of non-A, non-B hepatitis [1–6]. The HCV genome encodes a large polyprotein precursor. Comparative analysis of the genomes of several HCV strains indicated the virus to be closely related to both the pestivirus and flavivirus genera within the family *Flaviviridae*. Further studies of protein processing as well as hydropathy profile analysis of each viral protein suggested that HCV belongs to a new genus of the *Flaviviridae* [6,7]. The genomic organization of HCV, illustrated schematically in Figure 1, is homologous with those of related viruses, particularly, the pestiviruses [8].

## Translational strategy of HCV precursor polyprotein

The HCV genome has an untranslated region (UTR) at the 5′ end of the genome. It has been shown that polyprotein synthesis is initiated at nucleotide position 342 [9]. Because this region has a characteristic resemblance to the picornavirus 5′ UTR – such as the presence of several AUG codons scattered in this region and the possible formation of extensive secondary structure – it is suspected that the machinery translating the HCV proteins utilizes the internal ribosome entry site (IRES)-dependent system. In fact, it was demonstrated using *in vitro* expression systems that the HCV 5′ UTR could regulate translational initiation in a cap-independent manner [10].

## Proteolytic cleavage of the precursor polyprotein by signal peptidases

Apart from analysing precise mechanism of IRES-dependent translation, we have developed a system for the analysis of protein production using an *in vitro* microsomal processing system. We showed that a microsomal membrane-dependent proteinase activity processes the putative HCV proteins from the N-terminal half of a precursor viral protein [11]. Virus proteins produced by this mechanism include core, E1, E2 and E2-p7. A core protein of 21 kDa (p21) is released from the viral polyprotein by nascent proteo-lytic cleavage at amino acid 191 by host proteases [11]. However, it was shown that a second species of 19 kDa (p19) is generated by a secondary cleavage at amino acid 173 in mammalian cells [12–13]. Both p21 and p19 are located in the endoplasmic reticulum (ER) membrane and the conversion of p21 to p19 is presumably mediated by membrane-associated cellular enzymes. Both p21 and p19 have a cluster of hydrophobic amino acids at their C-terminal ends that act as translocation and stop-transfer signals to the membrane, and thus retain these proteins on the membrane. A further truncated form of the core protein, an approximately 151 amino acid protein, has also been detected in expression studies [14] and appears to be located in the nucleus.

E1 and E2 are major viral structural proteins and are glycosylated at N-linked glycosylation sites. These proteins are released from the viral precursor polyprotein by cleavage of host cell signal peptidases. Analysis of the amino termini of E1 (gp35) and E2 (gp70) indicated that they are cleaved at amino acids 383 and

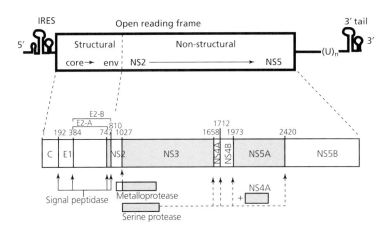

**Figure 1.** Schematic structure of HCV-1b genome and HCV polyprotein processing

Upper panel: structure of HCV-1b genome; lower panel: HCV polyprotein processing. Cleavage sites by signal peptidases, virus metalloprotease and virus serine protease are indicated by arrows and numbers of the N-terminal amino acid of each virus protein in the HCV precursor polyprotein.

746, respectively [11,15–17]. Some E2 is extended at its carboxyl terminus to include a smaller protein known as p7 [16–21]. The proteolytic cleavage between E2/p7 and p7/NS2 appears to occur post-translationally.

## Production of NS2 and involvement of a specific virus protease

The C terminus of NS2 is generated by cleavage with a virus-encoded protease that is distinct from another virus-encoded serine protease. This second virus-encoded protease was first reported by Hijikata et al. [22] who found that the protease responsible for the cleavage between NS2 and NS3 is derived from regions of both NS2 and NS3. Detailed analysis of the results of mapping studies [18,22] delineated the proteolytic domain for this activity from amino acids 827 to 1207, which encompasses the carboxyl terminus of NS2 and the amino terminus of NS3. Thus, the C-terminal region overlaps the domain for the serine protease in NS3. The activity of this protease is inhibited by EDTA and is restored by zinc ions.

## Production of non-structural virus proteins

NS3 is a 70 kDa protein with two different biochemical functions: serine protease and helicase. The N-terminal one-third of the molecule possesses the serine protease activity and the remainder the helicase activity. His-1083, Asp-1107 and Ser-1165 in NS3 constitute the catalytic triad present in all serine proteases analysed to date, and the spatial arrangement between these residues is also conserved suggesting that this region of the NS3 protein constitutes a serine protease. The NS3 protease mediates proteolysis at NS3/NS4A, NS4A/NS4B, NS4B/NS5A and NS5A/NS5B junctions to release NS3, NS4A, NS4B, NS5A and NS5B proteins. Cleavage at

NS3/NS4A is conducted in a *cis*-acting manner, whereas cleavage at the other sites occurs in *trans*. The efficient cleavage at these *trans*-cleavage sites is dependent on the presence of another HCV protein, NS4A, which acts as a cofactor for NS3. Mutagenesis experiments showed that the site of association between NS3 and NS4A lies in the amino-terminal region of the NS3 molecule [23,24], and the central region of NS4A is important for the association [23–29]. There are characteristic motifs of amino acids in the C-terminal region of NS3 for NTPase and RNA helicase activities. The presence of NTPase activity was confirmed by D'Souza et al. [30] and Suzich et al. [31]. Subsequently, other groups showed the presence of the RNA helicase activity [32]. Detailed biochemical and kinetic analyses were conducted by Preugschat et al. [33].

NS4A is a small protein with 54 amino acid residues. This protein is likely to play an important regulatory role in virus replication such as functioning as a cofactor for NS3 and as a modulator of phosphorylation of NS5A. NS4B is a hydrophobic protein the function of which in virus replication is not yet clear.

Plasmid-based expression of NS5A revealed production of two proteins which differ in SDS–PAGE mobility. The difference in size of these proteins was reflected by the different degrees of phosphorylation, which was in turn affected by the presence of NS4A. NS5B has RNA polymerase activity and is believed to be a key enzyme for viral RNA replication.

In total, at least 11 virus proteins are produced from the virus precursor polyprotein.

## Post-translational modification of HCV proteins

Four of these HCV proteins – core, E1, E2 and NS5A – are modified after translation. Core and NS5A are phosphorylated and E1 and E2 are glycosylated. Gylcosylation of E1 and E2 occurs in the endoplasmic reticulum, and modification of the glycosylation to so-called complex form occurs during the process of virus maturation.

Core protein is phosphorylated on its serine residues. Both the longest core protein (21 kDa) and its processed forms (19 and 15 kDa) were phosphorylated in insect cells in which these proteins were transiently expressed using the baculovirus expression vector.

Using the glutathione S-transferase fusion protein expression system and an in vitro coupled transcription–translation system, the phosphorylation of HCV core protein was shown to be carried out by protein kinase A (PKA) and protein kinase C (PKC) in vitro. The potential phosphorylated sites in core protein were identified as residues Ser-53 and Ser-116 for PKA and Ser-53 and Ser-99 for PKC. Comparison of the phosphorylation intensities of the wild-type and variants with mutations on serine residues suggested that Ser-99 and Ser-116 were the major phosphorylation sites for PKC and PKA, respectively [34]. It was also shown that phosphorylation of Ser-99 and Ser-116 is essential for the suppressive activity of HCV core protein on HBV gene expression.

The NS5A region produces two proteins; a faster-migrating form, the 56 kDa protein (p56), and a slower-migrating form, of 58 kDa (p58), which are distinguishable by SDS–PAGE [35–39]. Both forms are phosphorylated [36]. Detailed analysis of phosphorylation sites indicated that both proteins were phosphorylated at serine residues in the C-terminal region of NS5A and that p58 is additionally phosphorylated at serine residues in the central region [40]. When only the NS5A region of the HCV genome is expressed in cultured cells, most of the product is p56 with a trace amount of p58. In the presence of NS4A, however, the production of p58 is augmented strongly and both forms of NS5A are produced. The physiological role of NS5A phosphorylation in virus replication remains to be clarified.

By analysing the NS4A-dependent phosphorylation of a variety of N-terminally deleted and internally deleted forms of NS5A by examination of electrophoretic mobility, we determined that one region in the N-terminal portion of NS5A had an important role in phosphorylation of the central region of NS5A. When this region was deleted, phosphorylation of the central region of NS5A was no longer augmented by NS4A. The association of NS5A with NS4A was found to be important for phosphorylation of serine residues on the central region of NS5A. Precisely how

NS4A affects phosphorylation in the central region of NS5A remains to be clarified. A cellular serine kinase is involved in phosphorylation of NS5A. Therefore, one role of NS4A may be as a modulator which directly affects the kinase activity. Also, NS4A may facilitate NS5A phosphorylation through an interaction that results in exposure of phosphorylation sites to cellular serine kinases.

## Effects of HCV protein on cell proliferation: interaction of NS5A with PKR

There have been several reports that expression of HCV proteins modifies proliferation of cells [41–43]. These proteins include core, NS3 and NS5A. We were interested in clarifying the effects of NS5A on cell proliferation because this protein is highly mutated among virus proteins and also it has been reported that this protein might affect the efficacy of interferon treatment. In a previous study using the yeast assay system, it was reported that NS5A interacts with interferon-induced double-stranded RNA-dependent protein kinase (PKR) and the kinase activity of PKR is abolished [44]. We confirmed the association of NS5A with PKR in mammalian Saos-2 cells expressing the NS5A gene.

To identify the region in NS5A that is important for association with PKR, N- and C-terminally deleted NS5A proteins fused with E-tag (Pharmacia) were produced in Saos-2 cells. NS5A which lacks amino acid residue 163 still formed a complex with PKR. However, deletion of a further six amino acid residues severely impaired the association with PKR (Fig. 2a). The interaction of the C-terminally deleted NS5A with PKR was also analysed. In this case, deletion of 69 amino acid residues impaired the association (Fig. 2b). These results indicated that the region from amino acid 164 to the C terminus of NS5A was important for the association with PKR.

Trans-phosphorylation of PKR is an important step for activation of this protein to function as an antiviral mediator [45]. Many mechanisms are employed to block this activation process. Of these, viral and cellular inhibitors of PKR such as vaccinia virus K3L, HIV-1 Tat, and the cellular protein p58, block trans-phosphorylation of PKR mediated through the direct interaction with PKR [46–48]. To test whether NS5A inhibits trans-phosphorylation of PKR through the association with PKR in Saos-2 cells, we analysed the phosphorylation state of PKR in the PKR/NS5A complex. When cells which produce NS5A were metabolically labelled with [$^{35}$S]methionine and [$^{32}$P]orthophosphate, the methionine-labelled PKR co-precipitated with NS5A.

**Figure 2.** Determination of the region in HCV NS5A responsible for the association with PKR

**(a)**

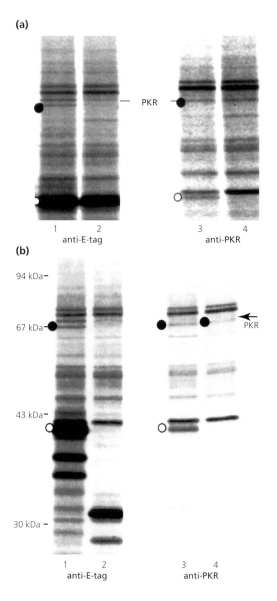

**(b)**

94 kDa–

67 kDa–

43 kDa–

30 kDa –

| 1 | 2 | 3 | 4 |
| anti-E-tag | | anti-PKR | |

(a) Analysis of the association of N-terminal-deleted NS5A with PKR by co-immunoprecipitation. ³⁵S-labelled Saos-2 cells transfected with a plasmid which produces the N-terminal-deleted NS5A (deletion from 1973 to 2134 of NS5A shown in Fig. 1) with an E-tag at the C-terminal end (lanes 1 and 3) or with a plasmid which produces the N-terminal-deleted NS5A (deletion from 1973 to 2139 of NS5A shown in Fig. 1) with an E-tag at the C-terminal end (lanes 2 and 4), were immunoprecipitated with anti-E-tag antibody (lanes 1 and 2) or with anti-PKR antibody (lanes 3 and 4). The immunoprecipitants were analysed by SDS–PAGE followed by radioimaging anlaysis. (b) An experiment similar to that shown in (a) was conducted except using a plasmid which produces the same N-terminal-deleted NS5A (from 1973 to 2134) (lanes 1 and 3) or the C-terminal-deleted derivative derived from the N-terminal-deleted NS5A (from 1973 to 2134) (lanes 2 and 4). Closed circles indicate PKR and open circles NS5A derivatives.

**Figure 3.** PKR complexed with NS5A is hypophosphorylated

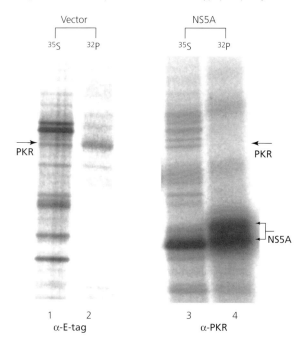

Saos-2 cells were transfected with an empty vector (lanes 1 and 3) or E-tagged-NS5A expression vector (lanes 3 and 4), and then ³⁵S- or ³²P-radiolabelled. Immunoprecipitation with anti-PKR antibody (lanes 1 and 2) or anti-E-tag antibody was analysed by SDS–PAGE.

However, no incorporation of ³²P radioactivity in the PKR was detected in the same fractions (Fig. 3). This result indicated that NS5A associated with unphosphorylated PKR suggesting that NS5A impaired the function of PKR through this association. Interaction of HCV NS5A with PKR, and inactivation of PKR by this interaction was recently demonstrated by Gale *et al.* using biochemical and yeast genetic approaches [44]. It is likely that phosphorylation of PKR is blocked by the association with NS5A. Thus, inhibition of PKR activity by HCV NS5A could be one of the mechanisms to prevent the effects of interferon (IFN) on viral replication in cells. Conversely, it is also possible that PKR may interfere with the role of NS5A on virus replication through this association. We identified the region of NS5A important for the interaction with PKR. This region spanned more than two-thirds of the C-terminal region of NS5A. Previously, we showed that HCV NS4A interacts with the N-terminal region of NS5A and that this interaction is important for phosphorylation of serine residues in the central region of NS5A. One such region in NS5A (interacting with NS4A) mapped to the very N-terminal region essential for the interaction with PKR.

Recently, a molecular epidemiological study suggested that the region responsible for determining interferon sensitivity was present in the HCV NS5A gene and this region was designated as interferon sensitivity determining region (ISDR) [49,50]. Amino acid sequence variations in this region have been proposed to affect the efficacy of IFN treatment [49,50]. However, conflicting results were also reported recently [51]. Nevertheless, we are interested in analysing the effects of amino acid variations in NS5A ISDR on PKR association. The interactions with PKR were examined in Saos-2 cells using several NS5A proteins with different amino acid sequences in the ISDR. All mutated NS5As associated with PKR (data not shown). Moreover, NS5A derivatives lacking the ISDR still interacted with PKR, and therefore the ISDR is not required for the association. This is in contrast to the results of Gales *et al.* who reported that the deletion of ISDR abolished interaction with PKR in yeast [44]. The reason for this discrepancy is not known. However, this may have been due to the use of different clones of NS5A with different ISDR sequences and different assay techniques.

The effects of HCV infection on cell proliferation are not known. Although the interaction of NS5A with PKR suggests that there may be interesting effects on cell proliferation, it will be necessary to examine the growth of cells constitutively producing NS5A.

# REFERENCES

1. Choo QL, Kuo G, Weiner AJ, Overby LR, Bradley DW & Houghton M. Isolation of a cDNA clone derived from a blood-borne non-A, non-B viral hepatitis genome. *Science* 1989; **244**:359–362.
2. Choo QL, Richman KH, Han JH, Berger K, Lee C, Dong C, Gallegos C, Coit D, Medina-Selby R, Barr PJ, Weiner AJ, Bradlry DW, Kuo G & Houghton M. Genetic organization and diversity of the hepatitis C virus. *Proceedings of the National Academy of Sciences, USA* 1991; **88**: 2451–2455.
3. Kato N, Hijikata M, Ootsuyama Y, Nakagawa M, Ohkoshi S, Sugimura T & Shimotohno K. Molecular cloning of the human hepatitis C virus genome from Japanese patients with non-A, non-B hepatitis. *Proceedings of the National Academy of Sciences, USA* 1990; **87**:9524–9528.
4. Okamoto H, Okada S, Sugiyama Y, Kurai K, Iizuka H, Machida A, Miyakawa Y & Mayumi M. Nucleotide sequence of the genomic RNA of hepatitis C virus isolated from a human carrier: comparison with reported isolates for conserved and divergent regions. *Journal of General Virology* 1991; **72**:2697–2704.
5. Okamoto H, Kurai K, Okada S, Yamamoto K, Lizuka H, Tanaka T, Fukuda S, Tsuda F & Mishiro S. Full-length sequence of a hepatitis C virus genome having poor homology to reported isolates: comparative study of four distinct genotypes. *Virology* 1992; **188**: 331–341.
6. Takamizawa A, Mori C, Fuke I, Manabe S, Murakami S, Fujita J, Onishi E, Andoh T, Yoshida I & Okayama H. Structure and organization of the hepatitis C virus genome isolated from human carriers. *Journal of Virology* 1991; **65**:1105–1113.
7. Kato N, Hijikata M, Nakagawa M, Ootsuyama Y, Muraiso K, Ohkoshi S & Shimotohno K. Molecular structure of the Japanese hepatitis C viral genome. *FEBS Letters* 1991; **280**:325–328.
8. Miller RH & Purcell RH. Hepatitis C virus shares amino acid sequence similarity with pestiviruses and flaviviruses as well as members of two plant virus supergroups. *Proceedings of the National Academy of Sciences, USA* 1990; **87**:2057–2061.
9. Han JH, Shyamala V, Richman KH, Brauer MJ, Irvine B, Urdea MS, Tekamp-Olson P, Kuo G, Choo QL & Houghton M. Characterization of the terminal regions of hepatitis C viral RNA: identification of conserved sequences in the 5′ untranslated region and poly(A) tails at the 3′ end. *Proceedings of the National Academy of Sciences, USA* 1991; **88**:1711–1715.
10. Tsukiyama-Kohara K, Iizuka N, Kohara M & Nomoto A. Internal ribosome entry site within hepatitis C virus RNA. *Journal of Virology* 1992; **66**:1476–1483.
11. Hijikata M, Kato N, Ootsuyama Y, Nakagawa M & Shimotohno K. Gene mapping of the putative structural region of the hepatitis C virus genome by in vitro processing analysis. *Proceedings of the National Academy of Sciences, USA* 1991; **88**:5547–5551.
12. Moradpour D, Englert C, Wakita T & Wands JR. Characterization of cell lines allowing tightly regulated expression of hepatitis C virus core protein. *Virology* 1996; **222**:51–63.
13. Santolini E, Migliaccio G & La Monica N. Biosynthesis and biochemical properties of the hepatitis C virus core protein. *Journal of Virology* 1994; **68**:3631–3641.
14. Lo SY, Masiarz F, Hwang SB, Lai MM & Ou JJ. Differential subcellular localization of hepatitis C virus core gene products. *Virology* 1995; **213**: 455–461.
15. Grakoui A, McCourt DW, Wychowski C, Feinstone SM & Rice CM. Characterization of the hepatitis C virus-encoded serine proteinase: determination of proteinase-dependent polyprotein cleavage sites. *Journal of Virology* 1993; **67**:2832–2843.
16. Mizushima H, Hijikata M, Tanji Y, Kimura K & Shimotohno K. Analysis of N-terminal processing of hepatitis C virus nonstructural protein 2. *Journal of Virology* 1994; **68**:2731–2734.
17. Mizushima H, Hijikata M, Asabe S, Hirota M, Kimura K & Shimotohno K. Two hepatitis C virus glycoprotein E2 products with different C termini. *Journal of Virology* 1994; **68**:6215–6222.
18. Grakoui A, McCourt DW, Wychowski C, Feinstone SM & Rice CM. A second hepatitis C virus-encoded proteinase. *Proceedings of the National Academy of Sciences, USA* 1993; **90**:10583–10587.
19. Lanford RE, Notvall L, Chavez D, White R, Frenzel G, Simonsen C & Kim J. Analysis of hepatitis C virus capsid, E1, and E2/NS1 proteins expressed in insect cells. *Virology* 1993; **197**:225–235.
20. Lin C, Lindenbach BD, Pragai BM, McCourt DW & Rice CM. Processing in the hepatitis C virus E2-NS2 region: identification of p7 and two distinct E2-specific products with different C termini. *Journal of Virology* 1994; **68**:5063–5073.
21. Selby MJ, Glazer E, Masiarz F & Houghton M. Complex processing and protein:protein interactions in the E2:NS2 region of HCV. *Virology* 1994; **204**: 114–122.

22. Hijikata M, Mizushima H, Akagi T, Mori S, Kakiuchi N, Kato N, Tanaka T, Kimura K & Shimotohno K. Two distinct proteinase activities required for the processing of a putative nonstructural precursor protein of hepatitis C virus. *Journal of Virology* 1993; **67**:4665–4675.

23. Koch JO, Lohmann V, Herian U & Bartenschlager R. In vitro studies on the activation of the hepatitis C virus NS3 proteinase by the NS4A cofactor. *Virology* 1996; **221**:54–66.

24. Satoh S, Tanji Y, Hijikata M, Kimura K & Shimotohno K. The N-terminal region of hepatitis C virus nonstructural protein 3 (NS3) is essential for stable complex formation with NS4A. *Journal of Virology* 1995; **69**:4255–4260.

25. Bartenschlager R, Lohmann V, Wilkinson T & Koch JO. Complex formation between the NS3 serine-type proteinase of the hepatitis C virus and NS4A and its importance for polyprotein maturation. *Journal of Virology* 1995; **69**:7519–7528.

26. Butkiewicz NJ, Wendel M, Zhang R, Jubin R, Pichardo J, Smith EB, Hart AM, Ingram R, Durkin J, Mui PW, Murray MG, Ramanathan L & Dasmahapatra B. Enhancement of hepatitis C virus NS3 proteinase activity by association with NS4A-specific synthetic peptides: identification of sequence and critical residues of NS4A for the cofactor activity. *Virology* 1996; **225**:328–338.

27. Failla C, Tomei L & De Francesco R. An amino-terminal domain of the hepatitis C virus NS3 protease is essential for interaction with NS4A. *Journal of Virology* 1995; **69**:1769–1777.

28. Lin C & Rice CM. The hepatitis C virus NS3 serine proteinase and NS4A cofactor: establishment of a cell-free trans-processing assay. *Proceedings of the National Academy of Sciences, USA* 1995; **92**:7622–7626.

29. Shimizu Y, Yamaji K, Masuho Y, Yokota T, Inoue H, Sudo K, Satoh S & Shimotohno K. Identification of the sequence on NS4A required for enhanced cleavage of the NS5A/5B site by hepatitis C virus NS3 protease. *Journal of Virology* 1996; **70**:127–132.

30. D'Souza EDA, Grace K, Sanger DV, Rowlands DJ & Clarke BE. *In vitro* cleavage of hepatitis C virus polyprotein substrate by purified recombinant NS3 protease. *Journal of General Virology* 1995; **76**:1729–1736.

31. Suzich JA, Tamura JK, Palmer-Hill F, Warrener P, Grakoui A, Rice CM, Feinstone SM & Collett MS. Hepatitis C virus NS3 protein polynucleotide-stimulated nucleoside triphosphatase and comparison with the related pestivirus and flavivirus enzymes. *Journal of Virology* 1993; **67**:6152–6158.

32. Kim DW, Gwack Y, Han JH & Choe J. C-terminal domain of the hepatitis C virus NS3 protein contains an RNA helicase activity. *Biochemical & Biophysical Research Communications* 1995; **215**:160–166.

33. Preugschat F, Averett DR, Clarke BE & Porter DJT. A steady-state and pre-steady-state kinetic analysis of the NTPase activity associated with the hepatitis C virus NS3 helicase domain. *Journal of Biological Chemistry* 1996; **271**:24449–24457.

34. Shih CM, Chen CM, Chen SY & Lee YH. Modulation of the trans-suppression activity of hepatitis C virus core protein by phosphorylation. *Journal of Virology* 1995; **69**:1160–1171.

35. Hijikata M, Mizushima H, Tanji Y, Komoda Y, Hirowatari Y, Akagi T, Kato N, Kimura K & Shimotohno K. Proteolytic processing and membrane association of putative nonstructural proteins of hepatitis C virus. *Proceedings of the National Academy of Sciences, USA* 1993; **90**:10773–10777.

36. Kaneko T, Tanji Y, Satoh S, Hijikata M, Asabe S, Kimura K & Shimotohno K. Production of two phosphoproteins from the NS5A region of the hepatitis C viral genome. *Biochemical & Biophysical Research Communications* 1994; **205**:320–306.

37. Tanji Y, Hijikata M, Hirowatari Y & Shimotohno K. Hepatitis C virus polyprotein processing: kinetics and mutagenic analysis of serine proteinase-dependent cleavage. *Journal of Virology* 1994; **68**:8418–8422.

38. Tanji Y, Hijikata M, Hirowatari Y & Shimotohno K. Identification of the domain required for trans-cleavage activity of hepatitis C viral serine proteinase. *Gene* 1994; **145**:215–219.

39. Tanji Y, Hijikata M, Satoh S, Kaneko T & Shimotohno K. Hepatitis C virus-encoded nonstructural protein NS4A has versatile functions in viral protein processing. *Journal of Virology* 1995; **69**:1575–1581.

40. Tanji Y, Kaneko T, Satoh S & Shimotohno K. Phosphorylation of hepatitis C virus-encoded nonstructural protein NS5A. *Journal of Virology* 1995; **69**:3980–3986.

41. Fujita T, Ishido S, Muramatsu S, Itoh M & Hotta H. Suppression of actinomycin D-induced apoptosis by the NS3 protein of hepatitis C virus. *Biochemical & Biophysical Research Communications* 1996; **229**:825–831.

42. Ray RB, Lagging LM, Meyer K & Ray R. Hepatitis C virus core protein cooperates with Ras and transforms primary rat embryo fibroblasts to tumorigenic phenotype. *Journal of Virology* 1996; **70**:4438–4443.

43. Sakamuro D, Furukawa T & Takegami T. Hepatitis C virus nonstructural protein NS3 transforms NIH 3T3 cells. *Journal of Virology* 1995; **69**:3893–3896.

44. Gale MJ, Korth MJ, Tang NM, Tan S-L, Hopkins DA, Derver TE, Polyak SJ, Gretch DR & Katze MG. Evidence that hepatitis C virus resistance to interferon is mediated through repression of the PKR protein kinase by the nonstructural 5A protein. *Virology* 1997; **230**:217–227.

45. Galabru J & Hovanessian AG. Autophosphorylation of the protein kinase dependent on double-stranded RNA. *Journal of Biological Chemistry* 1987; **262**:15538–15544.

46. Carroll K, Elroy-Stain O, Moss B & Jagus R. Recombinant vaccinia virus K3L gene product prevents activation of double-stranded RNA-dependent, initiation factor 2a-specific protein kinase. *Journal of Biological Chemistry* 1993; **268**:12837–12842.

47. McMillian NAJ, Chun RF, Siderovski DP, Galabru J, Toone WM, Samuel CE, Mak TW, Hovanessian AG, Jeang KT & Williams BRG. HIV-1 Tat directly interacts with the interferon-induced, double-stranded RNA-dependent kinase, PKR. *Virology* 1995; **213**:413–424.

48. Polyak SJ, Tang N, Wambach M, Barber GN & Katze MG. The p58 cellular inhibitor complexes with the interferon-induced, double-stranded RNA-dependent protein kinase, PKR. *Journal of Biological Chemistry* 1996; **271**:1702–1707.

49. Enomoto N, Sakuma I, Asahina Y, Kurosaki M, Murakami T, Yamamoto C, Izumi N, Marumo F & Sato C. Comparison of full-length sequences of interferon-sensitive and resistant hepatitis C virus 1b. Sensitivity to interferon is conferred by amino acid substitutions in the NS5A region. *Journal of Clinical Investigation* 1995; **96**:224–230.

50. Enomoto N, Sakuma I, Asahina Y, Kurosaki M,

Murakami T, Yamamoto C, Ogura Y, Izumi N, Marumo F & Sato C. Mutations in the nonstructural protein 5A gene and response to interferon in patients with chronic hepatitis C virus 1b infection. *Acta Gastroenterologica Latinoamericana* 1996; **26**:301–303.

51. Squadrito G, Leone F, Sartori M, Nalpas B, Berthelot P, Raimondo G, Pol S & Brechot C. Mutations in the nonstructural 5A region of hepatitis C virus and response of chronic hepatitis C to interferon alfa. *Gastroenterology* 1997; **113**:567–572.

# Section VI

## DRUG DISCOVERY

## Part A

### PRECLINICAL INVESTIGATION

# 30

# The mechanism of action and cellular pharmacology of anti-hepatitis B virus agents

## Phillip A Furman* and Raymond F Schinazi

## INTRODUCTION

Vaccination against hepatitis B virus (HBV) is one way to effectively prevent HBV infection [1]. However, even with a safe and effective vaccine available, millions of people worldwide are still being infected annually. Vaccination is not an effective measure for those who are chronic carriers, and about 5% of persons vaccinated do not produce protective antibodies [1]. Furthermore, the response among adults decreases with age. There are close to 350 million people infected worldwide, and in the USA, HBV incidence is currently 6.3 cases per 100 000 of the population. The Centers for Disease Control and Prevention has estimated that the direct cost of HBV infection exceeds $500 million annually in the USA [1], which makes this virus an important human pathogen for therapeutic approaches. The major therapeutic option for carriers of HBV is interferon α, which even in the most successful studies has shown disappointing response rates and high relapse rates [2,3]. Discontinuation of therapy owing to side effects has also contributed to the low response rate. Recently, the discovery of several nucleoside analogues that suppress HBV replication *in vitro* and *in vivo* offers promising new directions in the treatment of HBV disease [2,4]. While these new compounds have demonstrated very promising efficacy and tolerability in the clinic, short-term monotherapy is not sufficient to clear viral infection. Successful treatment of the disease on a long-term basis is likely to require combination therapy. We review below the major antiviral agents currently being developed for HBV infections. We focus on chemical agents and will not discuss immunotherapeutic or interferon intervention.

## Famciclovir

Famciclovir (Fig. 1a) is the oral prodrug of the guanine nucleoside analogue penciclovir. Famciclovir is converted to penciclovir by deacetylation of the side chains by esterases in the small intestine followed by oxidation of the purine base by aldehyde oxidase in the portal vein and liver [5,6]. Early on, penciclovir was shown to be an inhibitor of herpes simplex virus type 1 (HSV-1) and HSV-2 *in vitro* [7]. More recently, penciclovir was shown by Korba and Boyd [8] to be a potent and selective antiviral agent against intracellular HBV replication ($EC_{90}=1.6$ μM) and extracellular virion release ($EC_{90}=0.7$ μM) by the 2.2.15 assay. Penciclovir showed little toxicity towards the 2.2.15 cells with a $CC_{50}$ value of 450 μM. *In vivo*, Tsiquaye *et al.* [9] showed that oral treatment of ducks infected with duck hepatitis B virus (DHBV) with famciclovir resulted in the inhibition of intrahepatic replication of DHBV. In a 4 week study in the duck model, Lin *et al.* [10,11] demonstrated that treatment with famciclovir resulted in an inhibition of viral DNA replication as well as a suppression of the levels of intrahepatic viral covalently closed circular DNA (cccDNA), RNA, and viral antigens. The antiviral activity of famciclovir was likely to be the result of conversion to penciclovir, followed by phosphorylation to penciclovir 5′-triphosphate (PCV-TP).

The antiviral activity of penciclovir appears to be dependent on the intracellular phosphorylation of penciclovir to the 5′-triphosphate, which is entirely catalysed by cellular enzymes, as HBV does not encode enzymes capable of initiating the phosphorylation of penciclovir. The initial phosphorylation of penciclovir is probably catalysed by the phosphotransferase activity associated with inosine monophosphate-guanosine monophosphate 5′-nucleotidase (IMP-GMP-5′-nucleotidase [12,13]. This enzyme has been shown to phosphorylate a number of guanine nucleoside analogues including acyclovir, ganciclovir and ara-G, as well as several purine 2′,3′-dideoxynucleoside analogues. Vertebrate livers contain high levels of IMP-GMP-5′-nucleotidase, implying that this enzyme is the most likely candidate for phosphorylating penciclovir. The enzymes that phosphorylate penciclovir 5′-monophosphate to the 5′-di- and triphosphate have not been

Figure 1. Chemical structures of nucleoside anti-HBV agents

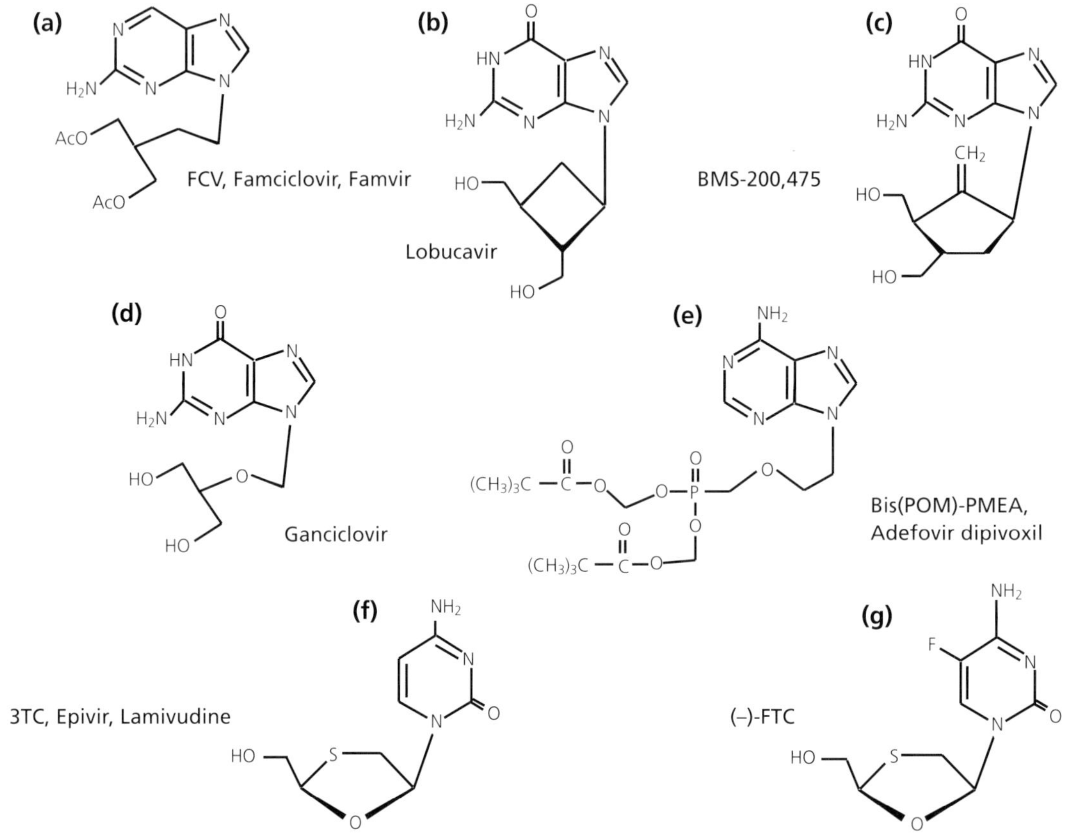

(a) FCV, Famciclovir, Famvir

(b) Lobucavir

(c) BMS-200,475

(d) Ganciclovir

(e) Bis(POM)-PMEA, Adefovir dipivoxil

(f) 3TC, Epivir, Lamivudine

(g) (–)-FTC

identified. Likely candidates to carry out these reactions are guanylate kinase, which could catalyse the phosphorylation of penciclovir 5′-monophosphate to the diphosphate, and several kinases or phosphotransferases capable of converting the 5′-diphosphate to the corresponding triphosphate [14,15].

Mechanistically, the 5′-triphosphate of penciclovir was shown to function as an alternative substrate inhibitor of the HBV polymerase. Shaw et al. [16] reported an apparent $K_i$ value for PCV-TP of 0.05 µM for HBV polymerase. In contrast, cellular DNA polymerases were not as sensitive to inhibition by PCV-TP. A $K_i$ value of 175 µM was obtained using the human DNA polymerase α, and IC$_{50}$ values of 120 and 373 µM were obtained for DNA polymerases β and γ, respectively. At present, the enantiomeric specificity of PCV-TP is unknown. The demonstration that (R)-PCV-TP inhibited hepadnaviral reverse transcription by inhibiting the synthesis of the short DNA primer, and that both R- and S-enantiomers inhibit elongation, gives further insight into the mode of action of penciclovir against HBV and the stereospecificity of the 5′-triphosphate. Interestingly, the R-enantiomer of PCV-

TP is markedly more effective than the S-enantiomer against the human immunodeficiency virus (HIV) reverse transcriptase [17]. Shaw et al. [16] estimated that peak intracellular levels of penciclovir 5′-triphosphate were 0.7 pmol/10$^6$ cells after incubation with 1 µM penciclovir for 24 hours. Based on these and other data, the concentration of penciclovir 5′-triphosphate produced in hepatocytes is sufficient to inhibit HBV replication without affecting DNA polymerases α, β, γ, δ and ε. Incorporation of penciclovir into actively replicating HBV DNA has not been demonstrated, although the R-enantiomer of PCV-TP can cause DNA chain termination [18,19]. Although it possesses the equivalent of a 3′-hydroxyl group, penciclovir has been demonstrated to cause premature, but not immediate chain termination of HSV DNA synthesis [6,20]. Therefore, it can be speculated that a similar mechanism may function in HBV DNA synthesis.

## Lobucavir

Lobucavir (LBV; Fig. 1b) is a guanosine analogue with a broad spectrum of activity against HBV and most members of the herpesvirus family [HSV; varicella-zoster virus (VZV); and human cytomegalovirus (HCMV)], including acyclovir-resistant HSV and ganciclovir-resistant HCMV [21–25].

Previous reports have shown that LBV inhibits HSV-1 DNA synthesis and that the 5′-triphosphate of LBV is an alternative substrate inhibitor of the HSV-1 and HSV-2 DNA polymerases *in vitro* [26]. The initial phosphorylation of LBV to the 5′-monophosphate is catalysed by the herpesvirus-encoded thymidine kinase (TK). TK-deficient HSV-1, HSV-2, and VZV have reduced sensitivities to LBV. From these results it is clear that the mechanism of action of LBV against members of the herpesvirus family involves phosphorylation by the virally encoded TK and inhibition of the viral DNA polymerase. What is not known is which cellular enzymes are responsible for phosphorylating the 5′-monophosphate to the 5′-diphosphate and its subsequent phosphorylation to the 5′-triphosphate.

For HBV, the mechanism of action of LBV is not as well defined. LBV 5′-triphosphate is a potent inhibitor of the HBV DNA polymerase with a $K_i$ value of 1.4 nM, however, the enzyme responsible for the phosphorylation of LBV to the 5′-monophosphate is not known. Since HBV encodes neither a homologue of the HSV TK nor a protein that has the ability to phosphorylate a nucleoside analogue, the phosphorylation of LBV is probably catalysed by a cellular enzyme. Tenney *et al.* [25] showed that uninfected WI38 cells were capable of phosphorylating LBV. Several guanine nucleoside analogues are known to be phosphorylated to the 5′-monophosphate by IMP-GMP-5′-nucleotidase. Whether this enzyme or another is responsible remains to be determined.

In a study in the woodchuck model [27], 20 mg/kg oral LBV was given once daily for 12 weeks to chronically infected animals, LBV rapidly produced undetectable levels of woodchuck hepatitis virus (WHV) in all six treated animals. LBV was well tolerated except for alopecia. No evidence of liver toxicity was detected by serum chemistries or liver biopsies. During the 12 week post-dosing period, four animals returned to baseline levels while the levels in the two remaining animals remained undetectable. In a subsequent study, animals were dosed once daily with 5 mg/kg of LBV for 6 weeks. Using this regimen, serum WHV DNA levels were reduced by 90–99% compared to placebo. Alopecia was not observed in this study.

## BMS200,475

BMS200,475 (BMS; Fig. 1c), is a guanosine analogue in which the sugar moiety is modified by the replacement of the tetrahydrofuran ring of 2′-deoxyguanosine with a methylene-cyclopentane [28,29]. This compound was originally developed as an antiherpetic agent. BMS displayed potent activity against HBV in the 2.2.15 assay, with an $EC_{50}$ value of 3 nM. Similar to lobucavir, BMS was also active against members of the herpesvirus family. Various human cell lines were used to measure the cytotoxicity of BMS. The concentration of BMS that gave 50% cytotoxicity ($CC_{50}$) varied with cell type, ranging from a $CC_{50}$ of 20 μM for CEM cells to >90 μM for WI38 cells. *In vitro* metabolism studies showed that BMS was taken up by cells and phosphorylated to the 5′-mono-, di- and triphosphate derivatives. There was no apparent difference in the phosphorylation of BMS with different cell lines, indicating that the anabolism was due to cellular kinases. In HepG2 cells, the uptake of BMS was linear between 1 μM and 25 μM, but the accumulation of intracellular triphosphate was most efficient at the lower concentrations, suggesting saturation of the transport mechanism and/or the anabolic enzymes involved in the uptake and phosphorylation of BMS. When cells were incubated in the presence of 1 μM BMS, the 5′-triphosphate accumulated slowly, but with linear kinetics for 3 days. An intracellular half-life of >15 hours was measured for the 5′-triphosphate in both HepG2 and 2.2.15 cell lines. Studies with the HBV polymerase indicated that the 5′-triphosphate of BMS acts as a non-obligate chain terminator.

The *in vivo* efficacy of BMS was evaluated in the woodchuck model using chronically infected animals. Animals were dosed orally at 0.02 to 0.5 mg/kg per day for 28 days [29]. At all doses used, BMS caused a 2–3 log decrease in serum viral DNA and endogenous DNA polymerase activity. In this same experiment 5 mg/kg per day of lamivudine resulted in only a 1 log decrease. Following cessation of therapy, WHV DNA serum levels returned to pretreatment levels within 2 to 3 weeks in both the BMS and lamivudine groups. In a subsequent experiment, animals were dosed orally with 0.1 and 0.02 mg/kg per day for 12 weeks. This dosing regimen proved to be extremely effective in reducing viral DNA levels. In the animals that received the 0.1 mg/kg per day dose, undetectable levels of WHV DNA were achieved within 1 to 5 weeks of dosing, and remained undetectable at the 2 week follow-up. Ten weeks after cessation of therapy, WHV DNA levels in some animals remained undetectable. Four of six animals that received the 0.02 mg/kg per day dose also had undetectable serum levels of HBV DNA. In a separate ongoing study to determine the efficacy of daily therapy followed by a weekly maintenance dose, animals were dosed orally for 8 weeks with 0.5 mg/kg per day and then given 0.5 mg/kg per week for 36 weeks. Virus levels in eleven of thirteen animals became undetectable and remained undetectable on maintenance therapy. The viral load of the two remaining animals returned to undetectable levels during maintenance therapy.

## Ganciclovir

Ganciclovir (Fig. 1d), a congener of acyclovir, an analogue of guanosine, was originally developed as an inhibitor of herpesviruses. More recently, ganciclovir has proven useful in the management of cytomegalovirus infections, especially in the immunocompromised patient [31]. Locarnini et al. demonstrated that ganciclovir could inhibit HBV DNA replication in patients also infected with HIV [32]. Ganciclovir also effectively inhibited DHBV replication in persistently infected hepatocytes [33–35]. This observation was subsequently confirmed by Yokota et al. [36] and others [37–40]. Wang et al. [33] found that treating ducks congenitally infected with DHBV with 10 or 30 mg/kg per day i.p. in two equally divided doses of ganciclovir for 21 days resulted in a rapid lowering of DHBV levels in the serum and liver. By the end of the treatment period, replicative intermediates, with the exception of the supercoiled DNA, form could no longer be detected. Within 2 weeks of cessation of treatment viral replication returned and, in some instances, rebound occurred.

As with other nucleoside analogues, the activity of ganciclovir is dependent upon it being phosphorylated to the active 5′-triphosphate. In HSV-infected cells, the primary phosphorylation is catalysed by the viral TK [41]. However, the activation of ganciclovir in HCMV-infected cells or cells infected with TK-deficient HSV requires that ganciclovir be phosphorylated by other enzymes. In HCMV-infected cells, a protein kinase encoded by the UL-97 gene has been shown to be responsible for phosphorylating ganciclovir to the 5′-monophosphate. The phosphorylation of ganciclovir to the 5′-triphosphate occurs in uninfected cells. IMP-GMP-5′-nucleotidase is probably the enzyme responsible for the activation of ganciclovir in uninfected cells. The rapid conversion of the 5′-monophosphate of ganciclovir to the corresponding diphosphate was shown by Boehme to be catalysed by guanylate kinase [42].

## PMEA and bis(POM)-PMEA (adefovir dipivoxil)

9-(2-Phosphonylmethoxyethyl)adenine (PMEA Fig. 1e) is an acyclic monophosphonate analogue of adenine with a broad spectrum of antiviral activity against RNA and DNA viruses [43–45]. In particular, PMEA has potent anti-HIV-1 activity and therefore was developed as a therapy for HIV-1 infection. Because the phosphonyl group of PMEA exhibits a negative charge at physiological pH, and hence the cellular uptake and oral bioavailability of PMEA is poor, the bis(pivaloyloxymethyl) [bis(POM)] ester was synthesized and found to exhibit a more favourable pharmacokinetic profile [43]. Consequently, the bis(POM) ester of PMEA is currently in development as a therapy for HIV-1 and HBV infections.

The anti-HBV activity of PMEA was first described by Yokota et al. [36,46,47]. Using an HB611 human hepatoblastoma cell-derived assay, they reported an $EC_{50}$ value of 0.005 µg/ml against HBV and a selectivity index (ratio of the 50% cytotoxic concentration to the 50% HBV inhibitory concentration) of about 300. PMEA was also evaluated for its inhibitory effect on HBV replication in HepG2 2.2.15 cells and HB611 cells transfected with HBV by Heijtink et al. [48]. PMEA inhibited HBV release from 2.2.15 cells and HB611 cells with an $EC_{50}$ of 0.7 µM and 1.2 µM, respectively. Intracellular viral DNA synthesis was inhibited at concentrations equivalent to those required to inhibit virus release from the cells [48]. PMEA also inhibited the release of DHBV from primary duck hepatocytes with $EC_{50}$ of 0.2 µM [48]. The 50% cytotoxic concentration, determined by measuring [$^3$H]thymidine incorporation into cellular DNA, was 150 µM for the two human cell lines and 40 µM for primary duck hepatocytes [48]. Preliminary results in the live duck models showed that the activity of PMEA against DHBV in vitro translated to activity in vivo. In these studies, a dose of 30 mg/kg on alternate days demonstrated efficacy in the model [48].

The metabolic pathway responsible for the activation of PMEA is unclear. Robbins et al. investigated the metabolism of PMEA in human T-lymphoid cells (CEM-SS) and a PMEA-resistant subline [49]. Extracts of CEM-SS phosphorylated PMEA to its 5′-mono- and diphosphate in the presence of ATP as the phosphate donor. No other nucleotides or 5′-phosphoribosyl pyrophosphate functioned as a phosphate donor. Subcellular fractionation experiments showed that CEM-SS cells contained two nucleotide kinase activities capable of phosphorylating PMEA, one in the mitochondria and one in the cytosol. The PMEA-resistant CEM cells proved to have a deficiency in mitochondrial adenylate kinase activity, suggesting that this enzyme plays an important role in the activation of PMEA.

## Oxathiolane nucleosides

Oxathiolane analogues of cytosine, such as lamivudine (3TC; Fig. 1f) and (–)-FTC (Fig. 1g), represent a promising new class of compounds with potent and selective antiviral activity against HIV and HBV [50–53]. Lamivudine is currently in Phase III clinical trials for HBV infections, whereas (–)-FTC is in Phase I/II. In contrast to their activity against HIV, where (–)-FTC is clearly the more potent *in vitro* and in patients, lamivudine and (–)-FTC appear to be equipotent against HBV [52]. An $EC_{50}$ value of 4–10 nM has been estimated for both compounds against HBV in the HepG2 2.2.15 assay. Both compounds caused a dose-dependent decrease in the amount of extra- and intracellular HBV DNA. To date, both compounds have shown little or no cytotoxicity and no mitochondrial toxicity *in vitro*.

The mechanism of action of (–)-FTC has been well characterized. Furman, Paff and colleagues have described the uptake and metabolism of (–)-FTC [52,54]. (–)-FTC was found to readily permeate cells, where it was subsequently phosphorylated to the 5′-triphosphate derivative of (–)-FTC. The influx of (–)-FTC was only partly inhibited by inhibitors of nucleoside transport, indicating that multiple transport mechanisms may be involved. The transport mechanism(s) of lamivudine has not been characterized. A time course study using HepG2 2.2.15 cells showed that the 5′-phosphates of (–)-FTC were formed in a dose-dependent manner and reached steady-state intracellular concentrations by 3–6 hours of exposure. The intracellular half-life of (–)-FTC-TP in HepG2 2.2.15 cells was reported to be relatively long, because like all L-nucleotides, (–)-FTC-TP is at least fourfold more resistant to phosphodiesterases than its D-counterpart [55,56].

Similarly, metabolism studies in cell culture showed that lamivudine is readily phosphorylated to the 5′-triphosphate derivative which is an inhibitor of viral polymerases [57–60]. In human primary hepatocytes exposed to 5 µM lamivudine (3TC), 3TC-5′-triphosphate was found to be the predominant intracellular metabolite, reaching a maximum of 24.2 pmol/$10^6$ cells by 48 hours [61,62]. The intracellular half-life of 5.6 hours for the 5′-triphosphate of lamivudine in HepG2 2.2.15 cells was similar to that reported for (–)-FTC [59].

The enzyme responsible for phosphorylating (–)-FTC to the corresponding 5′-monophosphate is deoxycytidine kinase [56]. Shewach *et al.* showed that lamivudine was also phosphorylated to its corresponding 5′-monophosphate by 2′-deoxycytidine kinase [56]. Phosphorylation of the 5′-monophosphate of (–)-FTC to the corresponding 5′-diphosphate was catalysed by 2′-deoxycytidine monophosphate kinase. The efficiency with which enzyme purified from calf thymus phosphorylates (–)-FTC 5′-monophosphate was 32% of that observed when 2′-deoxycytidine-5′-monophosphate was used as substrate. Although the enzyme responsible for phosphorylating the 5′-monophosphate of lamivudine has not been identified, because of the structural similarity with (–)-FTC, it would seem likely that the enzyme is 2′-deoxycytidylate kinase. The enzyme responsible for the phosphorylation of 5′-diphosphate of (–)-FTC and lamivudine to the corresponding 5′-triphosphate has not been identified. The most likely candidate is the nucleoside diphosphate kinase, a cytosolic enzyme with a broad substrate specificity for phosphorylating a variety of nucleoside-5′-diphosphates. Interestingly, (–)-FTC is phosphorylated to a greater extent than lamivudine 5′-TP in human liver homogenates [63].

In addition to the 5′-phosphorylated derivatives of (–)-FTC, an additional metabolite was isolated from HepG2 2.2.15 cells [54]. A small amount of (–)-FTC was converted to the corresponding diphosphocholine derivative, analogous to CDP-choline. (–)-FTC was not detectably deaminated at either the nucleoside or nucleotide level [57]. Similarly, the diphosphocholine metabolite of lamivudine has been observed in various cell types, including primary human hepatocytes [61,62].

The 5′-triphosphates of (–)-FTC and lamivudine are alternative-substrate inhibitors of the HIV reverse transcriptase. The replication cycle of HBV includes the reverse transcription of an RNA template [64–66]. This process is carried out by a polymerase that shares significant sequence homology with the reverse transcriptase of retroviruses [67]. As a consequence of this relationship, experiments were performed to determine whether the site of action of (–)-FTC 5′-TP is the HBV polymerase. Because of the difficulty in purifying HBV polymerase from various sources and because of the lack of success in cloning and expressing the enzyme, an endogenous assay employing permeabilized virions was used to test the activity of (–)-FTC and lamivudine 5′-TP [68]. In the endogenous assay, both lamivudine 5′-TP and (–)-FTC 5′-TP inhibited product formation in a dose-dependent manner. Competition studies were performed to determine whether the 5′-triphosphates of lamivudine and (–)-FTC compete solely with dCTP for binding to the enzyme or with the other nucleoside 5′-triphosphate substrates as well. The ability of increasing concentrations of dCTP, dTTP and dGTP

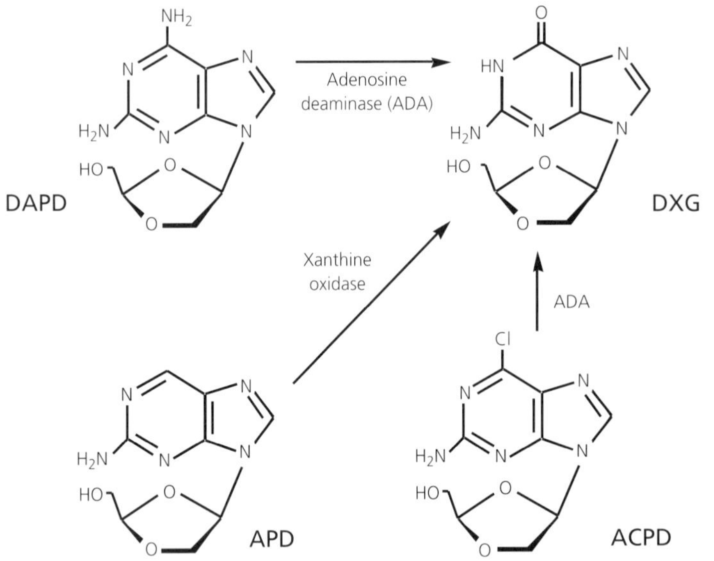

Figure 2. Structures and bioconversions of dioxolane nucleosides

to prevent inhibition of HBV DNA synthesis by (–)-FTC 5′-TP was examined. While dTTP and dGTP had no effect on inhibition by (–)-FTC 5′-triphosphate, a 10-fold excess of dCTP completely blocked the ability of (–)-FTC 5′-TP to inhibit HBV DNA synthesis. Similarly, inhibition of HBV polymerase activity by lamivudine 5′-TP was prevented by dCTP. Furthermore, (–)-FTC 5′-TP is incorporated into newly synthesized HBV DNA, resulting in chain termination. Taken together, these data suggest that both (–)-FTC 5′-TP and lamivudine 5′-TP are alternative substrate inhibitors of the HBV polymerase and compete with dCTP for incorporation into the growing HBV DNA chain.

## Dioxolane nucleosides

(–)-β-D-Dioxolane-guanine (DXG), (–)-β-D-2-amino-6-chloropurine dioxolane (ACPD), and (–)-β-D-2,6-diaminopurine dioxolane (DAPD) are three novel dioxolane nucleosides that were discovered to have anti-HBV activity *in vitro*. These compounds are active against HBV, HIV-1, HIV-2 and simian immuno-deficiency virus (SIV) [69–71]. Another compound being studied is (–)-β-D-2-amino purine dioxolane (APD). APD is not active against HIV-1 in culture, but is bioconverted to DXG *in vitro* and in animals by xanthine oxidase (Fig. 2). We have conducted a systematic study of the effect of the three dioxolane purines (ACPD, DAPD, and DXG) on various enzymes involved in pyrimidine and purine biosynthesis. Preliminary results indicate that these compounds have no effect on mouse liver adenosine deaminase, adenosine kinase, cytidine kinase, purine nucleoside phos-

phorylase, hypoxanthine-guanosine phosphoribosyl transferase (HGPT), xanthine oxidase and xanthine dehydrogenase (as inferred from formation of xanthine from inosine) when tested at concentrations of up to 1 mM. It also appears that these novel compounds are not inhibitors of these enzymes. However, studies using woodchuck and human liver homogenates confirmed that DAPD and the 6-deoxy analogue APD are readily converted to DXG.

In 2.2.15 cells, the order of decreasing potency of the (–)-β-dioxolanyl purine enantiomers against HBV was DAPD≈ACPD>(–)-FTC≥DXG≫DDC. The $EC_{50}$ for DAPD and ACPD for HBV DNA replication intermediates or HBV virion synthesis inhibition was close to 0.1 μM, making these purines some of the most potent anti-HBV agents yet seen. Complete cessation of viral replication occurred with these compounds at 3 μM. DXG and DAPD demonstrated no marked toxicity to myeloid and erythroid progenitor cells in clonogenic assays ($IC_{50}$ > 100 μM). In contrast, zidovudine had an $IC_{50}$ value close to 1 μM, as previously reported [72]. DAPD was shown not to affect mitochondrial DNA synthesis in HepG2 cells [73]. The high therapeutic indices of the dioxolane purines suggested that they should be further evaluated in animal models for HBV infection.

The woodchuck has proven to be a suitable animal model for studying HBV infection because of similarities between WHV and HBV infections. We conducted a pharmacokinetic study of DAPD in woodchucks (*Marmota monax*) as a prelude to studies in woodchucks chronically infected with WHV. DAPD and DXG (formed by deamination) were found to have half-lives of 6.7 hours and 17.6 hours, respectively, following intravenous administration. The oral bio-availability of DAPD ranged from 5-18%. The apparent availability of DXG following oral administration of DAPD was 18-68% [74]. Based on these studies, we initiated a 3 month treatment study in woodchucks comparing the potency of DAPD to lamivudine [75]. The results indicated that both compounds were tolerated at a dose of 2 mg/kg per day (twice daily – oral by gavage) over a period of 3 months. Statistically significant reductions in serum WHV DNA levels were noted for both compounds compared to the untreated control as early as 4 weeks after initiation of treatment. The viral DNA reductions for lamivudine and DAPD were almost identical [75]. When the drug treatments were discontinued at 3 months, a rebound in virus was noted for both compounds. This strongly suggests that a maintenance therapy approach should be considered for both lamivudine and DAPD. In addition, these results underline the importance of studying drug combinations for the treatment of HBV, since it is likely that drug-resistant virus will develop on prolonged therapy for a chronic disease such as HBV.

## L-FMAU

2′-Fluoro-5-methyl-β-L-arabinofuranosyl uracil (L-FMAU; clevudine; Fig. 3), first synthesized by Chu's group, was shown to be a potent inhibitor of HBV replication *in vitro*. L-FMAU produces a dose-dependent inhibition of virus replication in 2.2.15 cells and has an $EC_{50}$ value ranging from 0.02 to 0.15 μM, with a mean of 0.08 μM (four separate experiments) [76,77]. Compared with lamivudine and (–)-FTC, the $EC_{50}$ for L-FMAU was approximately four to seven-fold higher. In addition, L-FMAU was active against Epstein–Barr virus ($EC_{90}$ = 5 μM), but showed no significant activity against other herpesviruses or HIV. In the 2.2.15 assay, L-FMAU did not show toxicity ($CC_{50}$ ≥200 μM), whereas the D-enantiomer was toxic, with a $CC_{50}$ of 50 μM. L-FMAU also showed little or no toxicity towards H1 cells ($CC_{50}$ = 913±70 μM), CEM cells ($CC_{50}$≥200 μM), and MT-2 cells ($CC_{50}$ = 100 μM). In the human bone marrow progenitor cell assay, no significant toxicity was observed toward the CFU-GM or BFU-E stem cells at concentrations up to 100 μM. An assessment of the toxicity of L-FMAU towards mitochondria in HepG2 cells showed that L-FMAU was not toxic at concentrations up to 10 μM. The effect of L-FMAU on lactic acid production in HepG2 cells treated with compound was studied at concentrations of 100 μM and 200 μM. The levels of lactic acid produced in the L-FMAU-treated cells were com-

parable to those in untreated controls, whereas cells treated with D-FIAU and D-FMAU produced significant levels of lactic acid.

Phosphorylation of L-FMAU was examined in 2.2.15 cells [77]. The cells were treated with 5 μM [³H]-L-FMAU for 24 hours and assayed by HPLC for L-FMAU nucleotides formed intracellularly. Rapid conversion of L-FMAU to the corresponding mono-, di- and triphosphate forms could be seen as early as 2 hours, and maximal metabolite formation was observed at 8 hours. The major metabolite found in these studies was the 5′-triphosphate. In wash-out experiments, cells were treated for 24 hours; when compound was removed, the levels of mono-, di- and triphosphates dropped as a function of time. The clearance of the metabolites did not appear to follow first-order kinetics. In the initial phase, the levels of the metabolites dropped rapidly with about 50% of the triphosphate disappearing in 4–5 hours and 90% of the triphosphate disappearing in the first 8 hours. In the subsequent 16 hours, the triphosphate levels declined at a slower rate, with a small amount of triphosphate still present at 24 hours. The metabolic profile of L-FMAU was the same when experiments were conducted using HepG2 cells instead of the 2.2.15 cells. The enzymes responsible for phosphorylating L-FMAU to L-FMAU-MP are the cytosolic and mitochondrial TK, and the deoxycytidine kinase [77,78]. The 5′-triphosphate of L-FMAU competitively inhibits the HBV polymerase with an $K_i$ value of approximately 0.12 μM. In addition, it was shown that L-FMAU-5′-triphosphate is a weak inhibitor of and not a substrate for, human α, β, γ, δ, and ε DNA polymerases [77].

L-FMAU produced a sustained antiviral effect in chronically infected woodchucks [79]. The decline of virus load was rapid and, unlike other antiviral agents, virus rebound did not occur immediately after discontinuation of therapy. The compound was also effective in ducks infected with DHBV [80]. Unlike the D-enantiomer, no cytotoxicity was apparent with this compound, even when used up to 10 mg/kg per day for a prolonged treatment duration.

**Figure 3.** Structure of L-FMAU (clevudine)

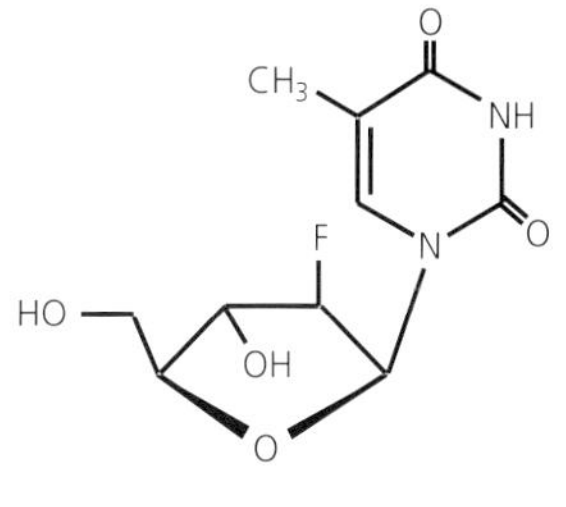

# PROSPECTS

Recently, investigators using the woodchuck model of chronic hepatitis B infection [79,81], demonstrated that treatment with lamivudine initiated early in the course of chronic WHV infection significantly reduced the risk for the development of hepatocarcinoma in a lifetime antiviral trial. This offers for the first time the possibility of preventing an important consequence of persistent HBV infection with antiviral agents. Since WHV recrudescence in serum of some woodchucks treated with lamivudine occurred at 80 weeks, it is clear that more potent agents or combined modalities are needed to prevent virus rebound and the development of resistant viruses [82–87]. The significance of these observations on the replication strategy and pathogenesis of infection requires further investigation. As more potent compounds or treatment modalities become available, they should be studied to determine whether they can completely prevent the emergence of resistant virus and hepatocellular carcinoma in animal models.

The potential toxicity of all antivirals directed against HBV will need to be determined in simple as well as highly sophisticated assays before their use in humans [73,88,89]. Advanced toxicological studies in woodchuck and duck models alone may not be adequate because long-term therapy is needed with these agents.

The next generation of compounds active against HBV are necessary for the treatment of patients already resistant to famciclovir and lamivudine [90, 91]. The focus should be on preventing the development of resistance of HBV to antiviral drugs and maximizing antiviral activity by using the highest possible safe dose of drug(s) and the most effective regimen early during infection. Based on the lessons learned from HIV medicine, the goal will also be to maximize the genetic barriers to resistance by selecting drugs that are not cross-resistant, and selecting combinations associated with phenotypic reversion. Combination chemotherapy with multiple non-toxic nucleoside analogues that act synergistically and require different activation pathways should produce highly effective regimens for controlling virus replication in the liver and in extrahepatic reservoirs.

# ACKNOWLEDGEMENTS

We acknowledge support from US Public Health Service Grant RO1-AI-41980 (RFS), and the Department of Veterans Affairs (RFS).

# REFERENCES

1. Hadler S & Margolis H. Hepatitis B immunization: vaccine types, efficacy, and indications for immunization. In: *Current Clinical Topics in Infectious Diseases.* 1992; pp. 283–308. Edited by J Remington & M Swartz. Boston, Massachusetts: Blackwell Scientific Publications.

2. Colacino J & Staschke K. *The identification and development of antiviral agents for the treatment of chronic hepatitis B virus infection,* 1998. (*Progress in Drug Research,* volume 50). pp. 259–322. Edited by E Jucker. Basel, Switzerland: Birkhauser Verlag.

3. Hoofnagle JH & Lau D. New therapies for chronic hepatitis B. *Journal of Viral Hepatitis* 1997; 4(Supplement 1):41–50.

4. Schinazi R. The impact of nucleosides on hepatitis viruses. In *Viral Hepatitis and Liver Disease,* 1997, pp. 736–742. Edited by M Rizzetto, R Purcell, J Gerin & G Verme. Torino, Italy: Edizioni Minerva Medica.

5. Vere Hodge RA & Cheng Y-C. The mode of action of penciclovir. *Antiviral Chemistry and Chemotherapy* 1993; 4(Supplement 1):13–24.

6. Vere Hodge RA. Famciclovir and penciclovir. The mode of action of famciclovir including its conversion to penciclovir. *Antiviral Chemistry and Chemotherapy* 1993; 4:67–84.

7. Bacon TH & Schinazi RF. An overview of the further evaluation of penciclovir against herpes simplex virus and varicella-zoster virus in cell-culture highlighting contrasts with acyclovir. *Antiviral Chemistry and Chemotherapy* 1993; 4 (Supplement 1):25–36.

8. Korba BE & Boyd MR. Penciclovir is a selective inhibitor of hepatitis B virus replication in cultured human hepatoblastoma cells. *Antimicrobial Agents and Chemotherapy* 1996; 40:1282–1284.

9. Tsiquaye KN, Sutton D, Maung M & Boyd MR. Antiviral activities and pharmacokinetics of penciclovir and famciclovir in Pekin ducks chronically infected with duck hepatitis B virus. *Antiviral Chemistry and Chemotherapy* 1996; 7:153–159.

10. Lin E, Luscombe C, Colledge D, Wang Y & Locarnini S. Long-term therapy with guanine nucleoside analog penciclovir controls chronic duck hepatitis B virus infection *in vivo. Antimicrobial Agents and Chemotherapy* 1998; 42:2132–2137.

11. Lin E, Luscombe C, Wang YY, Shaw T & Locarnini S. The guanine nucleoside analog penciclovir is active against chronic duck hepatitis B virus infection *in vivo. Antimicrobial Agents and Chemotherapy* 1996; 40: 413–418.

12. Locarnini SA, Civitico GM & Newbold JE. Hepatitis B: new approaches for antiviral chemotherapy. *Antiviral Chemistry and Chemotherapy* 1996; 7:53–64.

13. Shaw T & Locarnini SA. Hepatic purine and pyrimidine metabolism: implications for antiviral chemotherapy of viral hepatitis. *Liver* 1995; 15:169–184.

14. Miller WH & Miller RL. Phosphorylation of acyclovir (acycloguanosine) monophosphate by GMP kinase. *Journal of Biological Chemistry* 1980; 255: 7204–7207.

15. Miller W & Miller R. Phosphorylation of acyclovir diphosphate by cellular enzymes. *Biochemical Pharmacology* 1982; 31:3879–3884.

16. Shaw T, Mok S & Locarnini S. Inhibition of hepatitis B virus DNA polymerase by enantiomers of penciclovir triphosphate and metabolic basis for selective inhibition of HBV replication by penciclovir. *Hepatology* 1996; 24:996–1002.

17. Lesnikowski ZJ, Juodawlkis AS, Lloyd RM, Chu CK & Schinazi RF. Synthesis and anti-HIV-1 reverse transcriptase activity of triphosphates of penciclovir and β-D-dioxolane-guanine. *Phosphorus, Sulfur and Silicon* 1996; 111:83.

18. Lesnikowski ZJ, Juodawlkis AS, Lloyd RM, Jr & Schinazi RF. Stereoselective synthesis of (S)- and (R)-penciclovir triphosphate and their activity against viral enzymes. *Antiviral Research* 1995; **26**: A211–A362.

19. Schinazi RF, Juodawlkis AS, Lloyd RM, Jr & Lesnikowski ZJ. Differential inhibition of viral polymerases by enantiomers of penciclovir triphosphate. *35th Interscience Conference on Antimicrobial Agents and Chemotherapy.* San Francisco, California, September 17–19, 1995.

20. Vere Hodge RA, Darlison SJ, Earnshaw DL & Readshaw SA. Use of isotopically chiral [4'-¹³C]penciclovir and ¹³C NMR to determine the specificity and absolute configuration of penciclovir phosphate esters formed in HSV-1- and HSV-2-infected cells and by HSV-1-encoded thymidine kinase. *Chirality* 1993; **5**: 583–588.

21. Berenguer M & Wright TL. Hepatitis B and C viruses: molecular identification and targeted antiviral therapies. *Proceedings of the Association of American Physicians* 1998; **110**:98–112.

22. Maruyama T, Hanai Y, Sato Y, Snoeck R, Andrei G, Hosoya M, Balzarini J & De Clercq E. Synthesis and antiviral activity of carbocyclic oxetanocin analogues (C-OXT-A, C-OXT-G) and related compounds. II. *Chemistry and Pharmacology Bulletin (Tokyo)* 1993; **41**:516–521.

23. Hayashi S, Norbeck DW, Rosenbrook W, Fine RL, Matsukura M, Plattner JJ, Broder S & Mitsuya H. Cyclobut-A and cyclobut-G, carbocyclic oxetanocin analogs that inhibit the replication of human immunodeficiency virus in T cells and monocytes and macrophages *in vitro. Antimicrobial Agents and Chemotherapy* 1990; **34**:287–294.

24. Hung LF, Brumbaugh AE, Bhatia G, Marion PL, Hung PP, Norbeck DW, Plattner JJ & Robinson WS. Effects of purine nucleoside analogues with a cyclobutane ring and erythromycin A oxime derivatives on duck hepatitis B virus replication *in vivo* and in cell culture and HIV-1 in cell culture. *Journal of Medical Virology* 1991; **35**:180–186.

25. Tenney D, Yamanaka G, Voss S, Cianci C, Tuomari A, Sheaffer A, Alam M & Colonno R. Lobucavir is phosphorylated in human cytomegalovirus-infected cells and -uninfected cells and inhibits the viral DNA polymerase. *Antimicrobial Agents and Chemotherapy* 1997; **41**:2680–2685.

26. Terry BJ, Cianci CW & Hagen ME. Inhibition of herpes simplex virus type 1 DNA polymerase by [1R (1-alpha, 2-beta, 3-alpha)]-9-[2,3-bis(hydroxymethyl)-cyclobutyl] guanine. *Molecular Pharmacology* 1991; **40**:591–596.

27. Tennant B, Baldwin B, Hornbuckle W, Korba B, Cote P & Gerin J. Animal models in the preclinical assessment of therapy for viral hepatitis. *Antiviral Therapy* 1996; **1** (Supplement 4):47–52.

28. Bisacchi GS, Sundeen JE, Slusarchyk WA, Rinehart K, Innaimo S, Chao S, Jacobs G, Young MG, Kocy O, Merchant Z, Egli P, Lapointe P, Daris JP, Martel A, Colonno R & Zahler R. BMS-200475, a novel carbocyclic 2'-deoxyguanosine analog with potent and selective anti-hepatitis B virus activity *in vitro. 36th ICAAC.* New Orleans, Louisianna, September 15–18, 1996. Abstract F172.

29. Innaimo SF, Seifer M, Bisacchi GS, Standring DN, Zahler R & Colonno R. Identification of BMS-200475 as a potent and selective inhibitor of hepatitis B virus. *Antimicrobial Agents and Chemotherapy* 1997; **41**: 1444–1448.

30. Genovesi EV, Lamb L, Medina I, Clark JM, Taylor D, Standring D, Seifer M, Innaimo S, Sundeen JE, Bisacchi GS, Martel A, Zahler R & Colonno RJ. Efficacy of the novel nucleoside BMS-200475 in the woodchuck model of chronic hepatitis B infection. *36th ICAAC.* New Orleans, Louisiana, September 15–18,1996. Abstract F173.

31. Jacobson MA, Kramer F, Bassiakos Y, Hooton T, Polsky B, Geheb H, O'Donnell JJ, Walker JD, Korvick JA & Van der Horst C. Randomized phase trial of two different combination foscarnet and ganciclovir chronic maintenance therapy regimens for AIDS patients with cytomegalovirus retinitis: AIDS Clinical Trials. *Journal of Infectious Diseases* 1994; **170**:189–193.

32. Locarnini S, Guo K, Lucas R & Gust I. Inhibition of HBV DNA replication by ganciclovir in patients with AIDS. *Lancet* 1989; **ii**:1225–1226.

33. Wang Y, Bowden S, Shaw T, Civitico G, Chan Y, Qiao M & Locarnini S. Inhibition of duck hepatitis B virus replication *in vivo* by the nucleoside analogue ganciclovir (9-[2-hydroxy-1-(hydroxymethyl)ethoxymethyl]-guanine). *Antiviral Chemistry and Chemotherapy* 1991; **2**:107–114.

34. Shaw T, Amor P, Civitico G, Boyd M & Locarnini S. *In vitro* antiviral activity of penciclovir, a novel purine nucleoside, against duck hepatitis B virus. *Antimicrobial Agents and Chemotherapy* 1994; **38**: 719–723.

35. Locarnini S, Civitico G, Wang Y, Tachedjian G & Gust I. Mechanism of action of antiviral agents targeted against duck hepatitis B virus supercoiled DNA. In *The 1990 International Symposium on Viral Hepatitis and Liver Disease*, 1991; pp. 669–671. Edited by FB Hollinger, SM Lemon & HS Margolis. New York: Williams & Wilkins.

36. Yokota T, Konno K, Chonan E, Mochizuki S, Kojima K, Shigeta S & de Clercq E. Comparative activities of several nucleoside analogs against duck hepatitis B virus *in vitro. Antimicrobial Agents and Chemotherapy* 1990; **34**:1326–1330.

37. Civitico G, Wang Y, Luscombe C, Bishop N, Tachedjian G, Gust I & Locarnini S. Antiviral strategies in chronic hepatitis B virus infection: II. Inhibition of duck hepatitis B virus *in vitro* using conventional antiviral agents and supercoiled-DNA active compounds. *Journal of Medical Virology* 1990; **31**:90–97.

38. Civitico G, Shaw T & Locarnini S. Interaction between ganciclovir and foscarnet as inhibitors of duck hepatitis B virus replication in vitro. *Antimicrobial Agents and Chemotherapy* 1996; **40**:1180–1185.

39. Luscombe C, Pedersen J, Uren E & Locarnini S. Long-term ganciclovir chemotherapy for congenital duck hepatitis B virus infection *in vivo*: effect on intrahepatic-viral DNA, RNA, and protein expression. *Hepatology* 1996; **24**:766–773.

40. Wang Y, Luscombe C, Bowden S, Shaw T & Locarnini S. Inhibition of duck hepatitis B virus DNA replication by antiviral chemotherapy with ganciclovir-nalidixic acid. *Antimicrobial Agents and Chemotherapy* 1995; **39**:556–558.

41. Sullivan V, Talarico CL, Stanat SC, Davis M, Coen DM & Biron KK. A protein kinase homologue controls phosphorylation of ganciclovir in human cytomegalovirus-infected cells. *Nature* 1992; **358**:162–164.

42. Boehme R. Phosphorylation of the antiviral precursor 9-(1,3-dihydroxy-2-propoxymethyl)guanine mono-

phosphate by guanylate kinase isozymes. *Journal of Biological Chemistry* 1984; **259**:12346–12349.

43. Naesens L, Snoeck R, Andrei G, Balzarini J, Neyts J & De Clercq E. HPMPC (cidofovir), PMEA (adefovir) and related acyclic nucleoside phosphonate analogues: a review of their pharmacology and clinical potential in the treatment of viral infections. *Antiviral Chemistry and Chemotherapy* 1997; **8**:1–23.

44. Shigeta S, Konno K, Baba M, Yokota T & De Clercq E. Comparative inhibitory effects of nucleoside analogues on different clinical isolates of human cytomegalovirus *in vitro*. *Journal of Infectious Diseases* 1991; **163**: 270–275.

45. Starrett JE, Jr, Tortolani DR, Russell J, Hitchcock MJM, Whiterock V, Martin JC & Mansuri MM. Synthesis, oral bioavailability determination, and *in vitro* evaluation of prodrugs of the antiviral agent 9-[2-(phosphonomethoxy)ethyl]adenine (PMEA). *Journal of Medicinal Chemistry* 1994; **37**:1857–1864.

46. Yokota T, Mochizuki S, Konno K, Mori S, Shigeta S & De Clercq E. Inhibitory effects of selected antiviral compounds on human hepatitis B virus DNA synthesis. *Antimicrob Agents and Chemotherapy* 1991; **35**: 394–397.

47. Yokota T, Konno K, Shigeta S, Holy A, Balzarini J & De Clercq E. Inhibitory effects of acyclic nucleoside phosphonate analogues on hepatitis B virus DNA synthesis in HB611 cells. *Antiviral Chemistry and Chemotherapy* 1994; **5**:57–63.

48. Heijtink RA, De Wilde GA, Kruining J, Berk L, Balzarini J, De Clercq E, Holy A & Schalm SW. Inhibitory effect of 9-(2-phosphonylmethoxyethyl)adenine (PMEA) on human and duck hepatitis B virus infection. *Antiviral Research* 1993; **21**:141–153.

49. Robbins BL, Greenhaw J, Connelly MC & Fridland A. Metabolic pathways for activation of the antiviral agent 9-(2-phosphonylmethoxyethyl)adenine in human lymphoid cells. *Antimicrobial Agents and Chemotherapy* 1995; **39**:2304–2308.

50. Beach JW, Jeong LS, Alves AJ, Pohl D, Kim HO, Chang C-N, Doong S-L, Schinazi RF, Cheng Y-C & Chu CK. Synthesis of enantiomerically pure (2′R,5′S)-(−)-1-[2-(hydroxymethyl)oxathiolan-5-yl]cytosine as a potent antiviral agent against hepatitis B virus (HBV) and human immunodeficiency virus (HIV). *Journal of Organic Chemistry* 1992; **57**:2217–2219.

51. Doong S-L, Tsai C-H, Schinazi RF, Liotta DC & Cheng Y-C. Inhibition of the replication of hepatitis B virus *in vitro* by 2′,3′-dideoxy-3′-thiacytidine and related analogues. *Proceedings of the National Academy of Sciences, USA* 1991; **88**:8495–8499.

52. Furman PA, Davis M, Liotta DC, Paff M, Frick LW, Nelson DJ, Dornsife RE, Wurster JA, Wilson LJ, Fyfe JA, Tuttle JV, Miller WH, Condreay L, Averett DR, Schinazi RF & Painter GR. The anti-hepatitis B virus activities, cytotoxicities, and anabolic profiles of the (−) and (+) enantiomers of *cis*-5-fluoro-1-[2-(hydroxymethyl)-1,3-oxythiolan-5-yl]-cytosine (FTC). *Antimicrobial Agents and Chemotherapy* 1992; **36**: 2686–2692.

53. Schinazi RF, McMillan A, Cannon D, Mathis R, Lloyd RM, Peck A, Sommadossi J-P, St Clair M, Wilson J, Furman PA, Painter G, Choi W-B & Liotta DC. Selective inhibition of human immunodeficiency viruses by racemates and enantiomers of *cis*-5-fluoro-1-[2-(hydroxymethyl)-1,3-oxathiolan-5-yl]cytosine. *Antimicrobial Agents and Chemotherapy* 1992; **36**: 2423–2431.

54. Paff MT, Averett DR, Prus KL, Miller WH & Nelson DJ. Intracellular metabolism of (−)- and (+)-*cis*-5-fluoro-1-[2-(hydroxymethyl)-1,3-oxathiolan-5-yl]cytosine in HepG2 derivative 2.2.15 (subclone P5A) cells. *Antimicrobial Agents and Chemotherapy* 1994; **38**: 1230–1238.

55. Schinazi R. Development of enantiomerically enriched (−)-β-2′,3′-dideoxy-5-fluoro-3′-thiacytidine as an antiviral agent for HIV and HBV. In *Progress of Antiviral Research in Japan*, 1994; pp. 1–24. Edited by K Ono. Japanese Society of Antiviral Research.

56. Shewach DS, Liotta DC & Schinazi RF. Affinity of the antiviral enantiomers of oxathiolane cytosine nucleosides for human 2′-deoxycytidine kinase. *Biochemical Pharmacology* 1993; **45**:1540–1543.

57. Chang C-N, Doong S-L, Zhou JH, Beach JW, Jeong LS, Chu CK, Tsai C-H, Schinazi RF, Liotta DC & Cheng Y-C. Deoxycytidine deaminase-resistant stereoisomer is the active form of (±)-2′,3′-dideoxy-3′-thiacytidine in the inhibition of hepatitis B virus replication. *Journal of Biological Chemistry* 1992; **267**:13938–13942.

58. Hart GJ, Orr DC, Penn CR, Figueiredo HT, Gray NM, Boehme RE & Cameron JM. Effects of (−)-2′-deoxy-3′-thiacytidine (3TC) 5′-triphosphate on human immunodeficiency virus reverse transcriptase and mammalian DNA polymerases alpha, beta and gamma. *Antimicrobial Agents and Chemotherapy* 1992; **36**: 1688–1694.

59. Rahn J, Kieller D, Tyrrell L & Gati W. Modulation of the metabolism of β-L-(−)-2′,3′-dideoxy-3′-thiacytidine by thymidine, fludarabine, and nitrobenzylthioinosine. *Antimicrobial Agents and Chemotherapy* 1997; **43**: 918–923.

60. Schinazi RF. Competitive inhibitors of human immunodeficiency virus reverse transcriptase. *Perspectives in Drug Development and Design*, 1993; **1**:151–180.

61. Cretton-Scott E, Placidi L, Echoff D & Sommadossi J-P. Cellular pharmacology of lamivudine in hepatocyte primary cultures. *Second International Conference on Therapies for Viral Hepatitis*. Kona, Big Island, Hawaii, December 15–19, 1997: Abstract 16.

62. Cretton-Scott E & Sommadossi J-P. Cellular pharmacology of lamivudine in hepatocyte primary cultures. In *Therapies for Viral Hepatitis*. 1998; pp. 321–325. Edited by RF Schinazi, J-P Sommadossi & H Thomas. London: International Medical Press.

63. Schinazi RF, Hough L, Juodawlkis A, Marion P & Tennant B. Comparative activation of 2′-deoxycytidine and antiviral oxathiolane cytosine nucleosides by different mammalian liver extracts. *Antiviral Research* 1997; **34**:A65.

64. Ganem D, Pollack JR & Tavis J. Hepatitis B virus reverse transcriptase and its many roles in hepadnaviral genomic replication. *Infectious Agents and Disease* 1994; **3**:85–93.

65. Ganem D & Varmus HE. The molecular biology of the hepatitis B viruses. *Annual Review of Biochemistry* 1987; **56**:651–693.

66. Summers J & Mason W. Replication of the genome of a hepatitis B-like virus by reverse transcription of an RNA intermediate. *Cell* 1982; **29**:403–415.

67. McLachlan A. *Molecular Biology of the Hepatitis B Virus*, 1991. Boca Raton: CRC Press.

68. Condreay LD, Jansen RW, Powdrill TF, Johnson LC, Selleseth DW, Paff MT, Daluge SM, Painter GR, Furman PA, Ellis MN & Averett DR. Evaluation of the potent anti-hepatitis B virus agent (−)-*cis*-5-fluoro-1-[2-(hydroxymethyl)-1,3-oxathiolan-5-yl]cytosine in a novel *in vivo* model. *Antimicrobial Agents and Chemotherapy* 1994; **38**:616–619.

69. Schinazi RF, Chu CK, Korba BE & Sommadossi J-P. Selective inhibition of human immunodeficiency virus and hepatitis B virus by (–)-β-D-enantiomers of dioxolane-purines. *33rd Interscience Conference on Antimicrobial Agents and Chemotherapy.* 17–20 October 1993, New Orleans, Louisiana, USA. Abstract 43.

70. Schinazi RF, McClure HM, Boudinot FD, Jxiang Y & Chu CK. Development of (–)-β-D-2,6-diaminopurine dioxolane as a potential antiviral agent. *International Conference on Antiviral Research.* February 27–March 4, 1994, Charleston, SC, USA.

71. Schinazi RF, Korba BE, Belen'kii M, Chu CK & Gangemi JD. Evaluation of combinations of (–)-β-D-2,6- diaminopurine dioxolane with interferon or (–)-FTC against hepatitis B virus using multiple drug effect analyses with confidence intervals. *34th Interscience Conference on Antimicrobial Agents and Chemotherapy.* 4–7 October 1994, Orlando, Florida, USA. Abstract 13.

72. Sommadossi J-P, Schinazi RF, Chu CK & Xie M-Y. Comparison of cytotoxicity of the (–)- and (+)-enantiomer of 2′,3′-dideoxy-3′-thiacytidine in normal human bone marrow progenitor cells. *Biochemical Pharmacology* 1992; **44:**1921–1925.

73. Cui L, Schinazi R, Gosselin G, Imbach J-L, Chu C, Rando R, Revankar G & Sommadossi J-P. Effect of β-enantiomeric and racemic nucleoside analogues on mitochondrial functions in HepG2 cells. *Biochemical Pharmacology* 1996; **52:**1577–1584.

74. Rajagopalan P, Boudinot FD, Chu CK, Tennant BC, B.H. B & Schinazi RF. Pharmacokinetics of (–)-β-D-2,6-diaminopurine dioxolane and its metabolite dioxolane guanosine in woodchucks (*Marmota monax*). *Antiviral Chemistry and Chemotherapy* 1995; **7:**65–70.

75. Schinazi RF, Boudinot FD, Manouilov KK, Mellors JW, McMillan A, Schlueter-Wirtz S, Lloyd R, Jr, Korba BE, Tennant B & Chu CK. Anti-HBV and anti-HIV activities of dioxolane-purine nucleosides. *Ninth International Conference on Antiviral Research,* May 19–24 1996, Urabandai, Fukushima, Japan. Abstract 20.

76. Chu CK, Ma T, Shanmuganathan K, Wang C, Xiang Y, Pai SB, Yao G-Q, Sommadossi J-P & Cheng Y-C. Use of 2′-fluoro-5-methyl-β-L-arabinofuranosyluracil as a novel antiviral agent for hepatitis B virus and Epstein-Barr virus. *Antimicrobial Agents and Chemotherapy* 1995; **39:**979–981.

77. Pai S, Liu S, Zhu Y, Chu C & Cheng Y. Inhibition of hepatitis B virus by a novel L-nucleoside, 2′-fluoro-5-methyl-β-L-arabinofuranosyl uracil. *Antimicrobial Agents and Chemotherapy* 1996; **40:**380–386.

78. Liu S-H, Grove K & Cheng Y-C. Unique metabolism of a novel antiviral L-nucleoside analog, 2′-fluoro-5-methyl-β-L-arabinofuranosyluracil: a substrate for both thymidine kinase and deoxycytidine kinase. *Antimicrobial Agents and Chemotherapy* 1998; **42:** 833–839.

79. Peek S, Toshkov I, Erb H, Schinazi R, Korba B, Cote J, Gerin J & Tennant B. 3′-Thiacytidine delays development of hepatocellular carcinoma in woodchucks with experimentally induced chronic woodchuck hepatitis virus infection. Preliminary results of a lifetime study. *Hepatology* 1997; **26:**368A.

80. Aguesse-Germon S, Liu S, Chevallier M, Pichoud C, Jamard C, Borel C, Chu C, Trepo C, Cheng Y & Zoulim F. Inhibitory effect of 2′-fluoro-5-methyl-β-L-arabinofuranosyl-uracil on duck hepatitis B virus replication. *Antimicrobial Agents and Chemotherapy* 1998; **42:**369–376.

81. Tennant B, Peek S, Toshkov I, Erb H, Hornbuckle W, Schinazi R, Korba B, Core J & Gerin J. Treatment with (–)-β-L-2′-3′-dideoxy-3′-thiacytidine (3TC) delays development of hepatocellular carcinoma (HCC) in experimental woodchuck hepatitis virus (WHV) infection. *Second International Conference on Therapies for Viral Hepatitis,* 15–19 December 1997, Kona, Hawaii, USA; Abstract 030.

82. Bartholomew M, Jansen R, Jeffers L, Reddy K, Johnson L, Bunzendahl H, Condreay L, Tzakis A, Schiff E & Brown N. Hepatitis-B-virus resistance to lamivudine given for recurrent infection after orthotopic liver transplantation. *Lancet* 1997; **349:**20–22.

83. Allen M, Deslauriers M, Andrews C, Tipples G, Walters K-A, Tyrrell D, Brown N & Condreay L. Identification and characterization of mutations in hepatitis B virus resistant to lamivudine. *Hepatology* 1995; **27:**1670–1677.

84. Chayama K, Suzuki Y, Kobayashi M, Kobayashi M, Tsubota A, Hashimoto M, Miyano Y, Koike H, Kobayashi M, Koida I, Arase Y, Saitor S, Murashima N, Ireda K & Kumada H. Emergence and takeover of YMDD motif mutant hepatitis B virus during long-term lamivudine therapy and re-takeover by wild type after cessation of therapy. *Hepatology* 1998; **27:**1711–1716.

85. Allen MI, Deslauriers M, Andrews CW, Tipples GA, Walters KA, Tyrrell DL, Brown N & Condreay LD. Identification and characterization of mutations in hepatitis B virus resistant to lamivudine. Lamivudine Clinical Investigation Group. *Hepatology* 1998; **27:**1670–1677.

86. Niesters HG, Honkoop P, Haagsma EB, de Man RA, Schalm SW & Osterhaus AD. Identification of more than one mutation in the hepatitis B virus polymerase gene arising during prolonged lamivudine treatment. *Journal of Infectious Diseases* 1998; **177:**1382–1385.

87. Tipple M, Ma KP, Fischer KS, Gutfreund KS, Bain VG, Kneteman NM & Tyrrell D. Mutation in HBV RNA-dependent DNA polymerase confers resistance to lamivudine in vivo. *Hepatology* 1996; **24:**283A (Abstract #626).

88. Cui L, Yoon S, Schinazi RF & Sommadossi J-P. Cellular and molecular events leading to mitochondrial toxicity of 1-(2-deoxy-2-fluoro-1-β-D-arabinofuranosyl)-5-iodouracil in human liver cells. *Journal of Clinical Investigation* 1995; **95:**555–563.

89. Schinazi RF, Gosselin G, Faraj A, Korba BE, Liotta DC, Chu CK, Mathe C, Imbach J-L & Sommadossi J-P. Pure nucleoside enantiomers of β-2′,3′-dideoxycytidine analogues are selective inhibitors of hepatitis B virus and human immunodeficiency virus *in vitro. Antimicrobial Agents and Chemotherapy* 1994; **38:** 2172–2174.

90. Bartholomeusz A, Schinazi RF & Locarnini S. Significance of mutations in the hepatitis B virus polymerase selected by nucleoside analogues and implications for controlling chronic disease. *Viral Hepatitis Reviews* 1998; in press.

91. Bartholomeusz A & Locarnini S. Mutations in the hepatitis B virus polymerase gene that are associated with resistance to famciclovir and lamivudine. *International Antiviral News* 1997; **5:**123–124.

# 31

# Pathogenic effects of antiviral therapy in chronic hepatitis B virus infection

## Jia-Yee Lee, Danni Colledge and Stephen Locarnini*

## INTRODUCTION

Hepatitis B virus (HBV) infection is prevalent worldwide, causing both acute and chronic infections. Primary HBV infections can be self-limiting or can become persistent, with the clinical outcome generally dependent on the age at which the patient is infected, gender and the state of the individual's immune response. The major health concern with chronic HBV infection is that it can lead to the development of chronic active hepatitis, cirrhosis and hepatocellular carcinoma (HCC) [1,2]. It is estimated that there are 350 million chronic carriers of the virus worldwide, with one million dying each year from HBV-related diseases [3–5]. Although HBV infection may be prevented by vaccination, there is at present no effective therapy for the majority of individuals who are chronically infected. The only approved treatment for chronic HBV infection is interferon-α (IFN-α), but this is only effective in one-third of patients, and several significant side effects are associated with its use [6,7].

The goal of HBV antiviral therapy is to eliminate viral replication in the chronic HBV carrier and to prevent the progression to cirrhosis and HCC. In the past two decades, many antiviral agents that were active against hepadnaviruses in animal models have been unsuccessful in clinical trials because of problems with cytotoxicity or minimal efficacy. As a consequence the majority of these agents have been abandoned, and this has led to loss of interest in the treatment of chronic HBV infection. However, renewed interest in the treatment of chronic carriers has recently been stimulated by the discovery that several nucleoside analogues that have been developed for the treatment of human immunodeficiency virus (HIV) infection – such as lamivudine and adefovir – and herpesvirus infecton – such as penciclovir/famciclovir – exhibit potent anti-HBV activity with minimal cytotoxicity. While these nucleoside analogues have raised the level of optimism in treating chronic HBV infection, achieving treatment success with disease remission has proven to be a challenging task.

All anti-HBV agents to date have been found to be virustatic, whereby cessation of therapy results in the return of all viral replicative markers to at least pretreatment levels [8]. This relapse phenomenon appears to be due to the persistence of the viral covalently closed circular (ccc) DNA [9–11] and the presence of HBV-infected extrahepatic sites that are resistant to antiviral therapy [12–21]. The cccDNA representing the transcriptionally active template does not undergo semi-conservative replication and is therefore not a direct target for current antiviral agents. The eradication of chronic HBV infection either requires the inactivation of the viral cccDNA or the elimination of all infected cells [22]. In addition, further studies are required to determine the mechanism for antiviral persistence and replication at extrahepatic sites, as they constitute major reservoirs of the virus. Furthermore, the complex interplay between the virus and the host requires an understanding not only of the virus replication cycle but also of the viral dynamics involved in relation to the host and its immune response.

## NATURAL HISTORY OF CHRONIC HEPATITIS B VIRUS INFECTION

Chronic carriers who acquire HBV early in life have a higher risk of developing chronic active hepatitis, cirrhosis and HCC than those who acquire the virus later in life. Approximately 90% of chronic HBV infection is acquired through vertical transmission from the infected mother to the infant during the neonatal or perinatal stages [23]. The natural history of chronic HBV infection following acquisition of the virus early in life has been divided into three phases [6]; see Figure 1. The immunotolerant phase, the first phase of HBV chronicity, is characterized by the

---

*Corresponding author

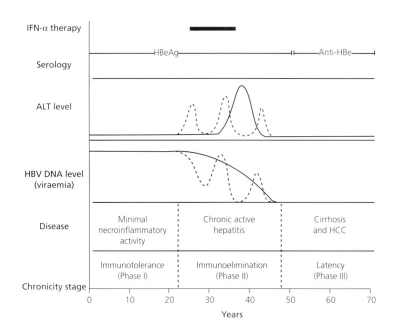

**Figure 1**. The natural history of chronic HBV infection acquired early in life

Adapted from [6].

presence of detectable HBV e antigen (HBeAg), and high levels of viraemia with minimal liver damage. The mechanism of immune tolerance is unclear, although it has been suggested that the secreted HBeAg plays an important role [24]. The function of HBeAg is largely unknown, as it is not required for virion production. However, studies in transgenic mice indicate that HBeAg may be a tolerogen, exerting a state of non-responsiveness at the T cell level in infected individuals. The tolerogenic potential of HBeAg may be advantageous for viral survival, as HBeAg and HBcAg share T-cell epitopes, which would target these proteins for immune-mediated viral clearance [24–27].

The immunotolerant phase can persist from a few weeks to more than 10 years until tolerance is lost. Carriers then enter an immunoelimination phase where significant necro-inflammatory liver damage becomes evident. Clearance of infected hepatocytes mediated by T cell killing is associated with fluctuations in alanine aminotransferase (ALT) levels (hepatic flares). The level of viraemia decreases during this stage until the HBV DNA in the serum becomes undetectable by hybridization analysis. The HBeAg also becomes undetectable in the serum and HBeAg seroconversion occurs. Some of these carriers who are serum HBeAg-negative enter into a third phase of chronic carrier state known as 'latency', which is characterized by the maintenance of serum HBsAg levels, very low levels of HBV DNA and normal ALT. During this phase, most of the viral DNA is integrated into the host cell genome. Individuals at this phase of chronicity are most at risk

of developing liver complications, including HCC.

A subgroup of chronic carriers has been reported with a different clinical profile. These patients have abnormal ALT levels, are HBeAg-negative and/or anti-HBe-positive, with low but detectable viral DNA [28]. Nucleic acid sequence analysis of the viral DNA extracted from these patients revealed that they have been infected with a HBV precore mutant virus. In such viral mutants, a point mutation within the precore region introduces a stop codon that results in the loss of HBeAg because the translated product is prematurely terminated. The production of HBcAg, however, is unaffected. These precore viral mutants are probably viruses that have mutated in order to escape immune clearance during HBeAg seroconversion.

The clinical management of chronic hepatitis B is best approached from an understanding of the natural history of the disease. Treatment strategies can be optimized according to the clinical profile of the infected individual. For example, IFN-α is not an effective treatment for patients in the immunotolerant phase, but is effective when used to treat carriers at the immunoelimination stage. Nevertheless, despite proper staging of chronicity, HBeAg seroconversion is reported in only 30% of cases [6].

## HBV REPLICATION CYCLE

HBV is the prototype member of the family *Hepadnaviridae*, which also includes three well-characterized animal hepadnaviruses – duck HBV

(DHBV), woodchuck hepatitis virus (WHV) and ground squirrel hepatitis virus [29]. Hepadnaviruses have a narrow host range; HBV infects only humans and chimpanzees [30,31] while DHBV infects Pekin ducks and domestic geese [32]. Each of the animal hepadnaviruses has been used as a model for the evaluation of anti-HBV agents [33–36]. However, the duck model is commonly used because DHBV establishes a persistent noncytopathic infection of hepatocytes, as seen in HBV-infected chronic carriers [37–48].

The replication cycle of HBV has been reviewed extensively [49–52], and is outlined in Figure 2. An understanding of the virus replication cycle is essential in light of the use of anti-HBV agents, such as nucleoside analogues, that act at the level of viral reverse transcription. HBV is an enveloped virus containing a 3.2 kilobase (kb), partially double-stranded (ds) open circular DNA genome that is encapsidated in a nucleocapsid together with a virally encoded polymerase. The compact HBV genome contains four overlapping open reading frames (ORFs) that encode: the viral polymerase (P); the core proteins, precore and core (HBcAg); three surface envelope proteins (HBsAg) – large (LHBs), medium (MHBs) and small (SHBs); and the X protein, a putative transcriptional transactivator that is only present in mammalian hepadnaviruses. The coordinated expression of HBV genes occurs by the regulation of HBV promoters located within two enhancer regions and other *cis*-acting promoter elements.

HBV infection of hepatocytes is mediated by receptor-mediated endocytosis [53,54]. Viral entry is preceded by the attachment of HBV virions to an as yet undefined cell surface receptor(s) via the pre-SI domain of the LHBs [55–57]. Following entry and uncoating of the virus in the cytoplasm, the viral nucleocapsid is translocated into the nucleus where the HBV genome is released and modified by the conversion of the single-stranded DNA region to a dsDNA [58–61]. The dsDNA genome undergoes further processing, whereby the terminal protein and the oligoribonucleotide attached to the 5′ end of the viral DNA strands are removed. Genomic DNA is then organized into nucleosomes to form a viral minichromosome where the viral DNA exists as a cccDNA molecule [62,63].

The viral cccDNA is unique in that it has several internal promoters, which mediate in the transcription of a 3.5 kb terminally redundant pregenomic mRNA, and three subgenomic mRNAs [64]. The pregenomic RNA is used both as a template for genomic replication by reverse transcription, and as an mRNA for the synthesis of the core, HBeAg and polymerase proteins. The subgenomic RNAs encode the HBV surface envelope proteins and the X protein [65,66].

Formation of the viral nucleocapsid occurs by the encapsidation of the pregenomic RNA along with the polymerase into core particles [66,67]. During maturation of the core particles, the pregenomic RNA is reverse transcribed into a relaxed circular (RC) partially dsDNA through a complex mechanism (reviewed in [52]). Viral assembly is initiated when the newly synthesized viral nucleocapsid buds into the endoplasmic reticulum where it acquires a lipid bilayer containing the viral surface proteins [68]. The resulting virions are then released from the cell via the constitutive pathway of secretion [69,70].

## PATHOGENESIS OF CHRONIC HBV INFECTION

It is now clear that the immunopathogenesis of HBV infection is due to an efficient cell-mediated immune (CMI) response [71–74]. Liver injury during acute HBV infection is mediated by cytotoxic T cells and natural killer (NK) cells that cause immune lysis of infected hepatocytes [71]. These events are mediated by cytokines that are primarily produced by CD4$^+$ T lymphocytes, and through the perforin and Fas lytic pathways, which induce apoptosis [75,76].

The CD4$^+$ T lymphocytes are divided into two subpopulations, termed T helper type 1 (Th1) and T helper type 2 (Th2), based on the cytokine secretion profile [77]. Th1 cells predominantly produce cytokines such as interleukin 2 (IL-2), IFN-γ and lymphotoxin (TNK-B), which induce CMI responses, while Th2 cells primarily produce IL-4, IL-5, and IL-10, which induce humoral responses. The predominance of Th1-type cytokine responses appears to play an important role in virus clearance of acute and chronic HBV infection [78]. The detection of human leucocyte antigen (HLA) class I and class II epitopes on HBeAg and HBcAg indicate that these viral proteins are the most likely targets for immune responses [71]. The role that these proteins play in the induction or maintenance of persistent infection is not well defined. Based on results from studies in transgenic mice, Milich has proposed that the induction or maintenance of the carrier state may be due to an imbalance in the HBcAg/HBeAg-specific Th1/Th2 cytokine responses [78]. A predominance of an HBV-specific Th2-type cytokine response during chronic infection would favour antibody production, whereas a predominance of the Th1-type response in acute infection would favour a CMI response. Milich

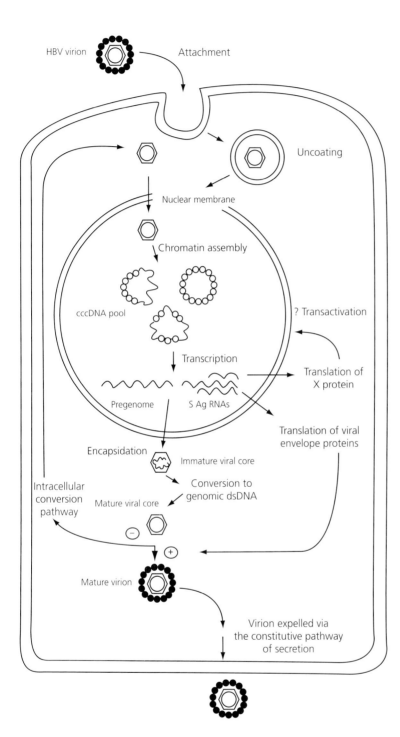

HBV virion

Attachment

Uncoating

Nuclear membrane

Chromatin assembly

cccDNA pool

? Transactivation

Transcription

Translation of
X protein

Pregenome

S Ag RNAs

Translation of viral
envelope proteins

Encapsidation

Immature viral core

Conversion to
genomic dsDNA

Intracellular
conversion
pathway

Mature viral core

−

+

Mature virion

Virion expelled via
the constitutive pathway
of secretion

**Figure 2**. Diagrammatic representation of the HBV replication cycle

Courtesy of G Civitico and T Shaw. The HBV virion enters the cell via receptor-mediated endocytosis. Following attachment, the virus is endocytosed into a coated vesicle where uncoating of the virus to release the viral nucleocapsid occurs. The viral nucleocapsid is then translocated to the nucleus where the viral genomic DNA is modified and converted into a viral minichromosome and the viral DNA exists as a covalently closed circular (ccc) DNA molecule. The cccDNA serves as template for viral RNA transcription to produce the pregenomic RNA and the three subgenomic mRNAs. The pregenomic RNA is encapsidated with the viral core protein to form a nucleocapsid or is used as a template for the translation of viral proteins. During maturation of the viral nucleocapid, the pregenomic RNA is converted to the genomic dsDNA. The translated envelope proteins play a role in regulating the amount of cccDNA in the nucleus. When low levels of viral envelope proteins are present within the cytoplasm, the mature nucleocapsid (core) is shunted back to the nucleus via the intracellular conversion pathway (−). However, when high levels of cytoplasmic viral envelope proteins are present, the mature viral core is targeted for virion assembly (+). The mature virion is then expelled via the constitutive pathway of secretion.

further suggests that cytokine therapy designed to shift a Th2-type response toward a Th1-type response may be beneficial for the treatment of chronic HBV infection [78].

Recently, studies in transgenic mice have shown that CD8[+] cytotoxic T lymphocytes (CTLs) secrete cytokines, such as IFN-γ and tumour necrosis factor-α (TNF-α), that may possess antiviral functions [79]. In contrast to the CTLs that are involved with direct killing of infected hepatocytes, thus causing liver injury, cytokines secreted by the CTLs exert a virucidal effect without causing cell death. It was found that TNF-α and IFN-γ eliminated viral nucleo-capsids and viral DNA replicative intermediates in one pathway, while in another pathway, they reduced the level of viral RNA in host cells [79]. More recent studies by this group have shown that IL-12 plays a significant role in the induction of IFN-γ, leading to the disappearance of HBV replicative intermediates from the liver and extrahepatic sites [80]. The reduction of viral replication markers in these cells has important implications for the maintenance of the cccDNA pool in the nucleus. However, this effect cannot be investigated in the transgenic mouse model as it does not produce cccDNA. The antiviral effect of IL-12 warrants further investigation as it may serve as an important antiviral agent in enhancing the Th1-type response in chronic HBV carriers.

## ROLE OF THE CELL CYCLE IN THE DISTRIBUTION OF HBcAg AND HBV REPLICATION

The key role that HBcAg plays in T-cell mediated lysis of infected hepatocytes has led several groups to investigate the intrahepatic distribution of HBcAg during chronic infection [81–83]. These investigators found that the distribution of HBcAg within infected hepatocytes changes depending on the stage of chronicity. In the early immunotolerant phase, the HBcAg is predominantly located in the nucleus. However, during the immunoelimination stage, there is significantly more HBcAg in the cytoplasm than in the nucleus. This shift in HBcAg distribution from the nucleus to the cytoplasm may present infected hepatocytes as targets for immune-mediated cell lysis [81]. The mechanisms that regulate the distribution of HBcAg within the hepatocytes are poorly understood. It appears that the intrahepatic distribution of HBcAg may be cell-cycle dependent [84,85]. These studies found that HBcAg was located primarily in the cytoplasm when cells were in S phase of the cell cycle, whereas the viral protein was found predominantly in the nucleus when cells were in G0/G1 phase. Thus, in quiescent infected cells, HBcAg is found predominantly in the nuclei, while in dividing cells, HBcAg is localized in the cytoplasm.

A role for cell cycle involvement in the replication of HBV was recently reported by Ozer and colleagues in *in vitro* and *in vivo* studies [86]. *In vitro* studies using an HBV-transfected hepatoma cell line have demonstrated an increase in the level of viral mRNA expression, viral DNA intermediates and virus production in cells arrested in the G1 or G2 phases of the cell cycle. In contrast, the levels of viral RNA

expression and viral DNA intermediates were reduced in cells in S phase. In *in vivo* studies, using liver tissue from HBV-infected patients with advanced chronic liver disease, little or no HBV DNA was detected in proliferating cells. Thus, these studies showed that in quiescent cells, there is enhanced viral replication, while during active cell proliferation, viral replication appeared to be suppressed.

It appears from the above studies that the cell cycle plays an important role in HBV replication and HBcAg distribution within the infected cell. However, the relationship between HBV replication and the distribution of viral proteins at various stages of the cell cycle remains to be defined.

## STABILITY OF THE cccDNA MOLECULE

Virus persistence in infected cells during chronic infection depends on the maintenance of the HBV cccDNA pool (reviewed in [50]). During antiviral treatment of HBV chronic carriers, this cccDNA is the most resistant viral DNA species and is probably the major cause for the relapse phenomenon commonly observed following cessation of therapy. The conversion of the relaxed circular viral genome into cccDNA represents a key step in the replication cycle of HBV. Thus, an understanding of the regulatory elements involved in this process may help elucidate the nature of cccDNA resistance to antiviral therapy.

Viral nucleocapsids from infecting virions or from mature intracellular nucleocapsids provide the source of cccDNA in the nucleus. During viral replication, the HBV nucleocapsid can be targeted for virion formation or transported into the nucleus, where the released viral genome is converted into cccDNA. The latter pathway is known as the intracellular conversion pathway and results in the amplification of the cccDNA pool [87,88]. Amplification of cccDNA occurs early in infection, until a pool of 10 to 50 copies of cccDNA per nucleus is achieved [87,88]. *In vitro* studies in the duck model have shown that the DHBV cccDNA has a finite half-life of 3–5 days [89]. These findings suggest that a mechanism must exist to maintain the cccDNA copy number in persistently infected cells. Indeed, studies by Summers and colleagues have demonstrated that the intracellular conversion pathway is, in part, regulated by the pre-S/S envelope proteins via negative feedback [90–92]. Thus, early in infection, when there are low amounts of surface envelope protein, mature nucleocapsids are shunted into the nucleus whereby the viral genome is converted into cccDNA. The number of cccDNA molecules increases as infection progresses and this leads to a rise in viral RNA synthesis. The viral envelope proteins are subsequently produced at high levels and exert a negative feedback on cccDNA amplification by redirecting the nucleocapsids into the pathway for virion formation. Interestingly, *in vitro* studies incorporating various forms of envelope-defective viruses demonstrated that failure in the regulation of the cccDNA copy number resulted in high levels of this DNA form; the increase in cccDNA levels led to the death of hepatocytes [91,92]. Thus, it appears that control to limit cccDNA amplification is an important feature in maintaining viral persistence in infected cells as failure to do so is detrimental to the cells.

## VIRAL DYNAMICS OF HBV INFECTIONS

An understanding of viral dynamics in infections was originally elucidated from mathematical modelling of data obtained from clinical drug trials of patients infected with HIV-1 [93–96]. These studies revealed that the rate of clearance of free virus, the lifespan of infected cells and the viral generation time are some of the important factors that need to be considered in developing effective antiviral therapeutic strategies.

Similarly, an understanding of viral dynamics in HBV infection is essential to achieve antiviral treatment success. Mathematical modelling of data obtained from short-term clinical trials using lamivudine on patients chronically infected with HBV is shedding some light on the relationship between viral kinetics and the pathogenesis of HBV [97,98]. The clinical data from these studies are derived from the measurement of the HBV DNA in the serum, which was sampled at regular intervals during therapy. The measurement of the HBV DNA level provides an indicator of the level of viraemia or viral load in the serum, which in turn reflects the extent of viral replication in the infected individual. Thus, in antiviral therapy, the decline in serum HBV DNA levels is indicative of the suppression of viral replication in the patient. This reduction in viral DNA level in the serum is caused by the clearance of free virus particles from the serum, and by the death of virus-producing infected cells.

By estimating the half-life of free virus particles and that of virus-producing infected cells in persistently infected patients, it is possible to determine the extent of antiviral treatment that may lead to complete suppression of viral replication. Nowak and colleagues calculated that HBV particles were cleared from the serum of persistently infected patients with a half-life of approximately 1 day [97]. In contrast, the half-life of infected cells was longer and more variable, with an estimated range of 10–100 days. It is assumed that this wide difference may reflect the level of immune responsiveness to the infected cells. Thus, at the stage of active disease during chronic HBV infection, the half-life of virus-producing infected cells would be about 10 days, whilst during the inactive phase of chronic infection, the half-life of these cells would be about 100 days. Based on this model, the authors predicted that in the active disease stage, 12 months treatment with lamivudine would reduce the total body viral burden by a factor of about $10^{11}$. However, in order to achieve this level of viral load reduction during the inactive phase of chronic disease, antiviral therapy would have to be extended to several years.

The estimated half-life for virus-producing cells in the active disease stage also provides a model to estimate the risk associated with the development of HCC. According to the model, during chronic HBV infection, about 1% of infected cells are killed per day. Thus, in the liver, which contains approximately $2 \times 10^{11}$ hepatocytes, there is a daily loss of $10^9$ cells. This massive loss of hepatocytes needs to be replenished to maintain a stable liver mass. According to Nowak and colleagues, the death and regeneration of hepatocytes is likely to be the driving force for the risk of developing HCC [97]. Presumably, inhibition of active viral replication through antiviral therapy would result in a reduced risk of developing HCC.

A similar short-term clinical trial using lamivudine to treat chronically infected HBV patients was also recently conducted by Zeuzem and colleagues [98]. However, their mathematical calculation of serum HBV virus particles with a half-life of 2–3 days appears to contradict that of Nowak and colleagues [97]. Interestingly, other investigators have also reported a half-life of 2–3 days for HBV virions [99] and WHV virions [100]. This discrepancy may be due to dose-dependent differences in drug efficacy [98]. The longer half-life of the virus-producing infected cells would significantly extend the duration of antiviral therapy should the active disease model of Nowak and colleagues [97] be applied.

Although mathematical calculations on clinical data cannot predict the clinical outcome of antiviral therapy, such predictions are useful if they are reflected in the clinical setting. However, as consistently observed in animal models and preliminary clinical trials using anti-HBV agents, cessation of therapy almost inevitably results in the relapse phenomenon, whereby HBV DNA levels return to pretreatment levels. The potential failure of antiviral therapy in eliminating viral replication may, in part, be due to the presence of extrahepatic sites, which represent a reservoir of HBV that is resistant to antiviral therapy, to the persistence of the viral cccDNA, or to the inability to affect the Th1/Th2 imbalance.

The return to pretreatment HBV DNA levels following cessation of antiviral therapy is an interesting phenomenon. While the mechanisms involved have not been elucidated, this rebound effect may be a reflection of the equilibrium reached between the virus and the host. Thus, in the absence of therapy, a steady state of viral persistence is maintained whereby there is a balance in the host–cell relationship. This phenomenon has been documented in viral kinetic analysis of viral load in HIV-infected patients [101–103]. These studies found that the levels of viraemia in HIV-infected individuals are maintained by a continuous cycle of replication and re-infection of the CD4+ cells. The level where viraemia is sustained in HIV-infected patients is defined as the virological setpoint. This virological setpoint or the steady state of viraemia varies between individuals and is predictive of clinical outcome. Thus, a high virological setpoint leads to a poor clinical outcome, whereas a low setpoint results in a more favourable prognosis. A similar phenomenon may be occurring during HBV replication in chronically infected individuals.

The viral dynamic studies of HBV infection have also demonstrated that the turnover rates of HBV are high [96,98]. This would result in the rapid generation of viral variants creating opportunities for immune evasion. Naturally occurring viral variants or quasi-species of HIV have been reported. Mutations in these variants occur in the gene encoding the HIV-1 polymerase because of the lack of proof-reading ability of the viral reverse transcriptase [104,105]. A similar lack of proof-reading ability for the hepadnaviral polymerase has been reported [106,107]. It has been calculated that the annual hepadnaviral polymerase mutation rate of about $2 \times 10^{-4}$ base substitutions per site is similar to that of the retroviral *gag* gene [108]. With a minimum virus production and clearance in HBV chronic carriers estimated at $10^{11}$ virions per day, it is possible that, like HIV [95,109], every mutation at every position in the HBV genome occurs numerous times each day in the infected patient [98]. Therefore, it appears that before commencement of therapy, a population of HBV variants resistant to antiviral agents already exists. As is the case with HIV infections, effective treatment would incorporate a combination of anti-HBV agents that would force the virus to be selected with mutations found simultaneously at several positions in one viral genome. Such mutations are more likely to be detrimental to the virus.

## ANTIVIRAL AGENTS
### Immunomodulating agents

IFN-α is the best studied antiviral agent to date and belongs to the type 1 IFN superfamily which also includes IFN-β. It is well established that these IFNs have broad antiviral and immunomodulatory properties [110]. The immunomodulatory properties of IFN-α that can alter the course of chronic HBV infection may include activation or induction of macrophages, NK cells and cytotoxic T cells, and modulation of antibody production. A corresponding antiviral effect is detected by the elimination of the virus, with subsequent loss of HBeAg and seroconversion to anti-HBe.

Results from clinical trials of IFN-α treatment for chronic HBV infection revealed that patients either exhibit a transient, partial or complete response to the agent [6,7]. A transient response to IFN-α is reported in 50% of treated patients and is characterized by a reduction in serum HBV DNA levels during therapy, which is not sustained upon its cessation. No accompanying improvement in the liver disease is observed during therapy. In contrast, during a partial response, an improvement in liver disease is observed with clearance of serum HBeAg and viral DNA replicative markers. However, serum HBsAg levels persist in these patients. Patients with this clinical profile have undergone a transition from chronic active hepatitis B carrier state to healthy asymptomatic hepatitis B carrier state (latent phase).

A complete response to IFN-α treatment is determined by a loss of serum HBV DNA, HBeAg and HBsAg, followed by seroconversion to anti-HBe, a reversal of liver disease and normalization of serum ALT. A complete response is only observed in 40–50% of patients who generally have low amounts of serum HBV DNA and HBeAg and have evidence of liver injury, as seen by the rise in ALT levels before commencement of treatment. For successful treatment of these patients, therapy with 5–10 million units given subcutaneously thrice weekly for 4–6 months is recommended [7]. Interestingly, a similar response to IFN-α was reported in studies in children with chronic HBV. It appears that children with elevated ALT levels responded to IFN-α at rates that were similar to those seen in adults, whereas those with normal ALT levels responded poorly to IFN-α [111,112]. The recommended treatment protocol for children who have elevated ALT levels is a thrice weekly dose of 6 million units per square metre of body surface area for 4–6 months [7]. To date, the best responses to IFN-α treatment are in patients who have been infected for a short period, have low amounts of serum HBV DNA but have elevated ALT levels with accompanying active liver disease. IFN-α treatment is not recommended for patients outside this narrow clinical profile, as they are generally poor-responders [6,113,114]. HBV chronic carriers not recommended for IFN-α treatment include those with underlying cirrhosis who are infected with a precore HBV mutant, HIV or hepatitis delta virus (HDV), or who are undergoing immunosuppressive therapy [7].

IFN-α therapy is not well tolerated in many patients. The side effects of IFN-α therapy include influenza-like symptoms such as fever, chills, myalgia, backache and headache during the first injection of IFN-α [6,7,115]. However, during chronic treatment, additional symptoms such as fatigue, anorexia, irritability, depression and bone marrow suppression have been reported [6,7,115]. These side effects are dose limiting and are resolved within a few weeks of discontinued therapy. Complications of IFN-α therapy including septicaemia and autoimmune disease have been shown to occur in a small proportion of patients [6,7,115].

Another immunomodulating agent, thymosin-alpha 1 (T-$\alpha_1$), a synthetic polypeptide of thymic origin, has undergone trials in a small group of patients with chronic active hepatitis who were anti-HBe-negative and HBV DNA-positive [116]. Preliminary results have indicated that T-$\alpha_1$ was well tolerated during therapy with no significant side effects and had similar efficacy to IFN-α treatment. This study found that, at the end of 6 months of treatment, T-$\alpha_1$ was effective in promoting disease remission and inhibition of viral replication in about 29% of patients, compared with 43% of patients who responded to IFN-α. However, a complete response at 6 months post-treatment follow-up was observed in 41% of patients treated with T-$\alpha_1$, compared with 25% of patients treated with IFN-α. The higher rate of complete response in the IFN-α group at the end of treatment, and in the T-$\alpha_1$ group at the end of the follow-up period, suggests that T-$\alpha_1$ may be exerting a delayed antiviral effect by stimulating the host immune response [116].

The mechanism of action of T-$\alpha_1$ is not well defined. However, it appears to enhance a Th1 response, as studies have shown that T-$\alpha_1$ is able to act synergistically with endogenous IFN-α and IFN-β in stimulating NK activity [117–119]. Thus, it is likely that a combination therapy with T-$\alpha_1$ and IFN-α may provide a better clinical outcome. Future trials with T-$\alpha_1$ will determine whether this agent can produce long-term inhibition of HBV replication.

## Nucleoside analogues

Nucleoside analogues exhibit their antiviral activity at the level of reverse transcription [120, 121]. For most of these compounds, intracellular phosphorylation to the monophosphate level is the major prerequisite for activity. Ultimate conversion of the analogue to the triphosphate level produces a biologically active form that competes with the natural nucleotides for polymerase binding sites. Some nucleoside analogues that lack the 3′-hydroxyl group on the (deoxy)-ribose also act as elongating viral DNA chain terminators. Moreover, recent studies have shown that different isomers of the same structure may differ in specific activities [122–124].

Three nucleoside analogues, lamivudine (3TC), famciclovir (FCV) and adefovir (PMEA), are currently undergoing Phase II/III clinical trials as potential anti-HBV agents.

## Famciclovir (FCV)

FCV, a purine nucleoside analogue, is the prodrug for penciclovir (PCV) and is structurally related to acyclovir, which was originally developed as an inhibitor of herpesvirus replication [125]. FCV is well absorbed and is rapidly converted to PCV by cellular esterases and oxidases [125]. *In vitro* and *in vivo* studies have shown that PCV is a potent and specific inhibitor of hepadnaviral replication [19,43,126,127]. PCV-triphosphate (PCV-TP) is the biologically active form that exhibits anti-hepadnaviral activity and is exceptionally stable with a half-life of 12–18 hours [43,125]. The precise mechanism of action of PCV-TP has not been determined. However, studies suggest that PCV-TP acts at the level of reverse transcription by preventing extension of the minus strand hepadnaviral DNA or by preventing priming of reverse transcription [43,128,129].

*In vivo* studies in ducks has revealed that PCV and FCV successfully reduced the level of viraemia and all intracellular viral replicative intermediate markers including the cccDNA [8,19,44,127]. A recent long-term *in vivo* study in ducks revealed that PCV suppressed intrahepatic DNA and RNA replication by 92% and 70%, respectively, after 6 months of treatment [130]. These studies also demonstrated a 50% reduction in cccDNA by the end of PCV treatment. However, bile duct epithelial cells and pancreatic cells were resistant to the antiviral activity of PCV. As seen with other nucleoside analogues, the antiviral effect of PCV was not sustained, as all viral replicative markers returned to pretreatment levels upon cessation of treatment. The relapse phenomenon is most likely due to the persistence of cccDNA or the resistance of PCV in extrahepatocyte and extrahepatic sites [130].

FCV has been shown to be effective in reducing HBV DNA replication in patients with recurrent HBV after orthotopic liver transplantation (OLT). In these settings, a reduction in HBV DNA levels of up to 30-fold was reported in some treated patients [131,132]. In clinical trials, FCV was shown to reduce HBV DNA replication with a dose-dependent antiviral response in patients with chronic HBV [133,134]. In a multicentre Phase II study in 333 patients treated with 125 mg, 250 mg or 500 mg FCV three times a day for 16 weeks, a rapid, dose-dependent reduction of serum HBV DNA levels was reported within 1 week of treatment and lasted throughout the treatment period [134]. All doses of FCV contributed to a significant reduction in ALT levels within 8 weeks of starting therapy. Notably, patients on the 500 mg FCV dosage maintained reduced ALT levels over the 8 months of follow-up period, despite a relapse in serum HBV DNA levels. In addition, 14% of patients in this treatment group demonstrated HBeAg seroconversion, which reached statistical significance.

FCV was found to be well tolerated in treated chronic HBV carriers [133,134]. The safety profile of FCV from its clinical use in herpes simplex virus and varicella zoster virus infections indicates that the drug is generally well tolerated. Over 5000 patients have received FCV in completed clinical trials and this agent has been found to have a similar safety profile to that of the placebo [135,136].

## Lamivudine (3TC)

3TC is the (–)-β-enantiomer of 2′,3′-dideoxy-3′-thia-cytidine (3TC) and lacks the 3′ hydroxyl group necessary for DNA chain extension [137]. It inhibits the production of HBV DNA and its replicative inter-mediates by blocking reverse transcriptase and DNA polymerase activity. Similar to PCV, intracellular phosphorylation is required to obtain the biologically active form [120].

The effects of 3TC on hepadnaviral replication are not as well documented as for FCV/PCV. *In vitro* studies in human hepatoma cells [138] and *in vivo* studies in chimpanzees [139] have shown that 3TC is a potent inhibitor of HBV replication. Recently, *in vitro* studies by Colledge and colleagues using primary duck hepatocytes demonstrated that 3TC can inhibit DHBV replication significantly, but was unable to reduce the viral cccDNA levels in hepato-

cytes [48]. However, its effect on bile duct epithelial cells and cells from extrahepatic sites that have been shown to support hepadnaviral replication is not known.

Preliminary results from clinical trials indicate that 3TC is well tolerated [140,141]. In a double-blind trial, 32 HBeAg-positive chronic HBV carriers were treated daily with 25, 100 or 300 mg 3TC orally for 12 weeks [142]. The patients were then followed up for an additional 24 weeks following cessation of therapy. The serum HBV DNA levels were undetectable in 70% and 100% of patients treated with the 100 mg or 300 mg dosage, respectively. Upon cessation of therapy, serum HBV DNA levels re-emerged in most patients. However, 16% of patients continued to experience sustained suppression of viraemia with normalization of ALT levels. The HBeAg levels were undetectable in 12% of patients with fluctuations in ALT levels during and after therapy in some patients.

A similar 3TC treatment dosage was employed in a single-blind, placebo-controlled trial involving a small group of Chinese HBsAg carriers [143]. These patients underwent 4 weeks of treatment and were followed up for another 4 weeks upon cessation of therapy. In this study, a dose of 25 mg was sufficient to suppress HBV replication in 94% of patients with no changes in HBeAg status or in ALT levels. Not surprisingly, viral replication returned to the pretreatment levels during the drug-free period.

## Adefovir (PMEA)

PMEA (9-(2-phosphonylmethoxyethyl) adenine) is a phosphonated acyclic purine nucleoside analogue that has previously been shown to be effective against cytomegalovirus, herpes simplex virus (HSV) and retroviruses [144]. PMEA does not require the initial phosphorylation step that is essential for other nucle-oside analogues for intracellular activation before subsequent conversion to the active form [120,145]. The rate limiting and initial phosphorylation step by adenine kinase is therefore not required for PMEA. For PMEA, adenylate kinase, a nucleotide kinase that converts PMEA to the active diphosphate form (PMEA-DP) is the rate-limiting factor [120,145].

PMEA inhibits hepadnaviral DNA replication at the level of reverse transcription by acting as a DNA chain terminator [145]. In addition to its antiviral activity, PMEA has the potential to exert immunomodulatory properties, including enhancement of NK activity and induction of IFN-α and IFN-β production [146,147]. The anti-HBV activity of PMEA was first established in stably transfected human hepatoma cell lines and in

DHBV-infected primary duck hepatocytes [148,149]. Recent *in vivo* studies in ducks showed that a 4 week treatment of congenitally infected ducks resulted in a 95% reduction in the total viral DNA level, with a 30% reduction in viral RNA and protein levels [150]. The cccDNA was reduced by PMEA treatment by almost 50%, but this did not reach statistical significance. Of particular significance was the reduction in the proportion of bile duct epithelial cells that were positive for viral markers. These findings demonstrated that PMEA is the first nucleoside analogue to inhibit hepadnaviral replication in bile duct epithelial cells.

Adefovir dipivoxil, an orally bioavailable prodrug of PMEA, has currently completed a Phase I/II clinical trial for chronic HBV infection [151]. Viral load was significantly reduced following 4 weeks treatment with this antiviral agent. Phase III studies are currently in progress.

## PATHOGENIC ISSUES IN ANTIVIRAL TREATMENT

### Drug toxicity

Nucleoside analogues can induce mitochondrial toxicity with clinical outcomes such as myopathy, neuropathy, lactic acidosis, pancreatitis, and hepatic failure [152]. A Phase II trial with fialuridine (FIAU) for patients suffering chronic HBV infection was terminated prematurely because of severe clinical multisystemic toxicity that eventually led to five deaths. The toxicity was attributed to mitochondrial damage [153], due to the incorporation of FIAU triphosphate into mitochondrial DNA (mtDNA) and the consequent inhibition of mtDNA synthesis. Such a tragedy was unforeseen, as *in vitro* studies indicated that FIAU had only minimal effect on mtDNA levels [154].

Recently, a study by Honkoop and his colleagues reported a case of severe HBV reactivation after a 6 month course of 3TC in a 29-year-old Chinese man with chronic HBV [155]. Within 4 weeks after cessation of therapy, patient serum ALT rose to 100 times the upper normal limit. Laparoscopy with liver biopsy at this stage showed hepatic collapse, and HBV serology revealed a resurgence of active viral replication. These investigators further reported that in 83 chronic carriers undergoing 3–6 months of 3TC treatment, post treatment ALT levels were elevated in 16% of the patients within 8 to 24 weeks after cessation of therapy.

The safety profile of 3TC to date has been very favourable and 3TC is well tolerated in HIV patients [156,157]. In contrast to the findings in the FIAU studies, recent studies on mitochondrial function and morphology found no evidence of subclinical signs of mitochondrial toxicity in 15 patients undergoing a 6 month course of 3TC [158]. Interestingly, in these patients, 3TC treatment appeared to restore mitochondrial enzyme activity. As observed by these investigators, this is probably due to the decrease in viral replication and general hepatocellular injury. These studies provide preliminary evidence indicating that the activity of 3TC *per se* may not be responsible for the reported liver toxicity in these patients. The sudden hepatic flares observed following the end of 3TC treatment might be due to the imbalance in HBV protein levels caused by 3TC treatment. Studies on the long-term ganciclovir (GCV) treatment of ducks congenitally infected with DHBV have demonstrated such an effect [20]. At the end of therapy, DHBV DNA replicative intermediates in the hepatocytes were reduced but the viral surface envelope proteins had increased and aggregated in the cytoplasm of hepatocytes. These envelope aggregates may represent precursors to the ground glass hepatocytes. As these envelope proteins are involved in the regulation of viral replication, an imbalance in their production could have potential pathological consequences. Interestingly, initial studies by Luscombe and colleagues have found evidence of an increase in Fas antigen expression indicative of apoptosis in hepatocytes containing high levels of the viral envelope proteins [20].

### Extrahepatic sites

Although the major source of virus production comes from HBV-infected hepatocytes, several studies in humans, Pekin ducks and woodchucks have demonstrated the presence of viral DNA and protein in other cell types. Within the liver, bile duct epithelial cells that form part of the biliary system have been shown to support viral replication [18–21]. Extrahepatic sites such as the pancreas, kidney, spleen, peripheral blood mononuclear cells and lymphoid tissues have been found to harbour HBV [12–17]. The presence of HBV genomes in these nonhepatic cells may have important implications in antiviral therapy and liver transplantation settings, as they constitute a potential reservoir for the virus.

*In vivo* studies have been performed to investigate the effect of DHBV replication in extrahepatic sites during antiviral therapy [19,20]. No significant reduction in viral replication was observed in intrahepatic bile duct epithelial cells and cells in the pancreas and kidney during short- or long-term monotherapy with GCV or PCV, despite significant reductions in the level of viral replicative intermediates and viral proteins in infected hepatocytes. The resistance of bile duct epithelial cells to treatment may be due to poor drug uptake, resulting in inadequate intracellular concentrations of the antiviral agent or the inability of cellular enzymes to convert the agent to its active form. However, recent *in vivo* studies in ducks have demonstrated the potential of PMEA to suppress viral replication in bile duct epithelial cells [150]. In these studies, PMEA was shown to inhibit all viral replication markers, including the normally recalcitrant cccDNA form in hepatocytes and bile duct epithelial cells. Interestingly, in this study, DHBV replication in pancreatic islet cells was unaffected by PMEA treatment [150]. Further studies are required to determine the basis for the lack of antiviral effect in these cells.

## EMERGENCE OF NUCLEOSIDE ANALOGUE RESISTANCE

Monotherapy with 3TC or FCV has resulted in the emergence of HBV mutants that are resistant to these compounds. These mutants were first detected in liver transplantation settings where 3TC or FCV were administered to HBV patients at pre- and post-OLT in order to prevent recurrence of HBV infection [159–162]. The emergence of drug-resistant HBV mutants is not unexpected in the light of the reports of 3TC and FCV resistance in HIV and HSV infections, respectively [163–165]. While complete resistance to 3TC in HIV-infected patients was detected [164,165], partial resistance to FCV was reported in HSV-infected individuals [163]. Interestingly, similar 3TC and FCV resistance profiles have been reported in liver transplantation settings where patients have undergone long-term therapy to prevent or manage recurrent HBV infection [159–162].

For both 3TC and FCV, the appearance of resistant HBV mutants was associated with a rise in serum HBV DNA and ALT levels, indicative of breakthrough in therapy [159–162]. Molecular analysis of the viral DNA extracted from patient sera revealed that all mutations associated with 3TC and FCV monotherapy have been located within the viral DNA polymerase gene. For 3TC mutants, mutations have been found within the tyrosine–methionine–aspartate–aspartate (YMDD) amino acid motif, which is involved in the nucleotide binding in the catalytic domain of the polymerase [160,166,167]. Mutation of the methionine at amino acid position 550 to either

isoleucine (I) [160,162,166,168] or valine (V) [162,166,167] was sufficient to confer virus resistance to 3TC. The dominant mutation detected was the M550V change, which was also associated with a domain B change, typically the L526M mutation. The M550I mutation found with 10–15% of cases seems to occur in isolation during antiviral therapy. Recently, a multicentre study in Asia has reported that 14% of chronic HBV patients treated with 100 mg of 3TC for 12 months developed the M550I or M550V mutation [169]. The YMDD catalytic domain is conserved with other RNA-dependent DNA polymerases and similar mutations have been reported for the HIV reverse transcriptase in patients treated with 3TC [164,165,170].

In contrast, HBV polymerase mutations generated from FCV monotherapy are not located within the YMDD motif, but in a region upstream from the YMDD. The valine to leucine change at amino acid position 519 (V519L) and a leucine to methionine change at position 526 (L526M) represent the two selected dominant mutations [161]. The location of these mutations corresponds broadly to the locations found in PCV-resistant HSV DNA polymerase [163]. Interestingly, the two dominant FCV-selected mutations have also been detected in some 3TC-resistant mutants. It is not surprising that in these 3TC-resistant mutants reduced sensitivity to FCV has been reported [171].

The effect of the 3TC- and FCV-selected polymerase mutants on the pathogenesis of the virus is unclear. As the surface ORF overlaps with the polymerase ORF, mutations in the polymerase region may affect expression and antigenicity of the HBsAg [160,166,171]. Interestingly, the neutralization domain of HBsAg overlaps with the domains A and B of the viral polymerase. Drug selected-mutations within these domains of the polymerase could affect the neutralization domain of the HBsAg, leading to potential vaccine escape mutants [171].

## FUTURE PROSPECTS

The emergence of antiviral-resistant HBV mutants, the presence of extrahepatic sites, the persistence of cccDNA and the dynamic interplay between the virus, the hepatocyte and the immune response (see Fig. 3) indicate that no single antiviral agent can effectively combat the problems outlined. Thus, monotherapy with an antiviral agent is unlikely to gain acceptance as the treatment regime of choice for chronic HBV infection. Combination therapy is more likely to offer advantages over monotherapy in reducing the rate of

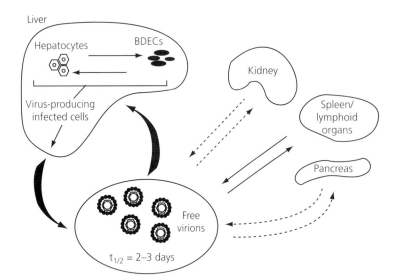

**Figure 3**. Diagrammatic representation of the role hepatic and extrahepatic sites play on viral dynamics during chronic HBV infection

While hepatocytes are the major source of HBV virions, bile duct epithelial cells (BDECs) and cells from extrahepatic sites such as the spleen, lymphoid organs, pancreas and kidney are reservoirs for the virus. The minimum virus production and clearance per day in an individual with chronic HBV has been calculated to be approximately $10^{11}$ virions/day [98]. Infectious virions produced from the various sites have an estimated half life ($t_{1/2}$) of 2–3 days [98]. In contrast, the half-life of virus-producing infected cells has been calculated to be 10–100 days [97,98].

emergence of drug-resistant mutants, in targeting different reservoirs of virus and in inducing an appropriate immune response that may have been suppressed or impaired. In addition, it is possible to reduce toxicity without sacrificing efficacy by choosing drug combinations that act in an additive or synergistic manner but display different spectra of toxicity. Indeed, recent *in vitro* studies have demonstrated a synergistic inhibition of DHBV replication using a combination therapy of PCV and 3TC [48]. More importantly, this drug combination was more effective in reducing the viral cccDNA [48]. Presently, there are a variety of anti-HBV agents such as BMS 200,475 [172], FTC (2′,3′-dideoxy-5-fluoro-3′-thiacytidine)[173], cytallene [174] and nucleosides conjugated to arabinogalactan [175] that are at various stages of antiviral testing. It remains to be determined which combination of nucleoside analogues will be most effective in reducing the levels of viral cccDNA.

Immunomodulatory agents such as IFN-α, recombinant human IL-12 and T-α$_1$ have been shown to play an important role in stimulating a Th1 response. Inclusion of such agents in a cocktail of nucleoside analogues may be clinically beneficial. Thus, the development of effective treatment strategies for chronic hepatitis B infection will depend on the proper staging of chronicity, an understanding of the immunopathogenesis of disease, a knowledge of the viral dynamics and the choice of combination antiviral therapy.

## ACKNOWLEDGEMENTS

Jia-Yee Lee is supported by the National Health & Medical Research Council of Australia.

## REFERENCES

1. Beasley RP & Huang LY. Epidemiology of hepatocellular carcinoma. In *Viral Hepatitis and Liver Disease*, 1984; pp. 209–224. Edited by GN Vyas, JL Dienstag and JH Hoofnagle. New York: Grune and Stratton.
2. Beasley RP. Hepatitis B virus: the major etiology of hepatocellular carcinoma. *Cancer* 1988; **61**:1942–1956.
3. Locarnini S & Gust ID. *Hepadnaviridae*: hepatitis B virus and delta virus. In *Laboratory Diagnosis of Infectious Diseases. Principles and Practice: II Viral, Rickettsial and Chlamydial diseases*, 1988; pp. 750–796. Edited by EH Lennette, P Halonen & F Murphy. New York: Springer-Verlag.
4. Lau JY & Wright TL. Molecular virology and pathogenesis of hepatitis B. *Lancet* 1993; **342**:1335–1340.
5. Kane M. Global programme for control of hepatitis B infection. *Vaccine* 1995; **13** (Supplement 1):S47–49.
6. Lok A. Treatment of chronic hepatitis B. *Journal of Viral Hepatitis* 1994; **1**:105–124.
7. Hoofnagle JH. The treatment of chronic viral hepatitis. *Drug Therapy* 1997; **336**:347–356.
8. Locarnini SA & Cunningham A. Clinical treatment of viral hepatitis. In *Antiviral Chemotherapy* 1995; pp. 441–530. Edited by E De Clercq & D Jeffries. Chichester: John Wiley.
9. Yokosuka O, Omata A, Imazeki F, Ocuda K & Summers J. Changes of hepatitis B virus DNA in liver and serum caused by recombinant leukocyte interferon treatment: analysis of intrahepatic replicative hepatitis B virus DNA. *Hepatology* 1985; **5**:728–734.
10. Sherker AH, Hirota K, Omata M & Okuda K. Foscarnet decreases serum and liver duck hepatitis B virus DNA in chronically infected ducks. *Gastroenterology* 1986; **92**:818–824.
11. Wang Y, Bowden S, Shaw T, Civitico G, Chan Y, Qiao M & Locarnini S. Inhibition of duck hepatitis B virus replication *in vivo* by the nucleoside analogue ganciclovir 9-(2-hydroxy-1{[hydroxymethyl]}guanine). *Antiviral Chemistry & Chemotherapy* 1991; **2**:107–114.
12. Blum HE, Stowring L, Figus A, Montgomery CK, Haase AT & Vyas GN. Detection of hepatitis B virus DNA in hepatocytes, bile duct epithelium, and vascular

elements by in situ hybridization. *Proceedings of the National Academy of Sciences, USA* 1983; **80**: 6685–6688.

13. Lie-Injo L, Balasegaram M, Lopez C & Herrera A. Hepatitis B virus DNA in liver and white blood cells of patients with hepatoma. *DNA* 1983; **2**:301–307.

14. Romet-Lemone JL, McLane MF, Elfassi E, Haseltine WA, Azocar J & Essex M. Hepatitis B virus infection in cultured human lymphoblastoid cells. *Science* 1983; **221**:667–669.

15. Halpern MS, Egan J, MacMahon S & Ewert DL. Duck hepatitis B virus is tropic for exocrine cells of the pancreas. *Virology* 1985; **146**:157–161.

16. Tagawa M, Omata M, Yokosuka O, Uchima K, Imazeki F & Okuda K. Early events in duck hepatitis B virus infection: sequential appearance of viral deoxyribonucleic acid in liver, pancreas, kidney and spleen. *Gastroenterology* 1985; **89**:1224–1229.

17. Walter E, Teubner H, Blum HE, Offensperger W-B, Offensperger S & Gerok W. Duck hepatitis B virus infection in non-hepatocytes. *Liver* 1991; **11**:53–62.

18. Luscombe C, Pedersen J, Bowden S & Locarnini S. Alterations in the intrahepatic expression of duck hepatitis B viral markers with ganciclovir chemotherapy. *Liver* 1994; **14**:182–192.

19. Lin E, Luscombe C, Wang Y, Shaw T & Locarnini S. The guanine nucleoside analog penciclovir is active against chronic duck hepatitis B virus infection *in vivo*. *Antimicrobial Agents and Chemotherapy* 1996; **40**:413–418.

20. Luscombe C, Pedersen J, Uren E & Locarnini S. Long term ganciclovir chemotherapy of congenital duck hepatitis B virus infection *in vivo*: effect on intrahepatic viral DNA, RNA, and protein expression. *Hepatology* 1996; **24**:766–773.

21. Nicoll A, Locarnini S, Chou S, Smallwood R & Angus P. Human hepatitis B virus infection in bile duct epithelium. *Hepatology* 1996; **24**:221A.

22. Averett DR & Mason W. Evaluation of drugs for antiviral activity against hepatitis B virus. *Viral Hepatitis Reviews* 1995; **1**:129–142.

23. Stevens CE, Beasley RP, Tsui J & Lee WC. Vertical transmission of hepatitis B antigen in Taiwan. *New England Journal of Medicine* 1975; **292**:771–774.

24. Milich DR, Jones JE, Hughes JL, Price J, Raney AK & McLachlan A. Is a function of the secreted hepatitis Be antigen to induce immunological tolerance *in utero*? *Proceedings of the National Academy of Sciences, USA* 1990; **87**:6599–6603.

25. Mondelli M, Vergani G, Alberti A, Vergani D, Portmann B, Eddleston AL & Williams R. Specificity of T lymphocyte cytotoxicity to autologous hepatocytes in chronic hepatitis B virus infection: evidence that T cells are directed against HBV core antigen expressed on hepatocytes. *Journal of Immunology* 1982; **129**:2773–2777.

26. Ferrari C, Penna A, Giuberti T, Tong MJ, Ribera E, Fiaccadori F & Chisari FV. Intrahepatic, nucleocapsid antigen-specific T cells in chronic active hepatitis B. *Journal of Immunology* 1987; **139**:2050–2058.

27. Bertoletti A, Ferrari C, Fiaccadori F, Penna A, Margolskee R, Schlict HJ, Fowler P, Guilhot S & Chisari FV. HLA class I-restricted human cytotoxic T cells recognize endogenously synthesized hepatitis B virus nucleocapsid antigen. *Proceedings of the National Academy of Sciences, USA* 1991; **88**:10445–10449.

28. Hadziyannis S. Hepatitis Be antigen negative in chronic hepatitis B: from clinical recognition to pathogenesis and treatment. *Viral Hepatitis Reviews* 1995; **1**:7–36.

29. Howard C. The structure of hepatitis B envelope and molecular variants of hepatitis B virus. *Journal of Viral Hepatitis* 1995; **2**:165–170.

30. Maynard JE, Berquist KR, Krushak DH & Purcell RH. Experimental infection of chimpanzees with the virus of hepatitis B. *Nature* 1972; **237**:514–515.

31. Barker LF, Chisari FV, McGrath PP, Dalgard DW, Kirschstein RL, Almeida JD, Edington TS, Sharp DG & Peterson MR. Transmission of type B hepatitis to chimpanzees. *Journal of Infectious Diseases* 1973; **127**:648–662.

32. Marion PL, Cullen JM, Azcarraga RR, Van Davelaar MJ & Robinson WS. Experimental transmission of duck hepatitis B virus to Pekin ducks and domestic geese. *Hepatology* 1987; **7**:724–731.

33. Smee DF, Knight SS, Duke AE, Robinson WS, Matthews TR & Marion PL. Activities of arabinosyladenine monophosphate and 9-(1,3-dihydroxy-2-propoxymethyl) guanine against ground squirrel hepatitis virus *in vivo* as determined by reduction in serum virion-associated DNA polymerase. *Antimicrobial Agents and Chemotherapy* 1985; **27**:277–279.

34. Mason WS & Taylor JM. Experimental systems for the study of hepadnavirus and hepatitis delta virus infections. *Hepatology* 1989; **9**:635–645.

35. Roggendorf M & Tolle T. The woodchuck: an animal model for hepatitis B virus infection in man. *Intervirology* 1995; **38**:100–112.

36. Fourel I, Hantz O, Watanabe KA, Jacquet C, Chomel B, Fox JJ & Trepo C. Inhibitory effects of 2'-fluorinated arabinosyl-pyrimidine nucleosides on woodchuck hepatitis virus replication in chronically infected woodchucks. *Antimicrobial Agents and Chemotherapy* 1990; **34**:473–475.

37. Hirota K, Sherker AH, Omata M, Yokosuka O & Okuda K. Effects of adenine arabinoside on serum and intrahepatic replicative forms of duck hepatitis B virus in chronic infection. *Hepatology* 1987; **7**:24–28.

38. Haritani H, Uchida T, Okuda Y & Shikata T. Effect of 3'-azido-3'-deoxythymidine on replication of duck hepatitis B virus *in vivo* and *in vitro*. *Journal of Medical Virology* 1989; **29**:244–248.

39. Kassianides C, Hoofnagle JH, Miller RH, Doo E, Ford H, Broder S & Mitsuya H. Inhibition of duck hepatitis B virus replication by 2',3'-dideoxycytidine: a potent inhibitor of reverse transcriptase. *Gastroenterology* 1989; **97**:1275–1280.

40. Niu J, Wang Y, Qiao M, Gowans E, Edwards P, Thyagarajan SP, Gust I & Locarnini S. Effect of Phyllanthus amarus on duck hepatitis B virus replication *in vivo*. *Journal of Medical Virology* 1990; **32**:212–218.

41. Fourel I, Li J, Hantz O, Jacquet C, Fox JJ & Trepo C. Effects of 2' fluorinated arabinosyl-pyrimidine nucleosides on duck hepatitis B virus DNA level in serum and in liver of chronically infected ducks. *Journal of Medical Virology* 1992; **37**:122–126.

42. Mason WS, Cullen J, Saputelli J, Wu TT, Liu C, London WT, Lustbader E, Schaffer P, O'Connell AP, Fourel I *et al.* Characterization of the antiviral effects of 2' carbodeoxyguanosine in ducks chronically infected with duck hepatitis B virus. *Hepatology* 1994; **19**:398–411.

43. Shaw T, Amor P, Civitico G, Boyd M & Locarnini S. *In vitro* antiviral activity of penciclovir, a novel purine nucleoside, against duck hepatitis B virus. *Antimicrobial Agents and Chemotherapy* 1994; **38**:719–723.

44. Tsiquaye KN, Slomka MJ & Maung M. Oral famciclovir against duck hepatitis B virus replication in

hepatic and nonhepatic tissues of ducklings infected in ovo. *Journal of Medical Virology* 1994; **42**:306–310.

45. Dean J, Bowden S & Locarnini S. Reversion of duck hepatitis B virus DNA replication *in vivo* following cessation of treatment with the nucleoside analogue ganciclovir. *Antiviral Research* 1995; **27**:171–178.

46. McMillan JS, Shaw T, Angus PW & Locarnini S. Effect of immunosuppressive and antiviral agents on hepatitis B virus replication *in vitro*. *Hepatology* 1995; **22**:36–43.

47. Civitico G, Shaw T & Locarnini S. Interaction between ganciclovir and foscarnet as inhibitors of duck hepatitis B virus replication *in vitro*. *Antimicrobial Agents and Chemotherapy* 1996; **40**:1180–1185.

48. Colledge D, Locarnini S & Shaw T. Synergistic inhibition of hepadnaviral replication by lamivudine in combination with penciclovir *in vitro*. *Hepatology* 1997; **26**:216–225.

49. Ganem D & Varmus HE. The molecular biology of hepatitis B viruses. *Annual Review of Biochemistry* 1987; **56**:651–693.

50. Locarnini S, Civitico G & Newbold JE. Hepatitis B: new approaches for antiviral chemotherapy. *Antiviral Chemistry & Chemotherapy* 1996; **7**:1–12.

51. Nassal M & Schaller H. Hepatitis B virus replication – an update. *Journal of Viral Hepatitis* 1996; **3**:217–226.

52. Tavis JE. The replication strategy of hepadnaviruses. *Viral Hepatitis Reviews* 1996; **2**:205–218.

53. Offensperger W-B, Offensperger S, Walter E, Blum HE & Gerok W. Sulphated polyanions do not inhibit duck hepatitis B virus infection. *Antimicrobial Agents and Chemotherapy* 1991; **35**:2431–2433.

54. Riggs RJ & Schaller H. Duck hepatitis B virus infection of hepatocytes is not dependent on low pH. *Journal of Virology* 1992; **66**:2829–2836.

55. Neurath AR, Seto B & Strick N. Antibodies to synthetic peptides from the preS1 region of the hepatitis B virus (HBV) envelope (env) protein are virus neutralizing and protective. *Vaccine* 1989; **7**:234–236.

56. Pontisso P, Ruvoletto MG, Gerlich WH, Heerman KH, Bardini R & Alberti A. Identification of an attachment site for human liver plasma membranes on hepatitis B virus particles. *Virology* 1989; **173**:522–530.

57. Dash S, Rao VS & Panda SK. Receptor for the Pre-S1 (21–47) component of hepatitis B virus on the liver cell: role in virus cell interaction. *Journal of Medical Virology* 1992; **37**:115–121.

58. Eckart SG, Milich DR & McLachlan A. Hepatitis B virus core antigen has two nuclear localization sequences in the arginine rich carboxy terminus. *Journal of Virology* 1991; **65**:575–582.

59. Robinson WS & Greenman R. DNA polymerase in the core of the human hepatitis B virus candidate. *Journal of Virology* 1974; **14**:384–391.

60. Hruska JF, Clayton DA, Rubenstein JLR & Robinson WS. Structure of hepatitis B Dane particle DNA before and after the Dane particle DNA polymerase reaction. *Journal of Virology* 1977; **21**:666–672.

61. Koch J & Schlict H-J. Analysis of the earliest steps of hepadnaviral replication: genome repair after infectious entry into hepatocytes does not depend on viral polymerase activity. *Journal of Virology* 1993; **67**:4867–4874.

62. Bock C-T, Schranz P, Schroder CH & Zentgraf H. Hepatitis B virus genome is organized into nucleosomes in the nucleus of the infected cell. *Virus Genes* 1994; **8**:215–229.

63. Newbold JE, Xin H, Tencza M, Sherman G, Dean J, Bowden DS & Locarnini S. The covalently closed duplex form of the hepadnaviral genome exists *in situ* as an heterogeneous population of viral minichromosomes. *Journal of Virology* 1995; **69**:3350–3357.

64. Schaller H & Fischer M. Transcriptional control of hepadnavirus gene expression. *Current Topics in Microbial Immunology* 1991; **168**:21–39.

65. Standring DN, Rutter WJ, Varmus HE & Ganem D. Transcription of hepatitis B surface antigen in cultured murine cells initiates within the presurface region. *Journal of Virology* 1984; **50**:563–571.

66. Junker-Neipmann M, Bartenschlager R & Schaller H. A short *cis*-acting sequence is required for hepatitis B virus pregenome encapsidation and sufficient for packaging foreign RNA. *EMBO Journal* 1990; **9**:3389–3396.

67. Hirsch RC, Loeb DD, Pollack JR & Ganem D. *Cis*-acting sequences required for encapsidation of duck hepatitis B virus pregenomic RNA. *Journal of Virology* 1991; **65**:3309–3316.

68. Huovila AJ, Eder AM & Fuller SD. Hepatitis B surface antigen assembles in a post-ER, pre-Golgi compartment. *Journal of Cell Biology* 1992; **118**:1305–1320.

69. Patzer EJ, Nakamura GR, Simonsen CC, Levinson AD & Brands R. Intracellular assembly and packaging of hepatitis B surface antigen particles occur in the endoplasmic reticulum. *Journal of Virology* 1986; **58**:884–982.

70. Simon K, Lingappa VR & Ganem D. Secreted hepatitis B surface antigen polypeptides are derived from a transmembrane precursor. *Journal of Cell Biology* 1988; **107**:2163–2168.

71. Chisari FV & Ferrari C. Hepatitis B virus immunopathogenesis. *Annual Review of Immunology* 1995; **13**:29–60.

72. Löhr, HF, Gerken G, Schlicht HJ, Meyer zum Buschenfelde KH & Fleischer B. Low frequency of cytotoxic liver-infiltrating T lymphocytes specific for endogenous processed surface and core proteins in chronic hepatitis B. *Journal of Infectious Diseases* 1993; **168**:1133–1139.

73. Waters JA, O'Rourke S, Schlicht H-J & Thomas HC. Cytotoxic T cell responses in patients with chronic hepatitis B virus infection undergoing HBe antigen/antibody seroconversion. *Clinical and Experimental Immunology* 1995; **102**:314–319.

74. Tsai SL & Huang SN. T cell mechanisms in the immunopathogenesis of viral hepatitis B and C. *Journal of Gastroenterology and Hepatology* 1997; **12** (Supplement):S227–235.

75. Kagi D, Vignaux F, Ledermann B, Burki K, Depraetere V, Nagata S, Hengartner H & Golstein P. *Fas* and perforin pathways as major mechanisms of T cell-mediated cytotoxicity. *Science* 1994; **265**:528–530.

76. Lowin B, Hahne M, Mattmann C & Tschopp J. Cytolytic T-cell cytotoxicity is mediated through the perforin and *Fas* lytic pathways. *Nature* 1994; **270**:650–652.

77. Mosmann TR, Cherwinski H, Bond MW, Giedlin MA & Coffman RL. Two types of murine helper T cell clone. I. Definition according to profiles of lymphokine activities and secreted proteins. *Journal of Immunology* 1986; **136**:2348–2357.

78. Milich DR. Influence of T-helper cell subsets and cross-regulation in hepatitis B virus infection. *Journal of Viral Hepatitis* 1997; **4** (Supplement 2):48–59.

79. Guidotti LG, Ishikawa T, Hobbs MV, Matzke B, Schreiber R & Chisari FV. Intracellular inactivation of the hepatitis B virus by cytotoxic T lymphocytes.

*Immunity* 1996; **4**:25–36.

80. Cavanaugh VJ, Guidotti LG & Chisari FV. Interleukin-12 inhibits hepatitis B virus replication in transgenic mice. *Journal of Virology* 1997; **71**:3236–3243.

81. Chu CM & Liaw YF. Intrahepatic distribution of hepatitis B surface and core antigens in chronic hepatitis B virus infection. Hepatocyte with cytoplasmic/membranous hepatitis B core antigen as a possible target for immune hepatocytolysis. *Gastroenterology* 1987; **92**:220–225.

82. Hsu HC, Su IJ, Lai MY, Chen DS, Chang MH, Chuang SM & Sung JL. Biologic and prognostic significance of hepatocyte hepatitis B core antigen expression in the natural course of chronic hepatitis B virus infection. *Journal of Hepatology* 1987; **5**:45–50.

83. Yoo JY, Howard R, Waggoner JG & Hoognagle JH. Peroxidase–antiperoxidase detection of hepatitis B surface and core antigens in liver biopsy specimens from patients with chronic type B hepatitis. *Journal of Medical Virology* 1987; **23**:273–281.

84. Yeh CT, Wong SW, Fung YK & Ou JH. Cell cycle regulation of nuclear localization of hepatitis B virus core protein. *Proceedings of the National Academy of Sciences, USA* 1993; **90**:6459–6463.

85. Chu CM, Yeh CT, Sheen IS & Liaw YF. Subcellular localization of hepatitis B core antigen in relation to hepatocyte regeneration in chronic hepatitis B. *Gastroenterology* 1995; **109**:1926–1932.

86. Ozer A, Khaoustov VI, Mearns M, Lewis DE, Genta RM, Darlington GJ & Yoffe B. Effect of hepatocyte proliferation and cellular DNA synthesis on hepatitis virus replication. *Gastroenterology* 1996; **110**:1519–1528.

87. Tuttleman JS, Pourcel C & Summers J. Formation of the pool of covalently closed circular viral DNA in hepadnavirus-infected cells. *Cell* 1986; **47**:451–460.

88. Wu T-T, Coates L, Aldrich CE, Summer J & Mason WS. In hepatocytes infected with duck hepatitis B virus, the template for viral RNA synthesis is amplified by an intracellular conversion pathway. *Virology* 1990; **175**:255–261.

89. Civitico G & Locarnini S. The half-life of duck hepatitis B virus supercoiled DNA in congenitally infected primary hepatocyte cultures. *Virology* 1994; **203**:81–89.

90. Summers J, Smith PM & Horwich AL. Hepadnavirus envelope proteins regulate covalently closed circular DNA amplification. *Journal of Virology* 1990; **64**:2819–2824.

91. Summers J, Smith PM, Huang M & Yu M. Morphogenetic and regulatory effects of mutations in the envelope proteins of an avian hepadnavirus. *Journal of Virology* 1991; **65**:1310–1317.

92. Lenhoff RJ & Summers J. Co-ordinate regulation of replication and virus assembly by the large envelope protein of an avian hepadnavirus. *Journal of Virology* 1994; **68**:4566–4571.

93. Wei X, Ghosh SK, Taylor ME, Johnson VA, Emini EA, Deutsch P, Lifson JD, Bonhoeffer S, Nowak MA, Hahn BH, Saag MS & Shaw GM. Viral dynamics in human immunodeficiency virus type 1 infection. *Nature* 1995; **373**:117–122.

94. Ho DD, Neumann AU, Perelson AS, Chen W, Leonard JM & Markowitz M. Rapid turnover of plasma virions and CD4 lymphocytes in HIV-1 infection. *Nature* 1995; **373**:123–126.

95. Perelson AS, Neumann AU, Markowitz M, Leonard JM & Ho DD. HIV-1 dynamics *in vivo*: virion clearance rate, infected cell life span, and viral generation time. *Science* 1996; **271**:1582–1585.

96. Herz AVM, Bonhoeffer S, Anderson RM, May RM & Nowak MA. Viral dynamics *in vivo*: limitations on estimates of intracellular delay and virus decay. *Proceedings of the National Academy of Sciences, USA* 1996; **93**:7247–7251.

97. Nowak MA, Bonhoeffer S, Hill A, Boehme R, Thomas HC & McDade H. Viral dynamics in hepatitis B virus infection. *Proceedings of the National Academy of Sciences, USA* 1996; **93**:4398–4402.

98. Zeuzem S, de Man RA, Honkoop P, Roth WK, Schalm SW & Schmidt JM. Dynamics of hepatitis B virus infection *in vivo*. *Journal of Hepatology* 1997; **27**:431–436.

99. Drouet J, Courouce-Pauty AM, Thevenoux AM, Soulier JB, Chanard J, Vallee G & Funch-Brentano JL. Kinetic of HBsAg in man. *Biomedicine* 1975; **22**:158–166.

100. Tencza MG & Newbold JE. Heterogeneous response for a mammalian hepadnavirus infection to acyclovir: drug arrested intermediates of minus-strand viral DNA synthesis are enveloped and secreted from infected cells as virion-like particles. *Journal of Medical Virology* 1997; **51**:6–16.

101. Mellors JW, Kingsley LA, Rinaldo CR, Hoo BS, Kokka RP & Gupta P. Quantitation of HIV-1 RNA in plasma predicts outcome after seroconversion. *Annals of Internal Medicine* 1995; **112**:573–579.

102. Mellors JW, Rinaldo C, Gupta P, White RM, Todd JA & Kingsley LA. Prognosis in HIV-1 infection predicted by the quantity of virus in plasma. *Science* 1996; **272**:1167–1170.

103. Ho DD. Viral counts in HIV infection. *Science* 1996; **272**:1124–1125

104. Cornelissen M, van der Burg R, Zorgdrager F, Lukashov V & Goudsmit J. Pol gene diversity of five human immunodeficiency virus type 1 subtypes: evidence for naturally occurring mutations that contribute to drug resistance, limited recombination patterns, and common ancestry for subtypes B and D. *Journal of Virology* 1997; **71**:6348–6358.

105. Najera I, Holguin A, Quinones-Mateu ME, Munoz-Fernandez MA, Najera R, Lopez-Galindez C & Domingo E. Pol gene quasispecies of human immunodeficiency virus: mutations associated with drug resistance in virus from patients undergoing no drug therapy. *Journal of Virology* 1995; **69**:23–31.

106. Brown JL, Carman WF & Thomas HC. The clinical significance of molecular variation within the hepatitis B virus genome. *Hepatology* 1992; **15**:144–148.

107. Miller R, Kaneko S, Chung C, Girones R & Purcell R. Compact organization of the hepatitis B virus genome. *Hepatology* 1989; **9**:322–327.

108. Girone R & Miller RH. Mutation rate of the hepadnavirus genome. *Virology* 1989; **170**:595–597.

109. Coffin JM. HIV population dynamics *in vivo*: implications for genetic variation. pathogenesis, and therapy. *Science* 1995; **267**:483–489.

110. Peters M. Mechanisms of action of interferons. *Seminar in Liver Diseases* 1989; **9**:235–239.

111. Lai CL, Lok ASF, Lin HJ, Wu PC, Yeoh EK & Yeung CY. Placebo controlled trial of recombinant alpha-interferon in Chinese HBsAg-carrier children. *Lancet* 1987, **2**:877–880.

112. Ruiz-Moreno M, Rua MJ, Molina J, Moraleda G, Moreno A, Garcia-Aguado J & Carreno V. Prospective, randomized controlled trial of interferon-α in children with chronic hepatitis B. *Hepatology* 1991;

13:1035–1039.

113. Tine F, Liberati A, Craxi A, Almasio P & Pagliaro L. Interferon treatment in patients with chronic hepatitis B: a meta-analysis of the published literature. *Hepatology* 1993; **18**:154–162

114. Niederau C, Heintges T, Lange S, Goldmann G, Niederau CM, Mohr L & Haussinger D. Long-term follow-up of HBeAg-positive patients treated with interferon alfa for chronic hepatitis B. *New England Journal of Medicine* 1996; **334**:1422–1427

115. Renault PF & Hoofnagle JH. Side effects of alpha interferon. *Seminar in Liver Diseases* 1989; **9**:273–277.

116. Andreone P, Cursaro C, Gramenzi A, Zavaglia C, Rezakovic I, Altomare E, Severini R, Franzone JS, Albano O, Ideo G, Bernardi M & Gasbarini G. A randomized controlled trial of thymosin-$\alpha_1$ versus interferon $\alpha$ treatment in patients with hepatitis Be antigen antibody- and hepatitis B virus DNA-positive chronic hepatitis B. *Hepatology* 1996; **24**:774–777.

117. Mutchnick MG, Prieto JA, Schaffner JA & Weller FE. Thymosin modulation of regulatory T cell function. *Clinical Immunology and Immunopathology* 1982; 23:626–633.

118. Serrate SA, Schulof RS, Leondaridis L, Goldstein AL & Sztein MB. Modulation of human natural killer cytotoxic activity, lymphokine production and interleukin 2 receptor expression by thymic hormones. *Journal of Immunology* 1987; **139**:2338–2343.

119. Mastino A, Favalli C, Grelli S & Garaci E. Thymic hormones and cytokines. *International Journal of Immunopathology and Pharmacology* 1992; **5**:77–82.

120. Shaw T & Locarnini S. Hepatic purine and pyrimidine metabolism: implications for antiviral chemotherapy of viral hepatitis. *Liver* 1995; **15**:169–184.

121. Luscombe C & Locarnini S. The mechanism of action of antiviral agents in chronic hepatitis B. *Viral Hepatitis Review* 1996; **1**:1–35.

122. Mansour TS, Jin H, Wang W, Hooker EU, Ashman C, Cammock N, Salomon H, Belmonte AR & Wainberg MA. Anti-human immunodeficiency virus and anti-hepatitis B virus activities and toxicities of the enantiomers of 2′-deoxy-3′oxa-4′thiacytidine and their 5-fluoro analogues *in vitro*. *Journal of Medical Chemistry* 1995; **38**:1–4.

123. Chang CN, Doong SL, Zhou JH, Beach JW, Leong LS, Chu CK, Tsai CH, Cheng YC, Liotta S & Schinazi R. Deoxycytidine deaminase-resistant stereoisomer is the active form of (±)-2′,3′-dideoxycytidine-3′-thiacytidine in the inhibition of hepatitis B virus replication. *Journal of Biological Chemistry* 1992; **267**:13938–13942.

124. Chang CN, Skalski V, Zhou JH & Cheng YC. Biochemical pharmacology of (+) and (−)-2′,3′-dideoxy-3′-thiacytidine as antihepatitis B virus agents. *Journal of Biological Chemistry* 1992; **267**: 22414–22420.

125. Vere Hodge RA. Famciclovir and penciclovir. The mode of action of famciclovir including its conversion to penciclovir. *Antiviral Chemistry and Chemotherapy* 1993; 4:67–84.

126. Shaw T, Mok SS & Locarnini SA. Inhibition of hepatitis B virus DNA polymerase by enantiomers of penciclovir triphosphate and metabolic basis of selective inhibition of HBV replication by penciclovir. *Hepatology* 1996; **24**:996–1002.

127. Tsiquaye K, Sutton D, Maung M & Boyd M. Antiviral activities and pharmacokinetics of penciclovir and famciclovir in Pekin ducks chronically infected with duck hepatitis B virus. *Antiviral Chemistry and Chemotherapy* 1996; **7**:153–159.

128. Dannaoui E, Trepo C & Zoulim F. Inhibitory effect of penciclovir-triphosphate on duck hepatitis B virus reverse transcription. *Antiviral Chemistry and Chemotherapy* 1997; **8**:38–46.

129. Ilsley DD, Lee S-H, Miller WH & Kuchta RD. Acyclic guanosine analogs inhibit DNA polymerases $\alpha$, $\delta$ and $\epsilon$ with very different potencies and have unique mechanisms of action. *Biochemistry* 1995; **34**:2504–2510.

130. Lin E, Luscombe C, Colledge D, Wang YY & Locarnini S. Long term therapy with the guanosine nucleoside analogue penciclovir controls chronic duck hepatitis B virus infection *in vivo*. *Antimicrobial Agents and Chemotherapy* 1998; **42**: 2132–2137.

131. Böker KHW, Ringe B, Krüger M, Pichmayr R & Manns MP. Prostaglandin E plus famciclovir: a new concept for the treatment of severe hepatitis B after liver transplantation. *Transplantation* 1994; **57**:1706–1708.

132. Krüger M, Tillman HL, Trautwein C, Bode U, Oldhafer K, Maschek H, Böker KH, Broelsch CE, Pichmayr R & Mann MP. Famciclovir treatment of hepatitis B virus recurrence after liver transplantation: a pilot study. *Liver Transplantation and Surgery* 1996; **2**:253–262.

133. Main J, Brown J, Howells, Galassini R, Crossey M, Karayiannis P, Georgiou P, Atkinson G & Thomas HC. A double blind, placebo-controlled study to assess the effect of famciclovir on virus replication in patients with chronic hepatitis B virus infection. *Journal of Viral Hepatitis* 1996; **3**:829–836.

134. Trepo C. Efficacy of famciclovir in chronic hepatitis B: result of a dose finding study. *Hepatology* 1996; **24**:188A.

135. Saltzman R, Jurewicz R & Boon R. Safety of famciclovir in patients with herpes zoster and genital herpes. *Antimicrobial Agents & Chemotherapy* 1994; **38**:2454–2457.

136. Boon RJ, Saltzman R & Atkinson G. The clinical safety experience with famciclovir. *47th Annual Meeting of the American Association for the Study of Liver Diseases*, Chicago, USA, 11–14 November 1996; Abstract 623.

137. Severini A, Liu X-Y, Wilson JS & Tyrell DL. Mechanism of inhibition of duck hepatitis B virus polymerase by (−)-$\beta$-L-2′,3′-dideoxy-3′-thiacytidine. *Antimicrobial Agents and Chemotherapy* 1995; **39**:1430–1435.

138. Doong SL, Tsai CH, Schinazi RF, Liotta DC & Cheng YC. Inhibition of the replication of hepatitis B virus *in vitro* by 2′,3′-dideoxy-3′-thiacytidine and related analogues. *Proceedings of National Academy of Sciences, USA* 1991; **88**:8495–8499.

139. Tyrrell DLJ, Fischer K & Cameron J. 2′,3′ Dideoxy 3′ thiacytidine (lamivudine) treatment of chimpanzees chronically infected with hepatitis B virus (HBV) results in rapid suppression of HBV DNA in sera. In *Program and Abstract of the 18th International Symposium on Viral Hepatitis and Liver Disease*, 1993; p. 156. Tokyo: Viral Hepatitis Foundation of Japan.

140. Tyrrell DLJ, Mitchell MC, De Man RA, Schalm SW, Main J, Thomas HC, Fevery J, Nevens F, Beranek P & Vicary C. Phase II trial of lamivudine for chronic hepatitis B. *Hepatology* 1993; **18**:112A.

141. Schalm SW, de Man RA, Heijtink RA & Niesters HGM. New nucleoside analogues for chronic hepatitis B. *Journal of Hepatology* 1995; **22** (Supplement 1):52–56.

142. Dienstag JL, Perillo RP, Schiff ER, Bartholomew M, Vicary C & Rubin MA. Preliminary trial of lamivudine for chronic hepatitis B infection. *New England Journal of Medicine* 1995; 333:1657–1661.

143. Lai C-L, Chiing C-K, Tung AK-M, Li E, Young J, Hill A, Wong BC-Y, Dent J & Wu P-C. Lamivudine is effective in suppressing hepatitis B virus DNA in Chinese hepatitis B surface antigen carriers: a placebo-controlled trial. *Hepatology* 1996; 25:241–244.

144. Naesens L, Neyts J, Balzarini J, Holy A, Rosenberg I & De Clercq E. Efficacy of oral 9-(2-phosphonyl-methoxyethyl)-2,6-diaminopurine (PMEDAP) in the treatment of retrovirus and cytomegalovirus infections in mice. *Journal of Medical Virology* 1993; 39:167–172.

145. Balzarini J, Hao Z, Herdewijn P, Johns DG & De Clercq E. Intracellular metabolism and mechanism of anti-retrovirus action of 9-(2-phosphonyl-methoxyethyl) adenine, a potent anti-human immunodeficiency virus compound. *Proceedings of the National Academy of Sciences, USA* 1991; 88:1499–1503.

146. Del Gobbo V, Foli A, Balzarini J, De Clercq E, Balestra E, Villani N, Marini S, Perno C & Calio R. Immunomodulatory activity of 9-(2-phosphonyl-methoxyethyl) adenine (PMEA), a potent anti-HIV nucleoside analogue, on *in vivo* murine models. *Antiviral Research* 1991; 16:65–75.

147. Calio R, Villani N, Balestra E, Sesa F, Holy A, Balzarini J, De Clercq E, Perno CF & Del Gobbo V. Enhancement of natural killer activity and interferon induction by different acyclic nucleoside phosphonates. *Antiviral Research* 1994; 23:77–89.

148. Heijtink RA, De Wilde GA, Kruining J, Berk L, Balzarini J, De Clercq E, Holy A & Schalm SW. Inhibitory effect of 9-(2-phosphonylmethoxyethyl) adenine (PMEA) on human and duck hepatitis B virus infection. *Antiviral Research* 1993; 21:141–153.

149. Heijtink RA, Kruining J, De Wilde GA, Balzarini J, De Clercq E & Schalm SW. Inhibitory effects of acylic nucleoside phosphonates on human hepatitis B virus and duck hepatitis B virus infections in tissue culture. *Antimicrobial Agents and Chemotherapy* 1994; 38:2180–2182.

150. Nicoll AJ, Colledge DL, Toole JJ, Angus PW, Smallwood RA & Locarnini SA. Inhibition of duck hepatitis B virus replication by 9-(2-phosphonyl-methoxyethyl) adenine (PMEA), an acrylic phosphonate nucleoside analogue. *Antimicrobial Agents & Chemotherapy* 1998; in press.

151. Gilson R, Chopra K, Murray-Lyon I, Newell A, Nelson M, Tedder R, Toole J, Jaffe H, Hellmann N & Weller I. A placebo-controlled phase I/II study of adefovir dipivoxil (bis-POM PMEA) in patients with chronic hepatitis B infection. *Hepatology* 1996; 24:281A.

152. Lewis W & Dalakas MC. Mitochondrial toxicity of antiviral drugs. *Nature Medicine* 1995; 1:417–422.

153. McKenzie R, Fried MW, Sallie R, Conjeevaram H, Di Bisceglia AM, Park Y, Savarese B, Kleiner D, Tsokos M, Luciono C *et al.* Hepatic failure and lactic acidosis due to fialuridine (FIAU), an investigational nucleoside analogue for chronic hepatitis B. *New England Journal of Medicine* 1995; 333:1099–1105.

154. Colacino JM, Malcolm SK & Jaskunas SR. Effect of fialuridine on replication of mitochondria DNA in CEM cells and human hepatoblastoma cells in culture. *Antimicrobial Agents and Chemotherapy* 1994; 38:1997–2002.

155. Hookoop P, de Man RA, Heijtink RA & Schlam SW. Hepatitis B reactivation after lamivudine. *Lancet* 1995; 346:1156–1157.

156. Eron JJ. The treatment of antiretroviral-naive subjects with the 3TC/zidovudine combination: a review of North American (NUCA 3001) and European trials. *AIDS* 1996; 10 (Supplement 5):S11–19.

157. Styrt BA, Piazza-Hepp TD & Chikami GK. Clinical toxicity and antiretroviral nucleoside analogs. *Antiviral Research* 1996; 31:121–135.

158. Honkoop P, de Man RA, Scholte HR, Zondervan PE, Van Dem Berg JWO, Rademakers LHPM & Schalm SW. Effect of lamivudine on morphology and function of mitochondria in patients with chronic hepatitis B. *Hepatology* 1997; 26:211–215.

159. Aye TT, Bartholomeusz A, Shaw T, Bowden S, Breschkin A, McMillan J, Angus P & Locarnini S. Hepatitis B virus polymerase mutations during famciclovir therapy in patients following liver transplantation. *Hepatology* 1996; 24:285A.

160. Tipple GA, Ma MM, Fischer KP, Bain VG, Kneteman NM & Tyrrell DLJ. Mutation in HBV-RNA-dependent DNA polymerase confers resistance to lamivudine *in vivo*. *Hepatology* 1996; 24:714–717

161. Aye TT, Bartholomeusz A, Shaw T, Bowden S, Breschkin A, McMillan J, Angus P & Locarnini S. Hepatitis B virus polymerase mutations during antiviral therapy in a patient following liver transplantation. *Journal of Hepatology* 1997; 26:1148–1153.

162. Bartholomew MM, Jansen RW, Jeffers LJ, Reddy KR, Johnson CC, Bunzendahl H, Condreay LD, Tzakis AG, Schiff ER & Brwon NA. Hepatitis B virus resistance to lamivudine given for recurrent infection after orthotopic liver transplantation. *Lancet* 1997; 349:20–22.

163. Chiou HC, Kumura K, Hu A, Kerns KM & Coen DM. Penciclovir resistance mutations in the herpes simplex virus DNA polymerase gene. *Antiviral Chemistry and Chemotherapy* 1995; 6:281–288.

164. Schuurman R, Nijhuis M, van Leeuwen R, Schipper P, de Jong D, Collis P, Danner SA, Mulder J, Loveday C, Christopherson C, Kwok S, Sninsky J & Boucher CAB. Rapid changes in human immunodeficiency virus type 1 RNA load and appearance of drug resistant virus populations in persons treated with lamivudine (3TC). *Journal of Infectious Diseases* 1995; 171:1411–1419.

165. Wainberg MA, Salomon H, Gu Z, Montaner JS, Cooley TP, MacCaffey R, Ruedy J, Hirst HM, Cammack N, Cameron J & Nicholson W. Development of HIV-1 resistance to (–) 2′-deoxy-3′-thiacytidine in patients with AIDS or advanced AIDS-related complex. *AIDS* 1995; 9:351–357.

166. Ling R, Mutimer D, Ahmed M, Boxall E, Elias E, Dusheiko M & Harrison TJ. Selection of mutations in the hepatitis B virus polymerase during therapy of transplant recipients with lamivudine. *Hepatology* 1996; 24:711–713.

167. Naoumov NV, Chokski S, Smith HM & Williams R. Emergence and characterization of lamivudine resistant hepatitis B virus variant. *Hepatology* 1996; 24:282A

168. de Man RA, Bartholomeusz A, Locarnini S, Niesters HGM & Zondervan PE. The occurrence of sequential viral mutations in a liver transplant recipient re-infected with hepatitis B: primary famciclovir resistance followed by a lethal hepatitis acquired during lamivudine resistance. *Journal of Hepatology* 1997; 26 (Supplement 1):79.

169. Lai CL, Liaw YF, Leung NWY, Chang TT, Guan R, Tai

DI, Ng KY, Wu PC, Dent JC & Gray DF. A 12 month course of lamivudine (100 mg od) therapy improves liver histology: results from a placebo controlled multi-center study in Asia. *Journal of Hepatology* 1997; **26** (Supplement 1):79.

170. Tisdale M, Kemp SD, Parry NR & Larder BA. Rapid *in vitro* selection of human immunodeficiency virus type 1 resistant to 3′-thiacytidine inhibitors due to a mutation in the YMDD region of the reverse transcriptase. *Proceedings of the National Academy of Sciences, USA* 1993; **90**:5653–5656.

171. Locarnini S. Hepatitis B virus surface antigen and polymerase gene variants: potential virological and clinical significance. *Hepatology* 1998; **27**:294–297.

172. Innaimo SF, Seifer M, Bisacchi GS, Standring DN, Zahler R & Colonno RJ. Identification of BMS-200475 as a potent and selective inhibitor of hepatitis B virus. *Antimicrobial Agents and Chemotherapy* 1997; **41**:1444–1448.

173. Cullens JM, Smith SL, Davis MG, Dunn SE, Botteron C, Cecchi A, Linsey D, Linzey D, Frick L, Paff MT, Goulding A & Biron K. *In vivo* antiviral activity and pharmokinetics of (−)-cis-5-fluoro-1-[2-(hydroxymethyl)-1,3-oxathiolan-5-yl]cytosine in woodchuck hepatitis virus-infected woodchucks. *Antimicrobial Agents and Chemotherapy* 1997; **41**:2076–2082.

174. Zhu Y-L, Pai BS, Liu S-H, Grove KL, Jones BCNM, Simons C, Zemlicka J & Cheng Y-C. Inhibition of replication of hepatitis B virus by cytallene *in vitro*. *Antimicrobial Agents and Chemotherapy* 1997; **41**:1755–1760.

175. Fiume L, Di Stefano G, Busi C, Mattioli A, Bonino F, Torrani-Cerenzia M, Verme G, Rapicetta M, Bertini M & Gervasi GB. Liver targeting of antiviral nucleoside analogues through the asialoglycoprotein receptor. *Journal of Viral Hepatitis* 1997; **4**:363–370.

# 32

# Preclinical investigation of L-FMAU as an anti-hepatitis B virus agent

Chung K Chu*, F Douglas Boudinot, Simon F Peek, Joon H Hong, Yongseok Choi, Brent E Korba, John L Gerin, Paul J Cote, Bud C Tennant and Yung-Chi Cheng

## INTRODUCTION

Despite the fact that over 350 million individuals worldwide are chronically infected with hepatitis B virus (HBV) and significant numbers of these individuals will suffer from liver cancer in their lifetime, no safe and effective chemotherapeutic agent for the treatment of HBV infection is currently available. Although a number of synthetic and natural products have been found to possess anti-HBV activity *in vitro*, nucleosides are the only class of compounds thus far identified that appear to hold promise for the treatment of chronic HBV infection in humans. In this regard, several nucleoside analogues are currently undergoing preclinical and clinical investigation as potentially effective anti-HBV agents (Fig. 1). (–)-β-L-2′,3′ Dideoxy-3′-thiacytidine (lamivudine; 3TC) [1,2], a nucleoside with an oxathiolane ring system, which has been approved by the US Food and Drug Administration for the treatment of human immunodeficiency virus (HIV) infection since 1995, also exhibits potent anti-HBV activity *in vitro* and *in vivo* [3]. Lamivudine is currently undergoing Phase III clinical trials for the treatment of HBV infection and will probably be approved for human use in the near future, first in China. The 5-fluoro congener of lamivudine, *cis*-5-fluoro-1-[2-(hydroxymethyl)-1,3-oxathiolan-5-yl]-cytosine (FTC), has been shown to have potent anti-HBV activity *in vitro* (EC$_{50}$ 0.01 μM) [4]. It has also demonstrated potent activity against HIV in ongoing Phase I/II clinical trials [5]. Clinical studies of FTC for the treatment of chronic HBV infection are anticipated in the near future. (–)-β-D-2,6-Diaminopurine dioxolane (DAPD) [6], a purine analogue with a dioxolane ring system, exhibits potent *in vitro* activity against HBV and is currently undergoing preclinical toxicology evaluation. DAPD is converted to an active metabolite, dioxolane-

guanine [7]. A novel carbocyclic nucleoside, BMS-200475, has been reported to have potent anti-HBV activity in 2.2.15 cells, with an EC$_{50}$ value of 3 nM [8]. Biochemical studies indicate that BMS-200475 can be efficiently phosphorylated by cellular enzymes to its triphosphate, which is a potent inhibitor of HBV DNA polymerase, inhibiting both the priming and elongation steps of HBV DNA replication [9]. BMS-200475 is currently undergoing Phase II clinical trials. Another carbocyclic nucleoside, lobucavir, a deoxyguanine nucleoside analogue, has broad spectrum antiviral activity [10]. Lobucavir was previously shown to inhibit herpes simplex virus (HSV) DNA polymerase after phosphorylation by the HSV thymidine kinase. Lobucavir has also been shown to inhibit human cytomegalovirus DNA synthesis to a degree comparable to that of ganciclovir, a drug known to target the viral DNA polymerase [11].

An acyclonucleoside, PMEA (adefovir) exhibits potent inhibitory effects on HBV replication and viral antigen production in two human hepatoma cell lines transfected with HBV (HepG 2.2.15 and HB611), with IC$_{50}$ values of 0.7 μM and 1.2 μM, respectively [12]. PMEA also shows an inhibitory effect on duck HBV (DHBV) in primary duck hepatocytes (IC$_{50}$ 0.2 μM), as well as *in vivo* [13]. Another acyclonucleoside, famciclovir, the oral prodrug of penciclovir, can be readily absorbed and sequentially deacetylated in the intestinal wall and liver to yield 6-deoxypenciclovir [14]. The latter can be oxidized by xanthine oxidase in the liver to give rise to the parent drug, penciclovir [15]. Famciclovir is currently undergoing Phase II clinical trials as an anti-HBV agent.

As described above, a number of nucleoside analogues are in various stages of development as potential anti-HBV agents in humans. Recently, we have discovered 1-(2-fluoro-5-methyl-β-L-arabinofu-

Figure 1. Anti-HBV nucleosides under development

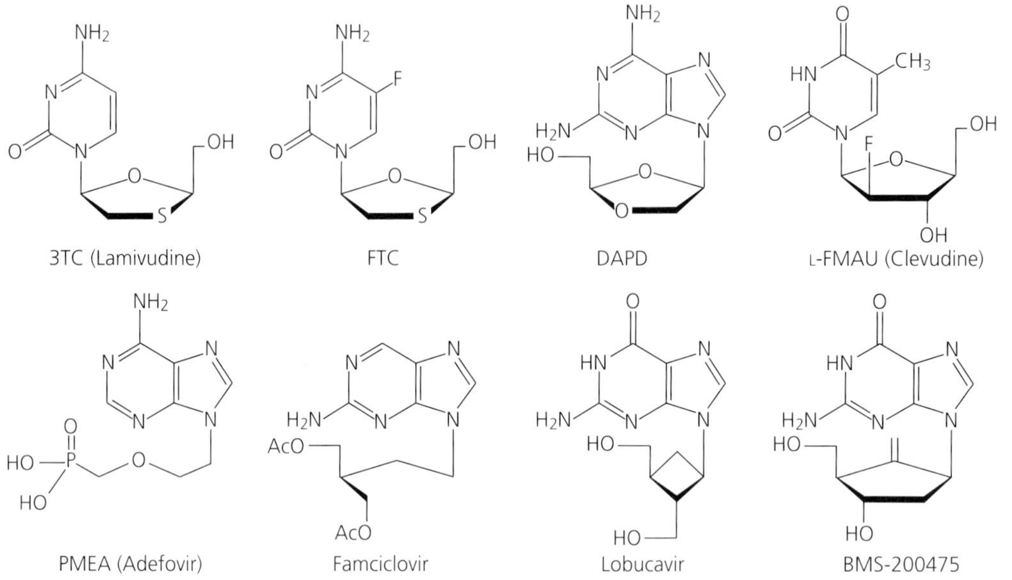

3TC (Lamivudine)  FTC  DAPD  L-FMAU (Clevudine)

PMEA (Adefovir)  Famciclovir  Lobucavir  BMS-200475

ranosyl)-uracil (L-FMAU) to be a potent antiviral agent against HBV *in vitro* and *in vivo*. This review briefly summarizes the preclinical evaluation of L-FMAU.

## SYNTHESIS

Since the key starting material for the synthesis of L-FMAU is L-ribose, which is expensive to purchase commercially, we attempted to identify a previously described method for the synthesis of L-ribose from readily available carbohydrates. Although several procedures have been reported [16–19], none of these appeared practical for large-scale preparation. We therefore decided to develop a preparative method for L-ribose. Two methods were considered, one from L-xylose and the other method using L-arabinose (Fig. 2).

The synthesis of L-FMAU was accomplished via the key intermediate 5, which was initially prepared from an L-ribose derivative following a procedure similar to that used for the synthesis of D-FMAU [20], as briefly summarized below. Previously, it was reported that D-ribose can be synthesized from D-xylose, the epimer of D-ribose, via a stereoselective oxidation–reduction procedure, albeit in low yield [21]. This strategy was used to prepare the L-ribose derivative 5 for the synthesis of L-FMAU [22–24]. Although various oxidizing agents have been described for the oxidation of the 3-OH of pento-furanose derivatives, it was found that pyridinium

dichromate (PDC) gave the best yield (96%) of ketone derivative 3. After a series of reactions, treatment of 5 with saturated hydrogen chloride in $CH_2Cl_2$ at 0°C followed by hydrolysis and treatment with $SO_2Cl_2$ and imidazole in $DMF:CH_2Cl_2$ gave the imidazolyl sulphonate in 73% yield. The imidazole derivative was fluorinated with $KHF_2$ and 48% HF: $H_2O$ to give 1,3,5-tri-O-benzoyl-2-fluoro-β-L-arabino-furanose (6). Activation to the bromo sugar coupled with silylated thymine in anhydrous $CHCl_3$ gave protected L-FMAU, which was treated with $NH_3$: $CH_3OH$ to give the desired L-FMAU.

Owing to the limited availability of L-xylose as the starting material, as well as the requirement for large amounts of L-FMAU for additional biological studies, we developed another procedure from L-arabinose. L-Arabinose is a natural sugar that is reasonably inexpensive. The anomeric position could be protected with a benzyl group in acidic conditions in the pyranose form and the vicinal diol group was protected with an isopropylidene group. In similar conditions as L-xylose, PDC was used for the oxidation reaction to obtain compound 4. Compound 4 was reduced with $NaBH_4$ in methanol with high stereoselectivity, because of the concave nature of the bicyclic system. After full deprotection with $CF_3COOH$, the resulting L-ribose was sequentially treated with 1% $HCl:MeOH$, BzCl: pyridine and $H_2SO_4:Ac_2O:AcOH$ to obtain compound 5. The remaining steps to L-FMAU were the same as described for the L-xylose procedure. A

**Figure 2.** Practical synthetic routes to L-FMAU

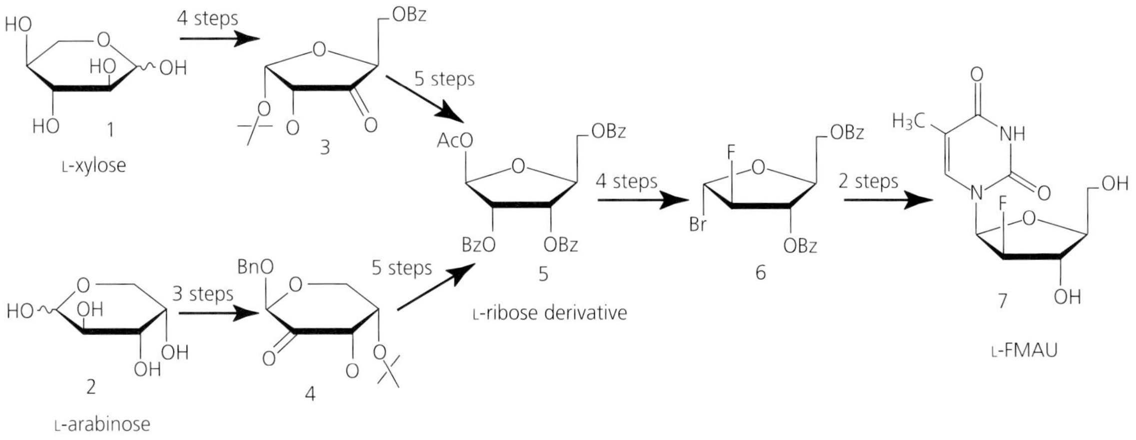

full account of the synthetic procedure for L-FMAU from L-arabinose will be published elsewhere.

## *IN VITRO* ANTIVIRAL ACTIVITY AND BIOCHEMISTRY

Although we synthesized a series of 2'-F-L-nucleosides according to the procedures discussed above, L-FMAU was found to be the most active against HBV *in vitro* [25]. Unlike β-L-ddC analogues, L-FMAU was inactive against HIV. Interestingly, it also exhibits antiviral activity against Epstein–Barr virus (EBV), with an $EC_{90}$ value of approximately 5 μM [26]. This is the first example of an L-thymidine analogue having potent biological activity.

*In vitro*, L-FMAU inhibits HBV DNA replication with an $EC_{50}$ value of 0.1 μM in 2.2.15 cells and does not show any significant toxicity up to 1000 μM, with an $EC_{90}$ value of approximately 1.0 μM, whereas the D-enantiomer was toxic with an $IC_{50}$ value of 50 μM. Furthermore, *in vitro* growth inhibition studies in other cell lines, including MT2, CEM and H1, indicated no significant cellular toxicities (Table 1).

Additionally, L-FMAU did not inhibit growth of human bone marrow progenitor cells [25].

The *in vitro* efficacy data was also confirmed in two independent laboratories, which suggests that L-FMAU is indeed a potent anti-HBV agent [25,27].

L-FMAU is phosphorylated stepwise to L-FMAUMP, L-FMAUDP and L-FMAUTP in 2.2.15 cells (Fig. 3). The concentration of L-FMAU metabolites over a 24 hour period was analysed by HPLC [27]. Rapid conversion of the compound to its phosphorylated forms could be detected as early as 2 hours. With the drug concentrations used, maximum metabolite formation was observed at 8 hours. The results suggest that despite the unnatural sugar configuration of L-FMAU, it can be readily metabolized by cells. After 24 hours treatment, when the drug was withdrawn, the levels of mono-, di- and triphosphate decreased as a function of time. However, the clearance of the metabolites did not appear to follow first-order kinetics. In the initial phase in drug-free medium, the levels of the metabolites dropped rapidly, with about 90% of the triphosphate disappearing in the first 8 hours. In the

**Table 1.** Anti-HBV and anti-EBV activities of D- and L-FMAU analogues

| Compound | Anti-HBV activity in 2.2.15 cells ($EC_{50}$; μM) | Anti-EBV activity in H1 cells ($EC_{90}$; μM) | Growth inhibition ($ID_{50}$; μM) in: | | | | Selectivity | |
|---|---|---|---|---|---|---|---|---|
| | | | MT2 | CEM | H1 | 2.2.15 | 2.2.15/HBV | H1/EBV |
| L-FMAU | 0.1 | 5±0.8 | 100 | >100 | 913±70 | >200 | >2000 | 183 |
| D-FMAU | 2.0 | 0.1±0.02 | 8–9 | 0 | <10 | 50 | 25 | >100 |
| L-FEAU | >5.0 | >20 | 100 | >100 | >400 | ND | ND | >90 |
| D-FEAU | 5.0 | 1±0.05 | 100 | 90 | >400 | ND | ND | >90 |

ND, Not determined.

**Figure 3.** Proposed metabolism of L-FMAU

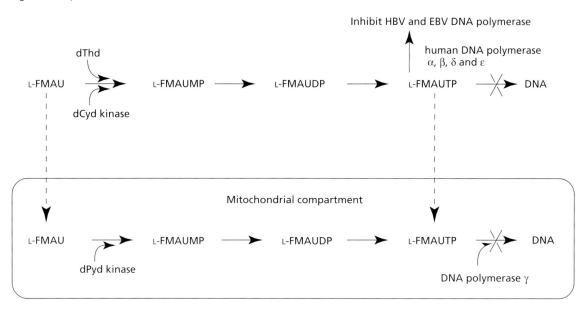

dThd, deoxythymidine; dCyd kinase, deoxycytidine kinase; dPyd kinase, deoxypyrimidine kinase

subsequent 16 hours, the triphosphate was removed at a lower rate, with 38% of the amount at 8 hours still present at 24 hours. This maintenance of triphosphate levels could be advantageous in the use of L-FMAU as a therapeutic agent, as it would exert the HBV-inhibitory effect for extended periods. The metabolism of L-FMAU was the same when the experiments were conducted in HepG2 instead of 2.2.15 cells, suggesting that the conversion of L-FMAU to various metabolites involved host cellular machinery.

L-FMAUTP acts as a potent inhibitor of HBV DNA polymerase, with a $K_i$ value of 0.12 μM. However, it is not utilize as a substrate by human α, β, γ or δ DNA polymerases. Unlike other deoxythymidine (dThd) or deoxycytidine (dCyd) analogues, L-FMAU was phosphorylated by cytosolic dThd kinase, cytosolic deoxycytidine kinase, as well as mitochondrial deoxypyri midine (dPyd) kinase. The phosphorylation of L-FMAU by these enzymes was also subject to inhibition by their feedback inhibitors. When the efficiency of L-FMAU as a substrate for all three enzymes was examined, it was found to be within the same order of magnitude as the natural substrate.

The uniqueness of L-FMAU among the known anti-HBV agents is that it is the first pyrimidine nucleoside analogue shown to have potent anti-HBV activity and it also has substrate properties different from those of all three cellular dPyd nucleoside kinases. In order to investigate whether L-FMAU could be phosphorylated by cytosolic dCyd kinase

and dThd kinase, the metabolism of L-FMAU was studied in cells that are deficient in these enzymes. L-FMAU was phosphorylated to a lesser extent but still substantially phosphorylated in both enzyme-deficient cell lines. dThd and dCyd influenced the degree of L-FMAU phosphorylation in these cell lines. There was a more pronounced inhibition of L-FMAU phosphorylation in cytosolic dCyd kinase-deficient cell lines by dThd than in those with all three enzymes. This is due to the fact that cytosolic dThd kinase is the only major enzyme responsible for its phosphorylation in these cells. Likewise, the phosphorylation of L-FMAU was much less influenced by dCyd in HeLa cells than in dThd kinase-deficient HeLa (Bu) cells. This observation was explained when the action of dCyd and/or dThd on L-FMAU metabolism was studied in HepG2 cells. Either dThd or dCyd could suppress L-FMAU phosphorylation to some extent. However, the combined effect of dThd and dCyd was the most effective.

Since L-FMAU can be readily metabolized to its phosphorylated products, the potential for these products to be incorporated into cellular DNA was examined [27]. With 5 μM [³H]L-FMAU treatment for 24 hours, there were no significant incorporation of radioactivity into DNA. The acid-insoluble fraction did not show any radioactivity, suggesting that this molecule may not be incorporated. In contrast, the positive control, thymidine, was incorporated. The presence of the D-FMAU metabolite in DNA could also be detected. However, L-FMAU metabolites were not inserted in the cellular DNA, as judged by the absence of radioactivity. Possible explanations for the lack of radioactivity could be either that the molecule is not utilized by the cellular polymerase or that the levels of radioactivity under the assay conditions were below the threshold of detection. However, data from this experiment indicated that L-FMAUTP is not a substrate or an inhibitor of isolated human DNA polymerases α, β, γ, δ or ε. This could explain the apparent lack of incorporation into DNA.

In addition to its potent anti-HBV activity, L-FMAU also exhibits potent anti-EBV activity. Thus far, no L-nucleoside analogues with anti-EBV activity have been reported in the literature. The $EC_{90}$ of L-FMAU is as potent as that of DHPG (5.0 μM in H1 cells), whereas the selectivity of L-FMAU is higher than that of DHPG (183 versus 15). However, the amount of L-FMAU nucleoside formed was three times larger in EBV-producing cells than in non-EBV-producing cells. The metabolic study of L-FMAU indicated that it is converted to its mono-, di- and triphosphates. The enzymes involved in this process are still under investigation. Given the differences in the formation of L-FMAUMP in H1 and L5 cells, it is possible that EBV-specified thymidine kinase in H1 cells could utilize L-FMAU as a substrate and could be responsible for the quantitative difference in L-FMAU phosphates formed. Since L-FMAUMP could also be formed in L5 cells as well as in other non-EBV containing cells, human enzymes may also be capable of utilizing L-FMAU as a substrate. One interesting feature of L-FMAU metabolism is that the major metabolite is L-FMAUMP. This finding suggests that the intracellular conversion to L-FMAUDP from L-FMAUMP could be the rate-limiting step in the L-FMAU phosphorylation pathway in L5 cells.

The detection of 3% of [³H]L-FMAU in the acid-insoluble fraction of cells raised the possibility that [³H]-L-FMAU could be incorporated into DNA. However, based on caesium sulphate gradient centrifugation, there was no detectable amount (less than 0.1 pmol/$10^6$ cells) of radioactivity in DNA. In contrast, D-FMAU was found to be incorporated into DNA in substantial amounts, even at 2% of the concentration of L-FMAU. Thus, the concern of toxicity manifested by D-FMAU resulting from its incorporation into DNA may not be an issue for L-FMAU. The lack of incorporation of L-FMAU into cellular DNA could be due to the inability of human DNA polymerases to use L-FMAU as a substrate. It is also interesting that L-FMAUTP is not a substrate of EBV DNA polymerase. This finding suggests that the anti-EBV activity of L-FMAU may not be due to its incorpo-

ration into EBV DNA. All of the antiviral nucleoside analogues studied thus far, with the exception of ribavirin, exert their antiviral action through their incorporation into viral DNA. Therefore, L-FMAU could have a very different mechanism of antiviral action from those antiviral compounds described [26].

## PHARMACOKINETICS

Initial preclinical pharmacokinetic studies of L-FMAU were conducted in rats [29]. Three doses of L-FMAU were administered intravenously (10, 25, and 50 mg/kg) to rats, and L-FMAU concentrations in plasma and urine were measured by HPLC. There were no significant differences in pharmacokinetic parameters between the three doses (Table 2). Thus, the disposition of L-FMAU was independent of dose over the dose range 10–50 mg/kg. Plasma concentrations of L-FMAU declined rapidly with a terminal phase half-life of 1.33±0.45 h (mean±SD). Total clearance of L-FMAU was moderate, averaging 1.15±0.28 l/h/kg. The fraction of compound excreted unchanged in urine was 0.59±0.13. No glucuronide metabolite was found in the urine. The steady-state volume of distribution was 1.12±0.26 l/kg, indicating intracellular distribution of the compound. The fraction of L-FMAU bound to plasma proteins was approximately 15% and was independent of nucleoside concentration. Bioavailability of L-FMAU following oral administration of 25 mg/kg averaged 63±13% [30].

Further preclinical pharmacokinetic studies characterized the disposition of L-FMAU in the woodchuck model. Woodchucks were given 25 mg/kg L-FMAU intravenously and orally. Following intravenous administration of 25 mg/kg L-FMAU to woodchucks, renal clearance and non-renal clearance averaged 0.13 ±0.08 l/h/kg and 0.10±0.06 l/h/kg, respectively. Steady-state volume of distribution averaged 0.99± 0.17 l/kg, indicating intracellular distribution of the nucleoside. The terminal phase half-life of L-FMAU following intravenous administration averaged 6.2± 2.0 h. Absorption of L-FMAU after oral administration was incomplete, and bioavailability ranged between 20

**Table 2.** Pharmacokinetic parameters of L-FMAU following intravenous and oral administration to rats

| CL (l/h/kg) | VSS (l/h.kg) | $t_{1/2}$ (h) | $f_e$ | F |
|---|---|---|---|---|
| 1.15 | 1.12 | 1.33 | 0.59 | 0.63 |
| (0.28)* | (0.26) | (0.45) | (0.13) | (0.13) |

*Values are given as mean (SD). CL, clearance; VSS, volume of distribution at steady state; $f_e$, fraction of excretion in urine; F, bioavailability.

and 40%. Slow absorption of L-FMAU resulted in an apparent terminal half-life of 16.2±12.1 hours following oral administration. Plasma concentrations of L-FMAU remained above the *in vitro* EC$_{50}$ value of 0.026 µg/ml for HBV for 24 hours after both intravenous and oral adminstration [32].

## TOXICITY

The effects of L-FMAU on growth in a variety of human cell lines, including HepG2, CEM and H1 indicated its lack of toxicity (Table 1). L-FMAU was also evaluated in bone marrow precursor cells (erythroid and granulocyte macrophage) [32], and no significant toxicity was detected up to 100 µM. Since L-FMAU is not an inhibitor or a substrate for DNA polymerase γ, toxicity for mitochondrial function is not expected. This is in contrast to other antiviral agents, such as D-FIAU, which is readily utilized as a substrate by DNA polymerases and is incorporated into cellular DNA [33]; this is believed to be responsible, at least in part, for FIAU-induced mitochondrial toxicity. A lack of incorporation of L-FMAU into DNA was also observed with Burkitt lymphoma HR1-derived cell lines H1 (EBV high-level producer) and L5 (EBV low-level producer), whereas D-FMAU was incorporated into DNA. In addition, when studies were conducted with isolated human DNA polymerases α, β, γ and δ, L-FMAU failed to be incor-

porated, whereas the D-enantiomer was readily incorporated. These results, especially with human DNA polymerase γ, which is responsible for mitochondrial DNA synthesis, suggest that L-FMAU may not induce mitochondrial toxicity or alter its function. The lack of lactic acid production in HepG hepatoma cells repeatedly treated with L-FMAU at concentrations up to 200 µM suggests that L-FMAU is unlikely to elicit adverse effects similar to those of D-FIAU and D-FMAU (Fig. 4) [34]. Toxicity studies performed with mice indicated no apparent toxicity after 30 days of continuous treatment with L-FMAU at 25 mg/kg twice daily.

Preliminary toxicity studies of L-FMAU were conducted in woodchucks for 12 weeks at 2 mg/day/kg, in comparison to D-FMAU. The results showed that there was no change in body weight in L-FMAU-treated animals, while there was marked decline in body weight in D-FMAU-treated woodchucks. These changes were only observed after 8 weeks of treatment, which is consistent with the clinical data for D-FIAU. By the end of the 12 week period of treatment, all D-FMAU-treated woodchucks either died or were euthanized because of drug toxicity. Delayed toxicity was associated with mixed microvesicular and macrovesicular steatosis and lactic acidaemia. No comparable toxicity was observed in L-FMAU-treated or placebo-treated animals [35].

## *IN VIVO* EFFICACY STUDIES IN ANIMAL MODELS

The administration of L-FMAU (40 mg/kg/day) for 5 days by the oral route in experimentally infected ducklings (EC$_{50}$ 0.1 µM) showed a potent inhibition of viral replication (72% compared to control) without any abnormalities [36] but was followed by a transient rebound of viraemia 5 days after drug withdrawal, as also observed with other drugs [37–40]. Interestingly, a more prolonged protocol with a 8 day administration of L-FMAU in ducklings did prevent a rebound of viraemia after drug withdrawal and was not associated with an increase of serum lactic acid levels. Statistical analysis showed that, although the number of animals was small, there was a significant trend for decreased viral production in L-FMAU-treated animals as compared with controls ($P<0.05$). Southern blot analysis of intrahepatic viral DNA, 2 weeks after drug withdrawal, showed the persistence of viral covalently closed circular DNA and replicative intermediates, as also observed in tissue culture, accompanied by the persistence of viral core protein expression as analysed by Western blot. This emphasizes the need for a prolonged therapy protocol in

**Figure 4.** Lactic acid production in HepG2 cell cultures treated with L-FMAU

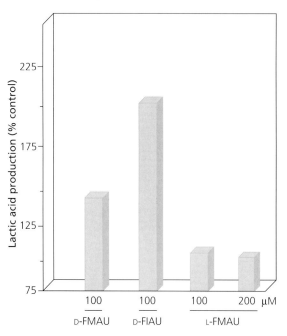

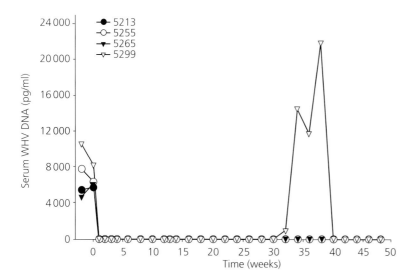

**Figure 5.** Serum WHV DNA in WHV carrier woodchucks treated with 10 mg/kg L-FMAU

Four woodchucks (5213, 5255, 5265 and 5299) were given 10 mg/kg/day L-FMAU orally for 50 weeks.

order to cure infected hepatocytes. Although DHBV *pol* gene mutants were not selected during short-term administration of L-FMAU, it remains to be determined whether this phenomenon could be observed during long-term therapy. After drug withdrawal, the persistence of viral DNA and proteins was associated with low level viraemia, under the limit of detection of a dot blot assay, which may suggest either a decrease in viral particle secretion from infected hepatocytes or an enhanced clearance of viral particles from serum. However, attempts to detect antibodies against envelope proteins in the serum of DHBV-infected ducklings during the course of experimental infection did not show any antibody response. Analysis of liver histology in infected ducklings showed the absence of significant signs of liver toxicity after short-term treatment with L-FMAU. With regards to toxicity, it is noteworthy that the drug was administered when the birds were rapidly growing and that cell division, including that of hepatocytes, was occurring at a significant rate [41].

Efficacy studies of L-FMAU were also conducted in woodchucks chronically infected with woodchuck hepatitis virus (WHV). L-FMAU was given orally to four chronic WHV carriers at a daily dose of 10 mg/kg for 50 weeks [42]. There was prompt and significant inhibition of viral replication compared to placebo-treated controls (Fig. 5). Within 2 weeks, the plasma WHV DNA of drug-treated woodchucks decreased more than 1000-fold and was undetectable by conventional blot hybridization [43]. The initial $t_{1/2}$ of plasma WHV DNA in drug-treated woodchucks was 17±1 hour. At the end of treatment, hepatic WHV DNA replicative intermediates were decreased more than 10-fold over pretreatment and control levels, and

decreased further following drug withdrawal.

Based on immunohistochemical analysis, hepatic expression of WHV was also diminished after 12 weeks of treatment and also decreased further after drug treatment ended. Decreases in body weight observed in L-FMAU-treated woodchucks were similar to those of controls, and no other physical or biochemical evidence of drug-related toxicity was observed. These results suggest that L-FMAU may be valuable for treatment of HBV infection and that the woodchuck model will be useful in assessing the long-term effects of treatment on the course of persistent hepadnavirus infection.

According to the dose escalation study (Fig. 6), a rapid and profound suppression in serum WHV DNA was observed at L-FMAU dosages varying between 0.3 mg/kg and 10 mg/kg orally once daily. The reduction in viral DNA was most marked at the 10 mg/kg dose and least at the lowest, 0.3 mg/kg dose. By comparison, WHV DNA levels were approximately 400-fold less after 3 weeks of treatment with L-FMAU at 10 mg/kg orally daily. L-FMAU at dosages of 1 mg/kg and 3 mg/kg resulted in a reduction in mean WHV DNA levels of 70-fold and 125-fold, respectively, when compared to pretreatment values. Viral recrudescence was observed following drug withdrawal within 4 weeks in those woodchucks receiving L-FMAU at 0.3 mg/kg and 1 mg/kg daily.

## SUMMARY

L-FMAU is a potent anti-HBV nucleoside in 2.2.15 cells with a favourable toxicity profile in various cell lines *in vitro*. L-FMAU is phosphorylated to its monophosphate by cellular dCyd kinase as well as dThd

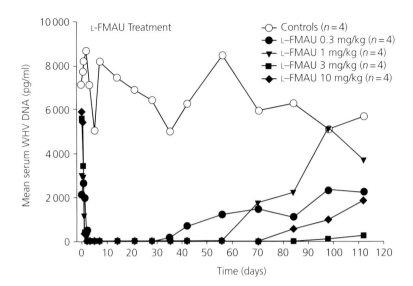

**Figure 6.** Dose escalation study of L-FMAU in WHV carrier woodchucks

kinase. Furthermore, it is also phosphorylated by mitochondrial dPyd kinase. The monophosphate is then phosphoryalted to di- and triphosphate. The triphosphate inhibits HBV and EBV DNA polymerases, which appears to be the mechanism of L-FMAU as an antiviral agent. Interestingly, L-FMAU is not incorporated into HBV or EBV DNA. Furthermore, the triphosphate does not interact with cellular DNA polymerases $\alpha$, $\beta$, $\gamma$, $\delta$ or $\epsilon$. This may explain the low toxicity of L-FMAU *in vitro* and *in vivo*. Pharmacokinetic studies in rats and woodchucks indicated that L-FMAU disposition is typical of nucleoside analogues. The compound is orally bioavailable. Preliminary toxicity studies conducted in mice and woodchucks suggest L-FMAU does not exhibit any marked toxicity in these animal models, whereas D-FMAU showed significant toxicity. *In vivo* efficacy studies conducted in chronically infected woodchucks at 10 mg/day/kg for 12 weeks indicated that L-FMAU is a potent anti-HBV agent and that no significant viral rebound was observed in three out of four animals even after the discontinuation of the drug up to 50 weeks. Therefore, potent *in vitro* and *in vivo* efficacy, favourable toxicity in animal models and various cell lines, as well as its unique structure, metabolism and mechanism make L-FMAU a promising candidate for an anti-HBV agent.

## ACKNOWLEDGEMENTS

This research was supported by US Public Health Service Research grants (AI 32351, AI 25899, NO1-AI-45195, NO1-AI-45179 and NO1-AI-35164) from the National Institutes of Health. We also thank Christopher Tseng for his help.

## REFERENCES

1. Coates, JAV, Cammack N, Jenkinson HJ, Mutton IM, Pearson BA, Storer R, Cameron JM & Penn CR. The separated enantiomers of 2′-deoxy-3′-thiacytidine (BCH-189) both inhibit human immunodeficiency virus replication *in vitro*. *Antimicrobial Agents and Chemotherapy* 1992; **36**:202–205.
2. Schinazi RF, Chu CK, Peck A, McMillan A, Mathis R, Cannon D, Jeong LS, Beach JW, Choi WB, Yeola S & Liotta DC. Activities of the four optical isomers of 2′,3′-dideoxy-3′-thiacytidine (BCH-189) against human immunodeficiency virus type 1 in human lymphocytes. *Antimicrobial Agents and Chemotherapy* 1992; **36**: 672–676.
3. Dienstag JL, Perillo RP, Schiff ER, Bartholomew M, Vacary C & Rubin M. A preliminary trial of lamivudine for chronic hepatitis B infection. *New England Journal of Medicine* 1995; **333**:1657–1661.
4. Furman PA, Davis M, Liotta DC, Paff M, Frick LW, Nelson DJ, Dornsife RE, Wurster JA, Wilson LJ, Fyfe JA, Tuttle JV, Miller WH, Condreay L, Averette DR, Schinazi RF & Painter GR. The anti-hepatitis B virus activities, cytotoxicities, and anabolic profiles of the (–) and (+) enantiomers of *cis*-5-fluoro-1-[2-(hydroxymethyl)-1,3-oxathiolan-5-yl]-cytosine. *Antimicrobial Agents and Chemotherapy* 1992;**36**:2686–2692.
5. Schinazi RF, McMillan A, Cannon D, Mathis R, Lloyd RM, Peck A, Sommadossi J-P, St Clair M, Wilson J, Furman PA, Painter G, Choi WB & Liotta DC. Selective inhibition of human immunodeficiency viruses by racemates and enantiomers of *cis*-5-fluoro-1-[2-(hydroxymethyl)-1,3-oxathiolan-5-yl]-cytosine. *Antimicrobial Agents and Chemotherapy* 1992; **36**: 2423–2431.
6. Schinazi RF, McClure HM, Boudinot FD, Xiang YJ & Chu CK. Development of (–)-β-D-2,6-diaminopurine dioxolane as a potential antiviral agent. *Antiviral Research* 1994; **23** (Supplement):81.
7. Rajagopalan PF, Boudinot FD, Chu CK, McClure HM & Schinazi RF. Pharmacokinetics of (–)-β-D-2,6-diaminopurine dioxolane as a potential antiviral agent. *Antiviral Research* 1994; **23** (Supplement):81.
8. Bisacchi GS, Chao ST, Bachard C, Daris JP, Innaimo S, Jacobs GA, Kocy O, Lapointe P, Martel A, Merchant

Z, Slusarchyk WA, Sundeen JE, Yong MG, Colonno R & Zahler R. BMS-200475, a novel carbocyclic 2′-deoxyguanosine analog with potent and selective anti-hepatitis B virus activity *in vitro*. *Bioorganic and Medicinal Chemistry Letters* 1997; **7**:127–132.

9. Colonno RJ, Innaimo SF, Seifer M, Genovesi E, Clark J, Yamanaka R, Hamatake B, Terry B, Standring D, Bisacchi G, Sundeen J & Zahler R. Identification of BMS-200475 as a novel and potent inhibitor of hepatitis B virus replication. *Antiviral Research* 1997; **34** (Suppl.):A51.

10. Dusheiko GM. Treatment and prevention of chronic viral hepatitis. *Pharmacology and Therapeutics* 1995; **65**:47–73.

11. Tenny DJ, Yamanaka G, Voss SM, Cianci CW, Tuomari AV, Sheaffer AK, Alam M & Colonno RJ. Lobucavir is phosphorylated in human cytomegalovirus-infected and uninfected cell and inhibits the viral DNA polymerase. *Antimicrobial Agents and Chemotherapy* 1997; **41**:2680–2685.

12. Heijtink RA, De Wilde GA, Kruining J, Berk L, Balzarini J, De Clercq E, Holy A & Schalm SW. Inhibitory effect of 9-(2-phosphanylmethoxyethyl)-adenine (PMEA) on human and duck hepatitis B virus infection. *Antiviral Research* 1993; **21**:141–153.

13. Nicoll AJ, Collede DL, Wang YY, Toole JJ, Dean JK, Angus PW, Smallwood RA & Locarnini SA. PMEA, an acyclic phosphate nucleoside analog with activity against duck hepatitis B virus *in vivo*. *Hepatology* 1996; **220A**:375.

14. Tsiquaye K, Slomka MJ & Maung M. Oral famciclovir against duck hepatitis B virus replication in hepatic and nonhepatic tissues of ducklings infected *in vivo*. *Journal of Medical Virology* 1994; **42**:306–310.

15. Perry CM & Wagstaff AJ. Famciclovir: a review of its pharmacological properties and therapeutic efficacy in herpes virus infections. *Drugs* 1995; **50**:396–415.

16. Walker TE & Hakgenkamp HPC. A new synthesis of L-ribofuranose derivatives. *Carbohydrate Research* 1974; **32**:413–417

17. Abe Y, Takizawa T & Kunieda T. Epimerization of aldoses catalyzed by dioxobis (2,4-pentanedionato-O.O′)-molybdenium (IV). An improved procedure for C-2 epimer preparation. *Chemical and Pharmaceutical Bulletin* 1980; **28**:1324–1326.

18. Kenneth JR & Edward MA. 9-β-L-ribofuranosyl-adenine (L-adenosine), configurational inversion within a furanoid ring. In *Synthetic Procedures in Nucleic Acids Chemistry,* 1968; vol. 1, pp. 163–167. Edited by WW Zorbach & RS Tipson. New York: John Wiley.

19. Batch A & Czernecki S. New synthesis of L-ribofuranose derivatives. *Journal of Carbohydrate Chemistry* 1994; **13**:935–940.

20. Tann CH, Brodfuehrer PR, Brundidge SP, Sapino C Jr & Howell HG. Fluorocarbohydrates in synthesis. An efficient synthesis of 1-(2-deoxy-2-fluoro-β-D-arabino-furanosyl)-thymine (β-D-FMAU). *Journal of Organic Chemistry* 1985: **50**:3644–3646.

21. Oka K & Wada H. Synthesis of D-ribose from D-xylose. *Yakugaku Zasshi* 1963; **83**:890–891.

22. Gosselin G, Bergogne M-C & Imbach J-L. 1,2-Di-O-acetyl-3,5-di-O-benzoyl-D-xylofuranose, a versatile precursor for the synthesis of various β-D-pentofuranosyl nucleosides and related analogs. In *Nucleic Acid Chemistry, Improved and New Synthetic Procedures, Methods and Techniques,* 1991; part 4, pp. 41–45. Edited by LB Townsent & RS Tipson. New York: John Wiley.

23. Ma T, Pai B, Zhu YL, Lin JS, Shanmuganathan K, Du J, Wang C, Kim H, Gary Newton M, Cheng YC & Chu CK. Structure–activity relationships of 1-(2-deoxy-2-fluoro-β-L-arabinofuranosyl)-pyrimidine nucleosides as anti-hepatitis B virus agents. *Journal of Medicinal Chemistry* 1996; **39**:2835–2843.

24. Ma T, Lin JS, Gary Newton M, Cheng YC & Chu CK. Synthesis and anti-hepatitis B virus activity of 9-(2-deoxy-2-fluoro-β-L-arabinofuranosyl)-purine nucleosides. *Journal of Medicinal Chemistry* 1997; **40**:2750–2754.

25. Chu CK, Ma TW, Shanmuganathan K, Wang CG, Xiang YJ, Pai SB, Yao GQ, Sommadossi J-P & Cheng Y-C. Use of 2′-fluoro-5-methyl-β-D-arabinofuranosyl-uracil as a novel antiviral agent for hepatitis B virus and Epstein–Barr virus. *Antimicrobial Agents and Chemotherapy* 1995; **39**:979–981.

26. Yao G-Q, Liu SH, Chou E, Kukhanova M, Chu CK & Cheng YC. Inhibition of Epstein–Barr virus replication by a novel L-nucleoside, 2′-fluoro-5-methyl-β-L-arabi-nofuranosyl uracil. *Biochemical Pharmacology* 1996; **51**:941–947.

27. Pai SB, Liu SH, Zhu YL, Chu CK & Cheng YC. Inhibition of hepatitis B virus: a novel L-nucleoside, 2′-fluoro-5-methyl-β-L-arabinofuranosyl uracil. *Antimicrobial Agents and Chemotherapy* 1996; **40**: 380–386.

28. Liu SH, Grove KL & Cheng YC. Unique metabolism of a novel antiviral L-nucleoside analogue, L-FMAU: a substrate for both thymidine kinase and deoxycytidine kinase. *Antimicrobial Agents and Chemotherapy* 1998; **42**: 833–839.

29. Wright JD, Ma T, Chu CK & Boudinot FD. Pharmaco-kinetics of 1-(2-deoxy-2-fluoro-β-L-arabinofuranosyl)-5-methyluracil (L-FMAU) in rats. *Pharmaceutical Research* 1995; **12**:1350–1353.

30. Wright JD, Ma T, Chu CK & Boudinot FD. Discontinuous oral absorption pharmacokinetic model and bioavailability of 1-(2-fluoro-5-methyl-β-L-arabi-nofuranosyl)-uracil (L-FMAU) in rats. *Biopharmaceutics and Drug Disposition* 1996; **17**:197–207.

31. Witcher JW, Boudinot FD, Baldwin BH, Ascenzi MA, Tennant BC, Du JF & Chu CK. Pharmacokinetics of 1-(2-fluoro-5-methyl-β-L-arabinofuranosyl)uracil in woodchucks. *Antimicrobial Agents and Chemotherapy* 1997; **41**:2184–2187.

32. Sommadossi J-P, Schinazi RF, Chu CK & Xie M-Y. Comparison of cytotoxicity of the (–) and (+)-enan-tiomer of 2′,3′-dideoxy-3′-thiacytidine in normal human bone marrow progenitor cells. *Biochemical Pharmacology* 1992; **44**:1921–1925.

33. Lewis W, Meyer RR, Simpson JM, Colcacino JM & Perrino FW. Mammalian DNA polymerase α, β, and ε incorporate fialuridine (FIAU) monophosphate into DNA and are inhibited competitively by FIAU triphosphate. *Biochemistry* 1994; **33**:14620–14624.

34. Cui L, Yoon S, Schinazi RF & Sommadossi J-P. Cellular and molecular events leading to mitochondrial toxicity of 1-(2-deoxy-2-fluoro-1-β-D-arabinofuranosyl)-5-iodouracil in human liver cells. *Journal of Clinical Investigation* 1995; **95**:555–563.

35. Peek SF, Jacob JR, Tochkov IA, Korba BE, Gerin JL, Chu CK & Tennant BC. Sustained antiviral activity of 1-(2-fluoro-methyl-β-L-arabinofuranosyl)-uracil (L-FMAU) in the woodchuck model of hepatitis B virus (HBV) infection. *Hepatology* 1997; **26**:1187.

36. Zoulim F, Aguesse S, Borel C, Trepo C & Cheng Y-C. 2′-Fluoro-5-methyl-β-L-arabinofuranosyl, a novel L-nucleoside analogue, inhibits hepatitis B virus replica-

tion in primary hepatocytes and *in vivo*. *Antiviral Research* 1996; **30**:A24.

37. Bridges E & Cheng YC. Use of novel β-L-(–)-nucleoside analogs for treatment and prevention of chronic hepatitis B virus infection and hepatocellular carcinoma. *Progress in Liver Diseases*, 1995; **13**:231–245.

38. Fourel I, Cullen J, Saputelli C, Aldrich P, Schaffer D, Averett J & Mason W. Evidence that hepatocyte turnover is required for rapid clearance of duck hepatitis B virus during antiviral therapy of chronically infected ducks. *Journal of Virology* 1994; **68**:8321–8330.

39. Fourel I, Saputelli J, Schaffer P & Mason W. The carbocyclic analog of 2′-deoxyguanosine induces a prolonged inhibition of duck hepatitis B virus DNA synthesis in primary hepatocyte cultures and in the liver. *Journal of Virology* 1994; **68**:1059–1065.

40. Zoulim F, Dannaoui E, Borel C, Hantz O, Lin T, Liu C & Cheng YC. 2′,3′-Dideoxy-β-L-5-fluorocytidine inhibits duck hepatitis B virus reverse transcription and suppress viral DNA synthesis in hepatocytes, both *in vitro* and *in vivo*. *Antimicrobial Agents and Chemotherapy* 1996; **40**:448–453.

41. Stéphanie A-G, Lui SH, Chevallier M, Pichoud C, Jamard C, Borel C, Chu CK, Trepo C, Cheng Y-C and Zoulim F. Inhibition effect of 2′-fluoro-5-methyl-β-L-arabinofuranosyl-uracil on duck hepatitis B virus replication. *Antimicrobial Agents and Chemotherapy* 1998; **42**:369–376.

42. Tennant BC, Jacob J, Graham LA, Peek S, Du J & Chu CK. Pharmacokinetic and pharmacodynamic studies of 1-(2-fluoro-5-methyl-β-L-arabinofuranosyl)-uracil (L-FMAU) in the woodchuck model of hepatitis B virus (HBV) infection. *Antiviral Research* 1997; **34**:A52.

43. Cheng Y-C, Chu CK, Peek SF, Tennant BC, Korba BE & Boudinot FD. Preclinical investigation of L-FMAU (clevudine): chemistry, biochemistry and *in vivo* woodchuck studies. *Second International Conference on Therapies for Viral Hepatitis*, December 15–19 1997, Hawaii, USA; Abstract O27.

# 33

# A rational strategy for the design of anti-hepatitis B virus nucleotide derivatives

## Christian Périgaud, Gilles Gosselin and Jean-Louis Imbach*

## SUMMARY

The potential in antiviral chemotherapy of a pronucleotide approach using mononucleoside phosphotriesters which incorporate *S*-acyl-2-thioethyl (SATE) groups as esterase-labile transient phosphate protectors is discussed in detail. The use of this approach leads to an increase of the antiretroviral activity of two well-established anti-human immunodeficiency virus (HIV) drugs, namely 2′,3′-dideoxyadenosine (ddA) and 2′,3′-didehydro-2′,3′-dideoxythymidine (stavudine; d4T). Moreover, in the case of acyclovir, which is currently used as a therapeutic agent for the treatment of herpesvirus infections, the corresponding bis(SATE) pronucleotides have emerged as potent and selective inhibitors of the hepatitis B virus (HBV) replication.

## INTRODUCTION

The mechanism of action of nucleoside analogues, which represent the major chemotherapeutic approach to the treatment of viral infections, is characterized by a common feature. These compounds have no intrinsic antiviral activity and must be metabolized to their respective 5′-triphosphates by nucleotidases, kinases and/or other activating enzymes present naturally in cells. Of the three metabolic steps of nucleoside analogues, the monophosphorylation step is generally considered to be the most restrictive [1–5]. Moreover, the presence and activity of the intracellular enzymes involved in the monophosphorylation of nucleoside analogues are often dependent on the host species, the cell type and the phase in the cell cycle. The dependence on phosphorylation for activation of a nucleoside analogue may therefore be a problem in cells where the activity of phosphorylating enzymes is known to be low or even lacking [6–9]. Unfortunately, this problem cannot be resolved by the use of nucleotides, which cannot penetrate the cell membrane because of their polar nature and are rapidly dephosphorylated in extracellular fluids and on cell surfaces [10–12]. Therefore, to overcome this limitation, many strategies have previously been designed to mask or reduce the negative phosphate charges of nucleoside 5′-monophosphate analogues with neutral substituents, thereby forming more lipophilic derivatives (pronucleotides), which would be expected to revert back to the corresponding 5′-mononucleoside inside the cell [13,14]. To be effective *in vitro*, such a pronucleotide approach should fulfil the following features [15]: (i) neutral species (such as a mononucleoside phosphotriester), which would be expected to cross the cell membrane by passive diffusion, should be used; (ii) the phosphotriester must be stable under the usual experimental cell culture conditions (37°C and RPMI containing 10% heat-inactivated fetal calf serum), or possible extracellular decomposition to the parent nucleoside could lead to ambiguous biological results; and (iii) inside the cell, the phosphotriester must be selectively transformed to the nucleoside 5′-monophosphate. Consequently, to prove unambiguously the validity of an approach for the intracellular delivery of a 5′-mononucleotide analogue, the corresponding phosphotriester must be evaluated for its *in vitro* inhibitory effects on the replication of the virus in cell lines deficient in the nucleoside kinase responsible for the monophosphorylation of the corresponding nucleoside analogue. In this case, when a biological response is detected in cell cultures for such a pronucleotide, it can be assumed that it is caused only by the release of the 5′-mononucleotide.

As no evident phosphotriesterase activity has been reported to be present inside the cell, the transformation of a nucleoside phosphotriester into its corresponding 5′-monophosphate necessarily involves a chemical mechanism among the possible process of the first decomposition step (Fig. 1).

*Corresponding author

**Figure 1.** Transformation pathway of a nucleoside phosphotriester into its corresponding nucleoside monophosphate

Phosphotriester ··· Step 1 Chemical process ··· Phosphodiester ··· Step 2 Enzymatic process ··· Nucleoside monophosphate

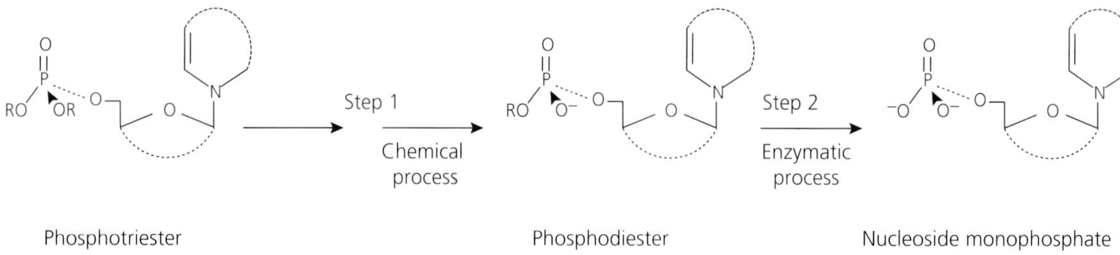

Once transformed into a phosphodiester, an enzyme-mediated release of the nucleoside 5′-monophosphate can be expected. This suggested the idea of generating intracellularly an unstable thioethyl phosphotriester, which will decompose spontaneously and selectively (C–O bond cleavage) into its parent nucleoside phosphodiester through an intramolecular nucleophilic substitution mechanism (Fig. 2).

The rate of this transformation is fast [16], and so such thioethyl phosphotriesters are unsuitable for a pronucleotide approach. Therefore, we decided to mask the thiol function temporarily with an enzyme-labile protecting group that could be selectively cleaved inside the cells. For this purpose, the thiol group has been masked with an acyl function in the expectation that a carboxylate esterase-dependent intracellular activation mechanism might ensue (Fig. 3).

With 3′-azido-3′-deoxythymidine (zidovudine; AZT) as a nucleoside model, several mononucleoside phosphotriesters incorporating SATE groups as enzyme-labile phosphate protectors have been synthesized [17]. It was demonstrated that the use of bis(SATE)phosphotriesters of zidovudine resulted in intracellular delivery of the parent 5′-monophosphate. This point was corroborated with the observation of an anti-HIV effect in thymidine kinase-deficient CEM cells and by decomposition data in culture medium and CEM cell extracts. Furthermore, it is noteworthy that the introduction of the SATE groups as esterase-labile transient phosphate protectors of 5′-mononucleoside (and their degradation products) does not induce additional toxicity *in vitro* [18].

Having shown the validity of a pronucleotide

approach using SATE groups as enzyme-labile transient phosphate protectors for zidovudine-MP, we decided to extend the investigation of the potential of these groups in the chemotherapy field. Consequently, we applied this approach to several other bioactive nucleoside analogue monophosphates.

## SATE PRONUCLEOTIDES
### 2′,3′-Dideoxyadenosine (ddA)

The nucleoside analogue ddA is a potent inhibitor of HIV replication [19–22]. The metabolism of ddA proceeds by a series of complex events (Fig. 4). Inside the cell, ddA can be directly phosphorylated to its corresponding 5′-monophosphate (ddAMP) by deoxycytidine kinase or adenosine kinase. Alternatively, ddA may be rapidly deaminated to 2′,3′-dideoxyinosine (didanosine; ddI) by adenosine deaminase, this latter being phosphorylated to ddI 5′-monophosphate (ddIMP) by 5′-nucleotidase and then converted to ddAMP by adenylosuccinate synthetase and adenylosuccinate lyase. This alternative mechanism appears to be the predominant pathway by which ddA is ultimately converted to the active metabolite ddA 5′-triphosphate (ddATP) which interacts with reverse transcriptase (RT). However, didanosine-MP conversion to ddAMP does not seem to be very efficient [23,24], which makes this the rate-limiting step for ddATP formation. In an effort to circumvent this limitation, the bis(S-acetyl-2-thioethyl)-phosphotriester derivative of ddA [bis(MeSATE)ddAMP; Fig. 5] has been synthesized [25,26] and evaluated in several cell culture systems, with ddA and zidovudine as reference compounds (Table 1).

**Figure 2.** Intramolecular nucleophilic mechanism involving selective C–O bond cleavage

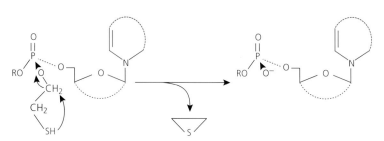

**Figure 3.** Decomposition pathway of a bis(SATE)phosphotriester derivative

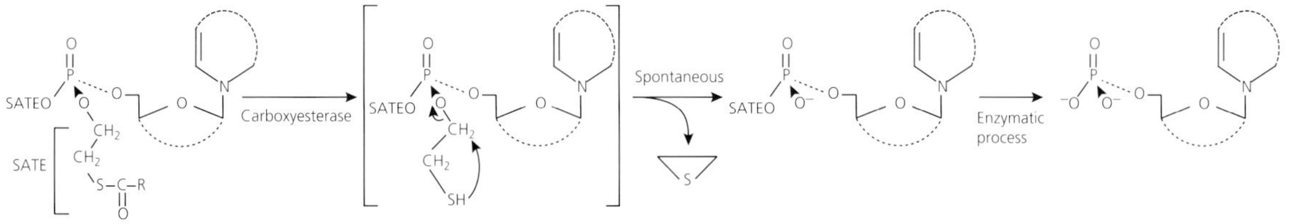

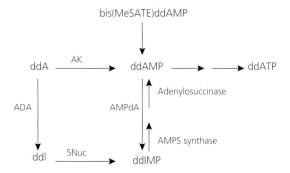

**Figure 4.** Metabolic pathway of ddA and expected metabolism of its corresponding bis(MeSATE)phosphotriester.

bis(MeSATE)ddAMP

ddA —AK→ ddAMP ——→ ddATP

ddA —ADA→ ddI

ddI —5Nuc→ ddIMP

ddAMP ↕ AMPdA (Adenylosuccinase, AMPS synthase) ddIMP

ADA, adenosine deaminase; AK, adenosine kinase; 5Nuc, 5'-nucleotidase; AMPdA, AMP deaminase; AMPS, adenylosuccinate; ddI, 2',3'-dideoxyinosine (didanosine); MeSATE, methyl SATE or S-acetyl-2-thioethyl.

In all cell lines, the bis(MeSATE)phosphotriester of ddA exhibited a very potent anti-HIV effect and proved to be superior to its parent nucleoside, with a decrease of between 3 and 4 logs in the 50% effective concentration ($EC_{50}$) values. The enhanced anti-HIV activity of the bis(MeSATE)ddAMP may be related to the direct intracellular delivery of ddAMP, thus circumventing the ddA/didanosine metabolism pathway. This may result in an increase of ddAMP concentration, which is subsequently transformed to ddATP (Fig. 4). In this respect, the slight increase in the cytotoxicity observed for the bis(MeSATE)phosphotriester of ddA, as compared with the parent nucleoside ddA, may reflect the intracellular accumulation of its corresponding phosphorylated forms, which possibly interact with host cellular enzymes (C Périgaud, G Gosselin and J-L Imbach, unpublished results). Nevertheless, the selectivity index of the bis(MeSATE)ddAMP remains very high and is in the same range as that of zidovudine. This last result does not reduce the potential interest in the SATE groups as transient protectors of 5'-mononucleotide of ddA but raises, in such approaches, the importance of the selectivity of the corresponding 5'-triphosphate derivative for the viral polymerase.

## 2',3'-Didehydro-2',3'-dideoxythymidine (stavudine; d4T)

Stavudine has been approved for the treatment of HIV-infected patients in an advanced stage of the disease who are not responding to other approved treatments [27,28]. The selective *in vitro* anti-HIV activity of stavudine is comparable with that of zidovudine [29,30]. Moreover, stavudine has been found to be less toxic than zidovudine for bone marrow stem cells [30,31] and to be less inhibitory to mitochondrial DNA replication [32]. The antiretroviral effects of stavudine involve its conversion by cellular nucleoside and nucleotide kinases to its corresponding 5'-triphosphate, which interacts with the HIV-associated RT. However, this dideoxynucleoside analogue is converted to its 5'-monophosphate much less efficiently than zidovudine in MT-4 cells [33,34]. In an effort to circumvent this limitation, the bis(S-acetyl-2-thioethyl)phosphotriester derivative of stavudine [bis(MeSATE)d4TMP; Fig. 6] has been synthesized [35] and evaluated for its inhibitory effects on the replication of HIV-1 in human T4 lymphoblastoid cell lines and human primary lymphocytes (Table 2).

The bis(MeSATE)phosphotriester of stavudine proved to be about 10-fold more effective than stavudine in inhibiting HIV-1 replication in human lymphocyte cell lines. As expected, stavudine proved to be completely inactive against HIV-1 replication in CEM/TK⁻ cells at concentrations up to 1 µM. In contrast, the bis(MeSATE)phosphotriester of stavudine emerged as a potent inhibitor with an $EC_{50}$ value of 0.01 µM in the CEM/TK⁻ cell line, which was in the

**Figure 5.** Structure of the bis(MeSATE)ddAMP

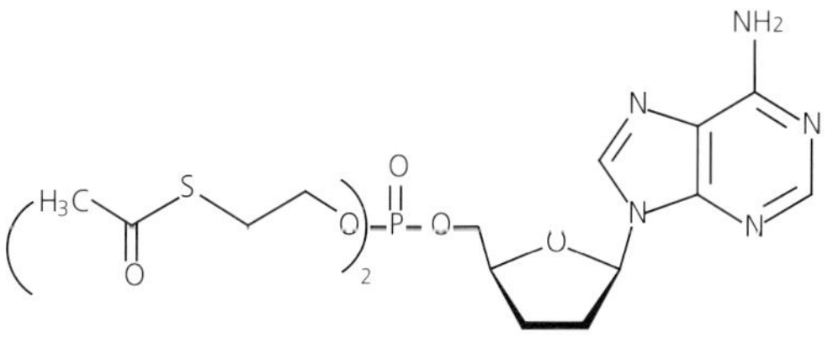

ddAMP, 2', 3'-dideoxyadenosine monophosphate

**Table 1.** Antiviral activity of the bis(MeSATE)phosphotriester derivative of ddA compared to its nucleoside parent and zidovudine in various cell lines infected with HIV-1

| | Cell type | | | | | | | |
| | MT-4 | | CEM-SS | | CEM/TK⁻ | | PBMC | |
| Drug | $EC_{50}$* | $CC_{50}$* | $EC_{50}$ | $CC_{50}$ | $EC_{50}$ | $CC_{50}$ | $EC_{50}$ | $CC_{50}$ |
|---|---|---|---|---|---|---|---|---|
| bis(MeSATE)ddA-MP | 0.011 | 16 | 0.00056 | 24 | 0.00077 | 10 | 0.00023 | 1.1 |
| ddA | 10 | >100 | 0.54 | > 100 | 1.1 | >100 | 0.09 | 22 |
| Zidovudine | 0.018 | >100 | 0.0048 | >100 | >100 | >100 | 0.0012 | 61 |

*$EC_{50}$, 50% effective concentration (μM) or concentration required to inhibit the replication of HIV-1 by 50%; $CC_{50}$, 50% cytotoxic concentration (μM) or concentration required to reduce the viability of uninfected cells by 50%.

**Figure 6.** Structure of the bis(MeSATE)d4TMP

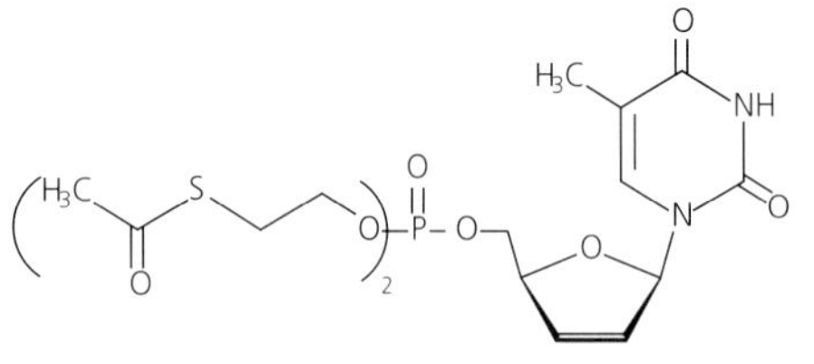

d4TMP, 2′,3′-didehydro-2′,3′-dideoxythymidine monophosphate (stavudine monophosphate); MeSATE, methyl SATE or S-acetyl-2-thioethyl.

same range as the $EC_{50}$ values observed for this pronucleotide in other cell lines.

These results strongly support the hypothesis that the enhanced anti-HIV activity of stavudine by the use of its corresponding bis(MeSATE)phosphotriester derivative is related, via the intracellular delivery of the 5′-mononucleotide, to an accumulation of the phosphorylated forms of stavudine inside the cell. Thus, applied to an antiviral nucleoside analogue which was hampered at the first phosphorylation step, the SATE pronucleotide approach leads to an enhanced *in vitro* antiviral efficiency.

## ACYCLOVIR

Acyclovir [9-(2-hydroxyethoxymethyl)guanine; ACV] is currently used as a therapeutic agent for the treatment of herpes simplex virus (HSV) and varicella-zoster virus (VZV) infections [36,37]. Its selectivity for HSV and

VZV is caused by its preferential monophosphorylation in virus-infected cells by a herpesvirus-encoded thymidine kinase. The resulting acyclovir 5′-monophosphate (ACVMP) is subsequently converted to the corresponding 5′-triphosphate derivative (ACVTP) by cellular enzymes. ACVTP inhibits herpesvirus DNA polymerase and its incorporation into viral DNA results in chain termination. Acyclovir remains essentially unchanged in uninfected cells; consequently, there is little interference with cellular DNA synthesis. Specificity for the herpesvirus-induced enzyme accounts for the wide therapeutic index of acyclovir but limits its activity spectrum, which is essentially confined to HSV and VZV and excludes important pathogens such as HBV that do not encode a thymidine kinase. Thus, acyclovir is of uncertain efficacy in the treatment of patients with chronic HBV [36], although ACVTP is a relatively good inhibitor of HBV DNA polymerase [38,39]. Randomized comparative studies of acyclovir alone [40,41] or in combination with interferon [42] have failed to show a statistically significant effect on the rate of seroconversion.

Consequently, the investigation of the SATE pronucleotide approach was extended to acyclovir. Two bis(SATE)phosphotriester derivatives [bis(MeSATE)ACVMP and bis(tBuSATE)ACVMP; Fig. 7] have been synthesized and evaluated for their inhibitory effects on the replication of human HBV in transfected human liver HepG2 (2.2.15) cells (Table 3).

As expected, acyclovir proved to be inactive against HBV replication in human liver HepG2 cells at

**Table 2.** Antiviral activity of the bis(MeSATE)phosphotriester derivative of stavudine compared with its nucleoside parent in various cell lines infected with HIV-1

| | Cell type | | | | | | | |
| | MT-4 | | CEM-SS | | CEM/TK⁻ | | PBMC | |
| Drug | $EC_{50}$ | $CC_{50}$ | $EC_{50}$ | $CC_{50}$ | $EC_{50}$ | $CC_{50}$ | $EC_{50}$ | $CC_{50}$ |
|---|---|---|---|---|---|---|---|---|
| bis(MeSATE)d4TMP | 0.016 | >100 | 0.006 | 68 | 0.012 | 60 | 0.007 | 22 |
| Stavudine | 0.28 | >100 | 0.059 | >100 | 10 | >100 | 0.050 | 42 |

**Figure 7.** Structures of the two studied bis(SATE)phosphotriester derivatives of acyclovir

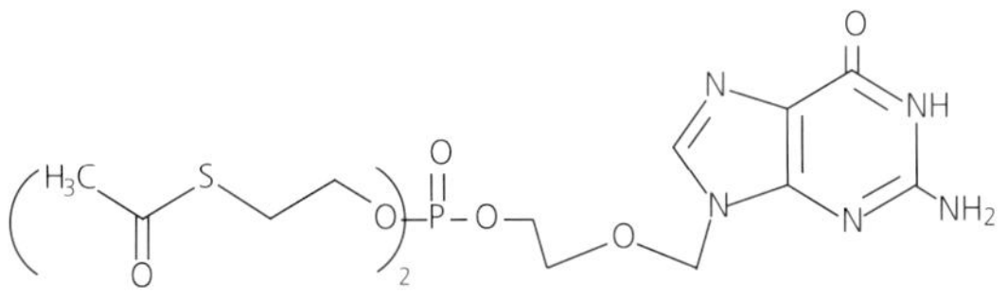

bis(MeSATE)ACVMP 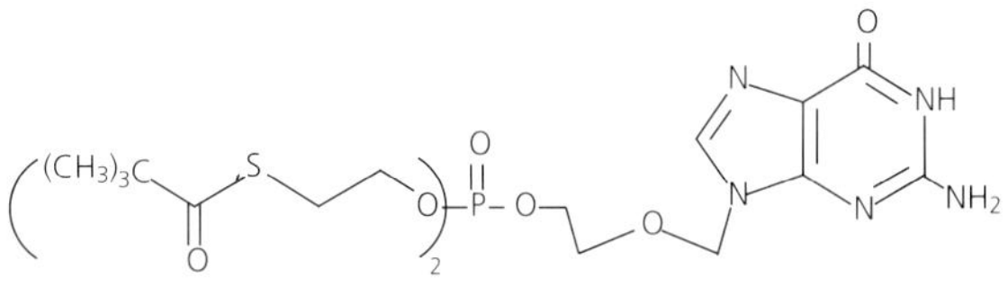                                    bis(tBuSATE)ACVMP

MeSATE, methylSATE or *S*-acetyl-2-thioethyl.

**Table 3.** Anti-HBV activity of two bis(SATE)phosphotriester derivatives of acyclovir compared with their nucleoside parent and 2′,3′-dideoxyguanosine (ddG) as reference compound in human liver HepG2 cells

| Drug | HBV replicative intermediate | | | HBV virions | |
|---|---|---|---|---|---|
| | $CC_{50}$ | $EC_{50}$ | SI* | $EC_{50}$ | SI |
| bis(MeSATE)ACVMP | 990 | 4.3 | 230 | 0.7 | 1410 |
| bis(tBuSATE)ACVMP | 1600 | 1.1 | 1450 | 0.2 | 8000 |
| Acyclovir | 630 | >100 | NA | 110 | 6 |
| ddG | 220 | 3.4 | 65 | 1.3 | 170 |

*SI, Selectivity index, ratio $CC_{50}/EC_{50}$; NA, not applicable.

concentrations up to 100 µM. These data illustrate the failure of acyclovir to undergo biotransformation to the active triphosphate form in HepG2 target cells [38]. Conversely, the two bis(SATE)phosphotriester derivatives of acyclovir emerged as potent inhibitors with $EC_{50}$ values that were in the same range as the $EC_{50}$ value observed for the reference compound 2′,3′-dideoxyguanosine (ddG). However, these pronucleotides exhibited low toxicity in mock-infected HepG2 cells and proved to be superior to ddG with regard to their selectivity index. Differences observed between the anti-HBV efficiencies of bis(MeSATE)ACVMP and bis(tBuSATE)ACVMP may be explained by the lipophilicity of these compounds or their kinetics of decomposition (in culture medium and inside the cell). More complete and detailed studies will be necessary to investigate the effect of the intracellular delivery of acyclovir 5′-monophosphate on the metabolism of the parent nucleoside.

The present results strongly support the hypothesis that the appearance of an anti-HBV activity of acyclovir by the use of its corresponding bis(SATE)-phosphotriester derivatives is related, via the intracellular delivery of the 5′-mononucleoside, to an accumulation of the phosphorylated forms of acyclovir inside the cell. Thus, applied to an antiviral nucleoside analogue which was hampered at the first phosphorylation step, the SATE pronucleotide approach has led to an extension of its antiviral spectrum.

## CONCLUSIONS

These results illustrate the potential of the SATE pronucleotide approach. Applied to anti-HIV nucleoside analogues, namely stavudine and ddA (which were hampered at the first metabolization step by, respectively, a dependence on kinase-mediated phosphorylation and a rate-limiting step in the anabolism pathway) this approach leads to markedly enhanced antiviral activity. Moreover, applied to the well-established anti-herpesvirus drug acyclovir, the activity of which is strictly dependent on a virus-encoded kinase, this approach gives rise to a potent anti-HBV activity without additional toxicity.

In summary, the SATE pronucleotide concept provides the drug designer with greater flexibility in approaching the development of optimal mononucleotide prodrug derivatives. Thus, by the variation of the acyl chain in the immediate vicinity of the thiol ester function, it should be possible to modulate their *in vivo* pharmacokinetics and to find an adequate balance between aqueous solubility, lipophilicity and stability. Currently, we are starting an *in vivo* implementation of the SATE pronucleotide approach in various animal models.

This article originally appeared in *Antiviral Therapy* 1996; **1** (Supplement 4):39–46.

# ACKNOWLEDGEMENTS

These investigations were supported by grants from the CNRS, Agence Nationale de Recherches sur le SIDA (ANRS, France) and Association pour la Recherche sur le Cancer (ARC, France). We are grateful to AM Aubertin (Institut de Virologie de la Faculté de Médecine, Strasbourg, France) and C Tseng (Department of Health & Human Services, NIH, Bethesda, Maryland, USA) for antiviral assays.

# REFERENCES

1. Balzarini J, Cooney DA, Dalal M, Kang GJ, Cupp JE, De Clercq E, Broder S & Johns DG. 2′,3′-Dideoxycytidine: regulation of its metabolism and anti-retroviral potency by natural pyrimidine nucleosides and by inhibitors of pyrimidine nucleotide synthesis. *Molecular Pharmacology* 1987; **32**:798–806.

2. Starnes MC & Cheng YC. Cellular metabolism of 2′,3′-dideoxycytidine, a compound active against human immunodeficiency virus in vitro. *Journal of Biological Chemistry* 1987; **262**:988–991.

3. Johnson MA, Ahluwalia G, Connelly MC, Cooney DA, Broder S, Johns DG & Fridland A. Metabolic pathways for the activation of the antiretroviral agent 2′,3′-dideoxyadenosine in human lymphoid cells. *Journal of Biological Chemistry* 1988; **263**:15354–15357.

4. Johnson MA & Fridland A. Phosphorylation of 2′,3′-dideoxyinosine by cytosolic 5′-nucleotidase of human lymphoid cells. *Molecular Pharmacology* 1989; **36**:291–295.

5. Hao Z, Cooney DA, Farquhar D, Perno CF, Zhang K, Masood R, Wilson Y, Hartman NR, Balzarini J & Johns DG. Potent DNA chain termination activity and selective inhibition of human immunodeficiency virus reverse transcriptase by 2′,3′-dideoxyuridine-5′-triphosphate. *Molecular Pharmacology* 1990; **37**:157–163.

6. Perno CF, Yarchoan R, Cooney DA, Hartman NR, Webb DSA, Hao Z, Mitsuya H, Johns DG & Broder S. Replication of HIV in monocytes: granulocyte–macrophage colony stimulating factor (GM–CSF) potentiates viral production yet enhances the antiviral effect mediated by AZT and other dideoxynucleoside congeners of thymidine. *Journal of Experimental Medicine* 1989; **169**:933–951.

7. Gao WY, Shirasaka T, Johns DG, Broder S & Mitsuya H. Differential phosphorylation of azidothymidine, dideoxycytidine, and dideoxyinosine in resting and activated peripheral blood mononuclear cells. *Journal of Clinical Investigation* 1993; **91**:2326–2333.

8. Sommadossi JP. Nucleoside analogs: similarities and differences. *Clinical Infectious Diseases* 1993; 16 (Suppl. 1):S7–S15.

9. Gao WY, Agbaria R, Driscoll JS & Mitsuya H. Divergent anti-human immunodeficiency virus activity and anabolic phosphorylation of 2′,3′-dideoxynucleoside analogs in resting and activated human cells. *Journal of Biological Chemistry* 1994; **259**:12633–12638.

10. Leibman KC & Heideberg C. The metabolism of $^{32}$P-labeled ribonucleotides in tissue slices and cell suspensions. *Journal of Biological Chemistry* 1955; **216**:823–830.

11. Roll PM, Weinfeld H, Caroll E & Brown GB. The util-

12. Lichtenstein J, Barner HD & Cohen SS. The metabolism of exogenously supplied nucleotides by Escherichia coli. *Journal of Biological Chemistry* 1960; **235**:457–465.

13. Alexander P & Holy A. Prodrugs of analogs of nucleic acid components. *Collection of Czechoslovak Chemical Communications* 1994; **59**:2127–2165.

14. Périgaud C, Girardet JL, Gosselin G & Imbach JL. Comments on nucleotide delivery forms. In *Advances in Antiviral Drug Design* 1995; pp. 147–172. Edited by E De Clercq. Greenwich: JAI Press.

15. Gosselin G & Imbach JL. The anti-HIV nucleoside phosphotriester approach: contorversial comments and complementary data. *International Antiviral News* 1993; **1**:100–102.

16. Eckstein F & Gish G. Phosphorothioates in molecular biology. *Trends in Biochemical Sciences* 1989; **14**:97–100.

17. Lefebvre I, Périgaud C, Pompon A, Aubertin AM, Girardet JL, Kirn A, Gosselin G & Imbach JL. Mononucleoside phosphotriester derivatives with S-acyl-2-thioethyl bioreversible phosphate protecting groups. Intracellular delivery of 3′-azido-2′,3′-dideoxythymidine 5′-monophosphate (AZTMP). *Journal of Medicinal Chemistry* 1995; **38**:3941–3950.

18. Périgaud C, Girardet JL, Lefebvre I, Xie MY, Aubertin AM, Kirn A, Gosselin G, Imbach JL & Sommadossi JP. Comparison of cytotoxicity of mononucleoside phosphotriester derivatives bearing biolabile phosphate protecting groups in normal human bone marrow progenitor cells. *Antiviral Chemistry & Chemotherapy* 1996; **7**:338–345.

19. McGowan JJ, Tomaszewski JE, Cradock J, Hoth D, Grieshaber CK, Broder S & Mitsuya H. Overview of the preclinical development of an antiretroviral drug, 2′,3′-dideoxyinosine. *Reviews of Infectious Diseases* 1990; **12**:S513–S521.

20. McLaren C, Datema R, Knupp CA & Buroker RA. Review: didanosine. *Antiviral Chemistry & Chemotherapy* 1991; **2**:321–328.

21. Faulds D & Brogden RN. Didanosine. *Drugs* 1992; **44**:94–116.

22. Shelton MJ, O'Donnell AM & Morse GD. Didanosine. *Annals of Pharmacotherapy* 1992; **26**:660–670.

23. Ahluwalia G, Cooney DA, Mitsuya H, Fridland A, Flora KP, Hao Z, Dalal M, Broder S & Johns DG. Initial studies on the cellular pharmacology of 2′,3′dideoxyinosine, an inhibitor of HIV infectivity. *Biochemical Pharmacology* 1987; **36**:3797–3800.

24. Nair A & Snells TB. Interpretation of the roles of adenylosuccinate lyase and of AMP deaminase in the anti-HIV activity of 2′,3′-dideoxyadenosine and 2′,3′-dideoxyinosine. *Biochemica et Biophysica Acta* 1992; **1119**:201–204.

25. Périgaud C, Aubertin AM, Benzaria S, Pelicano H, Girardet JL, Maury G, Gosselin G, Kirn A & Imbach JL. Equal inhibition of the replication of human immunodeficiency virus in human T-cell culture by ddA bis(SATE)phosphotriester and 3′-azido-2′,3′-dideoxythymidine. *Biochemical Pharmacology* 1994; **48**:11–14.

26. Benzaria S, Girardet JL, Périgaud C, Aubertin AM, Pelicano H, Maury G, Kirn A & Imbach JL. The SATE pronucleotide derivative of ddA: a more potent HIV inhibitor than AZT. *Nucleic Acids Symposium Series* 1994; **31**:129–130.

27. Casey R. Stavudine. *Drugs of the Future* 1994;

isation of nucleotides by the mammal. IV. Triply labeled purine nucleotides. *Journal of Biological Chemistry* 1956; **220**:439–454.

19:925–932.

28. Riddler SA, Anderson, RE & Mellors JW. Antiretroviral activity of stavudine (2′,3′-didehydro-3′-deoxythymidine, d4T). *Antiviral Research* 1995; **27**: 189–203.

29. Lin T, Schinazi RF & Prusoff W. Potent and selective in vitro activity of 3′-deoxythymidin-2′-ene (3′-deoxy-2′,3′-didehydrothymidine) against human immunodeficiency virus. *Biochemical Pharmacology* 1988; **36**: 2713–2718.

30. Mansuri MM, Starett JE Jr, Ghazzouli I, Hitchcock MJM, Sterzycki RZ, Brankovan V, Lin TS, August EM, Prusoff WH, Sommadossi JP & Martin JC. 1-(2,3-Dideoxy-β-D-*glycero*-pent-2-enofuranosyl)thymine. A highly potent and selective anti-HIV agent. *Journal of Medicinal Chemistry* 1989; **32**:461–466.

31. Mansuri MM, Hitchcock MJM, Buroker RA, Bregman CL, Ghazzouli I, Desiderio JV, Starett JE Jr, Sterzycki RZ & Martin JC. Comparison of biological properties *in vitro* and toxicity *in vivo* of three thymidine analogs (D4T, FddT, and AZT) active against HIV. *Antimicrobial Agents and Chemotherapy* 1990; **34**:637–641.

32. Simpson MV, Chin CD, Keilbaugh SA, Lin TS & Prusoff WH. Studies in the inhibition of mitochondrial DNA replication by 3′-azido-3′-deoxythymidine and other dideoxynucleoside analogues which inhibit HIV-replication. *Biochemical Pharmacology* 1989; **38**: 1033–1036.

33. Balzarini J, Herdewijn P & De Clercq E. Differential patterns of intracellular metabolism of 2′,3′-didehydro-2′,3′-dideoxythymidine and 3′-azido-2′,3′-dideoxythymidine, two potent anti-human immunodeficiency virus compounds. *Journal of Biological Chemistry* 1989; **264**: 6127–6133.

34. Ho HT & Hitchcock MJM. Cellular pharmacology of 2′,3′-dideoxy-2′,3′-didehydrothymidine, a nucleoside analog active against human immunodeficiency virus. *Antimicrobial Agents and Chemotherapy* 1989; **33**:

844–849.

35. Girardet JL, Périgaud C, Aubertin AM, Gosselin G, Kirn A & Imbach JL. Increase of the anti-HIV activity of d4T in human T-cell culture by the use of the SATE pronucleotide approach. *Bioorganic & Medicinal Chemistry Letters* 1995; **5**:2981–2984.

36. Wagstaff AJ, Faulds D & Goa KL. Aciclovir. *Drugs* 1994; **47**:153–205.

37. O'Brien JJ & Campoli-Richards DM. Acyclovir. *Drugs* 1989; **37**:233–309.

38. Littler E, Sangar D, Miller W, Ellis M, Parmer V, Alderton W & Lowe D. Studies on the *in vivo* biochemical properties of penciclovir triphosphate. *Antiviral Research* 1994; 23 (Suppl. 1):102.

39. Hantz O, Allaudeen HS, Ooka T, De Clercq E & Trepo C. Inhibition of human and woodchuck hepatitis virus DNA polymerase by triphosphates of acyclovir, 1-(2′-deoxy-2′-fluoro-β-D-arabinosyl)-5-iodocytosine and E-5-(2-bromovinyl)-2′-deoxyuridine. *Antiviral Research* 1984; **4**:187–199.

40. Guarascio P, De Felici AP, Migliorini D, Alexander GJM, Fagan EA & Visco G. Treatment of chronic HBeAg-positive hepatitis with acyclovir. *Journal of Hepatology* 1986; 3 (Suppl. 2):S143–S147.

41. Alexander GJM, Fagan EA, Hegarty JE, Yeo J, Eddleston ALWF & Williams R. Controlled clinical trials of acyclovir in chronic hepatitis virus infection. *Journal of Medical Virology* 1987; **21**:81–87.

42. Berk L, Schalm SW, De Man RA, Heytink RA, Berthelot P, Brechot C, Boboc B, Degos F, Marcellin P, Benhamou JP, Hess G, Rossol S, Meyer zum Büschenfelde KH, Chalumeau RAFM, Jansen PLM, Reesink HW, Meyer B, Beglinger C, Stadler GA, Den Ouden-Muller JW & De Jong M. Failure of acyclovir to enhance the antiviral effect of α lymphoblastoid interferon on HBe-seroconversion in chronic hepatitis B. *Journal of Hepatology* 1992; **14**: 305–309.

# 34 Cellular pharmacology of lamivudine in hepatocyte primary cultures

## Erika Cretton-Scott* and Jean-Pierre Sommadossi

## INTRODUCTION

Hepatitis B virus (HBV) is a leading cause of chronic hepatitis throughout the world. It is estimated that 5% of the world's population and up to one million people in the United States of America are chronic carriers of HBV. Chronic HBV infection can remain asymptomatic or progress to end-stage liver disease complicated by liver failure, portal hypertension and hepatocellular carcinoma. The development of an effective vaccine to prevent HBV infection should lead to the eventual eradication of HBV, however, antiviral therapy still remains the only therapeutic approach to delay or prevent the progression of this disease in chronic carriers. Currently, alpha-interferon represents the only drug approved for the treatment of chronic hepatitis, although only patients with high baseline aminotransferase levels and a low HBV DNA level, representing between 30 and 40% of chronic HBV patients, are responders. Furthermore, interferon therapy is associated with side-effects that can lead to discontinuation of therapy, further limiting its usefulness. In addition, transplanted livers can be re-infected with HBV, further emphasizing the need for the development of effective and non-toxic anti-HBV therapeutic agents.

Effective antiviral therapy against HBV infection has been hampered by its extremely narrow host range and, until recently, by limited access to culture systems with viral propagation. Animal hepadnaviruses such as woodchuck hepatitis virus (WHV) and duck hepatitis B virus (DHBV) are similar to the human HBV with regard to morphology, genomic structure and replication [1,2]. These animal hepadnaviruses provide useful experimental models for pre-clinical evaluation of potential anti-HBV candidates *in vivo* [3,4]. Currently, *in vitro* models include the HBV-producing human hepatoblastoma cell line, 2.2.15, and primary cultures of hepatocytes obtained from Pekin ducks infected with DHBV.

Among potential therapies being investigated, antiviral nucleoside analogues remain promising. With the observation that hepadnavirus replication occurs through an RNA template that requires reverse transcriptase activity, similar to the mechanism described for the replication of human immunodeficiency virus (HIV), several nucleoside analogues active against HIV were initially evaluated for potential anti-HBV activity. Among these analogues, lamivudine [(−)β-L-2′,3′-dideoxy-3′-thiacytidine; 3TC; (−)-BCH-189], has been demonstrated to be a potent inhibitor of HBV replication and is currently undergoing Phase III clinical trials.

## CELLULAR METABOLISM OF LAMIVUDINE

Lamivudine has no intrinsic activity against HBV and must first be metabolically activated to 3TC-5′-triphosphate (3TC-TP) by deoxycytidine kinase and pyrimidine nucleotide kinases [5]. It is through this 5′-triphosphate metabolite that inhibition of HBV DNA polymerase occurs. It should be noted that the moderate cytotoxicity exhibited by lamivudine is attributed to the weak inhibition of mammalian DNA polymerases by 3TC-TP [6]. The presence and activity of the cellular anabolic enzymes are highly dependent on host species (human or animal), cell type and stage in the cell cycle, hence cellular functions are important factors in the mechanism of action of nucleoside analogues [7]. In that context, the cellular activation of lamivudine has been studied primarily in cells in which it exerts antiviral activity, such as DHBV-infected duck hepatocytes and established cell lines including Hep G2 and 2.2.15. While these cells are adequate models for evaluating anti-HBV activity, they may not accurately predict the level of lamivudine activation in normal hepatocytes, the *in vivo* target cells for HBV infection. The recent development

Figure 1. Time course of intracellular lamivudine metabolites detected in Hep G2 cells, human hepatocytes and monkey hepatocytes after incubation with 5 μM lamivudine

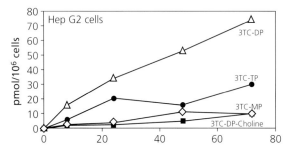

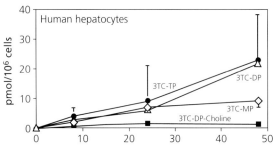

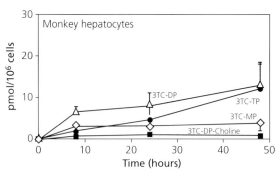

Each experimental value represents the mean±SD of four experiments with human and monkey hepatocytes. Values obtained with Hep G2 cells represent the mean of two experiments in duplicate.

## Lamivudine metabolism in hepatocytes primary cultures

Recently, the cellular metabolism of lamivudine, as related to both its activation (formation of 5′-phosphate metabolites) and potential deactivation (cytochrome P450/conjugation/deamination) was evaluated in normal human and monkey hepatocyte primary cultures.

### Lamivudine anabolism

The metabolite profiles obtained after a 0 to 48 hour exposure of cells to 5 μM lamivudine are illustrated in Figure 1. Lamivudine is rapidly phosphorylated to its 5′-monophosphate (3TC-MP), -diphosphate (3TC-DP) and -triphosphate (3TC-DP) metabolites in both monkey and human hepatocyte primary cultures. Profiles in monkey and human hepatocytes are similar, with 3TC-DP and 3TC-TP the predominant metabolites, although mean levels for both phosphates in human cells are 2-fold higher than in monkey cells. In parallel experiments with Hep G2 cells, levels of 3TC-TP were within the range observed in both monkey and human hepatocytes. However, levels of 3TC-DP were significantly higher in Hep G2 cells. High 3TC-DP levels have also been reported in phytohaemagglutinin-stimulated peripheral blood mononuclear cells (PHA-PBMC) and in the monocyte cell line U937 [5]. Accumulation of the 5′-diphosphate metabolite suggests that further conversion to the 5′-triphosphate is rate-limiting in these cells. This is in contrast to the profile observed in both human and monkey hepatocytes. In these cells there was no accumulation of 3TC-DP; in fact, for both monkey and human cells, the mean 3TC-DP and 3TC-TP levels were approximately equal (Table 1). This may suggest possible differences, related to cell type, in the activity of nucleoside diphosphokinase, the putative enzyme involved in the conversion of 3TC-DP to 3TC-TP. The 5′-DP-choline metabolite of lamivudine was also observed in hepatocyte primary cultures. Its formation appeared to be more consistent in human hepatocytes than in monkey cells, but in both cases, the mean levels of 3TC-DP-choline were approximately 3- to 6-fold lower than levels observed in Hep G2 cells (Table 1). This apparent difference in formation of the 5′-liponucleotide may reflect differences in cells. Similar differences in 5′-liponucleotide formation associated with cell type have been reported for β-L-2′,3′-dideoxy-5-fluorocytidine [11].

Of particular note is the substantial inter-individual variability in the formation of both 3TC-DP and 3TC-TP observed in human hepatocyte cultures

of culture conditions that maintain liver-specific functions for prolonged periods of time have lead to the increased use of human hepatocytes in primary culture. This culture system has been successfully used to evaluate both drug biotransformation and the regulation of drug-metabolizing enzymes. In many instances this culture system has been shown to be a good predictor of *in vivo* drug biotransformation in man [8,9]. More importantly, recent progress in the ability to infect adult human hepatocytes in culture with HBV has recently been reported [10], further emphasizing the potential usefulness of this system to evaluate cellular metabolism of potential antiviral candidates.

**Table 1.** Intracellular levels of lamivudine metabolites in Hep G2 cells, and human and monkey hepatocyte primary cultures following exposure to 5 μM lamivudine

| Cells | Period of incubation (h) | Concentration of intracellular metabolites (pmol/$10^6$ cells) | | | |
|---|---|---|---|---|---|
| | | 3TC-MP | 3TC-DP | 3TC-TP | 3TC-DP-choline |
| Human hepatocytes (*n*=4) | | | | | |
| | 8 | 2.11±1.19 | 2.86±0.84 | 4.14±2.63 | 0.85±0.36 |
| | 24 | 7.03±1.84 | 6.05±2.74 | 9.18±11.73 | 1.65±0.87 |
| | 48 | 9.30±1.90 | 21.82±16.56 | 22.75±15.27 | 1.42±0.80 |
| Monkey hepatocytes (*n*=4) | | | | | |
| | 8 | 3.14 (*n*=2) | 5.61 (*n*=2) | 0.8 (*n*=2) | Not Detected |
| | 24 | 3.26±1.01 | 8.19±3.01 | 4.69±3.44 | 1.23±1.16 |
| | 48 | 3.99±1.91 | 13.18±5.00 | 12.20±6.28 | 0.82 (*n*=2) |
| Hep G2 (*n*=2) | | | | | |
| | 8 | 2.39 | 15.81 | 6.15 | 2.01 |
| | 24 | 4.23 | 34.42 | 20.68 | 2.79 |
| | 48 | 11.37 | 52.97 | 16.01 | 4.93 |

(Table 1). Similar variation in the extent of lamivudine phosphorylation *in vitro* between donors has been reported in human peripheral blood lymphocytes [12]. Despite this variability, the levels of 5'-triphosphate, the active metabolite, achieved in normal human hepatocyte cultures should be sufficient for inhibition of HBV replication based on the reported $K_i$ for 3TC-TP against HBV replication *in vitro* [13]. Although the enzymes responsible for lamivudine phosphorylation to its active 5'-triphosphate have not been fully characterized, it is believed that the same anabolic enzymes involved in the phosphorylation of the endogenous nucleoside, deoxycytidine [5] mediate lamivudine activation. Whether the variability in lamivudine phosphorylation is related to differences among the four donor livers with respect to the level and/or activity of these anabolic enzymes was not examined.

## Lamivudine deactivation

It is well known that first-pass metabolism by the liver can markedly decrease the oral bioavailability of a large number of clinically important drugs, including nucleoside analogues [14] since the concentration of the major enzymes involved in their biotransformation are highest in the hepatocyte. Hence, an important component in drug development is the determination and evaluation of drug biotransformation. Such evaluation is routinely performed either *in vivo* or *in vitro* using various animal species including rats, rabbits, dogs and non-human primates. In hepatitis research, animals such as the woodchuck and Pekin duck are also used for pre-clinical evaluation. One of the major limitations of such studies is that important qualita-

tive and quantitative inter-species differences in metabolic pathways exist [15], making extrapolation to humans difficult. Similarly, use of permanent liver cell lines to evaluate drug biotransformation are of limited use as they either over-express or do not express several drug-metabolizing enzymes such as the cytochrome P450 (CYP 450) enzymatic system [16]. A possible exception to this is the Hep G2 cell line, although numerous discrepancies regarding their expression of CYP450 activities can be found in the literature.

As previously noted, advances in culture conditions have greatly enhanced the use of human hepatocytes as an *in vitro* model of drug biotransformation in man. In conjunction with the evaluation of lamivudine phosphorylation in hepatocyte primary cultures, potential metabolic pathways leading to lamivudine deactivation were examined in both human and monkey hepatocytes. Monkey hepatocytes were included in these studies because non-human primates are often utilized in the pharmacokinetic evaluation of antiviral candidates.

Deamination of lamivudine by deoxycytidine deaminase was not observed in either human or monkey hepatocytes, consistent with previous *in vitro* observations with partially purified human liver deoxycytidine deaminase [17]. In contrast, significant sulphoxidation of lamivudine was observed in both hepatocyte culture systems (Fig. 2). Levels of this metabolite represented as much as 50% of the total extracellular lamivudine concentration after 48 hours in monkey hepatocytes. Formation in human hepatocytes was significantly lower suggesting a possible inter-species variation in lamivudine sulphoxidation. Additionally, sulphoxide levels were highly variable

Figure 2. Extracellular levels of the 3'-sulphoxide of lamivudine in monkey and human hepatocyte primary cultures following incubation with 5 µM lamivudine

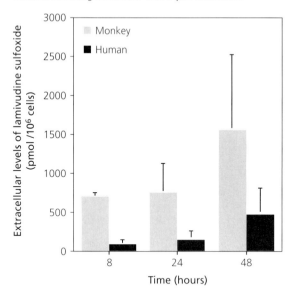

Values represent the mean±SD of four experiments.

among donors, for both monkey and human hepatocytes. Of particular note was the complete absence of lamivudine sulphoxidation in Hep G2 cells, suggesting that this human cell line lacks the enzyme(s) responsible for this reaction. Of interest, sulphoxidation of another unusual L(–)-configured cytidine analogue, (–)-β-L-2',3'-dideoxy-5-fluoro-3'-thiacytidine; (–)FTC, has been observed *in vivo* both in rhesus monkeys [18] and rodents [19].

The metabolic enzymes responsible for the formation of the 3'-sulphoxides of lamivudine and (–)FTC have not been identified, although CYP3A4 and microsomal flavin-dependent monooxygenase are likely candidates. Both enzymes have been implicated in the sulphoxidation of omeprazole [20] and *S*-methyl N,N-diethylthiolcarbamate [21]. Both inter-species and inter-individual differences in enzyme level, activity and substrate specificity involving CYP3A4 is well documented. Whether the differences in lamivudine sulphoxidation observed among different human hepatocyte cultures represent significant inter-individual variabilities among donors in CYP3A4 activity towards lamivudine is not clear. A larger donor pool will be needed to make this determination. In addition, the apparent inter-species difference in lamivudine sulphoxidation observed in hepatocyte primary cultures may be related to either low enzymatic activity in human cells or fundamental substrate specificity differences between the human

and monkey enzymes. Further elucidation of this reaction will be needed.

## CONCLUSION

The significant differences observed both in the activation (5'-phosphorylation) and deactivation (sulphoxidation) of lamivudine among three different cell culture models, specifically Hep G2 cells, monkey hepatocytes and human hepatocytes, emphasizes the importance of utilizing normal human cells in the intracellular investigations of anti-hepatitis agents. The extent of lamivudine sulphoxidation *in vivo* has not been reported. Since the closely related (–)FTC analogue undergoes some sulphoxidation *in vivo*, a similar metabolic fate for lamivudine may be observed. Pharmacokinetic studies indicate that as much as 32–59% and 60–80% of unchanged lamivudine is excreted in the urine of monkey and human subjects, respectively. Although no mention was made regarding the formation and/or detection of a metabolite, these levels of unchanged drug are consistent with the levels of unchanged lamivudine measured in media following exposure of monkey and human hepatocyte cultures. Whether formation of the sulphoxide is of significance regarding the efficacy or toxicity of lamivudine is not clear.

## REFERENCES

1. Summers J, Smolec JM & Snyder R. A virus similar to human hepatitis B virus associated with hepatitis and hepatoma in woodchucks. *Proceedings of the National Academy of Sciences, USA* 1978; **75**: 4533–4537.
2. Mason WS, Seal G & Summers J. Virus of Pekin ducks with structural and biological relatedness to human hepatitis B virus. *Journal of Virology* 1980; **36**: 829–836.
3. Zuckerman AJ. Screening of antiviral drugs for hepadnavirus infection in Pekin ducks: a review. *Journal of Virological Methods* 1987; **17**: 119–126.
4. Roggendorf M & Tolle TK. The woodchuck: an animal model for hepatitis B virus infection in man. *Intervirology* 1995; **38**: 100–112.
5. Kewn S, Veal GJ, Hoggard PG, Barry MG & Back DJ. Lamivudine (3TC) phosphorylation and drug interactions in vitro. *Biochemical Pharmacology* 1997; **54**: 589–595.
6. Hart GJ, Orr DC, Penn CR, Figueiredo HT, Gray NM, Boehme RE & Cameron JM. Effects of (–)-2'-deoxy-3'-thiacytidine (3TC) 5'-triphosphate on human immunodeficiency virus reverse transcriptase and mammalian DNA polymerases alpha, beta, and gamma. *Antimicrobial Agents and Chemotherapy* 1992; **36**:1688–1694.
7. Sommadossi J-P. Nucleoside analogs: similarities and differences. *Clinical Infectious Diseases* 1993; **16**:S7–S15.
8. Xin-Ru P, Cretton-Scott E, Zhou X-J, Xie M-Y, Rahmani R, Schinazi RF, Duchin K & Sommadossi J-P. Comparative metabolism of the antiviral dimer 3'-azido-3'-deoxythymidine-P-2',3'-dideoxyinosine and

the monomers zidovudine and didanosine by rat, monkey and human hepatocytes. *Antimicrobial Agents and Chemotherapy* 1997; **41**:2502–2510.

9. Guillouzo A, Morel F, Fardel O & Meunier B. Use of human hepatocyte cultures for drug metabolism studies. *Toxicology* 1993; **82**:209–219.

10. Gribon P, Diot C & Guguen-Guillouzo C. Reproducible high level infection of cultured adult human hepatocytes by hepatitis B virus: effect of polyethylene glycol on adsorption and penetration. *Virology* 1993; **192**:534–540.

11. Martin LT, Faraj A, Schinazi RF, Gosselin G, Mathe C, Imbach J-L & Sommadossi J-P. Effect of stereoisomerism on the cellular pharmacology of b-enantiomers of cytidine analogs in Hep G2 cells. *Biochemical Pharmacology* 1997; **53**:75–87.

12. Cammack N, Rouse P, Marr CLP, Reid PJ, Boehme RE, Coates JAV, Penn CR & Cameron JM. Cellular metabolism of (–) enatiomeric 2′-deoxy-3′-thiacytidine. *Biochemical Pharmacology* 1992; **43**:2059–2064.

13. Doong SL, Tsai C-H, Schinazi RF, Liotta DC & Cheng YC. Inhibition of the replication of hepatitis B virus in vitro by 2′3′-dideoxy-3′-thiacytidine and related analogs. *Proceedings of the National Academy of Sciences, USA* 1991; **88**:8495–8499.

14. Klecker RW, Collins JM, Yarchoan R, Thomas R, Jenkins JF, Broder S & Myers CE. Plasma and cerebralspinal fluid pharmacokinetics of 3′-azido-3′-deoxythymidine: a novel pyrimidine analogue with potential application for the treatment of patients with AIDS and related diseases. *Clinical Pharmacology and Therapeutics* 1987; **41**:407–412.

15. Rodrigues AD. Use of in vitro human metabolism studies in drug development. *Biochemical Pharmacology* 1994; **48**:2147–2156.

16. Schwarz LR & Wiebel FJ. Cytochrome P450 in primary and permanent liver cell cultures. In Cytochrome P450, vol. 105 1993; pp. 399–413. Edited by JB Schenkman & H Berlin. Heidelberg: Springer-Verlag.

17. Chang C-N, Doong S-L, Zhou JH, Beach JW, Jeong LS, Chu CK, Tsai C-H & Cheng Y-C. Deoxycytidine deaminase-resistant stereoisomer is the active form of (±)-2′,3′-dideoxy-3′-thiacytidine in the inhibition of hepatitis B virus replication. *Journal of Biological Chemistry* 1992; **267**:13938–13942.

18. Schinazi RF, Liotta DC, McClure H, Furman PA & Painter G. Cellular pharmacology and monkey pharmacokinetics of the antiviral (–)-2′,3′-dideoxy-5-fluoro-3′-thiacytidine [(–)-FTC]. *32nd Interscience Conference on Antimicrobial Agents and Chemotherapy*. Anaheim, California, USA, 11–14 October 1992; Abstract 1321.

19. Frick LW, St. John L, Taylor LC, Painter GR, Furman PA, Liotta DC, Furfine ES & Nelson DJ. Pharmacokinetics, oral bioavailability, and metabolic disposition in rats of (–)-cis-5-fluoro-1[2-(hydroxymethyl)-1,3-oxathiolan-5-yl] cytosine, a nucleoside analog active against human immunodeficiency virus and hepatitis B virus. *Antimicrobial Agents and Chemotherapy* 1993; **37**:2285–2292.

20. Bottiger Y, Tybring G, Gotharson E & Bertilsson L. Inhibition of the sulfoxidation of omeprazole by ketoconazole in poor and extensive metabolizers of S-mephenytoin. *Clinical Pharmacology and Therapeutics* 1997; **62**:384–391.

21. Madan A, Parkinson A & Faiman MD. Role of flavin-dependent monooxygenases and cytochrome P450 enzymes in the sulfoxidation of S-methyl N,N-diethylthiolcarbamate. *Biochemical Pharmacology* 1993; **46**:2291–2297.

# Section VI

## DRUG DISCOVERY

## Part B

### RESISTANCE AND QUASISPECIES

# 35 Influence of reverse transcriptase YMDD motif variants on replication and lamivudine resistance of hepatitis B virus

Suzane Kioko Ono-Nita, Naoya Kato*,
Yasushi Shiratori, Keng-Hsin Lan, Hideo Yoshida,
Flair José Carrilho and Masao Omata

## SUMMARY

Lamivudine is a reverse transcriptase inhibitor and has antiviral activity against hepatitis B virus (HBV). Recently the emergence of drug-resistant variants (Met to Ile or Val in the YMDD motif) of HBV has been reported. YMDD is a conserved reverse transcriptase motif present in various viruses, including HIV and hepadnaviruses. The aim of this study was to explore the consequences of mutations in the conserved motif of HBV reverse transcriptase with regard to replication ability and susceptibility to lamivudine.

We made seven variants by substituting the Met of the YMDD motif. Four variants with hydrophobic substitutions (Ile, Val, Ala and Leu) remained replication competent, whereas hydrophilic substitutions (Lys, Arg and Thr) impaired replication. Sensitivity to lamivudine was tested against the four replication-competent variants. Replication of mutants with YIDD and YVDD sequences was not reduced in the presence of lamivudine, while replication of the remaining two mutants was diminished.

The YIDD and YVDD mutants showed viral replication, and only one substitution (Met to Ile or Val) in the YMDD motif was enough to cause resistance to lamivudine. Because of replication incompetence or drug sensitivity, only viruses with YIDD or YVDD mutations survive in the presence of lamivudine, and both these HBV variants have been identified in clinical isolates of lamivudine-treated patients.

## INTRODUCTION

HBV infection is a major health problem and accounts for 1.2 million deaths per year worldwide, according to the 1997 WHO report [1]. Despite the existence of an effective vaccine, no effective antiviral treatment has been developed for patients chronically infected with HBV. The overall interferon response rate is less than 40% [2]. Because the replication of HBV DNA proceeds through reverse transcription of a pregenomic RNA intermediate [3], the use of reverse transcriptase inhibitors as antiviral drugs for hepatitis B has become an attractive option. Lamivudine $[(-)-\beta-L-2',3'-dideoxy-3'-thiacytidine; 3TC]$ is a reverse transcriptase inhibitor that is well tolerated and produces a rapid and profound decrease in serum HBV DNA levels in patients with chronic hepatitis B [4]. Histological improvement has also been reported [5]. However, the initial clinical trials to treat hepatitis B have shown that 14% of patients develop drug-resistant virus during long-term treatment [6]. These lamivudine-resistant viruses exhibit a mutation from Met to Iso/Val in the Tyr, Met, Asp, Asp (YMDD) motif of polymerase that is considered to be the catalytic centre of reverse transcriptase [7]. The present study was designed to further explore the consequences of mutations in the conserved motif of HBV reverse transcriptase with regard to replication ability and susceptibility to lamivudine.

*Corresponding author

# MATERIALS AND METHODS

## Extraction of DNA from serum

HBV DNA was extracted from 100 μl serum obtained from a 54-year-old male with hepatitis virus e antigen (HBeAg)-positive cirrhosis using the SepaGene kit (Sanko Junyaku, Tokyo, Japan) according to the manufacturer's instructions.

## Amplification and cloning of full-length HBV DNA

HBV DNA was amplified with the following primers having *Sac*I and *Sap*I restriction sites (the nucleotide positions in HBV adr4 [8] are shown in parenthesis): P1 (1821–1841), 5′-CCGGAAAGCTTGAGCTCTTCTT-TTTCACCTCTGCCTAATCA-3′, and P2 (1823–1806), 5′-CCGGAAAGCTTGAGCTCTTCAAAAAGTTGCA-TGGTGCTGG-3′ [9]. PCR was performed in 100 μl of reaction mixture containing specimen DNA, 20 mM Tris-HCl (pH 8.8), 10 mM KCl, 10 mM $(NH_4)_2SO_4$, 0.1% Triton X-100, 0.1 mg/ml bovine serum albumin, 200 mM dNTPs, 1 mM each of the amplification primers, 5 U of AmpliTaq DNA polymerase (Perkin Elmer) and 5 U of Taq extender PCR additive (Stratagene). The reaction was run in thin-walled tubes with GeneAmp PCR system 9600 (Perkin Elmer) and carried out as a hot-start PCR using a wax barrier (AmpliWax PCR gem, Perkin Elmer). The amplification was performed with denaturation at 94°C for 15 seconds, annealing at 56°C for 45 seconds, and elongation at 72°C for 3 minutes for the initial 5 cycles, followed for the last 40 cycles with denaturation at 94°C for 15 seconds and annealing and elongation at 68°C for 3 minutes. A 72°C final hold for 10 minutes was used for completion of strand synthesis. The PCR product was purified by phenol–chloroform (1:1) extraction, ethanol precipitated and digested with *Sac*I (Takara Shuzo, Kyoto, Japan). A fragment of 3.2 kbp was recovered from agarose gel, purified and cloned into *Sac*I site of pBluescript II SK+ (Stratagene). Plasmids were amplified in *E. coli* JM 109 (Toyobo, Tokyo, Japan) and purified by the Qiagen procedure (Qiagen).

## Site-directed mutagenesis

Seven variants were made by substituting the Met of the YMDD motif with Ile, Val, Ala, Leu, Lys, Arg and Thr with the Quickchange site-directed mutagenesis kit (Stratagene). These contain all possible variants (Ile, Val, Leu, Lys, Arg and Thr) produced by introducing one point mutation into codon ATG (encoding Met). For example, codon AT<u>T</u>, AT<u>C</u> and AT<u>A</u> (mutated

nucleotides are underlined) encode Ile, and codon <u>G</u>TG encodes Val. We added an Ala variant by introducing two point mutations (codon <u>GC</u>G) to cover all naturally existing variants (Ile, Val, Ala, Leu and Thr). The polymerase gene of variants was sequenced using a cycle DNA sequencing system (Applied Biosystems), as described previously [10], to confirm the introduction of mutations.

## Preparation of full-length HBV DNA for transfection

Plasmids containing wild-type and seven variants of HBV DNA were digested with *Sap*I (New England Biolabs) to make full-length HBV DNAs without additional sequences; complete digestion was confirmed by agarose gel electrophoresis. Full-length HBV DNAs were purified by phenol–chloroform (1:1) extraction, ethanol precipitated and dissolved in buffer containing 10 mM Tris-HCl and 1 mM EDTA.

## Transfection of full-length HBV DNA into HuH-7 cells

HuH-7 cells (Human Science Research Resource Bank, Osaka, Japan) [11] were cultured in RPMI 1640 supplemented with 0.5% FBS and 0.2% lactoalbumin. Approximately $1 \times 10^6$ cells were plated onto a 60 mm-diameter dish and 24 hours later transfected with 6 μg of full-length HBV DNA by using Lipofectamine (Gibco BRL). Twenty-four hours after transfection, medium was changed and reincubated with drug-free medium or medium containing lamivudine (Glaxo Welcome, Tokyo, Japan) at concentration of 2 μg/ml. Medium and cells (rinsed three times with ice-cold phosphate-buffered saline) were harvested 3 days later. The efficiency of transfection was monitored by co-transfecting the β-galactosidase expression plasmid, pCMV-β (Clontech Laboratories, Palo Alto, California, USA) and assays for β-galactosidase in extracts of HuH-7 cells were performed as described [12]. Experiments were performed in duplicate.

## Isolation of HBV DNA from transfected cells

Purification of HBV DNA from intracellular core particles was accomplished using a method described by Günther *et al.* [9] with minor modifications. In brief, cells were treated with 500 μl of lysis buffer containing 50 mM Tris-HCl (pH 7.4), 1 mM EDTA and 1% NP-40, transferred to eppendorf tubes, vortexed and allowed to stand on ice for 15 minutes. Nuclei were pelleted by centrifugation at 4°C, $15000 \times g$ for 1 minute.

**Figure 1.** Analysis of replication of YMDD variants of HBV

**(a)**

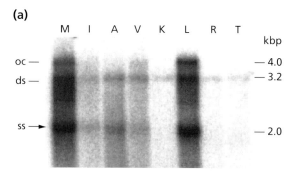

**(b)**

Replication-competent clones:

YMDD    FSY**M**DD<u>VVL</u>

YIDD    FSY**I**DD<u>VVL</u>

YVDD    FSY**V**DD<u>VVL</u>

YADD    FSY**A**DD<u>VVL</u>

YLDD    FSY**L**DD<u>VVL</u>

Replication-incompetent clones:

YKDD    FSY**K**DD<u>VVL</u>

YRDD    FSY**R**DD<u>VVL</u>

YTDD    FSY**T**DD<u>VVL</u>

(a) Southern blot hybridization analysis of HBV replication. Lanes correspond to DNA extracted from viral core particles derived from HuH-7 cells which were transfected with full-length HBV DNAs. The arrow indicates the single-stranded DNA band, representative of HBV replication intermediates. oc, open circular; ds, double-stranded; ss, single-stranded HBV DNA. (b) Hydrophobicity pattern of the YXDD box in the HBV sequences of replication-competent and -incompetent clones. Underlined letters designate hydrophobic amino acids.

The supernatant was transferred to a new tube, adjusted to 10 mM $MgCl_2$ and digested with 100 μg/ml of DNase I for 30 minutes at 37°C. To stop the reaction, EDTA was added to a final concentration of 25 mM. Then, 0.5 mg/ml proteinase K and 1% SDS were added and incubated at 50°C for 4 hours. Phenol–chloroform (1:1) extraction was performed and nucleic acids were ethanol precipitated with glycogen.

## Southern blot hybridization of HBV DNA

HBV DNAs were resolved in 1.5% agarose gel, transferred to a nylon membrane (Hybond N+, Amersham International) by Southern blotting, hybridized with a [32]P-labelled wild-type, full-length HBV DNA probe generated with Ready-To-Go DNA labelling kit (–dCTP) (Pharmacia Biotech). Autoradiography was performed and analysed using a BAS2000 image analyser (Fuji Photo Film).

## RESULTS

### Replication of seven YMDD motif variants

To test the replication ability of these seven variants, we performed Southern blot hybridization on DNA extracts (Fig. 1a). As previously reported [9,13,14], open circular, double-stranded and single-stranded HBV DNA bands were visualized at 4.0 kbp, 3.2 kbp and 2.0 kbp, respectively. A single-stranded HBV DNA band, previously shown to represent HBV replicative intermediates [3], was analysed to investigate whether lamivudine inhibits the reverse transcription of pregenomic RNA to single-stranded DNA during viral replication. Among the wild-type HBV DNA and seven variants tested, the single-stranded DNA band was found in samples from the wild-type virus and four of the variants (Ile, Val, Ala and Leu) (Fig. 1a), indicating that these were replication-competent. On the other hand, the single-stranded DNA band was not found in the other three variants (Lys, Arg and Thr), indicating these to be replication-incompetent.

The hydrophobicity profile of the YMDD motif of the variants was analysed and compared with replication ability, as shown in Figure 1b. Adequately replicating clones had a hydrophobic amino acid (Ile, Val, Ala and Leu) in place of the the Met residue of the YMDD motif, whereas non-replicating ones contained hydrophilic residues (Lys, Arg and Thr) at this position.

### Susceptibility of YMDD motif variants to lamivudine

To evaluate the effect of lamivudine on YMDD motif variants of HBV, we transfected HuH-7 cells with wild-type DNA and four replication-competent variants (Ile, Val, Ala and Leu), and added lamivudine to the medium. In the presence of lamivudine, the intensity of the single-stranded DNA bands of wild-type, YADD and YLDD variants were reduced by 67% to 96%, when compared with those of the untreated controls (Fig. 2). On the other hand, the intensity of the single-stranded DNA bands of YIDD and YVDD variants were unchanged, indicating that these variants are resistant to lamivudine.

**Figure 2.** Susceptibility of YMDD motif variants to lamivudine

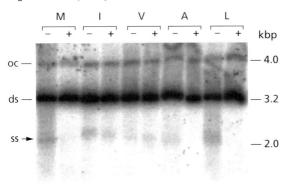

Southern blot hybridization analysis of HBV replication. Lanes correspond to DNA extracted from viral core particles derived from HuH-7 cells which were transfected with full-length HBV DNA without and with lamivudine treatment at a concentration of 2 μg/ml (indicated by – and +, respectively). The arrow indicates the single-stranded DNA band. oc, open circular; ds, double-stranded; ss, single-stranded HBV DNA. Amino acids are indicated by a single letter.

## DISCUSSION

Lamivudine has been developed as a potent treatment for HIV infection [15] and has more recently been used to treat patients with chronic hepatitis B [4] and HBV-infected liver transplant recipients [16–18]. Although it has a strong antiviral effect, the development of resistant virus has become a serious problem [19]. Lamivudine-resistant HIV was shown to have amino acid substitutions in the YMDD motif of reverse transcriptase [20–23], and recently these substitutions have also been reported in HBV [6,24–27]. As the number of new trials investigating nucleoside analogues for the treatment of hepatitis B increases, drug resistance may be a relevant problem in several clinical situations, such as in fulminant hepatitis, chronic hepatitis and orthotopic liver transplantation. We therefore decided to study the replication ability and lamivudine resistance of these YMDD motif variants of HBV.

The YMDD motif is a highly conserved domain in RNA-dependent DNA polymerases and is involved in nucleotide binding in the catalytic site of the polymerase. It was reported that the highly conserved Asp–Asp sequence of the YMDD motif was generally flanked by hydrophobic residues [7]. In the present study, adequately replicating clones actually contained hydrophobic amino acids (Ile, Val, Ala or Leu) at the Met position of the YMDD motif, whereas non-replicating ones contained hydrophilic residues (Lys, Arg or Thr) (see Fig. 1b). Although there are reports of a hydrophilic amino acid flanking the Asp–Asp sequence of the YTDD motif of HIV and feline

immunodeficiency virus, the enzyme activity of the HIV variant was less than 10% and the replication ability was severely reduced when compared with that of the wild-type virus [28,29].

To understand the mechanism of replication incompetence of YMDD motif variants, we referred to the HIV-1 reverse transcriptase structure [30]. The Tyr–Met sequence of the YMDD motif is believed to interact with template–primer complex. It appears that the Met residue has close interactions with the sugar moiety of the terminal nucleotide of the template strand and is also potentially in a position to directly affect dNTP binding. When the Met is substituted, this could alter the positioning of the template–primer complex and dNTP binding ability. This may cause replication-incompetence by changing the proper positioning of the template–primer complex or abolishing the ability to bind dNTP.

We investigated the susceptibility to lamivudine of our replication-competent HBV variants and showed that only one amino acid substitution (Met to Ile or Val) in the YMDD motif was enough to cause lamivudine resistance. These substitutions may cause lamivudine resistance by increasing the stringency of dNTP binding. Namely, amino acid substitutions from Met to Ile or Val in the YMDD motif may make it possible to distinguish lamivudine (a dCTP analogue) from dCTP. It seems reasonable to suppose that this result could explain why only those two variants have been found in HBV patients during lamivudine treatment. In other words, if many variants pre-exist or appear due to the selective pressure of lamivudine, only the resistant variants will be selected and will be able to outgrow the wild-type virus.

In conclusion, the YIDD and YVDD mutants showed viral replication, and only one substitution (Met to Ile or Val) in the YMDD motif was enough to cause resistance to lamivudine. Because of replication incompetence or drug sensitivity, only viruses having YIDD or YVDD mutations survive in the presence of lamivudine, and both these HBV variants have been identified in clinical isolates from lamivudine-treated patients.

## REFERENCES

1. World Health Organization warns of growing 'crisis of suffering'. http://www.who.ch/whr/1997/presse.htm.
2. Wong DK, Cheung AM, O'Rourke K, Naylor CD, Detsky AS & Heathcote J. Effect of alpha-interferon treatment in patients with hepatitis B e antigen-positive chronic hepatitis B. A meta-analysis. *Annals of Internal Medicine* 1993; **119**:312–323.
3. Summers J & Mason WS. Replication of the genome of a hepatitis B-like virus by reverse transcription of an RNA intermediate. *Cell* 1982; **29**:403–415.

4. Dienstag JL, Perrillo RP, Schiff ER, Bartholomew M, Vicary C & Rubin M. A preliminary trial of lamivudine for chronic hepatitis B infection. *New England Journal of Medicine* 1995; **333**:1657–1661.

5. Honkoop P, de Man RA, Zondervan PE & Schalm SW. Histological improvement in patients with chronic hepatitis B virus infection treated with lamivudine. *Liver* 1997; **17**:103–106.

6. Lai CL, Liaw YF, Leung NWY, Deslauriers M, Barnard J, Sanathan L, Gray DF & Condreay LD. Genotypic resistance to lamivudine in a prospective placebo-controlled multicenter study in Asia of lamivudine therapy for chronic hepatitis B infection: incidence, kinetics of emergence and correlation with disease parameters. *Hepatology* 1997; **26**:259A.

7. Kamer G & Argos P. Primary structural comparison of RNA-dependent polymerases from plant, animal and bacterial viruses. *Nucleic Acids Research* 1984; **12**:7269–7282.

8. Fujiyama A, Miyanohara A, Nozaki C, Yoneyama T, Ohtomo N & Matsubara K. Cloning and structural analyses of hepatitis B virus DNAs, subtype adr. *Nucleic Acids Research* 1983; **11**:4601–4610.

9. Günther S, Li B-C, Miska S, Krüger DH, Meisel H & Will H. A novel method for efficient amplification of whole hepatitis B virus genomes permits rapid functional analysis and reveals deletion mutants in immunosuppressed patients. *Journal of Virology* 1995; **69**:5437–5444.

10. Togo G, Toda N, Kanai F, Kato N, Shiratori Y, Kishi K, Imazeki F, Makuuchi M & Omata M. A transforming growth factor b type II receptor gene mutation common in sporadic cecum cancer with microsatellite instability. *Cancer Research* 1996; **56**:5620–5623.

11. Nakabayashi H, Taketa K, Miyano K, Yamane T & Sato J. Growth of human hepatoma cell lines with differentiated functions in chemically defined medium. *Cancer Research* 1982; **42**:3858–3863.

12. Sambrook J, Fritsch EF & Maniatis T. *Molecular Cloning. A Laboratory Manual.* 2nd edn 1989; pp. 16.56–16.67. New York: Cold Spring Harbor Laboratory Press.

13. Yokosuka O, Omata M, Imazeki F & Okuda K. Active and inactive replication of hepatitis B virus deoxyribonucleic acid in chronic liver disease. *Gastroenterology* 1985; **89**:610–616.

14. Yokosuka O, Omata M, Imazeki F, Okuda K & Summers J. Changes of hepatitis B virus DNA in liver and serum caused by recombinant leukocyte interferon treatment: Analysis of intrahepatic replicative hepatitis B virus DNA. *Hepatology* 1985; **5**:728–734.

15. Schinazi RF, Chu CK, Peck A, McMillan A, Mattis R, Cannon D, Jeong LS, Warren Beach J, Choi W-B, Yeola S & Liotta DC. Activities of the four optical isomers of 2′, 3′-dideoxi-3′-thiacytidine (BCH-189) against human immunodeficiency virus type 1 in human lymphocytes. *Antimicrobial Agents & Chemotherapy* 1992; **36**:672–676.

16. Bain VG, Kneteman NM, Ma MM, Gutfreund K, Shapiro JA, Fischer K, Tipples G, Lee H, Jewell LD & Tyrrell DL. Efficacy of lamivudine in chronic hepatitis B patients with active viral replication and decompensated cirrhosis undergoing liver transplantation. *Transplantation* 1996; **62**:1456–1462.

17. Grellier L, Mutimer D, Ahmed M, Brown D, Burrpughs AK, Rolles K, McMaster P, Beranek P, Kennedy F, Kibbler H, McPhillips P, Elias E & Dusheiko G. Lamivudine profilaxis against reinfection in liver transplantation for hepatitis B cirrhosis. *Lancet* 1996; **348**:1212–1215.

18. Ben-Ari Z, Shmueli D, Mor E, Shapira Z & Tur-Kaspa R. Beneficial effect of lamivudine in recurrent hepatitis B after liver transplantation. *Transplantation* 1997; **63**:393–396.

19. Lange JMA. Current problems and the future of anti-retroviral drug trials. *Science* 1997: **276**:548–550.

20. Wainberg MA, Drosopoulos WC, Salomon H, Hsu M, Borkow G, Parniak MA, Gu Z, Song Q, Manne J, Islam S, Castriota G & Prasad VR. Enhanced fidelity of 3TC-selected mutant HIV-1 reverse transcriptase. *Science* 1996; **271**:1282–1285.

21. Wainberg MA, Hsu M, Gu Z, Borkow G & Parnial MA. Effectiveness of 3TC in HIV clinical trials may be due in part to the M184V substitution in 3TC-resistant HIV-1 reverse transcriptase. *AIDS* 1996; **10** (Supplement):S3–S10.

22. Wakefield JK, Jablonski SA & Morrow CD. *In vitro* enzymatic activity of human immunodeficiency virus type 1 reverse transcriptase mutants in the highly conserved YMDD amino acid motif correlates with the infectious potential of the proviral genome. *Journal of Virology* 1992; **66**:6806–6812.

23. Back NKT, Nijhuis M, Keulen W, Boucher CAB, Essink BBO, van Kuilenburg ABP, van Gennip AH & Berkhout B. Reduced replication of 3TC-resistant HIV-1 variants in primary cells due to a processivity defect of the reverse transcriptase enzyme. *EMBO Journal* 1996; **15**:4040–4049.

24. Tipples GA, Ma MM, Fischer KP, Bain VG, Kneteman NM & Tyrrell DLJ. Mutation in HBV RNA-dependent DNA polymerase confers resistance to lamivudine *in vivo*. *Hepatology* 1996; **24**:714–717.

25. Fischer KP & Tyrrell DLJ. Generation of duck hepatitis B virus polymerase mutants through site-directed mutagenesis which demonstrate resistance to lamivudine [(−)-(-L-2′,3′-dideoxy-3′-thiacytidine] *in vitro*. *Antimicrobial Agents & Chemotherapy* 1996; **40**: 1957–1960.

26. Bartholomew MM, Jansen RW, Lennox JJ, Reddy KR, Johnson LC, Bunzendhal H, Condreay LD, Tzakis AG, Schiff ER & Brown NA. Hepatitis-B-virus resistance to lamivudine given for recurrent infection after orthotopic liver transplantation. *Lancet* 1997; **349**:20–22.

27. Ling R, Mutimer D, Ahmed M, Boxall EH, Elias E, Geoffrey MD & Harrison TJ. Selection of mutations in the hepatitis B virus polymerase during therapy of transplant recipients with lamivudine. *Hepatology* 1996; **24**:711–713.

28. Keulen W, Back NKT, van Wijk A, Boucher CAB & Berkhout B. Initial appearance of the 184Ile variant in lamivudine-treated patients is caused by the mutational bias of human immunodeficiency virus type 1 reverse transcriptase. *Journal of Virology* 1997; **71**:3 346–3350.

29. Smith RA, Kathryn MR, Lloyd Jr RM, Schinazi RF & North TW. A novel Met-to-Thr mutation in the YMDD motif of reverse transcriptase from feline immunodeficiency virus confers resistance to oxathiolane nucleosides. *Journal of Virology* 1997; **71**: 2357–2362.

30. Jacobo-Molina A, Ding J, Nanni RG, Clarck Jr AD, Lu X, Tantillo C, Williams RL, Kamer G, Ferris AL, Clarck P, Hizi A, Hughes SH & Arnold E. Crystal structure of human immunodeficiency virus type 1 reverse transcriptase complexed with double-stranded DNA at 3.0 resolution shows bent DNA. *Proceedings of the National Academy of Sciences, USA* 1993; **90**: 6320–6324.

*Therapies for Viral Hepatitis*
Edited by RF Schinazi, J-P Sommadossi and HC Thomas

# 36

# The consequences of quasispecies heterogeneity and within-host ecology for antiviral therapy of hepatitis B virus

Nigel J Burroughs*, David A Rand, Deenan Pillay, Elwyn Elias and David Mutimer

## SUMMARY

The emergence of drug-resistant strains in human immunodeficiency virus (HIV) and hepatitis B virus (HBV) therapy has a number of similarities, principally caused by their high mutation rates, which produce a dynamic and adaptable quasispecies. However, distinct differences in the within-host ecology of these viruses mean that combination therapy in HBV is likely to be more successful than with HIV. In an analysis of liver transplant patient data we emphasize the roles of the quasispecies structure and ecology in determining prophylaxis failure. The main results carry over to chronic HBV carriers and have important consequences in more general circumstances where the emergence of resistance limits the use of antiviral compounds. In the analysis we discuss the correlation between the emergence of resistant mutants and viraemia at various stages of treatment and interpret this in the context of whether single or double mutants are significant risk factors, specifically relating their survival through transplant to emergence of resistant strains. Our analysis of the dynamics indicates that mutants with a single mutation in the YMDD motif (lamivudine resistance mutation) are not capable of exponential growth and therefore are not the cause of prophylaxis failure. Additional mutations are required to achieve a mutant that is both resistant and sufficiently fit for growth.

## INTRODUCTION

The emergence of resistance to antiviral therapy is a serious problem for both HBV and HIV. Resistance emerges through evolution of the virus via mutation in response to the selection imposed by the presence of the antiviral compound. The probability of a resistant mutant emerging is determined by the *in vivo* dynamics of the virus, and therefore the problem of optimizing the use of antivirals and reducing the probability of resistance emergence can be reduced to an understanding of the dynamics of emergence and characterization of risk determinants. In an analyses of the emergence of lamivudine-resistant mutants in liver transplant patients with end-stage HBV-associated liver disease, we have developed a framework for the understanding of resistant mutant development and emergence that is generally applicable to other scenarios, such as antiviral treatment of chronic patients. In a cohort of nine patients undergoing liver transplant and lamivudine therapy, three developed lamivudine-resistant escape mutants; these three patients were those with the highest pretreatment viraemia. This is consistent with other studies where high pretreatment levels of viraemia have been associated with an increased frequency of emergence of resistant mutants to anti-HBV immunoglobulin [1] or lamivudine [2,3]. Examination of these patients through mathematical modelling indicates that the quasispecies structure of the viral population is significant in determining the risk of prophylaxis failure, principally through the existence of (resistant) mutant virions prior to treatment and their subsequent survival through transplant.

## MATERIALS AND METHODS

HBV DNA was measured (Genostics and Roche Amplicor HBV assay) in nine patients, each of whom survived at least 3 months after liver transplantation. Lamivudine treatment was started up to 4 months prior to transplant and continued post-transplant. The

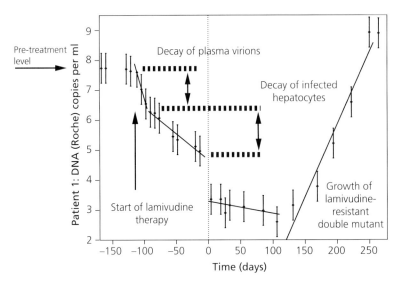

**Figure 1.** Observed viraemia and best fit log–linear lines in patient 1

The Genostics assay is used to extrapolate readings above $4\times10^7$ copies/ml. Transplant occurs at day 0, and lamivudine is administered prior to transplant as indicated by the arrow. Half-bars indicate readings above/below the limit of detection.

range of detection of the Amplicor assay is $400$–$4\times10^7$ copies per ml. A 95% confidence interval of $\pm0.5\,\log_{10}$ is assumed for this assay.

## RESULTS

The course of viraemia under lamivudine and transplant can be separated into a number of phases (Fig. 1). Upon administration of lamivudine, viraemia falls in a biphasic manner, initially with a rapid decline, possibly lasting 1 week, followed by a slower exponential decay. In non-transplant patients this decay reaches a plateau; however, in our study transplant is performed before this occurs. Immediately after transplant there is a rapid reinfection of the liver (1–4 days) followed by a gradual exponential decay. At 100–300 days post-transplant a resistant mutant may emerge, growing exponentially and increasing viraemia by five or more orders of magnitude. Viraemia eventually stabilizes at a level

higher than the initial chronic state. The presence of the mutant can be confirmed by sequencing [2]. Only three patients developed resistant mutants (Figs 1 and 2), while the other six had viraemia below detection limits (<400 copies/ml) a year after transplant. Reinfection of the transplanted liver was seen in three patients with viraemia above the detection limit for two months post-transplant, only one of which (patient 1) developed a resistant mutant. Thus, prophylaxis failure was not correlated with viraemia at transplant, or post-transplant, but with pretreatment viraemia (95% significance by rank of initial viraemia).

## ANALYSIS AND INTERPRETATION: BASIC SETUP

To analyse the time course of the infection, we use a simple model based on ordinary differential equations using ideas of mass action kinetics. Such systems have

**Figure 2.** Course of viraemia under lamivudine and transplant of the three patients with highest pretreatment viraemia after patient 1

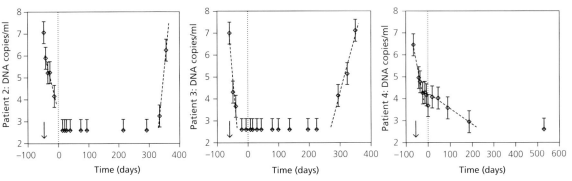

Note the extended time-scale in patient 4 relative to patients 1, 2 and 3.

**Figure 3.** Schematic illustration of the basic model incorporating virion production from infected hepatocytes and infection of susceptible hepatocytes by virions bathing the liver

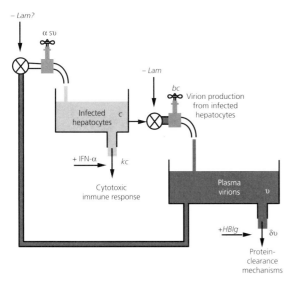

The equations are given by $\dot{c}=\alpha sv - kc$, $\dot{v}=bc - \delta v$

been successfully employed in HIV and HBV studies of drug treatment [4–6]. Our basic model incorporates the number of infected hepatocytes, denoted $c$, the number of susceptible hepatocytes $s$ and the density of virions $v$ in the plasma. Infected hepatocytes are lost by cellular immunity (rate constant $k$) and created by virion infection of susceptible hepatocytes (rate constant $\alpha$). Destruction of infected hepatocytes is assumed to occur at a constant rate $k$ corresponding to an established (chronic) infection. The virions are produced from infected hepatocytes (rate $b$ per cell) and cleared from the plasma (rate constant $\delta$), as shown schematically in Figure 3. The total number of hepatocytes in the liver, denoted $K$, limits the number of susceptible and infected cells ($s<K$, $c<K$).

Chronic infection is a steady state of the above equations, a state where the rate of destruction and production are balanced in both the plasma virion and infected hepatocyte compartments. The dynamics of the system during lamivudine treatment can be understood by using the fact that lamivudine reduces the rate of production of virions from infected cells by inhibiting the activity of the virus-encoded reverse transcriptase, and that the two compartments have very different response times (the time taken for the compartment to respond to a perturbation). Previous studies have indicated that the half-life of plasma virions is about 24 hours [5] which means that production and clearance of plasma virions equalize on the scale of days, while the

relatively long half-life of infected hepatocytes, 10–100 days [5], means that after initiation of antiviral therapy the chronic steady state is re-established on a time-scale of months.

The sudden fall in virion production by infected hepatocytes under administration of lamivudine results in a rapid decay of plasma DNA, thereby revealing the decay kinetics of the virion destruction process. This decline continues until the balance between production and destruction of virions is restored. A fall in the plasma virion level means that the rate of infection events by virions also declines; the infected hepatocyte compartment is also out of equilibrium. However, the slower turnover of infected hepatocytes dictates the time-scale over which the steady state is re-established, or virus cleared if no steady state exists. The decay in the number of infected hepatocytes is mirrored as a second decline phase of plasma viraemia (Fig. 1), because the plasma virion compartment is in balance. Log–linear plots of the biphasic decay give estimates for $k$, $\delta$ and the drug efficiency $\rho$ (Table 1); where the *drug efficacy for inhibition of virion output* is defined by the change in the virion production rate $b$, i.e. $b$ changes to a value $(1-\rho)b$ under lamivudine. These estimates (patient 1) correspond to a virion half-life of 2.8 days in plasma and an infected hepatocyte half-life of 17 days, consistent with previous estimates [5], and $\rho=93\%$ (95% confidence interval 83–97%). The other patients in Figure 2 have a viraemia fall of 10–10000 over the first phase of decay, indicating that drug efficiency is highly variable.

Liver transplant removes the infected hepatocytes. However, virus still exists in the body in the form of virions in the plasma (and extracellular spaces), and in extra-hepatic sites of infection. Reinfection of the liver from the plasma will be a very fast process because the half-life of virions is short. Each virion has a probability of infecting a hepatocyte, a probability given by the ratio of the rate of infection of hepatocytes to the rate of total virion clearance (including both adsorption by hepatocytes and destruction in the plasma) and is estimated to be in the range 0.017–1.0 for the double mutant (patient 1, using $K$ in the range $10^{11}$–$10^{12}$ hepatocytes). Our analysis suggests that it is unnecessary to invoke extra-hepatic sites to explain the observed reinfection of the liver. In order to reduce the reinfection of the liver by the wild-type virus post-transplant to a single infected hepatocyte, the viraemia at transplant must be reduced to about $10^{-2}$ copies/ml; whereas a 95% confidence level for no reinfection requires viraemia to be further reduced by a factor of 20. This is currently well below detection levels but is not an unreasonable target for therapy given the rapid

Table 1. Lamivudine-resistant mutant growth *in vivo*

| Patient* | Mutant sequence | Mutant growth rate§ | Time to appear[†] (days) viraemia reaches: | | Viraemia immediately post-transplant | | Plasma clearance§ δ (/day) | Cellular immunity§ k (/day) |
| | | | 400 copies/ml | $10^6$ copies/ml | Mutant‡ | Wild-type | | |
| --- | --- | --- | --- | --- | --- | --- | --- | --- |
| 1 ($5.5 \times 10^7$) | V550/M526 | 0.12 (0.007) | 146 | 210 | 0.006 | 2000 | 0.24 (0.05) | 0.040** (0.0026) |
| 2 ($1.2 \times 10^7$) | I550 | 0.31¶ | 329 | 354 | $4 \times 10^{-43}$ | <400 | 0.39 (0.014) | – |
| 3 ($1.0 \times 10^7$) | V550/M526 | 0.12 (0.005) | 268 | 332 | $3 \times 10^{-12}$ | <400 | 0.45¶ | 0.13 (0.01) |
| 4 ($2.9 \times 10^6$) | No mutant | – | – | – | – | 1000 | 0.25¶ | – |
| X | V550/M526 plus 1 | 0.166¶ | 210 | 260 | $10^{-13}$ | <400 | – | – |

*Patients are ordered by pretreatment viraemia (given in parentheses). The final patient, X, is from a different study.
†Two standardized measures for appearance are given based on the Genostics and Roche Amplicor assays, with appearance measured relative to the time of transplant. These give better comparisons than emergence at numerical dominance.
‡This is mutant viraemia extrapolated back to transplant from the observed exponential growth.
§SD are given in parentheses.
¶Based on two data points and therefore confidence intervals cannot be calculated.
**Cellular immunity falls to 0.009 (0.004) per day after transplant.

decline observed in some patients under lamivudine, and the possibility of using combination therapy. However, the wild-type is not a guide to the behaviour of all the strains present in the quasispecies; in particular strains that are (partially) resistant to lamivudine have very different dynamics.

## GENERATION OF LAMIVUDINE-RESISTANT STRAINS

HBV has a probability of point mutation per site per replication, $\mu_{pol}$, in the range $10^{-4}$–$10^{-5}$. Therefore the virion and infected hepatocyte populations are quasispecies of closely related strains about a master sequence. In patients with high viraemia the lamivudine resistant mutant is probably significantly represented in the virion and infected hepatocyte populations because of the large population size and mutation rate. For instance, with a population size of $10^{10}$ and a point mutation probability $10^{-4}$, specific single mutants occur with a population size of the order of $10^6$, while any specific double mutant occurs at $10^2$. Specific triple mutants are, however, unlikely to be represented. Sequencing of the lamivudine-resistant mutants indicates the presence of an essential mutation in the YMDD motif; however, in three of the four patients presented in Table 1 additional mutations are also observed, specifically a second mutation at position 526 [2]. Thus, both single and double mutants with (partial) resistance to lamivudine must be considered, which are very likely to exist pretransplantation.

The importance of pre-existence has been considered previously in HIV [7].

In patients where the lamivudine-resistant mutant grows exponentially, the infection event that lead to the mutant must precede the observed exponential growth phase by a few months to allow the mutant to grow to numerical dominance in the plasma. When a new infection occurs the number of infected cells are negligible relative to the liver capacity $K$. Therefore the infection grows exponentially at its maximum growth rate. The observed growth of the mutant can be used to extrapolate the growth back to the time of transplant. This gives a mutant virion plasma density of $\nu_m = 7.5 \times 10^{-6}$ copies/ml (95% confidence interval $5.5 \times 10^{-7}$–$1.0 \times 10^{-4}$) for patient 1. Thus, the mutant plasma density increases at most by a factor of $1.8 \times 10^{13}$ ($1.1 \times 10^{12}$–$2.7 \times 10^{14}$) over the maximum possible period of growth post-transplant (patient 1). This increase is also expected to be reflected in the number of mutant-infected hepatocytes and therefore should be compared to $K \sim 10^{11}$–$10^{12}$. Thus, allowing for a latent period of a couple of days before infected cells produce virions, there are at most two mutant-infected hepatocytes produced from Dane particles in the plasma at transplant in this patient (95% confidence). Thus, the mutant infection that caused prophylaxis to fail could have appeared a few days after infection from pre-existing mutants or, more probably, appeared by mutation up to 80 days post-transplant (95% confidence). In the latter case, the double mutant responsible for prophylaxis failure could have appeared by stepping through a

**Figure 4.** A two strain virus system consisting of a dominant wild-type and a mutant

**(a)**                                         **(b)**

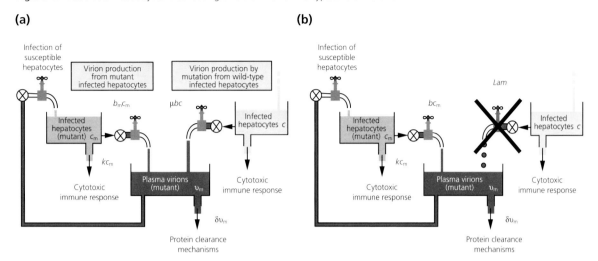

(a) The two strain virus system, consisting of a dominant wild-type with dynamics as in Fig. 3, and a mutant. (b) Administration of lamivudine to the system has an unequal effect on the two sources of mutant virions, the mutant-infected hepatocytes continuing to produce virions for a resistant strain, buffering the mutant viraemia against the effects of lamivudine. The equations for the mutant $\dot{c}_m = \alpha_m s v_m - k c_m$, $\dot{v}_m = \mu b c + b_m c_m - \delta v_m$.

single mutant intermediary, an intermediary that has a high probability of surviving transplant (since it is $10^4$ times more frequent than the double mutant). Thus, to evaluate the possible paths generating a double mutant the pretransplant dynamics of the possible resistant variants must be studied.

To model multiple strains, the model must be extended, and incorporate mutations from one strain to another. This is illustrated in Figure 4. Our discussion is in terms of a generic resistant mutant with a probability $\mu$ of generation from the wild-type per replication. Wild-type virus-infected hepatocytes producing virions $v$ at a rate $b$ also produce lamivudine-resistant mutant virions $v_m$ at rate $\mu b$. These infect susceptible hepatocytes at a rate $\alpha_m s v_m$, which then in turn produce mutant virions at a rate $b_m$ (using a subscript $m$ throughout to differentiate wild-type and mutant parameters). The effect of the mutant on the wild-type can be ignored, so the wild-type has identical dynamics to those described previously.

The strains compete for susceptible cells, and competition drives selection for the fittest strain and eradication of the other viral strains, which survive only as part of the quasispecies about the fittest strain. This quasispecies exists in both the virion and infected hepatocyte compartments; therefore mutant virions are produced from two sources – mutation from the fittest strain and from replication in mutant-infected cells. However, this only produces a minor correction to the expression for the relative frequency of a strain $v_m \sim \mu v$; that is the frequency of mutant virions is principally determined

by the mutation rate. The fitness $f$ of a strain is defined as the average number of virions produced from one virion through its life-cycle in a virgin liver; this takes into account the probability that the virion infects an hepatocyte which then produces virions until destroyed. This is the definition of $R_0$ used in epidemiology, where an epidemic grows if $R_0 > 1$, and dies out if $R_0 < 1$ [8]. Similarly, if the fitness $f > 1$, the virus grows in a naive liver, growth that ends in the formation of a chronic state with a susceptible cell population $s/K = f^{-1} < 1$. Thus, fitter viruses infect more hepatocytes since the number of susceptible cells remaining in the liver is reduced. The relative fitness of the strains can be estimated from the dynamic parameters; under lamivudine and immune suppression the ratio of wild-type to mutant fitness is 0.050 (95% confidence interval 0.017–0.15); that is, the mutant is approximately 20 times fitter in the presence of the drug (and immune suppression). A pretreatment estimate can be obtained by allowing for the effects of lamivudine giving $\varepsilon \sim 1$ (pretreatment) (or $\varepsilon \sim 20$ if lamivudine also affects the infectivity $\alpha$ with efficiency equal to $\rho$ as suggested in [9]). These pretreatment estimates should be compared to the estimate of the fitness of the corresponding mutant in duck hepatitis B virus, where the wild-type is 20 times fitter ($\varepsilon \sim 20$).

The resistant mutants are probably less fit than the wild-type in the absence of lamivudine because of differences in the efficacy of the polymerase ($b_m < b$), since the mutation principally affects the polymerase. However, the reading frames of *pol* and S antigen overlap, possibly causing differences in the clearance of virions and infected hepatocytes; the latter through indirect mechanisms such as processing/presentation or antibody-dependent cellular cytotoxicity that alter the immunogenicity of infected cells. These effects are expected to be weaker and as there is no quantification of these effects *in vivo* at present, they are ignored. We therefore assume that the cytotoxic immune response is the same against the resistant mutants and the wild-type.

## INFECTED CELL ECOLOGY

The ability of a resistant mutant to invade the wild-type virus-infected liver is a central problem in HBV therapy. Since the mutant is fitter in the presence of lamivudine and exists (in high load patients) at the start of therapy, the time-scale for it to be observable can be calculated. With a growth rate of 0.1–0.3 per day (Table 1), the mutant would numerically domi-nate on a time-scale $-\lambda^{-1}\log_e\mu = 60$–230 days (using $\mu = 10^{-8}$–$10^{-10}$). Resistant mutants in lamivudine-treated patients tend to appear over a longer time-scale [10], suggesting that mutant growth is initially inhibited. Growth will be inhibited by a lack of sus-ceptible cells caused by the high-level of wild-type infection still present in the liver; thus, the mutant is still competing with a high, but unsustainable, level of wild-type virus. This inhibition will in fact cause the level of mutant infection to decrease initially because the production via mutation from wild-type is reduced, and possibly lead to elimination of that strain if the inhibition period is of sufficient length. Growth inhibition has been discussed previously in HIV infection where a resistant mutant initially decreases in number prior to a growth phase brought on by the recovery of CD4+ cell numbers under the action of antiviral drugs [11]. The time-scale of the inhibition period is determined by the relative fitness of the mutant to the wild-type and the decay rate of the wild-type, so in HIV this is on a scale of days. In contrast, for HBV we propose that the inhibition period is extended over a period of weeks, partially due to the longer time-scales involved but also because of a localized immune response in the liver. This impor-tant consequences for therapy, especially therapies where high fitness resistant mutants do not pre-exist, since evolution and emergence of resistance in HBV to antivirals will be slower than in HIV and therefore we expect a higher success rate [12]. At present, the only possibilities for high fitness resistant mutants to not pre-exist is in combination therapies.

Immunohistological staining of HBV-infected liver sections with viral antigens indicates that infected hepatocytes appear as single isolated cells surrounded by uninfected cells, while under immune suppression all hepatocytes are infected. This implies that secreted virions are not infective immediately on secretion or the neighbouring cells are not susceptible to infection. Precedents exist for a localized protection of neigh-bouring cells since most animal cells secrete type I interferons when infected [13], and a non-cytotoxic clearance of HBV virus from infected cells has been observed [14,15], possibly mediated by cytokine secretion from T cells. This effectively separates the immune response into cytotoxic clearance (parame-tized by $k$) and a localized protection mediated by non-specific agents (probably cytokines), which is impaired under immune suppression. Local protection would reduce the availability of susceptible hepatocytes and thus determine the level of viraemia in chronic patients and extend inhibition times under administration of lamivudine. In contrast, a transplant allows the mutant to grow unrestrained, the mutant competing effectively (in the presence of lamivudine) for susceptible hepato-cytes since it is the fittest variant. Therefore, transplant patients are expected to develop resistant mutants sooner than non-transplant patients. If a resistant mutant emerges under immune suppression the liver is eventually saturated with virus-infected hepatocytes, which contrasts strongly with chronic patients. This suggests that immunosuppression has a significant effect on the spatial structure and dynamics of infected cells in the liver. We hypothesize that the neighbour-hood protection mechanism is inhibited under immune suppression, which has two consequences – the virus load is higher (as observed), and the virus grows faster in immunosuppressed patients.

## EFFECTS OF LAMIVUDINE ON THE QUASISPECIES

Although lamivudine is effective against the wild-type infection, it has a heterogeneous effect at the viral quasispecies level. Administration of lamivudine reduces virion production by wild-type virus-infected cells and therefore generation of mutants by mutation. However (partially) resistant mutant virions continue to be produced by mutant-infected hepatocytes. Consequently mutant viraemia falls but increases as a proportion of the total virion population; thus, mutant viraemia is buffered against the full effects of lamivudine because of production from mutant-infected hepatocytes. Mutant-infected hepatocytes in fact dominate production given that the mutant is fitter in the presence of lamivudine. Whereas wild-type viraemia during treatment is determined by the drug efficiency, mutant viraemia is determined by its fitness. Thus lamivudine decouples the mutant and wild-type infections at a population level because the drug efficiency is highly variable between patients. Provided susceptible cells remain limiting, the mutant and wild-type virus-infected hepatocyte populations decay identically, thereby retaining the frequency ratio $v_m/v$ over the second phase of decay. Thus, mutant viraemia at transplant is determined by the strain fitness and not the drug efficiency; the drug is therefore ineffective at reducing the mutant virion number. Thus, two patients that are identical except for a difference in drug efficacy, and undergo identical treatment, would have different plasma loads at transplant but identical mutant viraemia levels. Hence viraemia at transplant is not a good guide to the possible risk of developing a mutant. We further deduce that increasing the dose of lamivudine would probably not be effective, since its efficiency is limited by the presence of the fittest resistant mutant present at that time. Only if higher doses also reduce the fitness of that strain would dose increases be advised.

The frequency of mutant virions post-transplant (after reinfection from virions present at transplant) can be calculated. This can be used to obtain an upper boundary on the mutation probability μ by matching to the observed mutant growth of patient 1, giving $\mu < 2 \times 10^{-6}$, 95% confidence. This is only an upper boundary because of the possibility that the double mutant is lost at transplant, and generated later by remutation. However, it demonstrates that the dynamics have a double mutant signature. In particular, the nature of resistant mutants to an antiviral (single or double mutants) is captured in the dynamics of emergence. Dynamically, mutants that require only one mutation to escape will be observable far sooner than double mutants. In addition single mutants are present at a far higher frequency; therefore if a single mutation was sufficient to confer resistance to lamivudine without significant loss of fitness it would always appear (since it is present in all patients), and in fact would appear faster than the mutants observed in our patients. Thus we predict that all out-growing mutants observed under lamivudine treatment are at least double mutants; that is the mutant strain in patient 2 must have another mutation which has, as yet, not been found. These mutations are essential, whereas additional non-essential (random) mutations may occur which would differ between patients, the likelihood of additional mutations appearing being determined by the constraints on the genome. We ignore these non-specific mutations in the following.

## SINGLE AND DOUBLE MUTANTS

In Table 1, details of the three patients that developed a mutant infection are summarized, together with a patient from a separate study. Only patient 1 is consistent with the hypothesis that the mutant infection started from virions present in the plasma at transplant. The two other cases have an (extrapolated) mutant viraemia level immediately post-transplant that is too low by several orders of magnitude for this scenario, and have an emergence that is significantly later relative to that of patient 1. Thus, in these two patients the double mutant virions present at transplant failed to reinfect the liver. This correlates with the higher clearance rates of virions and infected hepatocytes for these patients, which would increase the probability of losing the double mutants at transplant.

If the double mutant strain fails to reinfect the liver after transplant the time-scale for its reappearance in the liver is inversely proportional to the viraemia of the generating strain. Double mutants would appear in the liver on a time-scale of 3200 days (range 35 days to 7.5 $\times 10^5$ days) when $v \sim 400$ copies/ml under generation from the wild-type (using the ranges $\mu \sim 10^{-8}$–$10^{-10}$, $K \sim 10^{11}$–$10^{12}$). Although the lower limit cannot rule out this path for the emergence of the double mutants, the mid-range value suggests that mutation directly from the wild-type is unlikely. Furthermore, this path would correlate emergence of the mutant with post-transplant viraemia, which is not observed. As viraemia continues to decay the probability of generating a mutant from this path falls over time.

In order to analyse the effects of the single mutant and its role in the generation of double mutants post-transplant, define $\varepsilon_1, \varepsilon_2, \varepsilon_{12}$ as the fitness ratios of the wild-type to the corresponding mutant (subscript 12 refers to the double mutant), $\rho, \rho_1, \rho_2$ as the drug efficacy against each mutant in reducing virion output ($\rho_{12} = 0$ for a resistant double mutant), and $\mu_1, \mu_2$ as the probabilities of producing (single) mutants 1 and 2 in a replication of the wild-type. Assuming the fidelity of the polymerase is not affected by the mutations, the probability per replication of producing the double mutant from the wild-type and single mutant $v_1$ are $\mu = \mu_1 \mu_2$ and $\mu_2$, respectively.

If the single mutant is fitter than the wild-type (under lamivudine), it is partially buffered against the effects of lamivudine (complete buffering if the single mutant is resistant) and dominates the production of double mutants via mutation relative to the wild-type post transplant. The time-scale for emergence of that double mutant from the single mutant is on the scale of hours if $v_1 \sim 400$ copies/ml. The importance of the differential effects of lamivudine on the different variants can now be clarified. Without buffering $v_1 \sim \mu_1 v$, and therefore this time-scale is similar to that for direct mutation from the wild-type. However, buffering increases the relative frequency of the single mutants, an increase that has a significant effect on the time-scale of double mutant generation because of its inverse relationship to $v_1$; for example, an increase in the relative frequency by 30 would reduce the mid-range time-scale estimate to 100 days, which is the appropriate order for patients 2 and 3.

The single mutant will grow in the transplanted liver if it is sufficiently fit, otherwise it will decay from transplant, reducing the risk of prophylaxis failure over time. In this case those patients that have failed to produce a mutant 2 years after transplant are very unlikely to develop the double mutant at this stage and can be considered cured. However, a single mutant chronic state capable of generating double mutants on a time-scale of days is below the sensitivity of available assays, and thus it is impossible at present to rule out single mutant growth post-transplant for these patients. There is also insufficient data to assess the possibility of discontinuing lamivudine since it is unknown whether our models are valid at low levels of viraemia (below 400 copies/ml), and whether other members of the quasi-species become important at lower levels of viraemia.

We conclude that prophylaxis failure in liver transplant patients has two main causes: (i) the double mutant pre-exists and survives transplant, growing in numbers immediately after transplant; and (ii) the double mutant is generated from a single mutant that survives transplant. The latter path is only important if the double mutant is lost at transplant, and requires that the single mutant infection is sufficient to give rise to a double mutant infection. Patient 1 is consistent with the first category; however this category is principally expected to be important for patients with initial pre-treatment viraemia higher than patient 1. The second category of events can explain the cases of prophylaxis failure observed in our cohort of nine patients. Although initial viraemia has emerged as the best guide to determine risk, this only reflects a combination of effects including the rates of clearance of virions and strength of the immune response (both cytotoxic and non-cytotoxic/neighbourhood protection responses); thus there is expected to be a correlation between high viraemia and poor rates of clearance.

## CONCLUSIONS

Viral quasispecies population structure has four principal implications for antiviral therapy:

(i) Resistant mutants that cause prophylaxis failure or (partially resistant) mutants in a sequence of mutation steps to the mutant causing prophylaxis failure may pre-exist, and therefore undergo positive selection upon administration of therapy.

(ii) The efficiency of therapy is limited by the fittest (partially) resistant strain in the quasispecies, which may be revealed after the wild-type has decayed as a plateau in the viraemia, particularly in treatment of chronic patients. Fitter strains may emerge through eventual growth to numerical dominance, or be produced through mutation.

(iii) Growth of resistant mutants to numerical dominance can take months because of the low frequency at which the resistant minority species are represented. Competition for resources and ecological considerations can extend the time of emergence through inhibition of growth of resistant strains at the initial stages of treatment. Therefore, evaluation of the efficiency of a drug must account for this emergence time; in HBV emergence takes 8–10 months in immunosuppressed patients (Table 1), therefore assessments of drugs based on clinical trials of less than 2 years duration probably under estimate the problem of resistance.

(iv) Determinants of risk must be robust against heterogeneous effects of antivirals on the quasispecies. Thus, viraemia at transplant and post-transplant are not good gauges of risk of prophylaxis failure because lamivudine decouples the resistant mutant viraemia (both single and double mutants) from the wild-type.

Improvements in therapy must recognize the fact that the virus acts as an heterogeneous population. The best strategy for reducing the probability of producing resistant mutants in liver transplant patients capable of growth is to use a therapy that reduces the number of single and double mutants in the plasma at transplant. For instance anti-HBV immunoglobulin administered prior to, and during transplant, would increase the clearance rate of virions from the plasma (presumably including lamivudine-resistant mutants) and therefore directly reduce the numbers of virions contributing to the risk. If combined therapy is used throughout the course of treatment the analysis presented above holds for the mutants resistant to the combined therapy. If a mutant capable of take-off requires three specific mutations, the risk of prophylaxis failure is correspondingly reduced by a factor of approximately $10^4$, effectively removing the possibility of failure. This case study also emphasises the difficulties of identifying risk determinants because of quasispecies heterogeneity – a strategy to improve therapy based on lowering viraemia at transplant is not necessarily optimum unless the levels of resistant mutants are also known to be correspondingly reduced.

# ACKNOWLEDGEMENTS

NJB is supported by EPSRC grant B/94/AF/1822. The research of DAR is supported by NERC and EPSRC. We gratefully acknowledge E Dragon, K O'Donnell, J Shaw in the Liver Unit (assay work), J King (viral loads), D Ratcliffe (sequencing) and P Cane in PHLS and colleagues at Glaxo Welcome R&D, Middlesex.

# REFERENCES

1. McMahon G, Ehrlich PH, Moustafa ZA, MaCarthy LA, Dottavio D, Tolpin MD, Nadler PI & Ostberg L. Genetic alterations in the gene encoding the major HBsAg: DNA and immunological analysis of recurrent HBsAg derived from monoclonal antibody-treated liver transplant patients. *Hepatology* 1992; **15**:757–766.

2. Ling R, Mutimer D, Ahmed M, Boxall EH, Elias E, Dusheiko GM & Harrison TJ. Selection of mutations in the hepatitis B virus polymerase during therapy of transplant recipients with lamivudine. *Hepatology* 1996; **24**:711–713.

3. Tipples GA, Ma MM, Fischer KP, Bain VG, Kneteman NM & Tyrrell DLJ. Mutation in HBV RNA-dependent DNA polymerase confers resistance to lamivudine in vivo. *Hepatology* 1996; **24**:714–717.

4. Ho DD, Neumann AU, Perelson AS, Chen W, Leonard JM & Markowitz M. Rapid turnover of plasma virions and CD4 lymphocytes in HIV-1 infection. *Nature* 1995; **373**:123–126.

5. Nowak MA, Bonhoeffer S, Hill AM, Boehme R, Thomas HC & McDade H. Viral dynamics in hepatitis B virus infection. *Proceedings of the National Academy of Sciences, USA* 1996; **93**:4398–4402.

6. Wei X, Ghosh SK, Taylor ME, Johnson VA, Emini EA, Deutsch P, Lifson JD, Bonhoeffer S, Nowak MA, Hak BH, Saag MS & Shaw GM. Viral dynamics in human immunodeficiency virus type 1 infection. *Nature* 1995; **373**:117–122.

7. Bonhoeffer S & Nowak MA. Pre-existence and emergence of drug resistance in HIV-1 infection. *Proceedings of the Royal Society of London Series B Biological Sciences* 1997; **264**:631–637.

8. Anderson RM & May RM. *Infectious Diseases of Humans*, 1991. Oxford: Oxford Science Publications.

9. Severini A, Liu XY, Wilson JS & Tyrrell DLJ. Mechanism of inhibition of duck hepatitis B virus polymerase by (–)-β-L-2′,3′-dideoxy-3′-thiacytidine. *Antimicrobial Agents and Chemotherapy* 1995; **39**: 1430–1435.

10. Brown N & Rubin M. Lamivudine therapy for hepatitis B: current worldwide results. *Second International Conference on Therapies for Viral Hepatitis*, Kona, Hawaii, December 15–19 1997; Abstract O2.

11. Nowak MA, Bonhoeffer S, Shaw GM & May RM. Anti-viral drug treatment: dynamics of resistance in free virus and infected cell populations. *Journal of Theoretical Biology* 1997; **184**:203–217.

12. Richman DD. Drug resistance and its implications in the management of HIV infection. *Antiviral Therapy* 1997; **2** (Suppl. 4):41–51.

13. Gresser I. Role of interferon in resistance to viral infection *in vivo*. In *Interferon 2: Interferons and the Immune System*, 1984; pp. 221–247. Edited by J Vilcek & E De Maeyer. Amsterdam: Elsevier.

14. Ando K, Guidotti LG, Cerny A, Ishikawa T & Chisari FV. CTL access to tissue antigen is restricted in vivo. *Journal of Immunology* 1994; **153**:482.

15. Guidotti LG, Ando K, Hobbs MV, Ishikawa T, Runkel L, Schreiber RD & Chisari FV. Cytotoxic T lymphocytes inhibit hepatitis B virus gene expression by a noncytolytic mechanism in transgenic mice. *Proceedings of the National Academy of Sciences, USA* 1994; **91**:3764–3768.

# Section VII

## CLINICAL AND THERAPEUTIC STRATEGIES

### Part A

#### THE IMMUNOCOMPETENT INDIVIDUAL

# 37 Mathematical modelling of chronic hepatitis B and C virus infection: a basis for planning new approaches to therapy

## Howard C Thomas

## INTRODUCTION

Intensive studies of the immunopathogenesis of persistent hepatitis B virus (HBV) and hepatitis C virus (HCV) infection have been undertaken over the last decade. Insights have derived from studies of transgenic mice as well as patients with the disease. It is from this basic understanding of the failures of the immune system which result in persistent HBV or HCV infection that future therapies must be planned.

## PERSISTENT HBV INFECTION

The time of exposure to HBV is a major factor determining the outcome of infection. Children born to HBV-infected mothers invariably become persistently infected [1] and approximately 30–50% of these individuals will die from the complications of cirrhosis or hepatocellular cancer. Those infected in adulthood, however, mainly recover and only 3–5% develop persistent infection, with the same incidence of liver-related death.

The clearance of HBV-infected cells is dependent on their recognition and lysis by cytotoxic T lymphocytes (CTLs), either directly or mediated by cytokines [2,3]. This response is probably amplified by hepatitis B core antigen (HBcAg)-sensitized CD4+ T helper lymphocytes (Th1 and Th2 cells) which, in addition, secrete antiviral cytokines including interferon γ (IFN-γ) and tumour necrosis factor α (Fig. 1). There follows a virus-neutralizing response to epitopes borne on the various envelope proteins of HBV.

In chronic HBV infection occurring at birth, the secretion of the hepatitis B e antigen (HBeAg), and possibly other viral proteins, induces T-cell tolerance which is an important factor contributing to viral persistence [4,5]. The nature of this T-cell tolerance has been the subject of elegant studies in mice using recombinant HBeAg and HBcAg, and trangenic mice expressing these proteins [6].

In adult-acquired infection, the reason for viral persistence is not entirely clear. The association of recovery with certain MHC class II alleles (for example HLA DRB1*1302) [7,8] suggests that MHC-restricted CD4+ T helper lymphocytes may have a

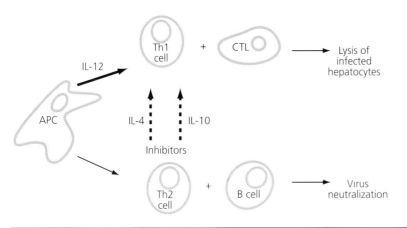

**Figure 1.** Induction of the immune response in acute HBV infection – the Th1 response is dominant

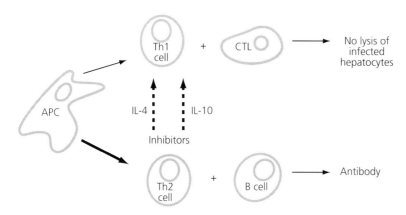

**Figure 2.** In chronic HBV infection the Th2 response is dominant

major influence on the outcome of infection. This raises the question of whether the efficacy of antigen presentation by MHC class II alleles is the reason for failure to clear the virus in those who develop persistent infection.

Whatever the initial defect resulting in viral persistence, once the infection is established, these patients have relatively minor CD4+ and CD8+ T lymphocyte responses to HBV antigens (Fig. 2). This is in marked contrast to the responses in acute infection, where there is induction of a strong CD4+ helper T cell and CTL response [9,10].

## Current therapy for persistent HBV infection

IFN-α amplifies the immune response by a variety of mechanisms. It increases the expression of MHC class I antigens [11], so enhancing viral antigen presentation to CTLs; it may directly activate CTLs [12]; it augments the activity of natural killer cells [13]; and recent data indicate that IFN-α induces the expression of the interleukin 12 receptor (IL-12R) β2 subunit on naive T helper cells during their differentiation along the Th1 pathway, but not the Th2 pathway [14]. Th1 cells are important in the induction of the inflammatory responses necessary for virus elimination, so this provides some insight into how IFN-α treatment may induce a response in HBV-infected patients. Sequential studies of patients undergoing IFN-induced seroconversion indicate an increased CD4+ proliferative response to HBcAg [15]; a CTL response to HBcAg also becomes detectable at the time of seroconversion [16]. It seems likely therefore that HBcAg induction of CD4+ T cell secretion of cytokines and amplication of the CD8+ T cell response resulting in lysis of infected cells are two components of the IFN-induced control of HBV replication. Currently this is seen in only 30–40% of patients with chronic hepatitis. Patients

who have minimal hepatitis or normal liver histology, often those who have been infected at birth, are non-responsive to IFN. This is consistent with the hypothesis that IFN can amplify an existing response but does not appear to be able to break the state of tolerance that may exist to HBV nucleocapsid proteins after exposure and infection at birth.

## Mathematical modelling of HBV infection

An alternative approach to clearance of HBV infection is suppression of HBV replication until such time as the residual infected cells are cleared from the liver, as part of the natural senescence process of liver cells. Lamivudine and famciclovir, both inhibitors of viral replication, have been shown to exhibit antiviral effects in persistent HBV infection and both are candidates for viral suppressive therapy [17,18].

Mathematical modelling in lamivudine-treated patients has shown that the half-life of the HBV virion in serum is about 1 day but HBV-infected cells have a half-life of between 10 and 100 days in different patients, indicating that treatment would need to be prolonged before the last HBV-infected cells might be expected to be cleared [19]. There was an inverse correlation between the calculated half-life of the infected cell and the serum concentration of alanine aminotransferase (ALT), an association that would be consistent with the idea that treatment responses may well occur earlier in those with more active antiviral immune responses.

The modelling data indicate that protracted periods of treatment may be necessary to clear residual HBV-infected cells after suppression of replication. This is consistent with the observation that clearance of hepatitis B surface antigen (HBsAg) and HBV DNA (detected by PCR) after successful HBeAg to anti-HBe seroconversion may not occur until 5–10 years after the end of antiviral therapy [20].

## Prospects for future management of persistent HBV infection

### Management of moderate/severe chronic hepatitis

IFN is still the mainstay of therapy in patients with moderate or severe chronic hepatitis, in whom the immune system appears to be already involved in the recognition and lysis of infected cells, albeit in a partially ineffective manner in that clearance of the virus does not occur. In such patients, IFN may induce clearance of the virus in up to 40% of cases. Studies of the immune response during this IFN-induced sero-conversion indicate that a Th1 response, albeit of lower intensity than that seen in acute hepatitis, has occurred [15]. This raises the prospect of amplification of the Th1 response to improve further response rates to IFN monotherapy. It is now clear that IL-12 has the capacity to amplify such a response (reviewed in [21]). It is currently undergoing clinical trials as monotherapy and should subsequently be tested in combination therapy, possibly combined with IFN-α in such patients.

### Management of minimal chronic hepatitis

In patients with minimal hepatitis, the results of therapy with IFN are poor: approximately 10% of patients respond. As a result, lamivudine has been suggested to have utility in a suppressive role. However, mathematical modelling predicts that this might need to be continued for a prolonged period (up to 10 years) before clearance of the last HBV-infected cells might be expected to occur. During this period, the possibility of emergence of drug-resistant virus variants arises and might thwart the ultimate goal of viral

clearance. With these agents, therefore, immunological stimulants that enhance the rate of clearance of infected cells offer substantial opportunities. Here again, IFN-α and IL-12 appear to have the correct immunological credentials, in that they either separately or together enhance the Th1 response, which should improve the rate of clearance of virus-infected cells. The existence of inhibitors of Th1 induction (IL-4 and IL-10) may negate a response to IL-12 and therefore therapy to inhibit this response may be required along with IL-12 (Fig. 3).

The future, therefore, appears to be in the development of regimens where antiviral compounds are combined with stimulants of the immune response, particularly those designed to stimulate a Th1 response, which current studies show to be deficient in those patients with persistent HBV infection. Combination of cytokines with vaccine therapy might further improve the efficacy of this type of therapeutic approach.

## PERSISTENT HCV INFECTION

In sharp contrast to the situation in HBV infection, after HCV exposure the majority of patients develop persistent infection, with only 20–25% clearing the virus in a 3 month period. Furthermore, the majority of patients are infected in adulthood as a result of exposure to blood during therapeutic procedures, intravenous drug use or as a result of sexual contact.

In HCV infection the virus is again not directly cytopathic and it would appear that immune recognition and destruction of infected hepatocytes is part of the hepatitic process. This is probably also part of the recovery process; as in many other viral diseases, the existence of protective immunity and tissue damaging immune responses occurring in parallel is seen in this infection.

Recovery from HCV infection is associated with certain MHC class II alleles, again suggesting a role for

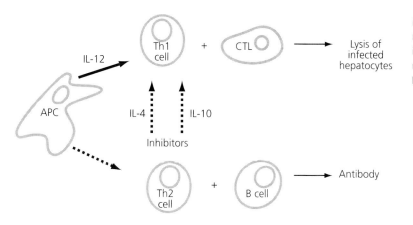

**Figure 3.** Administration of IL-12 may enhance the Th1 response, but inhibition of the Th2 response may be required to shut off the Th1 inhibitors IL-4 and IL-10

CD4+ T cells in the process [22,23]. In patients with persistent HCV infection, approximately 40% did not have detectable proliferative responses to HCV antigens [24,25]. However, patients with an acute infection who went on to normalize their ALT values had significantly more vigorous and more frequently detectable responses to HCV core and non-structural (NS) proteins than those whose ALT remained elevated [24,26]. This again suggests the importance of the CD4+ T cell response in control of viraemia.

CTLs have been identified in the liver and peripheral blood of patients with acute and persistent HCV infection [27,28]. Analysis of these cells does suggest an ongoing CTL response in persistent HCV infection and raises the question of why this is ineffective in clearing the virus [29].

HCV exhibits a high mutation rate, presumably because of a high rate of transcriptional errors occurring during viral genome replication. It is clear that antibodies directed to envelope proteins continually select envelope variants that have lost the epitopes targeted by the humoral immune response: certain areas of the E2 and NS1 regions of the viral genome have a high genetic variability among isolates in patients with a normal humoral immune system, but much lower rates in agammaglobulinaemic patients with no humoral immunity [30]. Whether any of the variants selected are capable of inhibiting the cellular immune response, as has been seen in other persistent viral infections, such as human immunodeficiency virus and HBV [31,32], remains to be established.

HCV may, under certain circumstances, infect B cells, monocytes and macrophages, and CD8+ lymphocytes (J Booth, JA Waters and HC Thomas, unpublished results); this may also have some effect on the ability of the immune system to destroy virus-infected lymphocytes.

## Current treatment of persistent HCV infection

The majority of patients with persistent HCV infection have minimal or mild hepatitis and do not need immediate treatment. Approximately 20% of patients have more severe disease and are at risk of progression to cirrhosis. These patients are currently offered IFN-α treatment for periods of 12 to 18 months and this results in approximately 20% of patients having sustained clearance of the virus (a clinical and virological cure). Cirrhotic patients have a much reduced response, and in many centres are not offered treatment. However, 3–5% of patients with cirrhosis develop hepatocellular cancer each year, and the treatment of this group of patients remains a major problem.

The method of action of IFN-α in HCV infection is unclear at present. Certainly it has an effect as a direct antiviral agent in that HCV titres in peripheral blood fall within the first few days of treatment. However, protracted periods of IFN treatment are necessary to produce the best response rates [33]. This suggests that after the direct antiviral effect evident over the first few weeks of treatment, there may be some contribution from the host immune response and that this may determine whether the initial response is sustained or otherwise. The selection of IFN-resistant quasispiecies of virus clearly occurs [34]. This is related to the C-terminal region of the NS5A antigen, and may also be related to the capacity of certain virus-encoded proteins to inhibit the antiviral response.

In a study in Japan, IFN treatment was shown to improve the inflammatory and fibrosis scores on liver biopsy and also to reduce the risk of hepatocellular carcinoma [35]. If this is confirmed, it raises the question of whether IFN has a stimulatory effect on immune surveillance as well as antiviral activity.

## Future prospects for treatment of persistent HCV infection

In this case, mathematical modelling studies are at an earlier stage and are limited by our inability to measure the half-life of infected liver cells. The half-life of the virus, however, is again short, approximately 1 day.

Clearly a better understanding of the process whereby HCV renders the infected hepatocyte resistant to IFN treatment is needed and may offer opportunities for improvements in IFN-α response rates.

Currently, ribavirin, a nucleoside analogue that appears not to have an antiviral effect when used alone [36], is being used in combination therapy with IFN-α, and in small uncontrolled trials has been shown to double sustained response rates to IFN [37]. How ribavirin operates in this setting is unclear.

In studies in cirrhotic patients, who after 3 months of IFN treatment are non-responsive, addition of ribavirin increases response rates to a significant degree (HC Thomas, unpublished results). This emphasizes that ribavirin, although not being directly antiviral, does appear to improve the response to IFN; studies of the mechanisms involved will hopefully lead to improved therapy.

Whether stimulants of Th1 cells or the CTL response will be beneficial in patients with chronic hepatitis C is less clear than in chronic HBV infection, because both of these immune responses are present in chronic hepatitis C patients.

# CONCLUSIONS

Knowledge of the process underlying viral persistence after HBV or HCV infection is providing useful information, allowing us to improve therapeutic options. Mathematical modelling shows us that, at least in HBV, immunostimulants added to antiviral drugs offer the best prospect of effective treatments. This is so, particularly when we consider that this approach will also minimize the rate of development of drug-resistant variants. The new cytokines with the capacity to amplify the Th1/CTL response offer major opportunities, combined with IFN-$\alpha$ or nucleoside analogues, particularly in HBV infection. Since Th2 cells secrete cytokines that inhibit the Th1 response, inhibition of this response at the time of stimulation of the Th1 response may be necessary. Whether similar opportunities exist in HCV will be dependent on more insight into the process of how HCV evades elimination. Current data suggest that there is a significant Th1/CTL response and why this is ineffective must be determined.

Finally, although the use of cytokines capable of amplifying the immune response is attractive, this is always second best compared to the possibility of antigen-specific manipulation of the immune response utilizing virus-encoded epitopes, possibly combined with cytokines.

Because of the relatively small size of HBV and HCV genomes and the detailed knowledge of the immunopathogenesis of these diseases, they are particularly attractive targets for antiviral and immunological approaches to therapy.

# REFERENCES

1. Stevens CE, Beasley RP & Tsu JWC. Vertical transmission of hepatitis B antigen in Taiwan. *New England Journal of Medicine* 1975; **292**:771–780.
2. Ando K, Guidotti LG, Wirth S, Ishikawa T, Missale G, Moriyama T, Schreiber RD, Schlicht HJ, Huang SN & Chisari FV. Class I-restricted cytotoxic T lymphocytes are directly cytopathic for their target cells *in vivo*. *Journal of Immunology* 1994; **152**:3245–3253.
3. Gilles PN, Fey G & Chisari FV. Tumour necrosis factor-alpha negatively regulates hepatitis B virus gene expression in transgenic mice. *Journal of Virology* 1992; **66**:3955–3960.
4. Thomas HC, Jacyna M, Waters J & Main J. Virus–host interaction in chronic hepatitis B virus infection. *Seminars in Liver Disease* 1988; **8**:342–349.
5. Milich DR, Jones J, Hughes J & Maruyama T. Role of T-cell tolerance in the persistence of hepatitis B virus infection. *Journal of Immunotherapy* 1993; **14**:226–233.
6. Milich DR. Immunogenetic factors influencing the outcome of HCV infection. *Journal of Viral Hepatitis* 1998 (Supplement); in press.
7. Thursz M, Kwiatkowski D, Allsopp CEM, Greenwood BM, Thomas HC & Hill AVS. Association between an MHC class II allele and clearance of hepatitis B virus in the Gambia. *New England Journal of Medicine* 1995; **332**:1065–1069.
8. Thursz M & Thomas HC. Genetic factors influencing the outcome of HBV infection. *Journal of Viral Hepatitis* 1998; in press.
9. Nayersina R, Fowler P, Guilhot S, Missale G, Cerny A, Schlicht HJ, Vitiello A, Chesnut R, Person JL, Redeker AG et al. HLA-A2 restricted cytotoxic T lymphocyte responses to multiple hepatitis B surface antigen epitopes during hepatitis B virus infection. *Journal of Immunology* 1993; **150**:4659–4671.
10. Ferrari C, Penna A, Bertoletti A, Valli A, Antoni AD, Giuberti T, Cavalli A, Petit MA & Fiaccadori F. Cellular immune response to hepatitis B virus-encoded antigens in acute and chronic hepatitis B virus infection. *Journal of Immunology* 1990; **145**: 3442–3449.
11. Harris H & Gill T. Expression of class I transplantation antigens. *Transplantation* 1986; **42**:109–117.
12. von Hoegan P. Synergistic role of type I interferons in the induction of protective cytotoxic T lymphocytes. *Immunology Letters* 1995; **47**:157–162.
13. Ortaldo JR, Herberman RB, Harvey C, Osheroff P, Pan YC, Kelder B & Pestka S. A species of human interferon that lacks the ability to boost natural killer cell activity. *Proceedings of the National Academy of Sciences, USA* 1984; **81**:4926–4929.
14. Rogge L, Barberis-Maino L, Biffi M, Passini N, Presky DH, Gubler U & Sinigaglia F. Selective expression of an interleukin-12 receptor component by human T helper 1 cells. *Journal of Experimental Medicine* 1997; **185**: 825–831.
15. Marinos G, Torre F, Chokshi S, Hussain M, Clarke BE, Rowlands DJ, Eddleston AL, Naoumov NV & Williams R. Induction of T-helper cell response to hepatitis B core antigen in chronic hepatitis B: a major factor in activation of the host immune response to the hepatitis B virus. *Hepatology* 1995; **22**:1040–1049.
16. Waters JA, O'Rourke S, Schlict H-J & Thomas HC. Cytotoxic T cell responses in patients with chronic hepatitis B virus infection undergoing HBe antigen/antibody seroconversion. *Clinical and Experimental Immunology* 1995; **102**:314–319.
17. Dienstag JL, Perrillo RP, Schiff ER, Bartholomew M, Vicary C & Rubin M. A preliminary trial of lamivudine for chronic hepatitis B infection. *New England Journal of Medicine* 1995; **333**:1657–1661.
18. Brown JL, Howels, C, Galassini R et al. A double blind placebo controlled study to assess the effect of famciclovir on viral replication in patients with chronic hepatitis B infection. *Journal of Viral Hepatitis* 1996; **3**:211–215.
19. Nowak AM, Bonhoeffer S, Hill AM, Boehme R, Thomas HC & McDade H. Viral dynamics in hepatitis B virus infection. *Proceedings of the National Academy of Sciences, USA* 1996; **93**:4398–4402.
20. Korenman J, Baker B, Waggoner J, Everhart JE, DiBisceglie AM & Hoofnagle H. Long-term remission of chronic hepatitis B after alpha-interferon therapy. *Annals of Internal Medicine* 1991; **114**:629–634.
21. Trincheri G. Interleukin-12: a proinflammatory cytokine with immunoregulatory functions that bridge innate resistance and antigen-specific adaptive immunity. *Annual Review of Immunology* 1995; **13**:251–276.
22. Congia M, Clemente MG, Dessi C, Cucca F, Mazzoleni

AP, Frau F, Lampis R, Cao A, Lai ME & De Virgiliis S. HLA class II genes in chronic hepatitis C virus-infection and associated immunological disorders. *Hepatology* 1996; **24**:1338–1341.

23. Tibbs C, Donaldson P, Underhill J, Thomson L, Manabe K & Williams R. Evidence that the HLA DQA1*03 allele confers protection from the chronic HCV-infection in North European Caucasoids. *Hepatology* 1996; **24**:1342–1345.

24. Lechmann M, Ihlenfeldt HG, Braunschweiger I, Giers G, Jung G, Matz B, Kaiser R, Sauerbruch T & Spengler U. T- and B-cell responses to different hepatitis C virus antigens in patients with chronic hepatitis C infection and in healthy anti-hepatitis C virus-positive blood donors without viremia. *Hepatology* 1996; **24**: 790–795.

25. Botarelli P, Brunetto MR, Minutello MA, Calvo P, Unutmaz D, Weiner AJ, Choo QL, Shuster JR, Kuo G, Bonino F *et al.* T-lymphocyte response to hepatitis C virus in different clinical courses of infection. *Gastroenterology* 1993; **104**:580–587.

26. Missale G, Bertoni R, Lamonaca V, Valli A, Massari M, Mori C, Rumi MG, Houghton M, Fiaccadori F & Ferrari C. Different clinical behaviors of acute hepatitis C virus infection are associated with different vigor of the anti-viral cell-mediated immune response. *Journal of Clinical Investigation* 1996; **98**:706–714.

27. Koziel MJ, Dudley D, Wong JT, Dienstag J, Houghton M, Ralston R & Walker BD. Intrahepatic cytotoxic T lymphocytes specific for hepatitis C virus in persons with chronic hepatitis. *Journal of Immunology* 1992; **149**:3339–3344.

28. Cerny A, McHutchison JG, Pasquinelli C, Brown ME, Brothers MA, Grabscheid B, Fowler P, Houghton M & Chisari FV. Cytotoxic T lymphocyte response to hepatitis C virus-derived peptides containing the HLA A2.1 binding motif. *Journal of Clinical Investigation* 1995; **95**:521–530.

29. Rehermann B, Chang KM, McHutchison JG, Kokka R, Houghton M & Chisari FV. Quantitative analysis of the peripheral blood cytotoxic T lymphocyte response in patients with chronic hepatitis C virus infection. *Journal of Clinical Investigation* 1996; **98**:1432–1440.

30. Kumar U, Monjardino J & Thomas HC. Hypervariable region of hepatitis C virus envelope glycoprotein (E2/NS1) in an agammaglobulinemic patient. *Gastroenterology* 1994; **106**:1072–1075.

31. Klenerman P, Rowland-Jones S, McAdam S, Edwards J, Daenke S, Lalloo D, Koppe B, Rosenberg W, Boyd D, Edwards A *et al.* Cytotoxic T-cell activity antagonized by naturally occurring HIV-1 Gag variants. *Nature* 1994; **369**:403–407.

32. Bertoletti A, Sette A, Chisari FV, Penna A, Levrero M, De Carli M, Fiaccadori F & Ferrari C. Natural variants of cytotoxic epitopes are T-cell receptor antagonists for antiviral cytotoxic T cells. *Nature* 1994; **369**:407–410.

33. Poynard T, Bedossa P, Chevallier M, Mathurin P, Lemonnier C, Trepo C, Couzigou P, Payen JL, Sajus M & Costa JM. A comparison of three interferon alfa-2b regimens for the long-term treatment of chronic non-A, non-B hepatitis. Multicenter Study Group. *New England Journal of Medicine* 1995; **332**:1457–1462.

34. Enomoto N, Sakuma I, Asahina Y, Kurosaki M, Murakami T, Yamamoto C, Izumi N, Marumo F & Sato C. Comparison of full-length sequences of interferon-sensitive and resistant hepatitis C virus 1b. Sensitivity to interferon is conferred by amino acid substitutions in the NS5A region. *Journal of Clinical Investigation* 1995; **96**:224–230.

35. Nishiguchi S, Kuroki T, Nakatani S, Morimoto H, Takeda T, Nakajima S, Shiomi S, Seki S, Kobayashi K & Otani S. Randomised trial of effects of interferon-alpha on incidence of hepatocellular carcinoma in chronic active hepatitis C with cirrhosis. *Lancet* 1995; **346**:1051–1055.

36. Dusheiko G, Main J, Thomas H, Reichard O, Lee C, Dhillon A, Rassam S, Fryden A, Reesink H, Bassendine M, Norkrans G, Cuypers T, Lelie N, Telfer P, Watson J, Weegink C, Sillikens P & Weiland O. Ribavirin treatment for patients with chronic hepatitis C: results of a placebo-controlled study. *Journal of Hepatology* 1996; **25**:591–598.

37. Braconier JH, Paulsen O, Engman K & Widell A. Combined alpha-interferon and ribavirin treatment in chronic hepatitis C: a pilot study. *Scandinavian Journal of Infectious Diseases* 1995; **27**:325–329.

*Therapies for Viral Hepatitis*
Edited by RF Schinazi, J-P Sommadossi and HC Thomas

# 38 Treatment of hepatitis B virus with lamivudine

## Winnie WS Wong and D Lorne J Tyrrell*

## INTRODUCTION

Chronic hepatitis B virus (HBV) infection affects more than 300 million people worldwide [1]. Interferon α (IFN-α) remains the only licensed antiviral treatment. However, since the response rate to IFN in selected patients is 30–45% [2–4], the search for more effective therapies continues. Nucleoside analogues such as vidarabine (9-β-arabinofuranosyladenine; ara-A) [5] and acyclovir [6] have been tried in the past but are limited by toxicity and poor efficacy, respectively. More recently tested nucleoside analogues include famciclovir (the orally available form of penciclovir), lobucavir, adefovir and lamivudine, the last of which will be discussed in detail in this chapter.

## PHARMACODYNAMIC PROPERTIES OF LAMIVUDINE

### Structure and historical background

Lamivudine (also known as 3TC) is the negative (*cis*) enantiomer of 2′-deoxy-3′-thiacytidine (SddC) (Fig. 1). It is a synthetic 2′-deoxycytidine analogue with the unnatural 2R,5S configuration [7]. The 3′ carbon is replaced by a sulphur atom with the loss of the 3′-OH group necessary for DNA chain elongation. Initially developed as an antiretroviral agent against human immunodeficiency virus (HIV) [8–10], the triphosphate form of lamivudine inhibits viral

reverse transcriptase by competing with dCTP for incorporation into HIV DNA and acting as a chain terminator [11–13]. It is currently one of the most commonly utilized therapies for HIV.

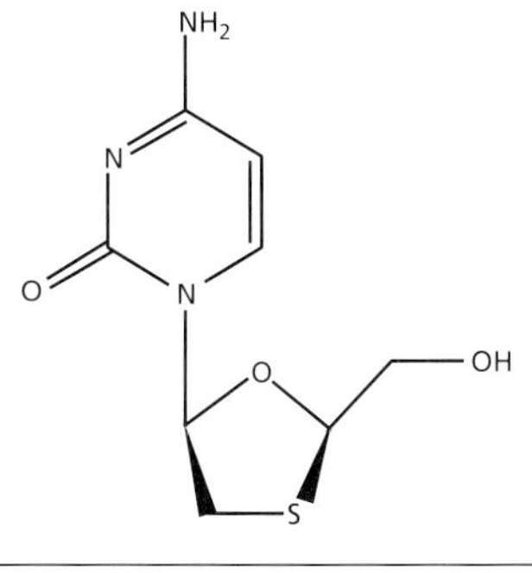

### Anti-HBV activity
#### *Replication of HBV*

HBV is a member of the family *Hepadnaviridae*, which includes woodchuck hepatitis virus (WHV), duck hepatitis B virus (DHBV) and ground squirrel hepatitis virus (GSHV) [14–17]. Although it is a DNA virus, it is remarkably similar to the retrovirus HIV, in that both utilize reverse transcription in their replicative cycle. Following entry into infected cells, HBV DNA is converted to covalently closed circular DNA (cccDNA) in the host cell nucleus. Transcription of cccDNA by host RNA polymerase generates the pregenomic RNA template which is transported to the cytoplasm for translation of gene products and encapsidation into virus cores for reverse transcription. In the virus core, the pregenomic RNA is copied by reverse transcriptase using a protein primer to initiate the first (minus) strand of DNA synthesis. Using the minus strand as template, the second (plus) strand of DNA is synthesized by the viral polymerase, resulting in the partially double-stranded viral DNA [18,19] (Fig. 2).

#### *Mechanism of action*

Following entry into cells, lamivudine is phosphorylated to its active metabolite, lamivudine-5′-triphosphate [20] by 2′-deoxycytidine kinase [21] and other cellular kinase enzymes [11,22]. Its mechanism of action involves inhibition of viral polymerase by DNA chain termination [23,24]. Using DHBV core particles prepared from DHBV-infected hepatocytes, lamivudine has been shown to compete with dCTP for binding to the viral polymerase, with kinetics consistent with irreversible competition and DNA chain termination at the C position [25].

**Figure 1.** Structure of lamuvidine

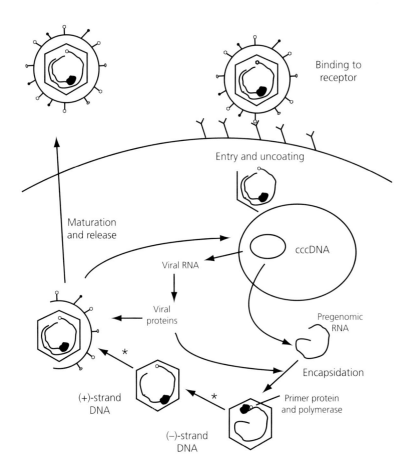

**Figure 2.** Replication of HBV

The asterisks indicate the site of action of lamivudine.

### In vitro antiviral activity

Lamivudine was initially synthesized as a racemic mixture of *cis*-isomers of 2′,3′-dideoxy-3′-thiacytidine (also known as BCH-189) [26]. In 2.2.15 cells (clonal cells derived from HepG2 cells transfected with a plasmid containing HBV DNA which secretes HBV virions), this mixture at 0.5 μM completely suppressed extracellular and intracellular episomal DNA. No effect was seen on the integrated HBV genome and hence HBV mRNA transcription remained unaffected [27]. Subsequent studies showed that the deoxycytidine deaminase-resistant (negative) stereoisomer of BCH-189, lamivudine (3TC), was the active form against HBV with an HBV $EC_{50}$ of 0.01 μM, 50 times more potent than the positive stereoisomer [26]. In primary duck hepatocytes infected with DHBV, the $EC_{50}$ of lamivudine is 0.1 μM [28].

### In vivo antiviral activity in animal models

In chimpanzees congenitally infected with HBV, lamivudine given orally at 0.3 mg/kg twice daily resulted in greater than 90% suppression of serum HBV DNA [28]. Similar suppression of serum DHBV in ducks was observed at an oral dose of 20 mg/kg twice daily [28]. However, even in prolonged therapy with lamivudine at 20 mg/kg twice daily given intramuscularly for greater than 1 year, viraemia reappeared when therapy was discontinued (DLJ Tyrrell, unpublished observations). In neonatally infected woodchucks given 5 to 15 mg/kg of lamivudine orally, there was prompt reduction of serum WHV DNA. After 19 months of treatment, 7 out of 20 woodchucks developed hepatocellular carcinoma (HCC) in the treated group, compared with 14 out of 20 HCCs, with seven deaths, in the placebo-treated group [29].

### In vitro combination therapy with other nucleoside analogues

Monotherapy with antiviral agents frequently leads to resistance. In an attempt to increase the efficacy and decrease the emergence of resistance, combination antiviral therapy against HBV has been studied. Combination therapy will probably be most effective when the antiviral agents have different mechanisms of action. For a DNA chain terminator such as lamivudine, the most effective combination will likely be with one of the purine analogues, which act by inhibiting the protein priming of viral DNA synthesis.

## Penciclovir

Penciclovir (9-[2-hydroxy-1-(hydroxymethyl)ethoxy methyl]guanine is a 2′-deoxyguanosine analogue which has anti-HBV activity [30–33]. It inhibits the priming step for reverse transcription [30]. Because of the difference in mechanism of action, penciclovir would be predicted to have an additive or synergistic effect when used in combination with lamivudine. Using drug-interaction modelling, the combination of penciclovir and lamivudine was tested over a wide range of clinically relevant concentrations and synergistic anti-DHBV effects in primary duck hepatocytes infected with DHBV were demonstrated [34].

## PMEA

9-(2-Phosphonylmethoxyethyl)adenine (PMEA) is an acyclic nucleotide analogue which has recently been identified as a potent inhibitor of HBV [35]. In primary duck hepatocytes from infected ducklings, the $EC_{50}$ of PMEA is 0.08 µM. Utilizing the same drug- interaction modelling as described for penciclovir, the anti-DHBV effect of PMEA in combination with lamivudine at clinically relevant concentrations was shown to be at least additive [36].

## β-L-ddAMP-bis(tbutylSATE)

The unnatural β-L-2′,3′-dideoxyadenosine (β-L-ddA) lacks anti-HBV activity [37], perhaps because it is not phosphorylated to its 5′-triphosphate intracellularly [38]. β-L-ddAMP-bis(tbutylSATE) is a β-L-ddAMP prodrug which has anti-DHBV activity in infected primary duck hepatocytes [39]. In 2.2.15 cells, β-L-ddAMP-bis(tbutylSATE) and lamivudine have been shown to have a synergistic effect [39].

Although the above *in vitro* data on combination therapy is promising, no clinical data is yet available. Such studies are much needed and will undoubtedly be planned as effective antiviral agents with different mechanisms of action receive approval for use in clinical trials in the future.

## Cytotoxicity

The cytotoxicity of lamivudine has been shown to be minimal in many well-established haematopoietic cell lines (C8166, CEM, H9, JM, U937, K562), in human peripheral blood lymphocytes, and in primary duck hepatocytes [9,34,40,41], with the $CC_{50}$ far exceeding the $EC_{50}$ for HBV. Compared with its positive stereoisomer, lamivudine is a much weaker inhibitor of mammalian DNA polymerases α, β and γ, which accounts for its lower cellular toxicity.

Because of the severe toxicity resulting from unrecognized mitochondrial effects of another nucleoside analogue, fialuridine [42,43], the effect of lamivudine on the mitochondria was studied in 15 patients with chronic HBV treated with lamivudine for 6 months. No abnormality in the morphology or enzymatic function of the mitochondria was observed [44].

## Pharmacokinetic properties of lamivudine

Pharmacokinetic studies were performed in two separate studies on 34 patients with asymptomatic HIV infection [45,46]. Following oral administration, lamivudine is rapidly absorbed, with a mean absorption time of 1–1.5 hours and a mean terminal half-life of 2.5–9 hours. The mean bioavailability is 82–88% and 70% of the given dose is excreted unchanged in the urine regardless of systemic bioavailability. Renal clearance of lamivudine exceeds the glomerular filtration rate, indicating active tubular secretion of the drug. All oral formulations (solution, capsule and tablet) are bioequivalent for absorption time, area under the serum concentration–time curve and maximum serum drug concentration.

Lamivudine is equally distributed into total body water with an observed volume of distribution of 1.3 l/kg [45]. In primates, lamivudine is found in the cerebrospinal fluid (CSF) and after an intravenous dose, the drug CSF:plasma ratio is 0.41 and 0.079 for lumbar and ventricular CSF, respectively. This is comparable to other 2′,3′-dideoxycytidine analogues and may suggest a transport mechanism for efflux of cytidine analogues from ventricular CSF [47]. Lamivudine has also been shown to cross the human placenta by simple diffusion *in vitro* [48].

The intracellular metabolism of lamivudine has been studied in different cell types [20,22]. In uninfected and mock HIV-infected human peripheral blood lymphocytes, the drug was metabolized to its triphosphate form (40% of total intracellular drug metabolites in 4 hours) with a half life of 10.5–15.5 hours [22]. A more recent study in monkey and human hepatocytes confirmed that the triphosphate form was the predominant intracellular metabolite but the inter-species variability was high [20].

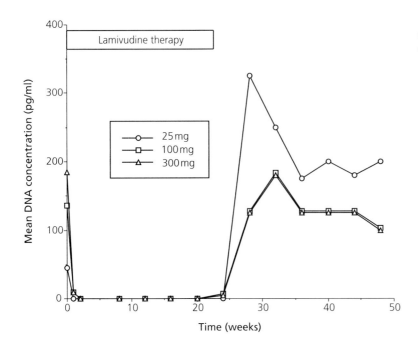

**Figure 3.** Representative graph of serum HBV DNA concentration by dose, during and after treatment with lamivudine

Modified from [57].

# CLINICAL STUDIES OF LAMIVUDINE
## Effect of lamivudine on HBV in HIV-infected individuals

HBV infection is not uncommon among HIV-infected individuals because of similar modes of transmission of the viruses. Lamivudine has known antiretroviral activity against HIV, which has been demonstrated in several clinical trials [49–51]. The effect of lamivudine on HBV replication was also examined in two of these studies.

In an open label prospective trial of lamivudine of 600 mg, then 300 mg daily for HIV infection, 40 patients with concurrent HIV and HBV were assessed during a 12 month treatment period. In the group with retrospectively determined high HBV replication (serum HBV DNA >5 pg/ml and HBeAg-positive), 96% had undetectable HBV DNA by molecular hybridization but 11.5% were still positive for HBV DNA by PCR. In the group with low pretreatment HBV replication (HBV DNA <5 pg/ml and anti-HBe-positive), all six patients with positive pretreatment HBV DNA by PCR became negative. Five of 27 patients positive for pretreatment HBeAg lost HBeAg (18.5%) and three of these developed anti-HBe [52].

In a randomized trial of the addition of lamivudine with or without loviride to zidovudine-containing regimens for patients with HIV infection (the CAESAR trial) [50], retrospective analysis of HBV markers of 118 HBsAg-positive patients showed a 2 $\log_{10}$ decrease in HBV DNA (no change in non-lamivudine-treated patients) and HBV DNA was negative by PCR (<400 copies/ml) in 40% (versus 10% in non-lamivudine-treated patients). HBeAg loss occurred in 22% with lamivudine treatment (versus none in the non-lamivudine-treated patients), but the number of patients retested for HBeAg was small and the difference between the two groups did not reach statistical significance [53].

## Effect of lamivudine on chronic hepatitis B
### HBV replication

The effect of lamivudine on HBV replication was initially assessed in 1 month [54], 3 month [55] and 6 month [56] dose-ranging studies of oral doses from 5 mg to 600 mg daily. Although HBV DNA became undetectable by hybridization in 74% of patients receiving doses greater than 20 mg/day [54], the efficacy was better with the higher doses, 93–100% and 88–100% with 100 mg and 300 mg lamivudine daily, respectively [54–56]. The efficacy was similar with the two higher doses but the time to HBV DNA suppression was shorter with the 300 mg dose. A total of 50% of patients became negative for HBV DNA in 2 and 4 weeks with the 300 mg and 100 mg dose, respectively. There were quantitative decreases in HBsAg and HBeAg during treatment [56], and HBeAg loss was 8–12% [55,56]. However, on cessation of lamivudine treatment, there was a prompt rebound (within 28 days) of HBV DNA to pretreatment levels in the majority of patients in all three studies (Fig. 3).

To date, the results of three randomized placebo-controlled trials of lamivudine 25–300 mg daily fo 4 [57], 32 [58] and 52 [59] weeks, involving 537 Asian subjects, have been published. The prompt HBV DNA suppression and reappearance on therapy cessation seen in previous dose-ranging studies were again evident. In the 52 week study, increased HBeAg seroconversion was seen in the lamivudine group (100 mg/day), 16% compared to 4% in the placebo-treated group.

## Necroinflammation and fibrosis

In the majority of patients treated with lamivudine, there is no significant increase in serum alanine aminotransferase (ALT) levels In patients with elevated pretreatment ALT, end of treatment normalization of ALT occurred in 33–72% of patients [55,56,60]. However, there have been observations of ALT elevations, and in one study, 40% of patients had a greater than twofold increase in serum ALT during or after therapy. The timing of the initial ALT peak appeared to be dose-related (more delayed with higher lamivudine doses). Most of the episodes of enzyme elevation were asymptomatic and drug withdrawal was necessary in only one patient. The significance of these enzyme elevations was not clear in general but in one patient was related to sustained HBV suppression [55]. There may be ethnic differences in the frequency and timing of ALT elevation [56].

Two studies examined the effect of lamivudine on histological features of HBV infection. In a 6 month study with 15 patients, there was a decrease in the Knodell histology activity index (HAI) in liver biopsies from 4.4 pre-treatment to 2.8 post-treatment. Further analysis of the components of the HAI showed a significant decrease in piecemeal necrosis with treatment [60]. Histological improvement with lamivudine was confirmed in a larger study conducted for 52 weeks in 358 patients. A 2 point reduction in HAI was seen in 67 and 59% of those treated daily with 100 mg and 25 mg of lamivudine, respectively, compared with 30% in the placebo group. The reduction in HAI was most marked in those with moderate/severe hepatitis at baseline. Progression of fibrosis was reduced with lamivudine treatment, 3% with 100 mg lamivudine compared to 15% with placebo [59].

## Retreatment with lamivudine

Twenty-four patients still positive for HBeAg/HBV DNA after earlier Phase II lamivudine trials were retreated for an additional 52 weeks. Treatment was effective, with HBV DNA suppression and HBeAg loss in 100% and 37.5% of the subjects, respectively [61]. In three patients with hepatitis flare after withdrawal of lamivudine, retreatment resulted in rapid decline in ALT, HBV DNA and HBeAg levels within 8 weeks [62].

## Atypical HBV serology

Treatment of nine patients, positive for HBV DNA but negative for HBeAg, with 100 mg lamivudine for 48 weeks resulted in negative HBV DNA (branched DNA, <0.7 Meq/ml) within 2 months, ALT normalization or near normalization in all patients at 6 months and reduction in HAI on repeat biopsy after 48 weeks [63].

## Decompensated HBV cirrhosis

In decompensated HBV cirrhosis, the treatment options are limited because interferon can result in serious clinical deterioration and is contraindicated in most cases. Lamivudine at 100 mg daily was given for 6 months to 12 patients with decompensated HBV cirrhosis. Three patients died of liver failure within 3 months and four underwent transplantation within 6 months. Of the five remaining patients, all showed slow but significant clinical and biochemical improvement in liver function [64].

# Lamivudine in orthotopic liver transplantation

## Pretransplant prophylactic treatment

In three separate studies, lamivudine at 100 mg daily given before orthotopic liver transplantation (OLT) for at least 4 weeks (until HBV DNA becomes undetectable) and continued post-OLT is effective in DNA suppression and clearance of HBeAg and HBsAg during the post-OLT period [65–67]. However, the major problem is recurrence of hepatitis associated with HBV DNA reappearance during both the pre- and post-OLT period, owing to the emergence of lamivudine-resistant HBV (see below).

## Post-transplant treatment for recurrent and de novo HBV

Initial studies of lamivudine for post-OLT recurrent HBV appeared promising when three patients with recurrent HBV were treated with a 100 mg daily dose for at least 20 weeks. HBV DNA became negative by hybridization after 6 weeks and by PCR after the tenth week [68]. In a larger study with 52 patients who had completed at least 6 months of therapy for post-OLT recurrent or *de novo* HBV infection, all became HBV DNA-negative by hybridization within 6 weeks. However, HBsAg, HBeAg and HBV DNA by PCR remained positive in 93, 62 and 23% of the patients, respectively. Emergence of resistant virus was also a problem in these patients, with 14 patients developing HBV DNA breakthrough after 8 months of therapy [69].

## Combination therapy with lamivudine and hepatitis B immunoglobulin

At the present time, combination therapy of lamivudine and hepatitis B immunoglobulin (HBIg) in the transplant setting has only been reported in preliminary studies with small numbers of patients. In one study, 13 patients received combination therapy with lamivudine and HBIg for HBV recurrence prophylaxis following OLT. Lamivudine (150 mg/day) was started pre-OLT in nine patients. HBIg was given at 10 000 IU during the anhepatic phase, daily during the first post-OLT week and monthly thereafter. The 1 year graft and patient survival was 92% [70]. In another study looking at residual HBV replication during lamivudine treatment, combination therapy with HBIg and lamivudine resulted in suppression of HBV DNA sooner than lamivudine alone, but the study was small with only five patients receiving combination therapy [71]. Conclusions on the efficacy of combination therapy during transplantation must await the results of larger clinical trials currently underway.

## Adverse effects of lamivudine

In general, lamivudine has been well tolerated in most clinical trials. Most adverse effects were mild and self-limiting and consisted of headache, dizziness and muscle ache [55,57]. In placebo-controlled trials, the frequency of most side-effects with lamivudine was not different from that with placebo. Transient elevations in lipase, amylase and creatinine kinase can occur during treatment with or after withdrawal of lamivudine and usually resolve despite continuation of therapy [55,56]. More serious adverse effects included hypoglycaemia in one diabetic patient requiring drug withdrawal [56] and several-fold elevations of serum ALT, which may represent reactivation of HBV [55,56]. Anaphylactoid reaction with angioedema and urticaria presumably related to lamivudine has also been reported [72].

## Lamivudine resistance

One serious problem with lamivudine treatment of HBV is the emergence of drug-resistant virus with prolonged therapy. Resistance to lamivudine is common during the treatment of HIV and is associated with mutations at the YMDD (tyrosine, methionine, aspartate, aspartate) motif of its reverse transcriptase [73–77] (see below). This motif is conserved in hepadnaviruses. When site-directed mutagenesis at this site in DHBV resulted in resistance to lamivudine in ducks, it was suggested that lamivudine resistance may also emerge in HBV [78]. Shortly thereafter, lamivudine resistance arising from mutations at the YMDD motif was recognized clinically; initially in association with transplantation [79–81], and subsequently with treatment of chronic hepatitis [82].

### Prophylactic therapy during OLT

In the study with 52 patients completing at least 6 months of lamivudine therapy for post-OLT recurrent and *de novo* HBV infection, 14 patients (27%) developed resistance with seven patients showing elevated serum ALT and two deaths [69]. The emergence of resistant virus with HBV is slower than in HIV, with all reported cases occurring at least 30 weeks post-OLT [79–81]. In most cases, resistance is only associated with an asymptomatic rise in serum ALT, without serious clinical deterioration. However, there have been three cases of liver failure owing to fibrosing cholestatic hepatitis resulting from the emergence of the resistant virus [83]. One patient died from gram-negative sepsis after developing hepatic insufficiency owing to lamivudine-resistant virus [69].

### Treatment of chronic HBV

In the study of 335 Asian patients receiving 52 weeks of therapy with lamivudine for chronic HBV infection, the rate of genotypic resistance was 4 and 14% at 36 and 52 weeks, respectively. With the emergence of resistance, the rise in HBV DNA and serum ALT was delayed and tended to be below pretreatment levels, perhaps suggesting that the resistant virus is less replication-competent and less pathogenic. Although patients with genotypic resistance were less likely to have HBeAg seroconversion and ALT normalization, they still had improvement in liver histology compared to placebo-treated patients [82]. HBeAg seroconversion may still be possible with the emergence of resistance and one case each of transient and stable HBeAg conversion has been reported in patients with genotypic resistance [84].

## Management of genotypic resistance

The natural history of genotypic resistance to lamivudine and the ideal strategy for its management are still unknown. As indicated above, although cases of liver failure have been reported, the majority of patients with lamivudine resistance do not seem to have significant clinical deterioration. There is indirect evidence of replication incompetence of the resistant virus [82,85] compared to wild-type. When lamivudine is withdrawn, wild-type virus rapidly becomes the predominant species over resistant virus with resultant clinical deterioration. Reinstitution of lamivudine is usually effective again for the suppression of viral DNA (N Brown, Glaxo Wellcome, personal communication). Treatment of the resistant virus with other nucleoside analogues has been tried with variable success. Introduction of famciclovir [83,86] infrequently suppressed viral DNA. Treatment with ganciclovir was more successful, with two out of three patients having a virological and clinical response [83]. However, the studies to date have been small and anecdotal. Until the results of larger studies on the effective therapy for resistant virus become available, the current strategy is to continue lamivudine treatment when genotypic resistance develops, since the lamivudine-resistant virus may be less virulent than wild-type.

### Identification and biological characterization of mutations

To date, all resistant isolates reported contain mutations in the YMDD motif, which is present in the catalytic site of the viral RNA-dependent DNA polymerase. Mutation at this motif in HIV can also lead to lamivudine resistance [73–77]. The emergence of resistance is slower and less frequent in HBV than in HIV, perhaps because of the lower mutation rates and higher genomic conservation in HBV, which is related to the multiple overlap of the open reading frames of viral proteins [18,19,87,88]. In early analyses, two patterns of mutation have been observed in association with lamivudine resistance; substitution of valine for methionine at residue 552 (YVDD) accompanied by substitution of methionine for leucine at residue 528, or a single substitution of isoleucine for methionine at residue 552 (YIDD) [80,81]. Constructs with both patterns of mutation have been found to be resistant to lamivudine *in vitro* [89] with a greater than 10 000-fold increase in EC$_{50}$ compared with wild-type. Multiple patterns of mutations have been constructed, and in transfection experiments, only constructs with a valine or isoleucine substitution have been found to be

replication-competent and resistant to lamivudine [90], albeit with lower levels of viral replication [85]. In the duck, lamivudine-resistant virus rapidly reverts to wild-type when the ducks are not treated with lamivudine. This reversion can be suppressed by institution of lamivudine treatment [91].

A number of nucleoside analogues have been tested for effectiveness against the lamivudine-resistant virus. Mutant human HBV DNA polymerases (YVDD and YIDD), showing resistance to lamivudine, remain sensitive to PMEA with inhibition constants ($K_i$) increasing by only two- to threefold compared to wild-type [92]. In the duck model, lamivudine-resistant virus remains susceptible to 2-amino-6-methoxy-2′,3′-dideoxypurine, a purine analogue which inhibits DHBV by blocking protein priming of viral DNA synthesis [93]. In contrast, the lamivudine-resistant virus remains resistant to other 2′-deoxycytidine analogues such as β-L dideoxy-5-fluorocytidine (FddC) [94].

## CONCLUSION

Lamivudine is expected to be licensed for the treatment of chronic HBV infection in the near future, based on promising antiviral studies showing prompt suppression of viral DNA in chronic hepatitis and post-transplant recurrent HBV infection. Despite effective suppression of viral DNA, HBeAg seroconversion remains low at 16% after 1 year. However, lamivudine appears to improve necroinflammation and fibrosis in the liver and is well tolerated with minimal adverse effects. The remaining unresolved issues include the optimum duration of treatment required to achieve HBeAg seroconversion and the natural history and management of drug-resistant virus. Taking into consideration all of the above factors, combination therapy with interferon plus nucleoside analogues or the simultaneous use of multiple nucleoside analogues with different mechanisms of action will probably be the most effective mode of antiviral treatment.

## REFERENCES

1. Purcell RH. The discovery of the hepatitis viruses. *Gastroenterology* 1993; **104**:955–963.
2. Carreno V, Castillo I, Molina J, Porres JC & Bartolome J. Long-term follow-up of hepatitis B chronic carriers who responded to interferon therapy. *Journal of Hepatology* 1992; **15**:102–106.
3. Perrillo RP, Schiff ER, Davis GL, Bodenheimer HC, Lindsay K, Payne J, Dienstag JL, O'Brien C, Tamburro C, Jacobson IM, Sampliner R, Feit D, Lefkowitch J, Kuhns M, Meschievitz C, Sanghvi B, Albrecht J, Gibas A & The Hepatitis Interventional Therapy Group. A randomized, controlled trial of interferon alfa-2b alone and after prednisone withdrawal for the treatment of

chronic hepatitis B. *New England Journal of Medicine* 1990; **323**:295–301.

4. Wong DKH, Cheung AM, O'Rourke K, Naylor CD, Detsky AS & Heathcote J. Effect of alpha-interferon treatment in patients with hepatitis B e antigen-positive chronic hepatitis B: a meta-analysis. *Annals of Internal Medicine* 1993; **119**:312–323.

5. Hoofnagle JH & Di Bisceglie AM. Antiviral therapy of viral hepatitis. In *Antiviral Agents and Viral Diseases of Man*, 3rd edn 1991; pp. 415–459. Edited by GJ Galasso, RJ Whitley & TC Merigan. New York: Raven Press.

6. Alexander GJ, Fagan EA, Hegarty JE, Yeo J, Eddleston AL & Williams R. Controlled clinical trial of acyclovir in chronic hepatitis B virus. *Journal of Medical Virology* 1987; **21**:81–87.

7. Soudeyns H, Yao XJ, Gao Q, Belleau B, Kraus JL, Nguyen-Ba N, Spira B & Wainberg MA. Anti-human immunodeficiency virus type 1 activity and *in vitro* toxicity of 2'-deoxy-3'-thiacytidine (BCH-189), a novel heterocyclic nucleoside analog. *Antimicrobial Agents and Chemotherapy* 1991; **35**:1386–1390.

8. Greenberg ML, Allaudeen HS & Hershfield MS. Metabolism, toxicity, and anti-HIV activity of 2'-deoxy-3'-thiacytidine (BCH-189) in T and B cell lines. *Annals of the New York Academy of Sciences* 1990; **616**:517–518.

9. Wainberg MA, Tremblay M, Rooke R, Blain N, Soudeyns H, Parniak MA, Yao XJ, Li XG, Fanning M, Montaner JSG, O'Shaughnessy M, Tsoukas C, Falutz J, Dionne G, Belleau B & Reudy J. Characterization of reverse transcriptase activity and susceptibility to other nucleosides of AZT-resistant variants of HIV-1. Results from the Canadian AZT Multicentre Study. *Annals of the New York Academy of Sciences* 1990; **616**:346–355.

10. Soudeyns H, Yao XJ, Gao Q, Belleau B, Kraus JL, Nguyen-Ba N, Spira B & Wainberg MA. Anti-human immunodeficiency virus type 1 activity and *in vitro* toxicity of 2'-deoxy-3'-thiacytidine (BCH-189), a novel heterocyclic nucleoside analog. *Antimicrobial Agents and Chemotherapy* 1991; **35**:1386–1390.

11. Hart GJ, Orr DC, Penn CR, Figueiredo HT, Gray NM, Boehme RE & Cameron JM. Effects of (–)-2'-deoxy-3'-thiacytidine (3TC) 5'-triphosphate on human immunodeficiency virus reverse transcriptase and mammalian DNA polymerases alpha, beta, and gamma. *Antimicrobial Agents and Chemotherapy* 1992; **36**:1688–1694.

12. Schinazi RF, Lloyd R, Oswald B & Manning C. Effect of AZT, AzddU, FDT, and BCH-189 nucleotides on DNA chain termination mediated by HIV-1 reverse transcriptase. *Antiviral Research* 1991; **15** (Supplement):97.

13. Wilson JE, Martin JL, Borroto-Esoda K, Hopkins S, Painter G, Liotta DC & Furman PA. The 5'-triphosphates of the (–) and (+) enantiomers of cis-5-fluoro-1-[2-(hydroxymethyl)-1,3-oxathiolane-5-yl]cytosine equally inhibit human immunodeficiency virus type 1 reverse transcriptase. *Antimicrobial Agents and Chemotherapy* 1993; **37**:1720–1722.

14. Summers J. Three recently described animal virus models for human hepatitis B virus. *Hepatology* 1981; **1**:179–183.

15. Summers J, Smolec JM & Snyder R. A virus similar to human hepatitis B virus associated with hepatitis and hepatoma in woodchucks. *Proceedings of the National Academy of Sciences, USA* 1978; **75**:4533–4537.

16. Mason WS, Seal G & Summers J. Virus of Pekin ducks

with structural and biological relatedness to human hepatitis B virus. *Journal of Virology* 1980; **36**:829–836.

17. Marion PL, Oshiro LS, Regnery DC, Scullard GH & Robinson WS. A virus in Beechy ground squirrels that is related to hepatitis B virus in humans. *Proceedings of the National Academy of Sciences, USA* 1980; **77**:2941–2945.

18. Ganem D & Varmus HE. The molecular biology of the hepatitis B viruses. *Annual Review of Biochemistry* 1987; **56**:651–693.

19. Nassal M & Schaller H. Hepatitis B virus replication. *Trends in Microbiology* 1993; **1**:221–228.

20. Cretton-Scott E, Placidi L, Echoff D & Sommadossi JP. Cellular pharmacology of lamivudine in hepatocytes primary cultures. *Second International Conference on Therapies for Viral Hepatitis*, Kona, Hawaii, 15–19 December 1997; Abstract O16.

21. Shewach DS, Liotta DC & Schinazi RF. Affinity of the antiviral enantiomers of oxathiolane cytosine nucleosides for human 2'-deoxycytidine kinase. *Biochemical Pharmacology* 1993; **45**:1540–1543.

22. Cammack N, Rouse P, Marr CL, Reid PJ, Boehme RE, Coates JAV, Penn CR & Cameron JM. Cellular metabolism of (–) enantiomeric 2'-deoxy-3'-thiacytidine. *Biochemical Pharmacology* 1992; **43**:2059–2064.

23. Coates JAV, Cammack N, Jenkinson HJ, Jowett AJ, Jowett MI, Pearson BA, Penn CR, Rouse PL, Viner KC & Cameron JM. (–)-2'-deoxy-3'-thiacytidine is a potent, highly selective inhibitor of human immunodeficiency virus type 1 and type 2 replication in vitro. *Antimicrobial Agents and Chemotherapy* 1992; **36**:733–739.

24. Coates JAV, Cammack N, Jenkinson HJ, Mutton IM, Pearson BA, Storer R, Cameron JM & Penn CR. The separated enantiomers of 2'-deoxy-3'-thiacytidine (BCH 189) both inhibit human immunodeficiency virus replication in vitro. *Antimicrobial Agents and Chemotherapy* 1992; **36**:202–205.

25. Severini A, Liu XY, Wilson JS & Tyrrell DLJ. Mechanism of inhibition of duck hepatitis B virus polymerase by (–)-β-L-2',3'-dideoxy-3'-thiacytidine. *Antimicrobial Agents and Chemotherapy* 1995; **39**:1430–1435.

26. Chang CN, Doong SL, Zhou JH, Beach JW, Jeong LS, Chu CK, Tsai CH & Cheng YC. Deoxycytidine deaminase-resistant stereoisomer is the active form of (–)-2',3'-dideoxy-3'-thiacytidine in the inhibition of hepatitis B virus replication. *Journal of Biological Chemistry* 1992; **267**:13938–13942.

27. Doong SL, Tsai CH, Schinazi RF, Liotta DC & Cheng YC. Inhibition of the replication of hepatitis B virus *in vitro* by 2',3'-dideoxy-3'-thiacytidine and related analogues. *Proceedings of the National Academy of Sciences, USA* 1991; **88**:8495–8499.

28. Tyrrell DLJ, Fischer K, Savani K, Tan W & Jewell L. Treatment of chimpanzees and ducks with lamivudine, 2'3' dideoxy 3' thiacytidine results in a rapid suppression of hepadnaviral DNA in sera. *Clinical and Investigative Medicine* 1993; **16** (Supplement):B77.

29. Peek SF, Toshkov IA, Erb HN, Schinazi RF, Korba BE, Cote PJ, Gerin JL & Tennant BC. 3'thiacytidine (3TC) delays development of hepato-cellular carcinoma (HCC) in woodchucks with experimentally induced chronic woodchuck hepatitis virus (WHV) infection. Preliminary results of a lifetime study. *Hepatology* 1997; **26**:368A.

30. Zoulim F, Dannaoui E & Trepo C. Inhibitory effect of penciclovir on the priming of hepadnavirus reverse transcription. In *Abstracts of the 35th Interscience*

*Conference on Antimicrobial Agents and Chemotherapy,* 1995; pp. 182. Washington, DC: American Society for Microbiology.

31. Shaw T, Amor P, Civitico G, Boyd M & Locarnini S. *In vitro* antiviral activity of penciclovir, a novel purine nucleoside, against duck hepatitis B virus. *Antimicrobial Agents and Chemotherapy* 1994; **38:**719–723.

32. Korba BE & Boyd MR. Penciclovir is a selective inhibitor of hepatitis B virus replication in cultured human hepatoblastoma cells. *Antimicrobial Agents and Chemotherapy* 1996; **40:**1282–1284.

33. Shaw T, Mok SS & Locarnini SA. Inhibition of hepatitis B virus DNA polymerase by enantiomers of penciclovir triphosphate and metabolic basis for selective inhibition of HBV replication by penciclovir. *Hepatology* 1996; **24:**996–1002.

34. Colledge D, Locarnini S & Shaw T. Synergistic inhibition of hepadnaviral replication by lamivudine in combination with penciclovir *in vitro*. *Hepatology* 1997; **26:**216–225.

35. Heijtink RA, De Wilde GA, Kruining J, Berk L, Balzarini J, De Clercq E, Holy A & Schalm SW. Inhibitory effect of 9-(2-phosphonylmethoxyethyl)-adenine (PMEA) on human and duck hepatitis B virus infection. *Antiviral Research* 1993; **21:**141–153.

36. Colledge D, Shaw T & Locarnini SA. Combination anti-hepadnaviral analysis of 9-(2-phosphonyl-meth-oxy-ethyl) adenine (PMEA) with either penciclovir or lamivudine *in vitro*: evidence for synergistic inhibition. *Second International Conference on Therapies for Viral Hepatitis*, Kona, Hawaii, 15–19 December 1997; Abstract P42.

37. Balzarini J, Kruining J, Wedgwood O, Pannecouque C, Aquaro S, Perno CF, Naesens L, Witvrouw M, Heijtink R, De Clercq E & McGuigan C. Conversion of 2′,3′-dideoxyadenosine (ddA) and 2′,3′-didehydro-2′,3′-dide-oxyadenosine (d4A) to their corresponding aryloxy-phosphoramidate derivatives markedly potentiates their activity against human immunodeficiency virus and hepatitis B virus. *FEBS Letters* 1997; **410:**324–328.

38. Placidi L, Perigaud C, Cretton-Scott E, Gosselin G, Pierra C, Schinazi RF, Imbach JL & Sommadossi JP. The intracellular pharmacology of β-L-ddA is responsible for the lack of potent anti-HBV activity. *Second International Conference on Therapies for Viral Hepatitis*, Kona, Hawaii, 15–19 December 1997; Abstract P21.

39. Loi AG, Faraj A, Pierra G, Gosselin G, Imbach JL, Locarnini SA, Groman EV, Schinazi RF & Sommadossi JP. Evaluation of the anti-HBV activity of β-D- and β-L-ddAMP-SATE prodrugs alone and in combination with lamivudine. *Second International Conference on Therapies for Viral Hepatitis*, Kona, Hawaii, 15–19 December 1997; Abstract P20.

40. Schinazi RF, Chu CK, Peck A, McMillan A, Mathis R, Cannon D, Jeong LS, Beach JW, Choi WB, Yeola S & Liotta DC. Activities of the four optical isomers of 2′,3′-dideoxy-3′-thiacytidine (BCH-189) against human immunodeficiency virus type 1 in human lymphocytes. *Antimicrobial Agents and Chemotherapy* 1992; **36:**672–676.

41. Sommadossi JP, Schinazi RF, Chu CK & Xie MY. Comparison of cytotoxicity of the (–)-enantiomer of 2′,3′-dideoxy-3′-thiacytidine in normal human bone marrow progenitor cells. *Biochemical Pharmacology* 1992; **44:**1921–1925.

42. McKenzie R, Fried MW, Sallie R, Conjeevaram H, Di Bisceglie AM, Park Y, Savarase B, Kleiner D, Tsokos M, Luciano C, Pruett T, Stotka JL, Straus SE & Hoofnagle JH. Hepatic failure and lactic acidosis due to fialuridine (FIAU), an investigational nucleoside analogue for chronic hepatitis B. *New England Journal of Medicine* 1995; **333:**1099–1105.

43. Swartz MN. Mitochondrial toxicity – new adverse drug effects. *New England Journal of Medicine* 1995; **333:**1146–1148.

44. Honkoop P, de Man RA, Scholte HR, Zondervan PE, VandenBerg JWO, Rademakers LHPM & Schalm SW. Effect of lamivudine on morphology and function of mitochondria in patients with chronic hepatitis B. *Hepatology* 1997; **26:**211–215.

45. van Leeuwen R, Lange JMA, Hussey EK, Donn KH, Hall ST, Harker AJ, Jonker P & Danner SA. The safety and pharmacokinetics of a reverse transcriptase inhibitor, 3TC, in patients with HIV infection: a phase I study. *AIDS* 1992; **6:**1471–1475.

46. Yuen GJ, Morris DM, Mydlow PK, Haidar S, Hall ST & Hussey EK. Pharmacokinetics, absolute bioavailability, and absorption characteristics of lamivudine. *Journal of Clinical Pharmacology* 1995; **35:**1174–1180.

47. Blaney SM, Daniel MJ, Harker AJ, Godwin K & Balis FM. Pharmacokinetics of lamivudine and BCH-189 in plasma and cerebrospinal fluid of nonhuman primates. *Antimicrobial Agents and Chemotherapy* 1995; **39:** 2779–2782.

48. Bloom SL, Dias KM, Bawdon RE & Gilstrap LC. The maternal–fetal transfer of lamivudine in the *ex vivo* human placenta. *American Journal of Obstetrics and Gynecology* 1997; **176:**291–293.

49. Lafeuillade A, Poggi C, Tamalet C, Profizi N, Tourres C & Costes O. Effects of a combination of zidovudine, didanosine, and lamivudine on primary human immunodeficiency virus type I infection. *Journal of Infectious Diseases* 1997; **175:**1051–1055.

50. CAESAR Coordinating Committee. Randomized trial of addition of lamivudine or lamivudine plus loviride to zidovudine-containing regimens for patients with HIV-1 infection: the CAESAR trial. *Lancet* 1997; **349:** 1413–1421.

51. Eron JJ. The treatment of antiretroviral-naive subjects with the 3TC/zidovudine combination: a review of North American (NUCA 3001) and European (NUCB 3001) trials. *AIDS* 1996; **10:**S11–19.

52. Benhamou Y, Katlama C, Lunel F, Coutellier A, Dohin E, Hamm N, Tubiana R, Herson S, Poynard T & Opolon P. Effects of lamivudine on replication of hepatitis B virus in HIV-infected men. *Annals of Internal Medicine* 1996; **125:**705–712.

53. Cooper DA, Dore G & Barrett C. Effect of lamivudine on hepatitis B/HIV co-infected patients from the CAESAR study. *Second International Conference on Therapies for Viral Hepatitis*, Kona, Hawaii, 15–19 December 1997; Abstract O37.

54. Tyrrell DLJ, Mitchell MC, De Man RA, Schalm SW, Main J, Thomas HC, Fevery J, Nevens F, Beranek P & Vicary C. Phase II trial of lamivudine for chronic hepatitis B. *Hepatology* 1993; **18:**112A.

55. Dienstag JL, Perrillo RP, Schiff ER, Bartholomew M, Vicary C & Rubin M. A preliminary trial of lamivudine for chronic hepatitis B infection. *New England Journal of Medicine* 1995; **333:**1657–1661.

56. Nevens F, Main J, Honkoop P, Tyrrell DL, Barber J, Sullivan MT, Fevery J, de Man RA & Thomas HC. Lamivudine therapy for chronic hepatitis B: a six-month randomized dose-ranging study. *Gastroenterology* 1997; **113:**1258–1263.

57. Lai CL, Ching CK, Tung AKM, Li E, Young J, Hill A, Wong BCY, Dent J & Wu PC. Lamivudine is effective in suppressing hepatitis B virus DNA in Chinese hepatitis B surface antigen carriers: a placebo-controlled trial. *Hepatology* 1997; **25**:241–244.

58. Tanikawa K, Hayashi N, Ichida F, Iino S, Kumada H, Ogawa N, Okita K, Omata M, Sata M & Suzuki H. A placebo-controlled phase III study of lamivudine in Japanese patients with chronic hepatitis B infection. *Hepatology* 1997; **26**:259A.

59. Lai CL, Chien RN, Leung NWY, Chang TT, Guan R, Tai DI, Ng KY, Wu PC, Dent JC, Barber J, Stephenson SL & Gray DF for the Asia Hepatitis Lamivudine Study Group. A one-year trial of lamivudine for chronic hepatitis B. *New England Journal of Medicine* 1998; **339**:61–68.

60. Honkoop P, de Man RA, Zondervan PE & Schalm SW. Histological improvement in patients with chronic hepatitis B virus infection treated with lamivudine. *Liver* 1997; **17**:103–106.

61. Dienstag JL, Schiff ER, Mitchell M, Gitlin N, Lissoos T, Condreay L, Garrett L, Rubin M & Brown N. Extended lamivudine retreatment for chronic hepatitis B. *Hepatology* 1996; **24**:188A.

62. Honkoop P, de Man RA, Niesters HGM & Schalm. Lamivudine withdrawal hepatitis flare successfully treated with lamivudine in patients with chronic hepatitis B. *Hepatology* 1997; **26**:429A

63. Lau DTY, Doo E, Ghany MG, Kleiner DE, Park Y, Condreay L, Herion D, Liang TJ & Hoofnagle JH. Lamivudine for chronic hepatitis B with typical and atypical serology. *Hepatology* 1997; **26**:429A.

64. Villeneuve JP, Bilodeau M, Fenyves D, Pomier G, Pilon D, Raymond G & Willems B. Suppression of hepatitis B virus replication by lamivudine results in improvement of liver function in patients with severe cirrhosis. *Hepatology* 1997; **26**:430A.

65. Grellier L, Mutimer D, Ahmed M, Brown D, Burroughs AK, Rolles K, McMaster P, Beranek P, Kennedy F, Kibbler H, McPhillips P, Elias E & Dusheiko G. Lamivudine prophylaxis against reinfection in liver transplantation for hepatitis B cirrhosis. *Lancet* 1996; **348**:1212–1215.

66. Bain VG, Kneteman NM, Ma MM, Gutfreund K, Shapiro JA, Fischer K, Tipples G, Lee H, Jewell LD & Tyrrell DLJ. Efficacy of lamivudine in chronic hepatitis B patients with active viral replication and decompensated cirrhosis undergoing liver transplantation. *Transplantation* 1996; **62**:1456–1462.

67. Perrillo R, Rakela J, Martin P, Wright T, Levy G, Schiff E, Dienstag J, Gish R, Dickson R, Adams P, Brown N & Self P. Lamivudine for suppression and/or prevention of hepatitis B when given pre/post liver transplantation (OLT). *Hepatology* 1997; **26**:260A.

68. Ben-Ari Z, Shmueli D, Mor E, Shapira Z & Tur-Kaspa R. Beneficial effect of lamivudine in recurrent hepatitis B after liver transplantation. *Transplantation* 1997; **63**:393–396.

69. Perrillo R, Rakela J, Martin P, Levy G, Schiff E, Wright T, Dienstag J, Gish R, Villeneuve JP, Caldwell S, Brown N & Self P. Long term lamivudine therapy of patients with recurrent hepatitis B post liver transplantation. *Hepatology* 1997; **26**:177A.

70. Markowitz JS, Martin P, Conrad AJ, Markmann JF, Seu P, Yersiz H, Goss JA, Pakrasi A, Artinian L, Holt C, Goldstein LI, Stribling R & Busuttil RW. Prophylaxis against hepatitis B recurrence following liver transplantation using combination lamivudine and hepatitis B immune globulin. *Hepatology* 1997; **26**:152A.

71. Petit MA, Buffello D, Roche B, Dussaix E, Aulong B, Bismuth H, Samuel D & Feray C. Residual hepatitis B virus (HBV) infection in liver transplant patients under treatment with lamivudine (3TC): assessment by quantitation of HBV DNA by PCR and assay of preS antigens. *Hepatology* 1997; **26**:315A.

72. Kainer MA & Mijch A. Anaphylactoid reaction, angioedema, and urticaria associated with lamivudine. *Lancet* 1996; **348**:1519.

73. Schuurman R, Nijhuis M, van Leeuwen R, Schipper P, de Jong D, Collis P, Danner SA, Mulder J, Loveday C, Christopher C, Kwok S, Sninsky J & Boucher CAB. Rapid changes in human immunodeficiency virus type 1 RNA load and appearance of drug-resistant virus populations in persons treated with lamivudine (3TC). *Journal of Infectious Diseases* 1995; **171**: 1411–1419.

74. Schinazi RF, Lloyd RM Jr, Nguyen M-H, Cannon DL, McMillan A, Ilksoy N, Chu CK, Liotta DC, Bazmi HZ & Mellors JW. Characterization of human immunodeficiency viruses resistant to oxathiolane-cytosine nucleosides. *Antimicrobial Agents and Chemotherapy* 1993; 37:875–881.

75. Gao Q, Gu Z, Parniak MA, Cameron J, Cammack N, Boucher C & Wainberg MA. The same mutation that encodes low-level human immunodeficiency virus type 1 resistance to 2′,3′-dideoxyinosine and 2′,3′-dideoxycytidine confers high-level resistance to the (–) enantiomer of 2′,3′-dideoxy-3′-thiacytidine. *Antimicrobial Agents and Chemotherapy* 1993; **37**:1390–1392.

76. Boucher CAB, Cammack N, Schipper P, Schuurman R, Rouse P, Wainberg MA & Cameron J. High-level resistance to (–) enantiomeric 2′-deoxy-3′-thiacytidine *in vitro* is due to one amino acid substitution in the catalytic site of human immunodeficiency virus type 1 reverse transcriptase. *Antimicrobial Agents and Chemotherapy* 1993; 37:2231–2234.

77. Tisdale M, Kemp SD, Parry NR & Larder BS. Rapid in vitro selection of human immunodeficiency virus type 1 resistant to 3′-thiacytidine inhibitors due to a mutation in the YMDD region of reverse transcriptase. *Proceedings of the National Academy of Sciences, USA* 1993; **90**:5653–5656.

78. Fischer KP & Tyrrell DLJ. Generation of duck hepatitis B virus polymerase mutants through site-directed mutagenesis which demonstrate resistance to lamivudine [(–)-β-L-2′,3′-dideoxy-3′-thiacytidine] in vitro. *Antimicrobial Agents and Chemotherapy* 1996; **40**:1957–1960.

79. Bartholomew MM, Jansen RW, Jeffers LJ, Reddy KR, Johnson LC, Bunzendahl H, Condreay LD, Tzakis AG, Schiff ER & Brown NA. Hepatitis-B-virus resistance to lamivudine given for recurrent infection after orthotopic liver transplantation. *Lancet* 1997; **349**:20–22.

80. Tipples GA, Ma MM, Fischer KP, Bain VG, Kneteman NM & Tyrrell DLJ. Mutation in HBV RNA-dependent DNA polymerase confers resistance to lamivudine *in vivo*. *Hepatology* 1996; **24**:714–717.

81. Ling R, Mutimer D, Ahmed M, Boxall EH, Elias E, Dusheiko GM & Harrison TJ. Selection of mutations in the hepatitis B virus polymerase during therapy of transplant recipients with lamivudine. *Hepatology* 1996; **24**:711–713.

82. Lai CL, Liaw YF, Leung NWY, Deslauriers M, Barnard J, Sanathanan L, Gray DF & Condreay LD. Genotypic resistance to lamivudine in a prospective, placebo-controlled multicentre study in Asia of lamivudine therapy for chronic hepatitis B infection: incidence,

kinetics of emergence and correlation with disease para-meters. *Hepatology* 1997; **26**:259A.

83. Shields PL, Ling R, Harrison T, Boxall E, Elias E & Mutimer DJ. Management and outcome of lamivudine (LAM)-resistant hepatitis B virus (HBV) infection after liver transplantation (LT). *Hepatology* 1997; **26**:260A.

84. Garrett L, Dienstag JL, Gauther J, Condreay L, Crowther L, Gelb L, Schiff ER & Brown N. Hepatitis B e-antigen (HBeAg) seroconversion in two patients with evidence of genotypic resistance following extended lamivudine treatment. *Hepatology* 1997; **26**:431A.

85. Melegari M, Scaglioni PP & Wands JR. Hepatitis B virus mutants associated with 3TC and famciclovir administration are replication defective. *Hepatology* 1997; **27**:628–633.

86. Naoumov NV, Chokshi S, Smith HM & Williams R. Emergence and characterization of lamivudine-resistant hepatitis B virus variant. *Hepatology* 1996; **24**:282A.

87. Girones R & Miller RH. Mutation rate of the hepadnavirus genome. *Virology* 1989; **170**:595–597.

88. Lee WM. Hepatitis B virus infection. *New England Journal of Medicine* 1997; **337**:1733–1745.

89. Allen MI, Deslauriers M, Andrews CW, Baldanti F, Tipples GA, Walters KA, Tyrrell DLJ & Brown N. Identification and biologic characterization of mutations in HBV resistant to lamivudine. *Hepatology* 1997; **26**: 430A.

90. Ono-Nita SK, Kato N, Shiratori Y & Omata M. Characteristic features among YMDD motif mutants of hepatitis B virus: replication and lamivudine resistance. *Hepatology* 1997; **26**:431A.

91. Fischer KP & Tyrrell DLJ. The lamivudine-resistant duck hepatitis B virus polymerase mutant, methionine 512 to valine (M512V), is susceptible to wild-type reversion *in vivo*. *Hepatology* 1997; **26**:430A.

92. Xiong X, Flores C, Gibbs C & Toole J. Lack of cross-resistance to PMEA for human hepatitis B DNA poly-merases which express lamivudine resistance codons. *Hepatology* 1997; **26**:431A.

93. Tyrrell DLJ, Robbins M, Condreay L & Fischer KP. Lamivudine-resistant virus in the duck model remains susceptible to 2-amino-6-methoxy-2',3'-dideoxypurine. *Hepatology* 1997; **26**:430A.

94. Fischer KP, Cheng YC & Tyrrell DLJ. The mutation in duck hepatitis B virus polymerase which confers resis-tance to lamivudine (beta-L-(–)-thiacytidine;-3TC) also confers cross-resistance to beta-L-dideoxy-5-fluorocyti-dine (FddC). *Hepatology* 1996; **24**:188A.

# 39 Treatment of chronic hepatitis B with famciclovir

## Christian Trepo* and Fabien Zoulim

## INTRODUCTION

Chronic hepatitis B virus (HBV) infection remains a major challenge since there is currently no safe or fully effective treatment. Interferon α (IFN-α) is the only antiviral compound licensed for the treatment of chronic hepatitis B [1], but clinical response rates are only 20–30% higher for IFN treatment than for placebo [2]. In addition, IFN-α treatment is associated with a range of dose-limiting side-effects, including bone marrow suppression, malaise and depression [3,4]. Furthermore, the need for parenteral administration of IFN-α means that therapy may be inconvenient for the patient. The majority of patients treated with IFN-α fail to respond [loss of hepatitis B e antigen (HBeAg)] and since HBV replication persists, these non-responders will be at risk of developing progressive liver disease and hepatocellular carcinoma.

Transplantation for endstage liver disease owing to chronic hepatitis B is frequently followed by recurrence of hepatitis B infection in the transplanted liver. The chronic hepatitis that develops in these patients follows a more aggressive course than is seen in non-immunocompromised subjects and this frequently results in graft failure. IFN-α therapy has limited clinical utility in these patients and may even be detrimental, since it may trigger graft rejection [5].

New therapies for chronic HBV infection are therefore required. New nucleoside analogues such as famciclovir (the prodrug of penciclovir), with proven efficacy against herpes simplex virus (HSV) and varicella-zoster virus (VZV), and lamivudine, with efficacy against human immunodeficiency virus (HIV), offer the most convenient, promising approaches to therapy [6] as oral alternatives to IFN-α.

Penciclovir, a purine nucleoside analogue [9-(4-hydroxy-3-hydroxymethylbut-1-yl)guanine; BRL 39123], is a highly selective antiviral agent, with potent activity against VZV and HSV-1 and HSV-2 [7–9]. Famciclovir is a diacetyl-6-deoxy oral derivative of penciclovir, and following oral administration is well absorbed (77% bioavailability) and converted by deacetylation to penciclovir as the major metabolite.

Penciclovir is then efficiently phosphorylated to the active metabolite, penciclovir-triphosphate, which has a prolonged intracellular half-life in VZV- and HSV-infected cells [10]. Famciclovir has been licensed in several countries for the treatment of acute herpes zoster and the treatment and suppression of recurrent genital herpes. Both famciclovir and the intravenous formulation penciclovir are currently undergoing regulatory review for treatment of herpesvirus infections in immunocompromised patients.

While clinical programmes for herpesvirus infections were underway, famciclovir was found to have activity against HBV in cell culture systems and in the Pekin duck infection model [11–14]. Preliminary observations in immunocompetent patients with chronic hepatitis B or HBV recurrence after liver transplant have shown encouraging results with famciclovir treatment in terms of antiviral activity and safety. This chapter will review the preclinical and clinical data on famciclovir in the treatment of chronic hepatitis B.

## PRECLINICAL STUDIES
### Cell culture

The HBV-producing human hepatoblastoma cell line, 2.2.15, was developed as an *in vitro* model of chronic HBV infection, and is established as a model that may predict an *in vivo* response to antiviral agents [15]. Penciclovir was found to be a potent and selective antiviral agent against intracellular HBV replication and extracellular virion release in this system [15]. Penciclovir also inhibited duck hepatitis B virus (DHBV) DNA replication *in vitro* in primary duck hepatocytes during continuous treatment of cultures [16]. In the same model, penciclovir also inhibited DHBV protein synthesis [16].

### Animal models

Results of *in vivo* experiments showed that the intraperitoneal administration of penciclovir induced a profound inhibition of viral DNA and protein

*Corresponding author

synthesis in Pekin ducks congenitally infected with DHBV [13]. Following 4 weeks of penciclovir treatment, molecular hybridization studies showed that intrahepatic viral DNA, RNA and protein levels were significantly reduced compared with those in placebo-treated controls. Synthesis of all viral replicative intermediates, including the recalcitrant viral supercoiled DNA species responsible for maintaining the replication cycle, was inhibited by penciclovir treatment [13]. These findings have also been confirmed in DHBV-infected Pekin ducks administered famciclovir [11–14].

Famciclovir treatment has also been shown to suppress HBV in chronically infected woodchucks at equivalent doses to those used in humans [17]. No significant toxicity was observed in either cell culture or in animal models of HBV infection.

## Mechanism of action

Penciclovir is a highly selective antiviral agent with activity against hepadnaviruses but which is non-toxic to replicating cells [8,18]. The mechanism of action involves transformation of penciclovir into the active triphosphate which subsequently interferes with HBV DNA synthesis. Penciclovir has multiple sites of action, inhibiting reverse transcription and the DNA polymerase at both the initiation and elongation steps [19]. Penciclovir-triphosphate has been shown to inhibit hepadnavirus reverse transcription by inhibiting the priming step for viral minus-strand DNA elongation [20]. In addition, penciclovir-triphosphate inhibits HBV replication by interfering with DNA chain elongation at the level of the viral DNA polymerase [14]. The action of penciclovir is highly selective, with a $K_i$ (inhibitory constant) for HBV DNA polymerase more than 4000 times that required to inhibit human cellular polymerases. In contrast to its anti-herpesvirus activity, (R)-penciclovir-triphosphate is a more efficient inhibitor of HBV polymerase than (S)-penciclovir-triphosphate [20].

## CLINICAL STUDIES

Early reports suggested that famciclovir may have clinical utility in the treatment of chronic hepatitis B in immunocompetent patients [21] and in liver transplant recipients with recurrent hepatitis B [22]. Additional studies have confirmed the initial findings and have found that famciclovir is well tolerated. The results from these clinical studies are discussed in detail below.

## Clinical studies of chronic hepatitis B

A placebo-controlled, double-blind pilot study showed a dose-dependent inhibitory effect on HBV replication, with a fall of HBV DNA levels by more than 90% following 1 week of treatment in six out of 11 evaluable patients receiving famciclovir at 250 mg or 500 mg three times daily. In contrast, no decrease in HBV DNA levels was observed in evaluable patients receiving placebo. Famciclovir was well tolerated and the fall in HBV DNA levels suggest a potential therapeutic benefit of more prolonged treatment in patients infected with HBV [21].

## Dose-finding studies

Following encouraging results in this pilot study, a large multicentre placebo-controlled dose-finding study was conducted, involving 64 centres and 333 patients [23]. A total of 41% of the patients had previously failed IFN-α treatment, and most had very high viral loads (median baseline viral DNA level 3600 pg/ml. During the 16 week course of famciclovir (125 mg, 250 mg or 500 mg three times daily), dose-dependent reductions in HBV DNA and serum alanine aminotransferase (ALT) were observed (Table 1). The effects of famciclovir on HBV DNA were apparent after 1 week of treatment. After cessation of therapy, viral replication resumed in the majority of patients, with a return of HBV DNA levels toward pretreatment values. In patients with baseline ALT levels (three times upper limit of normal) who received famciclovir 500 mg three times daily, median HBV DNA levels decreased by 92% ($P=0.007$, compared with placebo). A significant reduction in median ALT levels was also observed in the 500 mg treatment group at the end of the 8 month follow-up. In

**Table 1.** Percentage decrease from baseline in ALT levels during the double-blind phase in patients with screening values above the upper limit of normal

|  | Treatment group | |
|  | Famciclovir* | Placebo |
| --- | --- | --- |
| Treatment (week 12) | | |
| Median ALT decrease (%) | 31 | –4 |
| Number of patients | 53 | 51 |
| *P* value | 0.0001 | – |
| Follow-up week 52 | | |
| Median ALT decrease (%) | 36 | –8 |
| Number of patients | 44 | 47 |
| *P* value | 0.0043 | – |

*Dosage 500 mg three times daily.

addition, HBeAg seroconversion was observed in a significant number of patients receiving 500 mg three times daily compared with placebo ($P = 0.04$) (Table 2) [24]. Furthermore, Asian patients, patients infected at birth or during early childhood and non-responders to IFN-$\alpha$ treatment, responded as well as the total population. Famciclovir was well tolerated and there were no serious side-effects in the treatment groups compared with placebo. Most importantly, there were no episodes of severe hepatic decompensation following cessation of famciclovir treatment.

## Treatment and prevention of hepatitis B recurrence in liver transplant recipients

Following the initial favourable report by Boker *et al.* [22], describing famciclovir efficacy in a liver transplant recipient with fulminant recurrent hepatitis B, Krüger *et al.* [25] described 12 patients treated with famciclovir 500 mg three times daily for up to 30 months for HBV recurrence after orthotopic liver transplantation. Famciclovir treatment was associated with reductions from baseline in serum viral DNA levels of 90% at 6 months and 95% at 12 months. Serum ALT levels continuously decreased from baseline in six of the 12 treated patients. In addition, there were no clinically significant side-effects. The authors concluded that famciclovir was a promising antiviral strategy for the treatment of HBV in immunocompromised patients.

Encouraging results were also observed by Haller *et al.* [26], who described 18 patients receiving oral famciclovir 500 mg three times daily for the treatment of HBV reinfection after liver transplantation. HBV DNA values were decreased to undetectable levels in eight out of 18 patients studied. In addition, the clinical status improved in seven patients, based on normalization of transaminases, bilirubin and prothrombin time. Overall, when famciclovir was initiated early after reinfection, a response rate of approximately 66% was observed. Famciclovir was again well tolerated in all patients.

To determine whether famciclovir, administered prior to liver transplantation, was effective in inhibiting HBV replication in patients with end-stage liver disease caused by chronic hepatitis B with detectable HBV DNA levels, a pilot study was undertaken in eight patients. Following a 6 month course of famciclovir, an initial decline in HBV DNA titres occurred in all eight patients and 25% (2/8) of the patients became HBV DNA-negative and underwent liver transplantation. Both patients developed anti-HBs antibodies by the end of the 6 month treatment and remain HBV DNA-negative after nearly 2 years of

**Table 2.** Proportion of patients with HBe seroconversion during the double-blind phase

| HBe seroconversion | Famciclovir* | Placebo† |
|---|---|---|
| End of treatment | 0 | 0 |
| Total number of patients | 64 | 58 |
| End of follow-up | 4 (7%) | 0 |
| Total number of patients | 56 | 50 |
| End of open label phase | 5 | 2 |
| Total number of patients | 42 | 32 |
| Total‡ | 9/64 | 2/58 |

*Dosage 500 mg three times daily; $n = 83$.
†$n = 82$.
‡$P = 0.05$.

follow-up. Adverse effects attributable to famciclovir were not observed in any of the patients [27].

The initially reported experience for famciclovir treatment has now been extended to include 107 patients with HBV recurrence after orthotopic liver transplantation [28]. All patients received famciclovir at a dosage of 500 mg three times daily. Fifty-two patients received famciclovir for more than 1 year and 20 patients were under drug therapy for at least 2 years. In this cohort of patients, a median reduction of HBV DNA of 95% at 1 year and 99% at 2 years following the start of famciclovir treatment was observed, while the median reduction of ALT levels was 58% and 90% at 1 and 2 years, respectively. Famciclovir treatment was well tolerated, with some patients continuing treatment for up to 4 years.

## Other studies

HBV-associated periarteritis nodosa is another clinical situation where the patient may benefit from potent antiviral therapy, rather than traditional immunosuppressive therapy which may enhance viral replication [2,29]. Famciclovir combined with IFN-$\alpha$ was used successfully to treat a case of periarteritis nodosa that failed to respond to IFN-$\alpha$ and corticosteroid therapy [29]. A reduction in viral replication and an improvement in blood pressure, and symptoms of arthralgia and fatigue were noted within 4 weeks of starting famciclovir. Famciclovir therapy was continued for a total of 3–4 years and was found to be well tolerated.

## COMPARISON WITH OTHER NUCLEOSIDE ANALOGUES

Several nucleoside analogues have been evaluated or are being developed as potential therapies for chronic HBV infection [6]. Currently, famciclovir and lamivudine are at the most advanced stages of development for the treatment of chronic hepatitis B. In clinical studies, lamivudine has been shown to have potent antiviral activity in patients with chronic hepatitis B. Lamivudine inhibits reverse transcription and HBV replication, thus preventing translation of an RNA pre-genome to a complementary DNA molecule [30].

## Safety and post-treatment flares

Dose-finding clinical studies with lamivudine have found that short-term therapy (16–32 weeks) is well tolerated and induces a dose-dependent inhibition of viral replication [31]. Further studies have found lamivudine therapy to be well tolerated for longer dosing periods of up to 18 months [32,33]. However, reports of severe hepatic flares have been reported following discontinuation of lamivudine therapy [34,35]. In two cases, the post-treatment flare was associated with decompensation of liver disease and jaundice [36].

Famciclovir is well tolerated, with a safety profile comparable to that of placebo in studies of immunocompetent patients [23,37]. The overall incidence of serious adverse events was low and similar for the famciclovir and placebo groups. In addition, there were no reports of severe hepatic decompensation after discontinuing famciclovir treatment. These results are in agreement with the safety experience in liver transplant patients, where patients were treated with famciclovir at 500 mg three times daily for 1–4 years [28,29]. It has been proposed that differences in post-treatment flares between famciclovir and lamivudine may be due to differences in the mode of action, including balance between viral products and inhibition of supercoiled DNA for famciclovir (S Locarnini, personal communication). In addition, famciclovir did not result in the adverse events associated with fialuridine therapy (refractory lactic acidosis, hepatic and renal failure, pancreatitis or myopathy) [38].

## Rate of anti-HBe seroconversion

In the study by Trepo *et al.* [24], a significant proportion of patients treated with famciclovir at 500 mg three times daily lost HBeAg and developed HBeAb at the end of the study period compared with placebo ($P=0.04$). These results suggest that famciclovir has potential for HBV eradication in addition to viral suppression. This level of seroconversion is comparable to the seroconversion rates for patients treated with IFN-$\alpha$ and lamivudine for at least 1 year [32,34,36,39]. Seroconversion rates for famciclovir were especially encouraging considering that patients in this study were traditionally difficult to treat (low ALT levels, high HBV DNA levels, prior IFN-$\alpha$ treatment).

## Viral resistance to nucleoside analogues

The first cases of HBV breakthrough (resistance) were described in patients treated with lamivudine for at least 6 months for HBV recurrence after liver transplantation or as prophylaxis to prevent HBV recurrence on the liver graft [40–44]. Breakthrough rates for lamivudine have in general varied from 17–30% of treated patients [35].

HBV breakthrough has also been observed in transplant patients treated with famciclovir on compassionate use for HBV recurrence [45–47]. In contrast to the sites of mutations associated with lamivudine resistance, located in the catalytic site (the YMDD motif within domain C of the viral polymerase; M550 [40,48]), famciclovir breakthrough has mainly been associated with mutations in the B domain of the HBV polymerase. The mutations in domain B have occurred following long-term therapy in immunocompromised patients [44]. In addition, unlike lamivudine, famciclovir breakthrough has not been associated with sequence changes in the catalytic domain of the viral polymerase, such as M550I or M550V. A large programme is now in place to characterize more fully HBV resistance to famciclovir.

Following previous experience of antiviral therapy for HIV infection [49], combination therapy is being proposed as an approach for the management of chronic hepatitis B, by taking advantage of different modes of inhibition of the HBV DNA polymerase to produce an additive or synergistic antiviral effect. Combination therapy could therefore potentially prevent or delay the emergence of resistant mutants [49,50]. In this respect, a combination of two nucleoside analogues could be evaluated in clinical trials for their ability to prevent the emergence of resistant mutants and eradicate viral infection [51].

Strategies employing the manipulation of the host immune responses against HBV by IFN-$\alpha$ in combination with nucleoside analogues are also being studied [52,53].

## SUMMARY

Famciclovir is the oral prodrug of penciclovir, a purine nucleoside analogue with demonstrated efficacy for the

treatment of herpes simplex and herpes zoster infections, and potent *in vitro* and *in vivo* activity in cell culture and in the Pekin duck infection model. Famciclovir was highly effective at reducing HBV DNA and serum ALT levels in patients with chronic HBV infection, including those previously treated with IFN-α. Sustained normalization of ALT levels and/or significant rates of seroconversion were observed. In addition, famciclovir has been used to treat HBV recurrence in liver transplant recipients for up to 4 years.

Famciclovir was well tolerated, with an adverse event profile similar to placebo. In contrast to other nucleoside analogues, there was no evidence of liver decompensation post-treatment. Published data indicate that the clinical and molecular features of famciclovir resistance differ to those of lamivudine. Combination therapy with nucleoside analogues offers the potential for increased antiviral efficacy and prevention or delay in the emergence of resistant mutants.

# REFERENCES

1. Perrillo RP, Schiff ER, Davis GL, Bodenheimer HC Jr, Lindsay K, Payne J *et al.* A randomised, controlled study of interferon alfa-2b alone and after prednisone withdrawal for the treatment of chronic hepatitis B. *New England Journal of Medicine* 1990; **323**:295–301.
2. Wong DKH, Cheung AM, O'Rourke K, Naylor CD, Detsky AS & Heathcote J. Effect of alpha-interferon treatment in patients with hepatitis Be antigen-positive chronic hepatitis B: a meta-analysis. *Annal of Internal Medicine* 1993; **119**:312–323.
3. Carithers RL. Effect of interferon on hepatitis B. *Lancet* 1998; **351**:157.
4. Hoofnagle JH & Di Bisceglie AM. The treatment of chronic viral hepatitis. *New England Journal of Medicine* 1997; **336**:347–356.
5. Feray C, Samuel D, Gigou M, Paradis V, David MF, Lemonnier C *et al.* An open trial of interferon alfa recombinant for hepatitis C after liver transplantation: antiviral effects of risk of rejection. *Hepatology* 1995; **22**:1084–1089.
6. Zoulim F & Trepo C. Nucleoside analogs in the treatment of chronic viral hepatitis. Efficiency and complications. *Journal of Hepatology* 1994; **21**:142–144.
7. Boyd M, Bacon T, Sutton D & Cole M. Antiherpes virus activity of 9-(4-hydroxy-3-hydroxy-methylbut-1-yl)guanine (BRL 39123) in cell culture. *Antimicrobial Agents and Chemotherapy* 1987; **31**:1238–1242.
8. Vere Hodge R & Perkins R. Mode of action of 9-(4-hydroxy-3-hydroxymethylbut-1-yl) guanine (BRL 39123) against herpes simplex virus in MRC-5 cells. *Antimicrobial Agents and Chemotherapy* 1989; **33**:223–229.
9. Earnshaw D, Bacon T, Darlison S, Edmonds K, Perkins R & Vere Hodge R. Mode of antiviral action of penciclovir in MRC-5 cells infected with herpes simplex virus type 1 (HSV-1), HSV-2, and varicella-zoster virus. *Antimicrobial Agents and Chemotherapy* 1992; **36**:2747–2757.
10. Cirelli R, Herne K, McCrary M, Lee P & Tyring S.

Famciclovir: review of clinical efficacy and safety. *Antiviral Research* 1996; **29**:141–151.
11. Tsiquaye KN, Slomka MJ & Maung M. Oral famciclovir against duck hepatitis B virus replication in hepatic and nonhepatic tissues of ducklings infected in ovo. *Journal of Medical Virology* 1994; **42**:306–310.
12. Tsiquaye KN, Sutton D, Maung M & Boyd M. Antiviral activities and pharmacokinetics of penciclovir and famciclovir in Pekin ducks chronically infected with duck hepatitis B virus. *Antiviral Chemistry & Chemotherapy* 1996; **7**:153–159.
13. Lin E, Luscombe C, Wang Y, Shaw T & Locarnini S. The guanine nucleoside analog penciclovir is active against chronic duck hepatitis B virus infection *in vivo*. *Antimicrobial Agents and Chemotherapy* 1996; **40**:413–418.
14. Shaw T, Mok SS & Locarnini SA. Inhibition of hepatitis B virus DNA polymerase by enantiomers of penciclovir triphosphate and metabolic basis for selective inhibition of HBV replication by penciclovir. *Hepatology* 1996; **24**:996–1002.
15. Korba BE & Boyd M. Penciclovir is a selective inhibitor of hepatitis B virus replication in cultured human hepatoblastoma cells. *Antimicrobial Agents and Chemotherapy* 1996; **40**:1282–1284.
16. Shaw T, Amor P, Civitico G, Boyd M & Locarnini S. *In vitro* antiviral activity of penciclovir, a novel purine nucleoside, against duck hepatitis B virus. *Antimicrobial Agents and Chemotherapy* 1994; **38**:719–723.
17. Korba BE, Baldwin B, Cote P, Schinazi R, Gangemi D, Gerin JL *et al.* Effectiveness of combination therapies with 3TC, famciclovir, and alpha-interferon against woodchuck hepatitis virus replication in chronically-infected woodchucks: model for potential anti-HBV treatments. *37th Interscience Conference on Antimicrobial Agents and Chemotherapy*, Toronto, Canada, 28 September–1 October 1997; Abstract H-34.
18. Boyd MR. Update on famciclovir. In *Antiviral Chemotherapy: New Directions for Clinical Applications and Research*, 3rd edn, 1993; pp. 83–95. Edited by J Mills & L Corey. New Jersey: PTR Prentice Hall.
19. Zoulim F. Improving hepatitis B virus therapy– new inhibitors of reverse transcriptase. *International Antiviral News* 1997; **5**:110–112.
20. Dannaoui E, Trepo C & Zoulim F. Inhibitory effect of penciclovir-triphosphate on duck hepatitis B virus reverse transcription. *Antiviral Chemistry and Chemotherapy* 1997; **8**:38–46.
21. Main J, Brown JL, Howells C, Galassini R, Crossey M, Karayiannis P *et al.* A double blind, placebo-controlled study to assess the effect of famciclovir on virus replication in patients with chronic hepatitis B virus infection. *Journal of Viral Hepatitis* 1996; **3**:211–215.
22. Boker KH, Ringe B, Krüger M, Pichlmayr R & Manns MP. Prostaglandin E plus famciclovir– a new concept for the treatment of severe hepatitis B after liver transplantation. *Transplantation* 1994; **57**:1706–1708.
23. Trepo C, Jezek P, Atkinson GF & Boon RJ. Efficacy of famciclovir in chronic hepatitis B: results of a dose finding study. *Hepatology* 1996; **24** (Suppl. 4, Part 2): Abstract 247.
24. Trepo C, Jezek P, Atkinson GF & Boon RJ. Long term efficacy of famciclovir (FCV) in chronic hepatitis B: results of a Phase IIB study. *Journal of Hepatology* 1997; **26** (Suppl. 1): Abstract WP3/22.
25. Krüger M, Tillmann HL, Trautwein C, Bode U, Oldhafer K, Maschek H *et al.* Famciclovir treatment of

hepatitis B virus recurrence after liver transplantation: a pilot study. *Liver Transplantation Surgery* 1996; **2**:253–363.

26. Haller GW, Bechstein WO, Neuhaus R, Raakow R, Berg T, Hopf U *et al*. Famciclovir therapy for recurrent hepatitis B virus infection after liver transplantation. *Transplant International* 1996; **9** (Suppl. 1):S210–212.

27. Singh N, Gayowski T, Wannstedt CF, Wagener MM & Marino IR. Pretransplant famciclovir as prophylaxis for hepatitis B virus recurrence after liver transplantation. *Transplantation* 1997; **63**:1415–1419.

28. Neuhaus P, Manns M & Atkinson G. Safety and efficacy of famciclovir for the treatment of recurrent hepatitis B in liver transplant recipients. *Hepatology* 1997; **26** (Suppl. 4, Part 2): Abstract 528.

29. Krüger M, Böker KHW, Zeidler H & Manns M. Treatment of hepatitis B-related polyarteritis nodosa with famciclovir and interferon alfa-2b. *Journal of Hepatology* 1997; **26**:935–939.

30. Chang CN, Skalski V, Hua Zhou J & Cheng Y. Biochemical pharmacology of (+)- and (–)-2′,3′-dideoxy-3′-thiacytidine as anti-hepatitis virus agents. *Journal of Biological Chemistry* 1992; **267**:22414–22420.

31. Dienstag JL, Perillo R, Schiff ER, Bartholomew M, Vicary C & Rubin M. A preliminary trial of lamivudine for chronic hepatitis B infection. *New England Journal of Medicine* 1995; **333**:1657–1661.

32. Lai CL, Law YF, Leung NWY, Deslauriers M, Barnard J, Sanathanan L *et al*. Genotypic resistance to lamivudine in a prospective, placebo-controlled multicenter study in Asia of lamivudine therapy for chronic hepatitis B infection: incidence, kinetics of emergence and correlation with disease parameters. *Hepatology* 1997; **26** (Suppl. 4, Part 2): Abstract 522.

33. Dienstag JL, Schiff ER, Mitchell M, Gitlin N, Lisoos T, Condreay L *et al*. Extended lamivudine retreatment for chronic hepatitis B. *Hepatology* 1996; **24**: Abstract 245.

34. Honkoop P, de Man RA, Heijtink RA & Schalm SW. Hepatitis B reactivation after lamivudine. *Lancet* 1995; **346**:1156–1157.

35. Honkoop P, Niesters HGM, de Man RAM, Osterhaus ADME & Schalm SW. Lamivudine resistance in immunocompetent chronic hepatitis B: incidence and patterns. *Journal of Hepatology* 1997; **26**:1393–1395.

36. Nevens F, Main J, Honkoop P, Tyrrell DL, Barber J, Sullivan MT *et al*. Lamivudine therapy for chronic hepatitis B: a six month randomised dose-ranging study. *Gastroenterology* 1997; **113**:1258–1263.

37. Boon RJ, Saltzman R & Atkinson GF. The clinical safety experience with famciclovir. *Hepatology* 1996; **24** (Suppl. 4, Part 2): Abstract 623.

38. McKenzie R, Fried MW, Sallie R, Conjeevaram H, Di Bisceglie AM, Park Y *et al*. Hepatic failure and lactic acidosis due to fialuridine (FIAU), an investigational nucleoside analog for chronic hepatitis B. *New England Journal of Medicine* 1995; **333**:1099–1105.

39. Saracco G & Rozzetto M. A practical guide to the use of interferons in the management of hepatitis virus infections. *Drugs* 1997; **53**:74–85.

40. Ling R, Mutimer D, Ahmed M, Boxall EH, Elias E, Dusheiko GM *et al*. Selection of mutations in the hepatitis B virus polymerase during therapy of transplant recipients with lamivudine. *Hepatology* 1996; **24**:711–713.

41. Perillo R, Rakela J, Martin P, Wright T, Levy G, Schiff E *et al*. Lamivudine for suppression and/or prevention of hepatitis B when given pre-/post-liver transplantation (OLT). *Hepatology* 1997; **26** (Suppl. 4, Part 2): Abstract 526.

42. Perillo R, Rakela J, Martin P, Levy G, Schiff E, Wright T *et al*. Long-term lamivudine therapy of patients with recurrent hepatitis B post-liver transplantation. *Hepatology* 1997; **26** (Suppl. 4, Part 2): Abstract 196.

43. Locarnini SA & Newbold JE. Chronic hepatitis B: the therapeutic challenge. *Journal of Antimicrobial Chemotherapy* 1997; **39**:559–562.

44. Shields PL, Ling R, Harrison T, Boxall E, Elias E & Mutimer DJ. Management and outcome of lamivudine resistant hepatitis B virus infection after liver transplantation. *Hepatology* 1997; **26** (Suppl. 4, Part 2): Abstract 527.

45. Bartholomeusz A & Locarnini S. Mutations in the hepatitis B virus polymerase gene that are associated with resistance to famciclovir and lamivudine. *International Antiviral News* 1997; **5**:123–124.

46. Bartholomeusz A, Groenen LC & Locarnini SA. Clinical experience with famciclovir against hepatitis B virus and development of resistance. *Intervirology* 1997; (in press).

47. Aye TT, Bartholomeusz A, Shaw T, Bowden S, Breschkin A, McMillan J *et al*. Hepatitis B virus polymerase mutations during antiviral therapy in a patient following liver transplantation. *Journal of Hepatology* 1997; **26**:1148–1153.

48. Tipples GA, Ma MM, Fischer KP, Bain VG, Kneteman NM & Tyrrell DL. Mutation in HBV RNA-dependent DNA polymerase confers resistance to lamivudine *in vivo*. *Hepatology* 1996; **24**:714–717.

49. Zoulim F & Trepo C. Drug therapy for chronic hepatitis B: antiviral efficacy and influence of hepatitis B virus polymerase mutations on the outcome of therapy. *Journal of Hepatology* 1998; (in press).

50. Fontana RJ & Lok ASF. Combination therapy for chronic hepatitis B. *Hepatology* 1997; **26**:234–237.

51. McCaughan G, Angus P, Bowden S, Shaw T, Breschkin A, Sheil R & Locarnini S. Retransplantation for precore mutant-related chronic hepatitis B infection: prolonged survival in a patient receiving sequential ganciclovir/famciclovir therapy. *Liver Transplantation Surgery* 1996; **2**:472–474.

52. Marques AR, Lau D, McKenzie R, Straus S & Hoofnagle J. Combination therapy with famciclovir and interferon for the treatment of chronic hepatitis B. *37th Interscience Conference on Antimicrobial Agents and Chemotherapy*, Toronto, Canada, 28 September–1 October 1997; Abstract H-35.

53. Piqueras Alcoh B, Salcedo M, Banares R, Garcia-Duran F, Banos E, De Diego A, Roldan PP, Cos E & Clemente G. Famciclovir plus interferon in the management of a patient with chronic hepatitis B and severe liver failure. *Revista Espanola de Enfermedades Digestivas* 1997; **89**:217–221.

# 40 Treatment of chronic hepatitis C with interferon: 1998 update

Thierry Poynard\*, Joseph Moussali, Thierry Thevenot, Vlad Ratziu and Pierre Opolon

## SUMMARY

The standard regimen of interferon α (IFN-α) used to treat patients with chronic hepatitis C was initially 3 MU three times a week for 6 months, and then moved to a longer duration of at least 12 months. Recently, evidence has accumulated indicating a greater efficacy on the eradication of hepatitis C virus (HCV) when a combination of ribavirin and IFN is given. The results are clear for relapsers after a first treatment with IFN of 3 MU three times a week. In the next few months, results of this combination therapy will be known for therapy-naive patients. For patients without sustained virus eradication, several studies have suggested that IFN could block progression of fibrosis. Trials of combination therapies should now be performed in these non-responders.

## INTRODUCTION

Chronic hepatitis C is a major healthcare problem throughout the world. The disease is often asymptomatic, but may progress to cirrhosis in 20% of cases and thereafter to cirrhosis complications: hepatocellular carcinoma (HCC; 5% incidence per year), digestive haemorrhage and hepatocellular insufficiency. IFN-α is the only drug approved for the treatment of hepatitis C in Europe and North America. Since 1986 IFN-α has been evaluated thoroughly and has been confirmed as the basic treatment for hepatitis C [1]. Its effectiveness appears to be related to dose and duration of therapy. The best efficacy/risk ratio seems to be 3 MU three times per week on a 12 month schedule. With this regimen, a sustained alanine aminotransferase (ALT) response is achieved in nearly 35% of patients [2]. In the last few years, two concepts have emerged. The first is that in patients without prolonged viral eradication (non-responders), the fibrosis progression rate can be reduced by IFN in comparison to controls (Fig. 1). The second is that ribavirin has emerged as potentially the

second most effective drug. Disappointing in monotherapy, ribavirin appears very effective in combination with IFN.

The antiviral activity of IFN is based on the inhibition of all phases of viral interactions within cells, including viral entry, viral uncoating and synthesis of mRNA and proteins [3]. IFN-α may also have antifibrotic effects [4]. A decrease in perisinusoidal cell activation and an activation of collagenase should decrease collagen synthesis. Various patterns of response to treatment may be considered.

## BIOCHEMICAL RESPONSE

A complete biochemical response is defined as the normalization of serum ALT levels. The persistence of a response at least 6 months after arrest of therapy is generally defined as a sustained biochemical response. Early randomized trials have documented that a minimum dose of 3 MU of IFN given three times a

**Figure 1.** Progression of HCV-associated liver fibrosis in non-responders to IFN in comparison to responders and to matched controls

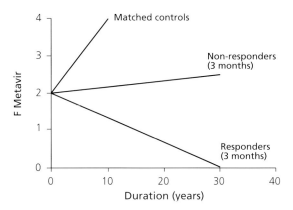

Adopted from [59]. F metavir scoring system: FO, no fibrosis; F1, portal fibrosis; F2, few septa; F3, many septa; F4, cirrhosis.

---

\*Corresponding author

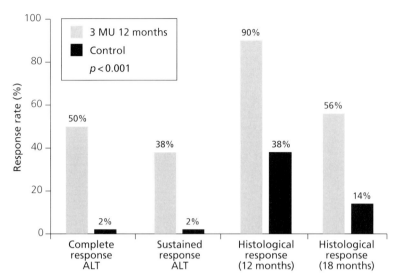

Figure 2. Meta-analysis of randomized trials comparing IFN at 3 MU three times a week for 12 months to controls

week for 6 months is effective in inducing a biochemical response, sustained remission and histological improvement in a significant proportion of patients. With this regimen, approximately half of the treated patients respond, with serum ALT values becoming normal; however only 20 to 25% maintain the response after stopping treatment. Further strategies tested higher doses of IFN or an extended duration of treatment or both. Although some studies described no benefit of escalating the dosage of IFN in increasing the response rates [5,6], other trials documented improvement in response rates with higher doses [7–11] or with high induction doses [12]. This was particularly true in patients infected with HCV genotype 1b, whose sustained response rate increased from 16% with 3 MU three times a week for 12 months to 28% with 6 MU [13]. The benefit of extended duration of treatment in increasing sustained response rates has been assessed in many studies [14–17]. Additional courses at the same dose in relapsers increased the sustained response rate [17]. Meta-analysis showed a significant dose effect (6 MU compared with 3 MU three times per week) upon the sustained response rate at 12 months, with a mean 18% increase (46% versus 28%; $P<0.001$), but not at 6 months [2]. There was a significant duration effect (12 months compared with 6 months) on the sustained response rate both at a dose of 3 MU three times a week, with a mean 21% increase (35% versus 14%; $P<0.001$) (Fig. 2), and at a dose of 6 MU three times per week, with a mean 20% increase (49% versus 29%; $P=0.003$). Finally, taking into account the side-effects of high-dose IFN therapy, the best efficacy/risk ratio seemed to favour 3 MU three times per week for at least 12 months in patients with

chronic hepatitis C who had never been treated with IFN [2]. With this regimen, the rate of sustained biochemical response was 38% [2] (Fig. 2).

## VIROLOGICAL RESPONSE

IFN therapy induces a significant decrease in HCV RNA titres compared to pretreatment values [18]. It was demonstrated among most responders that a decrease in viraemia was correlated with an ALT decrease [19]. Nevertheless, a discrepancy between biochemical and virological responses was observed. HCV RNA disappeared in 60% to 80% of complete ALT responders and in 60% to 100% of sustained ALT responders [13,18,20–22]. The persistence of HCV RNA in complete ALT responders was usually associated with relapse [13,21,22]. In contrast, elimination of viraemia generally predicted a sustained response. Undetectable HCV RNA at early time points between 4 and 12 weeks after the beginning of treatment forecast sustained virological responses after treatment with IFN [23,24]. The disappearance of HCV RNA from serum was usually associated with the disappearance from the liver and from peripheral blood mononuclear cells [25,26]. As demonstrated with the biochemical response, the duration and dose of IFN appeared to affect the virological response. The residual viraemia level after treatment was significantly lower in patients treated at 3 MU for 18 months than in patients treated at the same dose for 6 months or at a lower dose for 12 months ($P=0.008$) [14]. After 6 months of treatment, HCV RNA became undetectable in 48% of patients treated at 6 MU, as compared with 23% of patients treated at 3 MU ($P<0.05$) [19]. Among biochemical non-responders, it

**Figure 3.** Modelling of liver fibrosis progression in 1157 patients with chronic hepatitis C

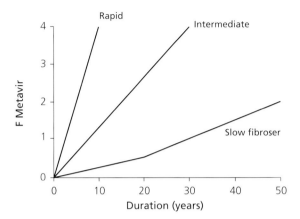

Adopted from [27]

seems likely that the viral load diminishes significantly, although it is not totally eradicated [13,18,19].

## HISTOLOGICAL FINDINGS

Subjects infected with HCV do not die from viraemia or elevated ALT, but rather from the complications of cirrhosis. We have identified three groups of patients (each of the same size) according to the fibrosis progression rate. Only one third of infected patients will not progress to cirrhosis (Fig. 3). Independent factors associated with an increased rate of fibrosis progression include: age at infection higher than 40 years, heavy alcohol consumption and male sex [27] (Fig. 4). Therefore, one further primary prognostic goal should be the reduction in fibrosis progression. Unfortunately, it was difficult in randomized trials to obtain a second biopsy in nearly half of the patients, even in trials that focused on histological criteria [2]. Nevertheless, it is clear that histological activity (necrosis and inflammation) and fibrosis are significantly improved in sustained biochemical responders to IFN therapy [9,16,21,22]. In the subgroup of transient biochemical responders, histological activity decreased significantly, while fibrosis remained stable or was slightly improved [13,16]. Controversy persists concerning the histological outcome of biochemical non-responders to IFN. Several studies have pointed out significant improvement in liver lesions and greater efficacy of long-term treatment with IFN, even in patients without normalization of ALT [14,28–30]. This may be explained by the reduction in viral load, although it is not totally eradicated [14,18] or by the antifibrotic effect of IFN. On the other hand, a recent meta-analysis [31] of 17

trials involving 1223 individuals has shown that patients treated with IFN as compared to controls had significant improvement in Knodell's total hepatitis activity index (–0.82; $P<0.0001$) and fibrosis score (–0.20; $P<0.01$). In the subgroup of trials reporting histological changes in biochemical non-responders, there was no significant histological improvement. From our point of view, this 'negative' observation on a small subgroup of patients is not proof of a lack of efficacy, since the statistical power is very low, the fibrosis scoring system by Knodell's index is not sensitive and linear, and patients with cirrhosis were not excluded. Thus, controversy remains concerning histological improvement in non-responders. Further studies with numerous patients undergoing pre- and post-treatment liver biopsies are needed to evaluate this important endpoint. As demonstrated for the biochemical response, it appears that reinforced regimens increase the histological response in treated patients and might significantly decrease the incidence of cirrhosis. In the large scale randomized study we published [19], 69% of patients treated at 3 MU for 18 months had improved histological activity as compared to 47% of patients ($P=0.02$) treated at a lower dose for the same duration and 38% of patients ($P<0.001$) treated at 3 MU for 6 months. In another large-scale randomized study [32], the incidence of cirrhosis in patients treated at 3 MU for 6 months was 10% as compared to 1% ($P=0.001$) in patients treated with a higher dose (6 MU followed by 3 MU) for 12 months. If a reinforced regimen decreases the incidence of cirrhosis when compared to 6 months of treatment, the result should be even better when compared to no treatment.

**Figure 4.** Risk groups among 1157 patients with chronic hepatitis C

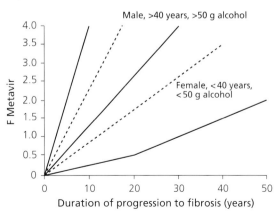

Adapted from [27]

## OTHER EFFECTS

In patients with chronic hepatitis C, HCC occurs in 5% of cases, almost all of which are associated with cirrhosis. Recent studies suggest that IFN treatment in patients with HCV infection and cirrhosis significantly decreases the incidence of HCC [33,34] and improves liver function [34] as compared to untreated patients. This occurs despite low biochemical response rates in cirrhotic patients as compared to patients without cirrhosis [34,35], and even in patients for whom IFN is judged ineffective according to the biochemical response [33,34]. In a prospective randomized controlled trial involving 90 patients with compensated HCV cirrhosis, the incidence of HCC was 4% in IFN-treated patients as compared to 38% in control patients ($P=0.002$), while the sustained ALT response rate was 8% in treated patients as compared to 0% in control patients [34]. Most retrospective studies also suggest that IFN decreases mortality related to primary liver cancer and to other complications of cirrhosis [36]. It has also been suggested that treatment for 18–24 months with IFN in patients with mild chronic hepatitis C might further prolong life expectancy as compared to a 6 month treatment or no treatment. In that study, the increase in life expectancy in patients younger than 70 years was achieved at a reasonable marginal cost-effectiveness ratio [37].

## PREDICTORS OF RESPONSE

Most predictors have been assessed in patients treated with short duration IFN therapy and using ALT normalization as the endpoint. Low pretreatment HCV RNA levels [38–41] and genotypes other than 1b [40,41] are predictive factors of a sustained ALT response. In patients with HCV genotype 1b infection, a substantial correlation between the ALT response to IFN and genomic diversity characterized by mutations in the NS5A gene was suggested [42,43], but this correlation was not shown in other studies [44]. In many 6 month studies, it has been shown that the presence of cirrhosis significantly decreases the sustained ALT response rate to less than 10% [3,35]. However, when the histological response is considered, long-term IFN treatment can improve inflammation and necrosis lesions in comparison to a short duration regimen [19]. To be of practical interest, predictors should also have high negative predictive values. Based on published studies, it is impossible to exclude patients from treatment according to these factors. Future studies should assess the predictive value of factors according to the reduction in liver fibrosis progression in patients treated for 12 months.

## RIBAVIRIN

Ribavirin, a synthetic purine nucleoside, exerts broad-spectrum antiviral activity against RNA and DNA viruses after intracellular phosphorylation, without an apparent development of resistance. The primary action of ribavirin seems to lead to intracellular virustasis of most susceptible viruses, rather than intracellular virucidal activity or induction of IFN. Antiviral effects are produced through three different mechanisms [45]: (i) depletion of the intracellular pool of GTP via inhibition of inosinate dehydrogenase; (ii) interruption of viral mRNA synthesis by incorporation of ribavirin metabolites into viral RNA; and (iii) direct inhibition of the virus-encoded RNA polymerases. Ribavirin may also have a mild inhibitory effect on host immune responses. Several studies have been conducted to evaluate ribavirin monotherapy in daily doses of 600–1200 mg in the treatment of chronic hepatitis C. The results consistently showed that ALT levels decreased in all patients [46,47] and fell into the normal range in about 30% of patients during treatment periods of 12 to 48 weeks, but relapsed quickly in almost all patients after treatment was stopped [46–48]. In addition, there was no effect on HCV RNA in treated patients as compared to untreated patients, and the disappearance of HCV RNA was not observed [49,50]. When given for more than 6 months, ribavirin was associated with minor histological improvement in liver biopsy samples [48,49]. In a randomized trial comparing ribavirin monotherapy to IFN in naive patients [51], there were significant differences in favour of IFN based on the complete ALT response rate (56% versus 22%), the sustained ALT response rate (22% versus 0%), and viral eradication (22% versus 0%). Thus, ribavirin alone had only an incomplete, transient beneficial effect on the ALT response. It had lower efficacy than IFN. Further studies are needed to evaluate its efficacy in terms of histology over a long-term regimen, specifically in patients with contraindication to IFN.

## COMBINATION THERAPY WITH IFN AND RIBAVIRIN

Four relatively small trials [50–54] and a meta-analysis strongly suggested that the sustained response rate was significantly higher for IFN plus ribavirin combination therapy than for IFN or ribavirin monotherapy. It has been estimated that the probability of a sustained response following IFN–ribavirin combination therapy is 51% for patients without previous IFN therapy, 52% for patients with previous IFN therapy and response–relapse and 16% for previous IFN non-responders. These results consistently indicated a syner-

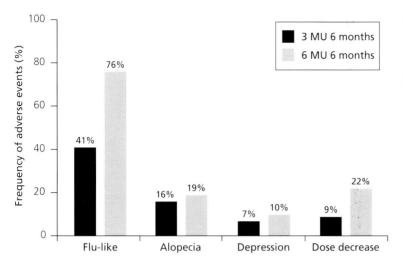

**Figure 5.** Adverse events according to the dose of IFN

Dose decrease refers to the percentage of patients for whom the dose was reduced during trials.

gistic effect between ribavirin and IFN in patients previously untreated with IFN or previously treated with no response or a only transient response. Furthermore, two large-scale randomized trials have recently confirmed the benefit of the IFN–ribavirin combination in relapsers with a 49% sustained response (HCV RNA disappearance and normal ALT and histological improvement) 6 months after the end of combination therapy versus 5% in the IFN group [55].

## SIDE-EFFECTS OF THERAPY

IFN is generally well tolerated at a standard regimen. Side-effects are dose- and duration-dependent (Fig. 5) and are generally reversible after arrest of therapy. The most commonly observed side-effects include fatigue, myalgia, mental disorders, alopecia, haematological changes (especially granulocytopenia and thrombopenia) and thyroid dysfunction [2]. Adverse reactions to ribavirin are generally mild and fully reversible. The most prominent side-effect is haemolytic anaemia, which is rarely severe and rapidly reversible after dose reduction or drug withdrawal. Nevertheless, the haemoglobin level may fall under 8 g/dl in 5% of patients. Therefore, patients with cardiovascular disease or impaired renal function should be managed with caution. Other side-effects include nausea, fatigue, myalgia, abdominal discomfort, pruritus, skin disorders, hyperuricaemia, cough, depression and nervousness [46,47,55–57]. Ribavirin may increase the platelet count [56], which might advantageously antagonize the thrombocytopenic effect of IFN. Female and male contraception is recommended, since significant teratogenic and embryocidal potential, as well as spermatogenesis impairment, have been demonstrated in animals.

## CONCLUSIONS

Unfortunately, the classical primary goal of antiviral therapy, sustained virus eradication, may not be universally reached with the presently available therapy. Therefore, a reduction in liver fibrosis progression should be considered as a primary prognostic goal in patients where virus is not eradicated. Treatment with IFN in chronic active hepatitis C should be considered for patients with a high likelihood of progressive disease or for patients who could transmit the virus. From recent analysis of the natural history of fibrosis progression, it seems that two-thirds of infected subjects are at significant risk of progression to cirrhosis. It is not known whether patients with persistently normal ALT levels or with a minor form of the disease may benefit from therapy. Despite a low sustained response rate, IFN therapy can be effective and safe in patients with compensated type C cirrhosis [58]. The IFN therapeutic modality may be important, since there is a dose effect and a duration effect upon sustained response rates. The best efficacy/risk ratio seems to be in favour of 3 MU three times per week for at least 12 months in patients who have never been treated with IFN. With this regimen, sustained remission is achieved in nearly 35% of patients. More aggressive regimens with higher doses or high induction doses may be considered in patients with HCV genotype 1b or with high viral load. The policy of stopping IFN therapy in patients who do not have an early ALT response can be debated. Controversy persists concerning the long-term benefit of IFN, particularly in transient responders and non-responders. The absence of a serum ALT response may not be a reliable predictor of a lack of benefit of treatment.

**Figure 6.** Potential impact of IFN-α on the natural history of chronic hepatitis C

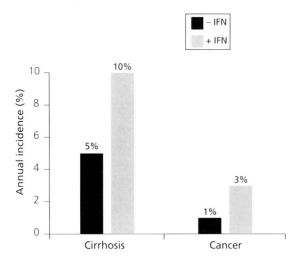

Some studies suggest that irrespective of the usual biochemical response criteria, IFN therapy may improve inflammatory lesions, stabilize fibrosis progression and prevent hepatocellular carcinoma, with greater efficacy of long-term treatment. Inflexion of the natural history of the disease and long-term benefits remain to be demonstrated in these patients. Ribavirin as monotherapy is quite disappointing. Therefore, it should be considered only when IFN is contraindicated, particularly in transplant patients with severe histological lesions. Combination therapy seems to exert a synergistic effect between ribavirin and IFN, achieving a sustained response in nearly 50% of previously untreated patients, 50% of relapsers and 15% of non-responders. In the future, combination therapy may also be considered in naive patients or early in the course of therapy in non-responders. From a clinical point of view, the goals expected from available therapy include a reduction, by half, of the annual incidence of cirrhosis and by two-thirds of the annual incidence of HCC (Fig. 6). Management of hepatitis C remains a considerable challenge over the next few years, and new drugs should be sought to improve the results of therapy.

# REFERENCES

1. Hoofnagle JH, Mullen KD, Jones DB, Rustgi V, Di Bisceglie A, Peters M, Waggoner JG, Park Y & Jones EA. Treatment of chronic non-A, non-B hepatitis with recombinant human alpha interferon. *New England Journal of Medicine* 1986; 315:1575–1578.
2. Poynard T, Leroy V, Cohard M, Thevenot T, Mathurin P, Opolon P & Zarski JP. Meta-analysis of interferon randomized trials in the treatment of viral hepatitis C: effects of dose and duration. *Hepatology* 1996; **24:**778–789.
3. Peters M. Actions of cytokines on the immune response and viral interactions: an overview. *Hepatology* 1996; **23:**909–916.
4. Mallat A, Preaux AM, Blazejewski S, Rosenbaum J, Dhumeaux D & Mavier P. Interferon alfa and gamma inhibit proliferation and collagen synthesis of human Ito cells in culture. *Hepatology* 1995; **21:**1003–1010.
5. Marcellin P, Pouteau M, Martinot-Peignoux M, Degos F, Duchatelle V, Boyer N, Lemonnier C, Degott C, Erlinger S & Benhamou JP. Lack of benefit of escalating dosage of interferon α in patients with chronic hepatitis C. *Gastroenterology* 1995; **109:**156–165.
6. Saez-Royuela F, Porres JC, Moreno A, Castillo I, Martinez G, Galiana F & Carreno V. High doses of recombinant α interferon or gamma interferon for chronic hepatitis C: a randomized, controlled trial. *Hepatology* 1991; **13:**327–331.
7. Hakozaki Y, Shirahama T, Katou M, Nakagawa K, Oba K & Mitamura K. A controlled study to determine the optimal dose regimen of interferon α 2b in chronic hepatitis C. *American Journal of Gastroenterology* 1995; **90:**1246–1249.
8. Poterucha JJ, Gossard JB, Gross JB Jr, Okaja AJ, Lindor KD, Batts KP, Persing DH, Zem NN & Rakela J. High dose interferon α 2b for patients with chronic hepatitis C who have failed standard treatment. *Gastroenterology* 1996; **110:**A1298.
9. Chemello L, Bonetti P, Cavalletto L, Talato F, Donadon V, Casarin P, Belussi F, Frezza M, Noventa F, Pontisso P *et al.* Randomized trial comparing three different regimens of alpha-2a-interferon in chronic hepatitis C. *Hepatology* 1995; **22:**700–706.
10. Shiratori Y, Yokosuka O, Imazeki F, Hashimoto E, Hayashi N, Nakamura A, Asada M, Kuroda H, Ohkuba H, Tanaka T, Arakawa Y, Kimura Y, Iwama A, Fujimura K, Iijima T, Shibuya A, Saito H, Yoshimasu H, Itakura S, Matsuzuki S, Sugimoto M, Ishiyama N, Saito S & Omata M. Viral eradication rate is proportional to the total doses of interferon; 'Tokyo–Chiba' hepatitis C multicentric, randomized and prospective study. *Gastroenterology* 1996; **110:**A1324.
11. Heathcote J, Keefe E, Lee S *et al.* Retreatment of chronic HCV infection with a higher dose of consensus interferon produces sustained responses in nonresponders and relapsers. *Gastroenterology* 1997; **112:** A1280.
12. Lam NP. Rapid HCV clearance with high induction interferon doses is important for sustained response. *Gastroenterology* 1997; **112:**A1312.
13. Reichard O, Foberg U, Fryden A, Mattsson L, Norkrans G, Sonnerborg A, Wejstal R, Yun ZB & Weiland O. High sustained response rate and clearance of viremia in chronic hepatitis C after treatment with interferon α 2b for 60 weeks. *Hepatology* 1994; **19:**280–285.
14. Poynard T, Bedossa P, Chevallier M, Mathurin P, Lemonnier C, Trepo C, Couzigou P, Payen JL, Sajus M & Costa JM. A comparison of three interferon α 2b regimens for long term treatment of chronic non-A non-B hepatitis. *New England Journal of Medicine* 1995; **332:**1457–1462.
15. Angelini G, Sgarbi D, Colombari R, Bezzi A, Castagnini A, de Berardinis F, Conti A, di Piramo D, Dolci L, Falezza G *et al.* Alpha-interferon treatment of chronic hepatitis C: a controlled, multicentre, prospective study. *Digestion* 1995; **56:**199–203.
16. Kasahara A, Hayashi N, Hiramatsu N, Oshita M, Hagiwara H, Katayama K, Kato M, Masuzawa M,

Yoshihara H, Kishida Y *et al.* Ability of prolonged interferon treatment to suppress relapse after cessation of therapy in patients with chronic hepatitis C: a multicenter randomized controlled trial. *Hepatology* 1995; **21:**291–297.

17. Marcellin P, Pouteau M, Boyer N, Castelnau C, Erlinger S & Benhamou JP. Retreatment with recombinant interferon-alpha in patients with chronic hepatitis C. *Journal of Infectious Diseases* 1993; **167:**780–781.

18. Hagiwara H, Hayashi N, Mita E, Takehara T, Kasahara A, Fusamoto H & Kamada T. Quantitative analysis of hepatitis C virus RNA in serum during interferon α therapy. *Gastroenterology* 1993; **104:**877–883.

19. Shindo M, Di Bisceglie AM, Cheung L, Shih JW, Cristiano K, Feinstone SM & Hoofnagle JH. Decrease in serum hepatitis C viral RNA during alpha-interferon therapy for chronic hepatitis C. *Annals of Internal Medicine* 1991; **115:**700–704.

20. Lau J, Mizokami M, Ohno T, Diamond D, Kniffen J & Davis GL. Discrepancy between biochemical and virological responses to interferon-α in chronic hepatitis C. *Lancet* 1993; **342:**1208–1209.

21. Saracco G, Rosina F, Abate ML, Chiandussi L, Gallo V, Cerutti E, Di Napoli A, Solinas A, Deplano A, Tocco A *et al.* Long-term follow-up of patients with chronic hepatitis C treated with different doses of interferon α 2b. *Hepatology* 1993; **18:**1300–1305.

22. Reichard O, Glaumann H, Fryden A, Norkrans G, Schvarcz R, Sonnerborg A, Yun ZB & Weiland O. Two-year biochemical, virological, and histological follow-up in patients with chronic hepatitis C responding in a sustained fashion to interferon α-2b treatment. *Hepatology* 1995; **21:**918–922.

23. Lee WM, Reddy KR, Van Leeuwen DJ *et al.* Undetectable HCV RNA concentrations at early time points predict sustained virological responses after treatment with consensus interferon. *Gastroenterology* 1997; **112:**A1317.

24. McHutchinson JG, Blatt LM, Russell J & Conrad A. Kinetics of changes in serum HCV RNA during interferon therapy in patients with chronic hepatitis C infection. *Gastroenterology* 1997; **112:**A1330.

25. Romeo R, Pol S, Berthelot P & Brechot C. Eradication of hepatitis C virus RNA after α-interferon therapy. *Annals of Internal Medicine* 1994; **121:**276–277.

26. Balart LA, Perrillo R, Roddenberry J, Regenstein F, Shim KS, Shieh YS, Taylor B, Dash S & Gerber MA. Hepatitis C RNA in liver of chronic hepatitis patients before and after interferon α treatment. *Gastroenterology* 1993; **104:**1472–1477.

27. Poynard T, Bedossa P & Opolon P. Natural history of liver fibrosis progression in patients with chronic hepatitis C. *Lancet* 1997; **349:**825–832.

28. Manabe N, Chevallier M, Chossegros P, Causse X, Guerret S, Trepo C & Grimaud JA. Interferon-α 2b therapy reduces liver fibrosis in chronic non-A non-B hepatitis: a quantitative histological evaluation. *Hepatology* 1993; **18:**1344–1349.

29. Craig JR, Bain VG, Ehrinpreis M, Foust R, Lee W, Smith CI, van Leeuwen DJ & the Consensus Interferon Study Group. Liver histology improves in both cirrhotic and non cirrhotic patients with chronic HCV infection following consensus interferon therapy. *Gastroenterology* 1997; **112:**A1248.

30. Jensen D, Shafritz D, Craig JR, Krawitt E & the CIFN Study Group. Nonresponders to CIFN show clinically relevant improvements in liver histology. *Gastroenterology* 1997; **112:**A1294.

31. Camma C, Giunta M, Linea C & Pagliaro L. The effect of interferon on the liver in chronic hepatitis C: a quantitative evaluation of histology by meta-analysis. *Journal of Hepatology* 1997; **26:**1187–1199.

32. Degos F, Daurat V, Gayno S, Bastie A, Riachi G, Bartolomei-Portal I, Barange K, Mousalli J, Navcau S, Bailly F, Chaumet-Riffaud P, Chastang C & the Multicentre GER-CYT-04 Group. Reinforced regimen of interferon alpha-a reduces the incidence of cirrhosis in patents with chronic hepatitis C: a multicentre randomised trial. *Journal of Hepatology* 1998; **29:**224–232.

33. Accogli E, Mazzella G, Somli S *et al.* Alpha interferon prevents hepatocellular carcinoma in responders with HCV-associated hepatic cirrhosis. *Gastroenterology* 1997; **112:**A1206.

34. Nishiguchi S, Kuroki T, Nakatani S, Morimoto H, Takeda T, Nakajima S, Shiomi S, Seki S, Kobayashi K & Otani S. Randomized trial of effects of interferon α on incidence of hepatocellular carcinoma in chronic active hepatitis C with cirrhosis. *Lancet* 1995; **346:**1051–1055.

35. Jouet P, Roudot-Thoraval F, Dhumeaux D & Metreau JM. Comparative efficacy of interferon α in cirrhotic and noncirrhotic patients with non-A non-B, C hepatitis. *Gastroenterology* 1994; **106:**686–690.

36. Davis G, Beck JR, Farrell G & Poynard T. Prolonged course versus 6 months of interferon α or no treatment in patients with histologically mild chronic hepatitis C: a decision analysis. *Gastroenterology* 1997; **112:**A1252.

37. Poynard T & Opolon P. Hepatitis C: somber views of natural history and optimistic views of interferon treatment? *Hepatology* 1998; **27:**1443–1444.

38. Lau JY, Davis GL, Kniffen J, Qian KP, Urdea MS, Chan CS, Mizokami M, Neuwald PD & Wilber JC. Significance of serum hepatitis C virus RNA levels in chronic hepatitis C. *Lancet* 1993; **341:**1501–1504.

39. Magrin S, Craxi A, Fabiano C, Simonetti RG, Fiorentino G, Marino L, Diquattro O, Di Marco V, Loiacono O, Volpes R *et al.* Hepatitis C viremia in chronic liver disease: relationship to interferon α or corticosteroid treatment. *Hepatology* 1994; **19:**273–279.

40. Tsubota A, Chayama K, Ikeda K, Yasuji A, Koida I, Saitoh S, Hashimoto M, Iwasaki S, Kobayashi M & Hiromitsu K. Factors predictive of response to interferon-α therapy in hepatitis C virus infection. *Hepatology* 1994; **19:**1088–1094.

41. Martinot-Peignoux M, Marcellin P, Pouteau M, Castelnau C, Boyer N, Poliquin M, Degott C, Descombes I, Le Breton V, Milotova V *et al.* Pretreatment serum hepatitis C virus RNA levels and hepatitis C virus genotype are the main and independent prognostic factors of sustained response to interferon α therapy in chronic hepatitis C. *Hepatology* 1995; **22:**1050–1056.

42. Enomoto N, Sakuma I, Asahina Y, Kurosaki M, Murakami T, Yamamoto C, Ogura Y, Izumi N, Marumo F & Sato C. Mutations in the nonstructural protein 5A gene and response to interferon in patients with chronic hepatitis C virus 1b infection. *New England Journal of Medicine* 1996; **334:**77–81.

43. Sakuma I, Enomoto N, Asahina Y, Kurosaki M, Marumo F & Sato C. Differential effect of interferon therapy on hepatitis C virus 1B quasispecies in the nonstructural 5A gene. *Gastroenterology* 1997; **112:**A1371.

44. Chung RT, Monto A, Dienstag JL & Kaplan LM. NS5A mutations do not predict response to interferon in American patients infected with genotype 1 hepatitis C virus. *Gastroenterology* 1997; **112**:A1244.

45. Patterson JL & Fernandez-Larson R. Molecular action of ribavirin. *Reviews of Infectious Diseases* 1990; **12**:1132–1146.

46. Reichard O, Andersson J, Schvarcz R & Weiland O. Ribavirin treatment for chronic hepatitis C. *Lancet* 1991; **337**:1058–1061.

47. Di Bisceglie AM, Shindo M, Fong TL, Fried MW, Swain MG, Bergasa NV, Axiotis CA, Waggoner JG, Park Y & Hoofnagle JH. A pilot study of ribavirin therapy for chronic hepatitis C. *Hepatology* 1992; **16**:649–654.

48. Bodenheimer HC Jr, Lindsay KL, Davis GL, Lewis JH, Thung SN & Seeff LB. Tolerance and efficacy of oral ribavirin treatment of chronic hepatitis C: a multicenter trial. *Hepatology* 1994; **20**:207A.

49. Di Bisceglie AM, Conjeevaram HS, Fried MW, Sallie R, Park Y, Yurdaydin C, Swain M, Kleiner DE, Mahaney K & Hoofnagle JH. Ribavirin as therapy for chronic hepatitis C. A randomized, double-blind, placebo-controlled trial. *Annals of Internal Medicine* 1995; **123**:897–903.

50. Brouwer JT, Nevens F, Michielsen P *et al.* What options are left when hepatitis C does not respond to interferon? Placebo-controlled Benelux multicentre retreatment trial on ribavirin monotherapy versus combination with interferon. *Journal of Hepatology* 1994; **21** (Supplement):S17.

51. Kakumu S, Yoshioka K, Wakita T, Ishikawa T, Takayanagi M & Higashi Y. A pilot study of ribavirin and interferon beta for treatment of chronic hepatitis C. *Gastroenterology* 1993; **105**:507–512.

52. Chemello L, Cavaletto L, Bernardinello E *et al.* The effect of interferon α and ribavirin combination therapy in naive patients with chronic hepatitis C. *Journal of Hepatology* 1995; **23** (Supplement 2):8–12.

53. Lai MY, Kao JH, Yang PM, Wang JT, Chen PJ, Chan KW, Chu JS & Chen DS. Long-term efficacy of ribavirin plus interferon α in the treatment of chronic hepatitis C. *Gastroenterology* 1996; **111**:1307–1312.

54. Weiland O, Schvarcz R, Yun Z & Sonneborg A. IFN relapsers and nonresponders: Scandinavian experience. In *Perspectives on a New Paradigm: Combination Antiviral Therapy in Chronic Hepatitis C*, 1995; pp. 441–450. London: European Association for the Study of the Liver.

55. Schalm SW, Hansen BE, Chemello L, Bellobuono A, Brouwer JT, Weiland O, Cavalletto L, Schvarcz R, Ideo G & Alberti A. Ribavirin enhances the efficacy but not the adverse effects of interferon in chronic hepatitis C. Meta-analysis of individual patient data from European centers. *Journal of Hepatology* 1997; **26**:961–966.

56. Davies G, Esteban-Mur R, Rustgi V, Hoefs J, Gordon S, Trepo C, Schiffman M, Zeuzen S, Coxsi A, Roffanel C, Reindollar R & Rizetto M. Retreatment of relapse after interferon for chronic hepatitis C: an international randomized controlled trial of interferon plus ribavirin vs interferon alone. *Hepatology* 1997; **26**:247A.

57. Thevenot T, Mathurin P, Moussalli J, Perrin M, Plassart F, Blot C, Opolon P & Poynard T. Effects of cirrhosis, interferon and azathioprine on adverse events in patients with chronic hepatitis C treated with ribavirin. *Journal of Viral Hepatitis* 1997; **4**:243–253.

58. Saito T, Shinzawa H, Kuboki M, Ishibashi M, Toda H, Okuyama Y, Nakamura T, Yamada N, Wakabayashi H, Togashi H *et al.* A randomized, controlled trial of human lymphoblastoid interferon in patients with compensated type C cirrhosis. *American Journal of Gastroenterology* 1994; **89**:681–686.

59. Sobetsky R, Mathurin P, Thevenot T, Charlotte F, Moussalli J, Vidsud M, Opolon P & Poynard T. Interferon alfa reduces fibrosis progression independently of genotype, viral load and 3 month ALT response in chronic hepatitis C. *Gastroenterology* 1997; **26**:413A.

# 41 Interferon plus thymosin α-1 treatment of chronic hepatitis C infection: a meta-analysis

## Kenneth E Sherman* and Susan N Sherman

## INTRODUCTION

Hepatitis C virus (HCV) infection leads to the development of chronic, progressive liver disease in a significant proportion of infected subjects. Current management of this infection is centred on the use of interferon (IFN), which has been demonstrated to reduce serum alanine aminotransferase (ALT) levels, improve histology and, in some individuals, induce a sustained loss of virus. Unfortunately, such responses occur in the minority of patients. Considerable effort has been expended in recent years to study new IFN dosing modalities and the use of IFN combined with other therapeutic interventions. These include ribavirin, phlebotomy, amantadine and thymosin α-1 (Tα-1).

Tα-1 is a synthetically produced 28 amino acid peptide that has been shown to have numerous *in vivo* and *in vitro* biological activities. Studies have demonstrated that it has a role in the maturation of CD4+ T helper cells, and that it increases activity of natural killer cells. Furthermore, in some systems, Tα-1 will increase the levels of interleukin 2 and its receptor, thus promoting a cascade of cytokine-mediated immmunological effects. There have been several small studies suggesting that the combination of IFN with Tα-1 is beneficial in terms of biochemical and virological outcomes in patients with HCV infection. Unfortunately, the relatively small numbers of treated patients has limited interpretation of the individual trials. Therefore, we undertook the performance of a meta-analysis based on the pooled data derived from reported studies.

## METHODS

A MEDLINE search was performed to identify published literature in which the combination of IFN and Tα-1 was utilized for the treatment of chronic hepatitis C infection. Cited literature was then reviewed to determine if other studies could be identi-

fied. In addition, abstracts from meetings about liver disease and hepatitis were obtained and reviewed. Finally, the manufacturer of Tα-1 was contacted to determine if unpublished, non-abstracted data were available from any other source. This step was performed to reduce bias introduced by negative studies that were not presented or published.

Response data were first pooled and analysed by $\chi^2$ or Fisher's exact tests as appropriate for subject number. Next, meta-analysis was performed using FastPro Software [1]. Combined analysis was calculated using a Baysean model, which permits conservative combination of studies with random effects. This permitted combinations of mildly heterogeneous patient study cohorts, as well as the creation of model controls for the studies that were not performed in a randomized, controlled manner. For uncontrolled studies, a 40% end-treatment response and a 20% sustained response were used to represent the control cohort. This is a generous estimate of response based on recent literature from large randomized controlled series and would tend to lead to an underestimation of response.

Definitions of response were determined prior to the analysis and the reported studies were then analysed to determine which outcome criteria could be directly obtained or deduced by calculation from information provided about the study cohorts. An end-treatment response was defined in both biochemical and virological terms as normalization of serum ALT or negative HCV RNA by PCR at the end of treatment, respectively. Sustained response was also subdivided into biochemical and virological outcome parameters.

## RESULTS

A review of available literature revealed three studies amenable to analysis that utilized the combination therapy described in the screening criteria. The char-

*Corresponding author

**Table 1.** Demographics and characteristics of the studies used in meta-analysis

| Study | Sherman et al. [2] | Moscarrella et al. [3] | Rasi et al. [4] |
|---|---|---|---|
| Design | Randomized | Randomized | Open label, historical controls |
| IFN plus Tα-1 (n) | 35 | 17 | 15 |
| IFN (n) | 37 | 17 | 15 |
| Mean age | 42 | 51 | 47 |
| Gender (M/F) | 54/18 | 24/10 | 7/8 |
| Cirrhosis (%) | 6 | ? | 40 |
| Prior IFN failure | 4 | 0 | 4 |

acteristics of these studies are shown in Table 1. One randomized controlled trial has been published in abstract format and the full manuscript is in press [2]. The full manuscript was available for analysis. A second randomized controlled trial was available in abstract form only [3]. The third study was published as a full article, and represents an open-label treatment study [4]. In all studies, patients were treated for a period ranging from 6 months to 1 year. The type of IFN varied and included IFN-α2b and lymphoblastoid IFN. Age and gender distributions were comparable, although the percentage of female subjects was slightly higher in the study by Rasi et al. [4]. Two studies included prior IFN failures, accounting for a total of eight patients. There was a high frequency of cirrhotic patients (40%) treated by Rasi et al. [4]. We were unable to determine the percentage of cirrhotic patients in the report of Moscarella et al. [3].

Pooled analysis was performed as the first phase of the analysis. A total of 121 patients were identified including 54 in the IFN alone arm and 67 in the IFN plus Tα-1 arm. The biochemical end-treatment response in the IFN plus Tα-1 combination arm was 44.7%. In contrast, the IFN alone treatment group had a pooled response of 22%. This difference was statistically significant ($\chi^2$ 6.71, $P=0.01$). Sustained

biochemical response was observed in 11.1% of the patients treated with IFN alone but increased to 22.4% with combination therapy. This trend did not reach full statistical significance ($P=0.10$). For this reason, we applied a Baysean model to combine the studies, in an effort to assess better the role of combination therapy with a relatively small patient cohort.

Figure 1 depicts the results of the meta-analysis in terms of biochemical end-treatment response. This type of analysis permits the calculation of the odds ratio of response, using the IFN alone arm as the baseline. The odds ratio is the measurement comparing the two treatment arms, with values greater than 1 suggesting increased efficacy, and those less than 1 indicating a treatment advantage for IFN alone. All individual studies had odds ratios greater than 1. The combination odds ratio was 3.1, suggesting that IFN plus Tα-1 was more than three times better at normalizing ALT at the end of treatment than IFN alone. The confidence interval (CI) demonstrates the statistical validity of this finding. Figure 2 shows the same graphical representation for biochemical sustained response. Again, all odds ratios are greater than 1, suggesting efficacy for this outcome. The 95% CI values show that there is a small chance that this could be due to random effects, as the lower limit of the combined data extends to

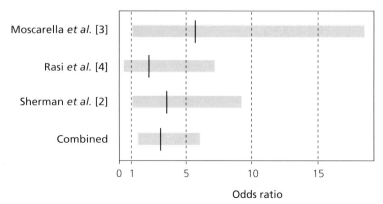

**Figure 1.** Odds ratio of biochemical (ALT) end-treatment response using IFN alone as the baseline measurement

Odds ratios greater than 1.0 indicate improved efficacy for combination therapy. The error bars represent 95% CI of the odds ratio. The last line in each group represents the combined efficacy based on the Baysean analysis, which includes the theoretical control group for the uncontrolled data sets as described in the Methods section.

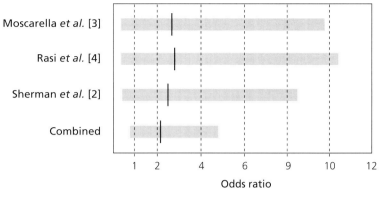

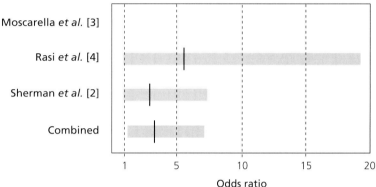

slightly less than unity (1.0).

The meta-analysis of viral response is shown in Figures 3 and 4. One of the studies [3] did not report viral response, and the analysis was therefore restricted to the other two studies. Here, combination analysis reveals a statistically significant benefit of combination therapy at the end of treatment, which was suggested but not definitively demonstrated in the individual study analyses (Fig. 3). Sustained response was also evaluated by the meta-analysis method. Data combination shows a probable benefit for this outcome in the combination therapy arm (Fig. 4).

Subset analysis was performed to evaluate the value of combination therapy among IFN-naive patients only. Meta-analysis produced a calculated odds ratio of 3.9 (95% CI=1.64–7.92) for biochemical end-treatment response. Sustained biochemical response was 2.38 times as likely among those receiving combination therapy (95% CI=0.84–5.53).

Data regarding side-effect profiles were not sufficient to perform a meta-analysis. It would be fair to conclude that the individual studies did not describe toxicities associated with combination therapy that were not observed at similar rates for patients taking IFN alone. Specifically, pooled total patient drop-out

was noted in 3/67 patients treated with IFN plus Tα-1 and 2/54 patients treated with IFN alone. These differences are not statistically significant.

## DISCUSSION

While IFN represents the current standard therapeutic intervention for chronic hepatitis C, efforts continue to study alternate treatment regimes. Adjunctive interventions such as phlebotomy, alteration of IFN dose or timing and combinations of complementary therapeutic agents may all increase efficacy. Tα-1 is an immunomodulatory agent that appears to have no intrinsic antiviral activity for hepatitis C when used as a monotherapy [5]. To date, three small studies have investigated the value of combining this peptide with IFN. Independently, these studies suggest that there may be some efficacy in terms of end-treatment response, but study size precludes adequate evaluation of other endpoints such as sustained response rates. Various mathematical methods exist to compensate for random diversity and variation and permit a more accurate assessment of pooled data. The Baysean approach allows for the incorporation of indirect evidence, and is thought to be helpful when little data from randomized trials exist [6].

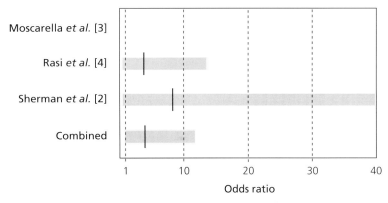

**Figure 4.** Odds ratio of virological sustained responses

See legend to Fig. 1 for details.

Odds ratio

End-treatment response was evaluated for biochemical and virological endpoints, and in the subset of patients who were previously naive to IFN. The results clearly demonstrate an end-treatment response benefit for both ALT normalization and HCV RNA clearance. The importance of these findings is unclear. Since hepatitis C infection is a slowly progressive disease in terms of development of cirrhosis, liver failure, hepatocellular carcinoma and death, it is difficult to evaluate the role of end-treatment response as a clinical outcome. Similarly, sustained response is at best a surrogate marker of desirable outcomes, but it has been the standard objective measure pending the results of large long-term studies that might better define the treatment results. There are data from early IFN trials demonstrating that primary response was associated with histological improvement in the liver [7]. Sherman *et al.* [2] described an improvement in this outcome in a trial with patients receiving combination therapy. The presented data did not permit meta-analysis of histological responses. If one assumes that most biochemical end-treatment responses are associated with histological improvement, then combination therapy might also benefit this outcome parameter. The significance of such a response, in terms of disease progression and development of hepatocellular carcinoma is unknown, but some studies suggest that it may be beneficial [8,9].

Another combination therapy that has garnered much interest includes ribavirin with IFN. Early results suggest that IFN plus ribavirin combination therapy improves sustained response in IFN responders, but may not affect the likelihood of primary response [10]. One might speculate that addition of thymosin to an IFN plus ribavirin treatment might increase the primary response and thus improve the subsequent sustained response.

IFN and Tα-1 seem to improve sustained biochemical and virological response. The calculated odds ratios support this interpretation and suggest an efficacy two to three times greater for these outcomes in the combined meta-analysis. However, small total numbers of these subsets result in a 95% CI that crosses unity, and therefore this result may have occurred by random variability of the responses, even though the trend towards significance is strong.

New or worsened toxicity profiles were not described in the three study cohorts that would raise concerns about combination therapy compared with IFN alone. Total patient drop-out from all causes was low. Higher rates of toxicity, secondary to haemolysis and other factors, was described for the combination of IFN plus ribavirin [10].

In conclusion, the current meta-analysis supports the hypothesis that IFN plus Tα-1 combination therapy has greater efficacy than IFN alone. Clearly, larger well controlled clinical trials are needed to determine the role that Tα-1 might play in hepatitis C treatments of the future.

## REFERENCES

1. Eddy DM & Hasselblad V. *Fast*Pro: Software for Meta-Analysis by the Confidence Profile Method*, 1991. San Diego: Academic Press.
2. Sherman KI, Sjogren M, Creager M, Damiano MA, Freeman S, Lewey S, Davis D, Root S, Weber FL, Ishak KG & Goodman ZD. Combination therapy with thymosin alpha-1 and interferon for the treatment of chronic hepatitis C infection: a randomized, placebo-controlled double-blind trial. *Hepatology* 1998; **27**:1128–1135.
3. Moscarrella S, Buzzelli G, Monti M, Gianni C, Careccia B, Marrocchi RG, Romanelli AL & Zignego AL. Treatment with interferon-alfa (IFNα) and thymosin-α1 (Tα1) of naive patients affected by chronic hepatitis C. *Fourth International Symposium on Hepatitis C and Related Viruses*, Kyoto, Japan, March 1997; Abstract 287.
4. Rasi G, DiVirgilio D, Mutchnick MG, Colella F, Sinibaldi-Vallebona P, Pierimarchi P, Valli B & Garaci E. Combination thymosin α1 and lymphoblastoid interferon treatment in chronic hepatitis C. *Gut* 1996; **39**:679–683.

5. Andreone P, Cursaro C, Gramenzi A, Buzzi A, Covarelli MG, DiGiammairno L, Miniero R, Arienti V, Bernardi M & Gasbarrini G. A double-blind, placebo-controlled, pilot trial of thymosin alpha1 for the treatment of chronic hepatitis C. *Liver* 1996; **16:**207–210.

6. Lau J, Ioannidis JPA & Schmid CH. Quantitative synthesis in systematic reviews. *Annals of Internal Medicine* 1997; **127:**820–826.

7. Davis GL, Balart LA, Schiff ER, Lindsay K, Bodenheimer HC Jr, Perrillo RP, Carey W, Jacobson IM, Payne J, Dienstag JL *et al.* Treatment of chronic hepatitis C with recombinant interferon alfa. A multicenter randomized, controlled trial. *New England Journal of Medicine* 1989; **321:**1501–1506.

8. Kuwana K, Ichida T, Kamimura T, Ohkoshi S, Ogata N, Harada T, Endoh K & Asakura H. Risk factors and the effect of interferon therapy in the development of hepatocellular carcinoma: a multivariate analysis in 343 patients. *Journal of Gastroenterology and Hepatology* 1997; **12:**149–155.

9. Nishiguchi S, Kuroki T, Nakatani S, Morimoto H, Takeda T, Nakajima S, Shiomi S, Seki S, Kobayashi K & Otani S. Randomised trial of effects of interferon-alpha on incidence of hepatocellular carcinoma in chronic active hepatitis C with cirrhosis. *Lancet* 1995; **346:**1051–1055.

10. Reichard O, Norkrans G, Fryden A, Braconier JH, Sonnerborg A & Weiland O. Randomised, double-blind, placebo-controlled trial of interferon alpha-2b with and without ribavirin for chronic hepatitis C. The Swedish Study Group. *Lancet* 1998; **351:**83–87.

# 42

# Primary response to interferon α plus ribavirin in non-responders and relapsers with chronic liver disease owing to hepatitis C virus

Antonio Ascione*, Carmine Canestrini, Silvia Astretto, Massimo De Luca, Alfonso Galeota Lanza, Filomena Morisco, Concetta Tuccillo, Nicola Caporaso, Francesca Froio, Piero Piergrossi and Carmelo D'Asero

## INTRODUCTION

A standard regimen of interferon (IFN) therapy for chronic liver disease caused by hepatitis C virus (HCV) infection is unsatisfactory because the long-term response is only 20–25% [1–3]. Previous pilot studies of the combination of IFN plus ribavirin in a relatively small number of patients confirmed a synergistic therapeutic benefit. A long-term biochemical [alanine aminotransferase (ALT) normalization] and virological (loss of serum HCV RNA) response was obtained after 6 months of treatment and 6 months of follow-up [4–6]. Recently, the results of two further trials [7,8] were very impressive. These studies focused on the effects of the combination therapy as far as virological, biochemical and histological endpoints are concerned. The preliminary data confirmed that retreatment of relapsers with IFN alone has a very low long-term response rate (20–30%) but the rate was much higher in the IFN–ribavirin group (50–60%) [7]. In non-responders, retreatment with IFN–ribavirin resulted in a loss of HCV RNA in 32.9% of patients, whereas in those treated with IFN alone only 12% obtained the same result ($P=0.0066$) [8]. Efficacy, safety and tolerability have also been confirmed by other studies [9–10].

The aim of this study was to evaluate the response to combination therapy with IFN plus ribavirin in patients with chronic HCV-associated liver disease, who did not respond to a previous cycle of standard IFN therapy (3 or 6 MU three times weekly for at least 6 months) or who subsequently relapsed on cessation of therapy.

## PATIENTS AND METHODS

A total of 81 patients with biopsy-proven chronic liver disease and out of therapy for at least 6 months were enrolled into the study. Thirty-two (39.5%) were relapsers with a mean age of 48±5 years and a male: female ratio of 4:1. Twenty patients (63%) had chronic hepatitis and 12 (37%) were cirrhotic. Mean viraemia before entering the study was $2.5\pm2.7\times10^6$ HCV RNA copies/ml. Most of the relapsers were infected with HCV genotype 1b (88%).

Forty-nine (60.5%) were non-responders with a mean age of 52±7 years and a male:female ratio of 11:1. Thirty-one (63%) had chronic active hepatitis and 18 (37%) were cirrhotic. Viraemia before entering the study was $4.3\pm9.1\times10^6$ HCV RNA copies/ml; 80% were infected with HCV genotype 1b.

Both groups were treated with intramuscular IFN-α at 3 MU three times weekly plus ribavirin at 1000 mg (body weight <75 kg) or 1200 mg. The first evaluation was planned at the third month of therapy; in patients who were non-responders the treatment was stopped, while the responders continued the combination treatment for a further 3 months and were then treated with IFN alone for an additional 6 months. All patients were followed up monthly for 1 year and bimonthly for a further 2 years after the end of treatment. Results were evaluated in an 'intention-to-treat' analysis. The end of therapy response was defined as normalization of ALT by the end of the third month and throughout the therapy, while a long-term response was defined as stable normalization of

Table 1. Results of therapy in relapsers

|  | Number of patients | Percentage |
|---|---|---|
| End of therapy response | 28 | 88 |
| Adverse events | 2 | 6 |
| Drop-outs | 2 | 6 |

Table 2. Results of therapy in non-responders

|  | Number of patients | Percentage |
|---|---|---|
| End of therapy response | 21 | 43 |
| Adverse events | 4 | 8 |
| Drop-outs | 0 | – |

ALT throughout the 2 years of follow-up after the end of therapy.

Serum HCV RNA was quantified by a branched DNA assay (Chiron Diagnostics) and HCV genotypes were detected by a Line Probe Assay (Innogenetics). Sera were stored at −80°C until tested.

## RESULTS

The end-treatment response of relapsers was 88% (28/32; Table 1), whereas the end-treatment response of non-responders was 43% (21/49; Table 2). Among the group of relapsers who did not respond, two dropped out and two had to stop treatment because of side-effects (pruritus and allergic reaction) and were considered to be non-responders according to the intention-to-treat analysis. Among the group of non-responders, none dropped out while four patients had adverse events (myalgia, asthenia, leukopenia and cardiac arrhythmia).

To date, the mean follow-up has been $13 \pm 5$ months. For this reason we have reported only data on the end-treatment response, because in our protocol long-term response is defined as stable normalization of ALT for 24 months after the end of therapy.

## CONCLUSION

IFN plus ribavirin is actually the treatment of choice for patients with HCV-associated chronic liver disease who are non-responders or relapsers on a previous cycle of IFN therapy. In patients who relapse after a first trial of IFN, this new treatment gives virtually 100% of end-treatment response if the patients do not develop side-effects. As far as the long-term response is concerned, it is necessary to wait until the end of follow-up before we can draw any conclusions. In non-responder patients, the end of therapy response is lower and so far 60% of them have already relapsed.

## REFERENCES

1. Carithers RL & Emerson S. Therapy of hepatitis C: meta-analysis of interferon alfa-2b trials. *Hepatology* 1997; **26** (Supplement 1):83–88.
2. Lee WM. Therapy of hepatitis C: interferon alfa 2-a trials. *Hepatology* 1997; **26** (Supplement 1):89–95.
3. Keefe EB, Hollinger FB and the Consensus Interferon Study Group. Therapy of hepatitis C: consensus interferon trials. *Hepatology* 1997; **26** (Supplement 1):101–107.
4. Porst H, Wiese M & Porst T. One year follow up of re-treatment with alpha-interferon in combination with ribavirin versus interferon for chronic hepatitis C. *Gastroenterology* 1997; **112**:A1361
5. Schvarcz R, Ando Y, Sonnerborg A & Weiland O. Combination treatment with interferon alfa-2b and ribavirin for chronic hepatitis C in patients who have failed to achieve sustained response to interferon alone: Swedish experience. *Journal of Hepatology* 1995; **23** (Supplement 2):17–21.
6. Schvarcz R, Yun ZB, Sonnerborg A & Weiland O. Combined treatment with interferon alpha-2b and ribavirin for chronic hepatitis C in patients with a previous non-response or non-sustained response to interferon alone. *Journal of Medical Virology* 1995; **46**: 43–47.
7. Davis GL, Esteban-Murr R, Rustgi V, Hoefs J, Gordon S, Trepo C, Shiffman M, Zeuzem S, Craxì A, Raffanel C, Reindollar R, Rizzetto M and The International Hepatitis Interventional Therapy Group. Retreatment of relapse after interferon therapy for chronic hepatitis C: an international randomized controlled trial of interferon plus ribavirin vs interferon alone. *Hepatology* 1997; **26** (Supplement 2):247A.
8. Ferenci P, Stauber R, Hackl W, Datz C, Gschwantler W & Steindl P. A prospective randomized controlled trial of high dose of interferon-α plus ribavirin in interferon-non responders with chronic hepatitis C. *Hepatology* 1997; **26** (Supplement 2):415A.
9. Bodenheimer HC, Lindsay KL, Davis GD, Lewis JH, Thung SW & Seef LB. Tolerance and efficacy of oral ribavirin treatment of chronic hepatitis C: a multicentric trial. *Hepatology* 1997; **26**:473–477.
10. Reichard O, Schvarcz R & Weiland O. Therapy of hepatitis C: alpha interferon and ribavirin. *Hepatology* 1997; **26** (Supplement 1):108–111.

# Section VII

## CLINICAL AND THERAPEUTIC STRATEGIES

### Part B

#### TRANSPLANT PATIENTS

# 43

# Hepatitis C virus in the transplant setting

## Marina Berenguer* and Teresa L Wright

## INTRODUCTION

End-stage liver disease secondary to hepatitis C virus (HCV) infection has become one of the leading indications for liver transplantation among adults in the US and Western Europe, accounting for approximately 20–25% of transplantations in many centres [1]. In addition, hepatitis C is a major cause of chronic hepatitis worldwide, affecting approximately 0.5–2% of the general population in developed countries [2]. Persistence of infection after acute infection is very frequent, with as many as 80% of patients continuing to be viraemic after 6 months of follow-up. Eventually, a proportion of these patients develop cirrhosis and a subset of them progress to hepatocellular carcinoma (HCC) [3,4]. Unfortunately, current treatment of chronic hepatitis C with interferon (IFN), either alone or in combination with ribavirin, appears to be of limited efficacy. Thus, if a new potent drug does not become available within the next few years, one can anticipate that the number of liver transplantations related to HCV infection will continue to rise.

Orthotopic liver transplantation provides a unique opportunity to study HCV infection for the following reasons: (i) the exact timing of the infection is known, as opposed to the immunocompetent patient where the timing of initial infection is often difficult to determine accurately because acute infection is typically subclinical; (ii) possible source(s) of infection can be identified (pre-transplantation infection and/or infection from the organ donor or from blood products transfused in the peri-operative period); in contrast, no clear risk factor for infection is present in a substantial proportion of immunocompetent patients infected with HCV; (iii) serial serum samples are frequently available since these patients are usually followed in a single centre; (iv) multiple liver biopsies are usually available which facilitates study of the histological evolution of HCV-associated liver disease.

Following liver transplantation, reinfection of the grafted liver with HCV occurs in the majority of patients [5,6], with subsequent development of hepatitis in the majority and progression to cirrhosis in some [7–10].

However, graft and patient survival are generally good, at least for the first 5–7 years, and comparable to those observed in other patients undergoing transplantation for non-viral end-stage liver disease [9,10].

Several questions remain to be answered at this point: (i) when should we consider liver transplantation as a therapeutical option and can pre-transplant treatment with IFN and/or ribavirin improve prognosis?; (ii) what is the long-term natural history of hepatitis C post-transplantation and can treatment alter it?; (iii) can we identify prognostic factors capable of accurately predicting variable rates of progression of HCV-related liver disease following transplantation?

## PRE-TRANSPLANT EVALUATION

Liver transplantation should be considered a therapeutic option when the course of the disease is sufficiently advanced that median-term survival is unlikely without transplantation. Thus, a major goal is to identify patients at a time at which they are in clinical need of transplantation, sufficiently compensated to tolerate surgery, yet with enough hepatic decompensation to be at risk for life-threatening complications.

When defining the optimum time to refer a patient for consideration of transplantation, several issues should be considered: (i) the prognosis with and without transplantation; (ii) the availability of therapy prior to transplantation that may modify the natural history of HCV-related end-stage liver disease; and (iii) factors such as organ availability and blood type which influence local waiting times for transplantation.

### Timing of liver transplantation for HCV-infected candidates

To date, a natural history model that can be used to predict survival without liver transplantation in HCV cirrhotic patients, which is similar to that used for primary biliary cirrhosis (PBC) [11], is lacking. It is therefore difficult to estimate the rate at which liver

*Corresponding author

disease will progress in an individual patient. Moreover, the prognosis of compensated and decompensated cirrhosis caused by HCV remains uncertain. A recent study has documented a 5 year survival rate of only 50% in patients with HCV-related decompensated cirrhosis [4]. This compares with survival rates of at least 60–65% after liver transplantation with the same duration of follow-up. Thus, liver transplantation appears to be a clear option for decompensated HCV-related end-stage liver disease.

Decisions regarding patients with compensated HCV cirrhosis are unfortunately less straightforward. The prognosis of compensated HCV-related cirrhosis has recently been assessed in 384 European patients [4]. Five year survival was 91%. Hepatic decompensation and HCC were observed in 18% and 7%, respectively. Thus, in the absence of controlled trials assessing the efficacy of liver transplantation, the 5 year outcome of compensated HCV cirrhotic patients favours observation in the absence of transplantation. The exponential rise of waiting times for liver transplantation further complicates decisions. The average waiting time and the number of patients dying on the waiting list have been steadily increasing in the past decade [12]. As a result, decisions regarding listing for transplantation must be made in advance, limiting even more the ability to choose the appropriate time-point for patient referral.

## Management of patients awaiting transplantation

Two approaches can be used in an attempt to decrease mortality in these patients. The first is to use effective antiviral therapy in order to reduce clinical disease progression. The second is to enlarge the pool of potential donors by including those who are anti-HCV positive. Each approach will be considered in turn.

### Pre-emptive antiviral therapy

Data from several trials of IFN have consistently shown a lower biochemical and virological sustained response rate in cirrhotic patients (9–16%) compared to non-cirrhotic patients (17–34%) [13]. Moreover, the clinical impact of IFN monotherapy in compensated cirrhotic patients is largely unknown. Although several preliminary studies have demonstrated a decreased incidence of HCC among HCV-infected patients treated with IFN compared to those who have never been treated [14], the beneficial effects of IFN in patients with cirrhosis have not been convincingly demonstrated [13].

### HCV-positive organ donors

The use of seropositive organ donors provides a mechanism for improving the shortage of suitable donors. It is well established that organs from anti-HCV (radioimmunoblot assay; RIBA2)-positive donors with virus detectable by PCR transmit infection almost universally, whereas organs from anti-HCV RIBA2-positive, PCR-negative donors transmit infection at a lower rate of approximately 50% [15]. PCR is, however, labour intensive and time consuming, and hence not a suitable screening method for donors. In the USA, a national collaborative study of 3078 cadaver organ donors reported a mean prevalence of anti-HCV (enzyme immunoassay; EIA2) and of HCV RNA (PCR) of 4.2% (range 2.3–8.3%) and 2.4% (range 0.8–4.2%), respectively [16]. Thus, approximately 50% of the seropositive donors are not viraemic, and present a reduced risk of transmitting infection. While discarding these organs would eliminate transmission, it would also lead to a waste of almost 2% of organs that transmit infection infrequently. Furthermore, whether the use of these organs is appropriate largely depends on the prognosis of recipients receiving HCV-infected grafts. Data regarding this issue remain controversial. With a prolonged follow-up of 6–7 years, no significant differences in graft loss or death were found between 24 recipients of anti-HCV-positive donors and 74 recipients of anti-HCV-negative donors [17]. These data, nevertheless, should be extrapolated with caution to patients undergoing liver transplantation, as the vast majority of patients included in the study were recipients of renal allografts and the minority received an allograft from a seropositive donor. An alternative option is to use seropositive organs for candidates who are already HCV-infected. Superinfection in that setting has been described [18]. In one series where 14 HCV cirrhotic patients received anti-HCV-positive organs, the viral genotype that prevailed after liver transplantation was the one from the donor in half the cases and the one from the recipients in the other half. Subtype 1b and type 1 became the predominant strains in all recipient/donor pairs in which they were present, suggesting that genotype 1/subtype 1b may have replicative advantages over other genotypes. Interestingly, after approximately 1 year of follow-up, patients retaining their own strain had more severe liver disease that those infected by the donor strain, suggesting different pathogenic capabilities of different HCV strains [18]. Studies are needed to evaluate the long-term consequences of HCV superinfection. Until these data become available, seropositive donors should continue to be used in patients with life-threatening disease, and the consequences of such infection should be carefully evaluated.

# POST-TRANSPLANTATION HCV INFECTION

## Source of infection

When the patient is infected at the time of transplantation, persistent HCV infection following transplantation is the rule [5]. The virus may be acquired in those without evidence of viral infection prior to transplantation by infected organ donors, blood and/or blood products, and by nosocomial acquisition of virus during the transplant hospitalization.

## HCV acquisition

HCV infection may be acquired in the peri-transplant period from infected donor organs or from blood products. The risk of acquiring HCV with liver transplantation, which was initially reported to be as high as 35% [5], currently ranges from 0% to 2.5% [19]. Several factors have contributed to this important drop: (i) the rates reported in early studies were most probably an overestimate due to the use of low sensitivity first generation assays to diagnose pre-transplantation infection. As a consequence, anti-HCV assays gave false-negative results in a large proportion of truly HCV-infected cirrhotic patients; (ii) the risk of acquiring HCV infection from blood products has declined substantially after screening of donors with specific serological tests for HCV, and is currently estimated to be extremely low (0.01–0.001% per unit transfused) [20]; (iii) blood requirements during surgery and in the immediate post-operative period have diminished with improvements in surgical techniques; (iv) different methods of organ preservation and perfusion may change the amount of virus transmitted by the organ. A reduction in viral load has been obtained with pulsatile perfusion of kidney allografts.

## *HCV recurrence*

HCV recurs in virtually all patients with pre-transplantation infection [5], with infection of the graft largely a result of reinfection of the donor liver with endogenous HCV [6]. While replication in extrahepatic sites may provide a source of allograft infection, the presence of extrahepatic replication is controversial. In a recent study [21], HCV RNA levels were measured at frequent time-points before, immediately after and up to 30 days following liver transplantation. A rapid and sharp decline in viral load was observed immediately after removal of the infected liver and low levels persisted for the first 48 hours after transplantation, suggesting that extrahepatic sites of virus contribute little to serum levels. HCV RNA levels at 72 hours after liver transplantation were higher than preoperative values, supporting the hypothesis that the liver is the preferential site for viral replication and that immunosuppression increases levels of viral replication. From the rapid turnover of serum virions, the authors were able to calculate a half-life of virus in plasma of approximately 4 hours (range 2–5.2 hours).

## Definition of HCV recurrence

The natural history of HCV infection in liver transplant recipients has been investigated by several centres. Results, however, are difficult to compare, mainly due to a lack of uniformity in defining recurrent hepatitis C. Recurrent HCV 'infection' should be clearly differentiated from recurrent HCV 'disease'. Recurrent infection is defined as persistence of virus detected by molecular techniques, such as PCR, while recurrent disease is defined as histological evidence of hepatitis of the graft. Other definitions based on biochemical or serological markers may be inaccurate, since altered liver function tests in the transplant setting clearly lack specificity [22], and serological assays are relatively insensitive. Evidence for the relative insensitivity of serological assays comes from extensive studies on antibody titres in the setting of immunosuppression, which have shown a fall of certain HCV antibody titres. Titres of antibodies to C22, C25, NE1 and NE2 are less affected, explaining the greater sensitivity of second generation assays [23]. Indeed, a positive RIBA2 result is a reasonably good marker of viraemia in the transplant population, and indeterminate RIBA2 results (defined by a single reactive band pattern), frequently found among immunocompromised patients, often indicate HCV infection in this setting [24].

## *Virological assays*

Nucleic acid detection techniques have enabled the identification of HCV infection in patients undergoing liver transplantation with a high degree of accuracy. The sensitivity and specificity of PCR as a diagnostic assay prior to and following liver transplantation is high. By PCR, the majority of anti-HCV (EIAII)-positive cirrhotic patients are found to be viraemic. Moreover, an additional 5–11% of seronegative patients are diagnosed prior to transplantation with HCV infection when PCR is used [5]. While antibody production is impaired in the transplant setting, serum HCV RNA is consistently detected and the level of viraemia after transplantation are 10- to 20-fold higher compared to pre-transplant values [25,26].

Although regarded as the 'gold standard' for diagnosis of HCV infection, PCR can produce inaccurate results and is subjected to wide variability [27]. Quantitative assays, such as the branched DNA assay, although less sensitive than PCR-based assays, accurately quantify the amount of viral RNA over a wide range, are standardized and are less labour-intensive than PCR-based methodologies [27].

Viraemia is nonetheless not always associated with disease. One year after transplantation, 30–50% of the recipients have evidence of HCV infection without evidence of histological disease [5,19,26,28].

## Natural history

With short-term follow-up, post-transplantation HCV infection is a relatively benign condition [28], yet with follow-up of 5–7 years, 8–12% of the patients develop cirrhosis [8,9]. Thus, while the disease course is benign in many patients, an accelerated course of liver injury leading to rapid development of cirrhosis is observed. Factors influencing the rate of progression are largely unknown, but likely relate to: (i) the intrinsic characteristics of the infecting viral strains; (ii) genetically determined characteristics of the infected individual; and (iii) environmental and/or iatrogenic influences on the infected individual such as immunosuppression [29] or alcohol consumption.

Knowledge of the natural history of HCV-related liver damage following liver transplantation and factors associated with disease progression may aid in: (i) patient selection for liver transplantation; (ii) management of recipients with severe HCV disease through rational modification of immunosuppression; and (iii) identification of patients most in need of therapy.

Long-term consequences of HCV infection (Table 1) remain to be defined and the results of short-term studies are conflicting. One study showed that moderate chronic hepatitis developed in 27% of patients after a median of 35 months and that disease progressed to cirrhosis in 8% after a median of 51 months [9]. In another recent study [10], with up to 12 years of follow-up, the majority of HCV-infected liver transplant recipients developed histological evidence of post-transplantation disease, but liver injury was mild in the majority and mortality in the first decade was identical to controls without HCV infection. No deaths related to viral hepatitis of the graft were observed.

Although median term survival of HCV-infected patients compared to uninfected controls appears to be similar, published series to date have not included sufficient patients to detect minor differences in outcome. In the USA, a large body of data from the United Network for Organ Sharing (UNOS) suggests that HCV infection adversely affects both patient and graft survival. Patient survival at 5 years was only 65% in those undergoing liver transplantation for HCV infection, whereas it reached 80% in patients undergoing liver transplantation for cholestatic or autoimmune liver disease [30]. These results suggest that we clearly need a longer period of observation to detect differences in outcome. The use of newer immunosuppressive agents may complicate the analysis even more. Studies will be under-powered if the endpoints chosen occur infrequently within the period of follow-up (typically 3–5 years post-transplantation). There are a number of difficulties in determining the influence of HCV infection on patient and graft survival: (i) it is unclear which is the most appropriate control group because there is a wide variation in outcomes depending on the initial diagnosis, with patients with cholestatic liver disease doing the best and patients with HCC doing the worst; (ii) other factors which may alter the outcome, such as age, Child's Pugh or UNOS status and donor age must be taken into account; (iii) the quality of the data can vary greatly depending on the method of data collection; (iv) post-transplantation factors that could potentially affect natural history (such as immunosuppression) are either unidentified or unmeasured and hence not controlled for in most published series; and (v) the number of patients included and the duration of follow-up is largely insufficient to determine small differences in outcome.

With time, the full impact of recurrent HCV infection will become apparent, although good short-term survival warrants continued transplantation of this group of patients.

## Factors influencing disease severity and disease progression

These factors are as yet not defined, with most of the emphasis placed on post-transplantation factors, mainly viral factors.

### Viral factors

Viral factors may be important in the pathogenesis of disease either directly, through cellular injury associated with accumulation of the intact virus or viral proteins, or indirectly through a differential immune response

**Table 1.** Median-term natural history of HCV infection following liver transplantation

| Study* | Histological hepatitis | Time to histological hepatitis | Follow-up | Graft | Survival Patients | Survival Controls |
|---|---|---|---|---|---|---|
| Feray et al. [8] (79; 106) | Acute 66%, Chronic 28%; Actuarial at 1, 2, 4 years: 57%, 62%, 72% | Acute: 4 months (1–48) | Patients 46 months (12–84); Controls 55 months (1–86) | Re-OLT: Patients 13%; Controls 10% | 95%, 90%, 80% at 1, 2, 5 years | 98%, 96%, 89% at 1, 2, 5 years |
| Gane et al. [9] (149; 623) | Acute 62%. Last biopsy: Normal 12% at 20 months; Mild chronic 54% at 35 months; Moderate chronic 27% at 35 months; Cirrhosis 8% at 51 months‡; No differences in the number of grafts without hepatitis (8.5% vs 5%); or with mild (62% vs 51%); moderate (29% vs 23%) at 1 and 5 years; No cirrhosis at 1 year, 8 at 5 years | Acute: 77 days (23–469) | 36 months (1–138) | Graft loss: 18% (29% due to HCV) | 79%, 74%, 70% at 1, 3, 5 years | 75%, 71%, 69% at 1, 3, 5 years |
| Boker et al. [10] (61; 474) | Inflammatory changes 88%; Fibrosis 24%; Serial biopsy: improvement in inflammatory changes/fibrosis (12 & 2); unchanged (22 & 14); worsening (22 & 14) | NA | Reinfected 1012±898 days; De novo HCV 2767±1018 days | Re-OLT: 21% (none for HCV disease) | 67%, 62%, 62% at 2, 5, 10 years§ | 62%, 57%, 52% at 2, 5, 10 years |

NA, Not available; OLT, orthotopic liver transplantation.

*The number of patients and controls, respectively, are given in parentheses.

In the control group, the actuarial rates of acute hepatitis were 10%, 18% and 20% at 1, 2 and 4 years, respectively. Progression to chronic hepatitis occurred in 85% of the patients who had previously developed acute hepatitis. All of these patients had acquired HCV infection.

‡30 patients had a biopsy at 1 and 5 years. Of 21 with mild hepatitis at 1 year, four progressed to moderate hepatitis and one to cirrhosis at 5 years. Of nine patients with moderate hepatitis at 1 year, six had cirrhosis at 5 year (P<0.05).

§In the HCV-infected group, survival was different depending on the presence or not of hepatocellular carcinoma at transplantation, with survival rates of 53% and 35% at 2 and 5 years, respectively, in the hepatocellular carcinoma group compared to 73% and 73% in the HCV group without hepatocellular carcinoma.

**Table 2.** Hepatitis C post-transplantation: relationship with HCV genotypes

| Study | No. of patients | Follow-up (months) | Genotype 1b (%) | Recurrent hepatitis (%); 1b/non-1b | Time to recurrent hepatitis (days); 1b/non-1b | 'Severe hepatitis post-OLT' (%); 1b/non-1b | Genotype–disease severity association |
|---|---|---|---|---|---|---|---|
| Feray et al. [31] | 60 | 42 (14–90) | 68 | 77.5/40 | NA | 60/20* | Yes |
| Zhou et al. [32] | 124 | 25 (1–75) | 27 | NA | NA | 23/21† | No |
| Gane et al. [9] | 100 | 36 (1–248) | 43 | NA | NA | 46/24‡ | Yes |
| Gayowski et al. [34] | 47 | 38 (6–74) | 25 | 67/49 | 198 (72–714)/ 301 (87–994)¶ | NA§ | No |

*Severe hepatitis was defined as the development of CAH or cirrhosis.
†Severe hepatitis was defined as a histological score higher than 4 (normal range: 0–16).
‡Severe hepatitis was defined as the development of moderate CAH or cirrhosis.
§Severity of HCV recurrence assessed by Knodell score was similar between genotype 1a-, 1b- and 2b-infected patients (mean Knodell score: 5, 5.8 and 2, respectively).
¶Non-1b refers to genotype 1a in this case.

associated with one viral strain but not with another.

*HCV genotypes.* Studies evaluating the relationship between severity of liver disease post-transplantation and HCV genotypes are conflicting [9,31–34] (Table 2). Some studies [9,31], mainly from Europe, have implicated genotype 1, and in particular subtype 1b, in causing aggressive post-transplantation disease compared with non-genotype 1. Other studies, in contrast, could not demonstrate such an association [10,32,33,34]. The similar genotype distribution among patients undergoing liver transplantation and patients with chronic hepatitis C seen at tertiary centres in the USA further supports the hypothesis that HCV genotype does not affect disease severity or disease progression [35]. Factors that could account for these discrepant results include differences in: (i) genotype distribution in the study population (Table 3) [33,35–38]; (ii) genotyping methods; (iii) the type and amount of administered immunosuppression; (iv) the length of histological follow-up; and (v) the methods of assessing disease severity.

*HCV RNA levels.* Circulating HCV RNA levels following liver transplantation are typically 10- to 20-fold higher than levels prior to transplantation, with a positive correlation between the pre- and post-transplant viraemia level [25,26], and no differences between patients with recurrent and acquired HCV infection [26]. As opposed to the conflicting results obtained in studies of immunocompetent patients, the studies carried out in liver transplant recipients have mainly, but not always, documented a lack of correlation between HCV RNA levels and disease severity, suggesting that the mechanism of liver injury is most likely not due to direct cytopathic effect of the virus, but

rather to a host immune response to the infection. Indeed, some patients have very high levels of virus with no histological evidence of hepatitis [5,25], suggesting the existence of a 'healthy carrier state', as has been described in immunocompetent patients with HCV infection [39]. A few studies, however, have described high levels of viraemia in patients with severe post-transplantation liver disease [26]. The reasons for these discordant results include: (i) small numbers of patients; (ii) study design cross-sectional rather than longitudinal in nature; (iii) methods used for viral quantification; (iv) differences in genotype distribution; (v) differences in timing of HCV quantification; (vi) differences in the definition and methods of assessing disease severity; and (vii) methods of handling and storage of serum samples [27].

An inherent assumption in all these studies is that HCV RNA quantified in serum is reflective of HCV RNA in liver, and that HCV RNA detected in a needle biopsy is representative of HCV RNA levels in the liver as a whole, both of which have been demonstrated [40,41]. In a recent study [42], although a positive correlation was found between liver and serum HCV RNA in the majority of patients, discrepant results were observed in 19% of cases. Multiple regression analysis showed that the level of HCV RNA in serum was independently correlated both to the level of liver HCV RNA and to the duration of serum conservation.

Only one study has longitudinally assessed liver HCV RNA in liver transplant recipients [42]. A long-term decline in intrahepatic HCV RNA, despite progression to severe liver disease, was observed. This progressive decline was more marked among genotype 1b patients, and it occurred at the same time as the decrease in the amount of immunosuppression. Furthermore, a strong correlation was observed

**Table 3.** Distribution of HCV genotypes in patients with chronic hepatitis C and in patients undergoing liver transplantation

| Study | Type/No. of population | Number of patients having genotype (%) | | | | | | | | | | Genotyping method |
|---|---|---|---|---|---|---|---|---|---|---|---|---|
| | | 1a | 1b | 1a+1b | 2a | 2b | 2c | 3a | 4 | Mixed | NT | |
| Lau et al. [35] | Tertiary referral centres (USA); 384 | 160 (36.5) | 131 (29.9) | 11 (2.5) | 16 (3.7) | 28 (6.6) | – | 24 (5.5) | 5 (1.1) | 16 (3.7) | 4 (0.9) | Line probe (5'UTR), RFLP (UTR), serotyping (NS4); concordance 98.2–100% |
| Zhou et al. [32] | Transplant centre (UCSF); 124 | 39 (32.2) | 33 (27.3) | – | 9 (7.5) | 10 (8.3) | – | 17 (14) | – | 4 (3.3) | 9 (7.5) | PCR with TSP (NS5/C), serotyping (NS4), RFLP (UTR); concordance 92.5% (~30% untypable with TSP and serotyping) |
| Vargas et al. [33] | Transplant centre (Pittsburg); 185 | 85 (46) | 52 (28.1) | – | 2 (1.1) | 14 (7.6) | – | 5 (2.7) | 13 (7) | – | 13 (7) | PCR with TSP (NS5/C), direct sequencing (NS5); concordance >95% |
| Gayowski et al. [34] | Transplant centre (Pittsburg); 68 | 31 (45) | 12 (18) | – | – | 4 (6) | – | – | – | – | 11 (16) | Sequencing (NS5), PCR with TSP |
| Nousbaum et al. [38] | Tertiary referral centres (France, Italy); 220 | 22 (10) | 136 (61.8) | – | 2 (0.9) | 2 (0.9) | – | 20 (9) | – | 12 (5.4) | 26 (12) | PCR with TSP |
| Guadagnino et al. [36] | General population survey (Italy); 148 | – | 75 (50.7) | – | | 1 (0.7) | 66 (44.6) | 4 (2.7) | 2 (1.3) | – | – | Line probe (5'UTR), PCR with TSP |
| Gane et al [9] | Transplant centre (UK); 100 | 20 (20) | 43 (43) | – | 8 (8) | – | – | 11 (11) | 14 (14) | 3 (3) | 1 (1) | Line probe (5'UTR) |
| Feray et al. [31] | Transplant centre (France); 60 | 12 (20) | 40 (68) | – | 6 (10) | – | – | 1 (1.5) | – | – | 1 (1.5) | PCR with TSP (C), line probe (UTR); concordance 100% for 1b, but only 42% for non-1b (then better line probe) |

RFLP, restriction fragment length polymorphism; TSP, type-specific primers. NT, not typeable.

between the first determination of intrahepatic HCV RNA at the time of acute hepatitis and the risk of subsequent progression to chronic active hepatitis (CAH). Multivariate analysis identified three independent factors associated with the development of CAH: lobular hepatitis on the first biopsy, the level of liver HCV RNA in the first biopsy and young age. From these data, the authors concluded that recurrent hepatitis C can be divided in two successive stages: (i) the first stage, where lobular acute hepatitis develops, is characterized by high levels of HCV RNA in liver independently of genotype, suggesting that the mechanism of liver injury is via a direct cytopathic effect; and (ii) the second stage is marked by progression to CAH, characterized by a decline in intrahepatic HCV RNA, which is more marked among genotype 1b patients than those with non-genotype 1b infection. This suggests that the mechanism of liver injury at this point is immune-mediated – that is, the host response, as the amount of immunosuprression decreases, is able both to control intrahepatic HCV replication and induce liver damage. This response may be stronger, and thus liver disease more severe, in patients with high levels of replication at the time of lobular hepatitis and in those infected with HCV genotype 1b.

*HCV diversity.* There have been data mainly in immunocompetent but also in immunocompromised patients suggesting that HCV diversity plays a role in the pathogenesis of progressive HCV infection, but findings are again controversial. In one report [43], where the degree of HCV complexity was determined by single-strand conformation polymorphism (SSCP) analysis in three patients undergoing liver transplantation, the number of SSCP bands decreased within 3 months of transplantation, but returned to similar levels as those present pre-transplantation after 3 months, suggesting that the limited immunological pressure of the first months post-transplantation results in an homogeneous HCV population that becomes more heterogeneous with time. In the only patient in which direct sequencing data were available, although the diversity was found also to diminish immediately after transplantation, the major variant pre-transplantation was also detected post-transplantation. In another report [44], heteroduplex assays were used to measure viral diversity before and after liver transplantation in five individuals, three of whom developed severe recurrent hepatitis C. In these three patients, the major variants present prior to transplantation were efficiently propagated following transplantation throughout the course of acute and

chronic hepatitis. In contrast, in the two patients with a mild course, there was a rapid depletion of the major variants present pre-transplantation while the minor variants present pre-transplantation became dominant post-transplantation.

## Non-viral factors

*HLA-matching.* Some, but not all studies [45,46], have suggested that while HLA-B sharing between the donor and the recipient reduces the incidence of acute cellular rejection, it also promotes the recurrence of viral hepatitis in the liver transplant recipients by augmenting cell-mediated immune responses towards HCV-infected liver allografts.

*Immunosuppression.* Results on the association between the type of administered immunosuppression and disease severity are conflicting [29,47,48], and warrant prospective studies comparing different types of immunosuppression-based regimens in HCV-infected recipients.

The findings of studies relating the amount of immunosuppression and disease severity have also been conflicting [47,48,49]. Furthermore, allograft rejection, but not increased immunosuppression therapy, has been shown to be associated with a severe liver disease. Two explanations for this association have been proposed: (i) rejection may activate immune-mediated virus-associated hepatocellular injury through immune activation; (ii) increased immunosuppression which results from treatment of rejection is directly deleterious. In a recent study [49] focusing on a homogeneous population of 63 genotype 1b liver transplant recipients treated with the triple standard immunosuppression regimen, the presence of rejection, mainly during the first year, and the number of methyl-prednisolone boluses were significantly more common in patients who subsequently developed severe disease than in those who did not. Among the former, there was also a trend towards higher cumulative steroid and azathioprine doses [49]. Although the association between high viral load related to immunosuppression and more severe graft damage may suggest a direct cytopathic effect, it does not exclude immune-mediated mechanisms of liver damage. An increase in hepatic expression of HCV antigens in patients with high viral load due to increased immunosuppression may enhance the immune response of the host, particularly when the latter is restored with prolonged follow-up. Similar findings have been observed in chronic carriers of HCV on withdrawal of chemotherapy or reduction of

**Table 4.** Recurrent hepatitis C: therapeutic approaches

| Study (n) | Study type | Time from OLT to treatment (months) | Type/total dose/duration of treament (months) | Post-treatment follow-up (months) | Baseline histology | Response at end of treatment: biochemical; virological | Sustained response after follow-up: biochemical; virological | Histological improvement after follow-up | Risk of rejection/adverse effects |
|---|---|---|---|---|---|---|---|---|---|
| Wright et al. [58] (18) | Uncontrolled | 15±2 (4–38) | IFN-α2b/205 MU (mean)/5.7±0.1 (4–6) | R 4 (2–5); NR 7 (1–19) | Knodell 6 (3–13) | BR 5 (28%); VR 1 (0.05%) | BR 4 (22%); VR 0 | 5 (28%) | 1/18 (0.05%) |
| Feray et al. [59] (14) | Control group (n=32), not randomized | 31±19 (7–60) | IFN-α2b/180 MU (mean)/5±1.8 (1–6) | 13 (5–24) | Knodell 7.5 (4–13); Fibrosis 2.2 (0–3) | BR 2/9 (22%); VR 2/9 (22%) | BR 1/9 (11%); VR 1/9 (11%) (Control 0%; 0%) | Treated 2/9 (22%); control 0% | Treated 5/14 (35%); control 1/32 (3%) |
| Vargas et al. [60] (7) | Control group (n=7) | 2–3 | IFN-α2b/216 MU/6 | 0 | Acute hepatitis | BR 0% vs 0%; VR 0% vs 0% | NA | Treated 0%; control NA | Acute response: treated 2/7 (28%); control 1/7 (14%); chronic response 2/7 (28%) vs 0% |
| Cattral et al. [62] (9) | Uncontrolled | 5±3.7 | RBV/1000–1200 mg per day/3 | 14–20 | Mean HAI 6.1±2.2 | BR 4 (44%); VR 0 | BR 0; VR 0 | 2/8 (25%) | No rejection, symptomatic reversible haemolytic anaemia in 3 |
| Bizollon et al. [63] (21) | Uncontrolled | 9 (3–24) | RBV+IFN-α2b/RBV 1000–1200 mg/day; IFN 216 MU/6 | 6 | Knodell 6.3±2 (3–12) | BR 21 (100%); VR 10 (48%) | During RBV maintenance: BR 17/18 (94%); VR 5/18 (28%) | 17/18 (94%) | No rejection, symptomatic reversible haemolytic anaemia in 3 |
| Mazzaferro et al. [64] (21) | Uncontrolled | 3 weeks | RBV+IFN-α2b/RBV 10 mg/kg/day; IFN 216 MU/12 | NA | NA | BR 21/21 (100%); VR 9/21 (43%) | NA | CAH 1/21 (4.7%) | No rejection, haemolytic anaemia (38%) |

NA, Not available; RBV, ribavirin; HAI, hepatic activity index; R, Response; NR, non-response; BR, biochemical response; VR, virological response.

glucocorticoids and in bone marrow transplantation.

The use of OKT3 (anti-lymphocyte MAbs) has also been associated with an earlier onset of lobular hepatitis and with a more severe chronic hepatitis than are seen with other immunosuppressive drugs [50].

*Histological assessment.* Necroinflammatory activity and fibrosis grading observed on the initial liver biopsy has been used by some authors as predictive of cirrhosis development in patients with chronic hepatitis C and an intact immune system. Studies addressing similar issues are lacking in the setting of liver transplantation.

*Others.* One study has reported that patients who develop human cytomegalovirus viraemia are at increased risk of severe HCV recurrence through the induction of immunodeficiency, trigger of production and release of tumour necrosis factor, or through the existence of cross-reactive immunological responses [51]. Coinfection with other viruses such as hepatitis B virus [52] or hepatitis G virus [53] does not seem to influence the post-transplantation course of HCV disease.

In conclusion, numerous host and viral factors have been implicated in the development of severe liver disease following transplantation, suggesting that this process is multifactorial.

## Pathology

The histology of post-transplantation HCV infection includes many of the features seen in non-immunocompromised patients, such as portal-based mononuclear cell infiltrates, lymphoid aggregates, fatty changes, bile duct damage and patchy parenchymal lymphocytic aggregates. Additional features that appear to be unique to the transplant recipient include progressive fibrosis and marked periportal and parenchymal inflammation with hepatocyte necrosis [28,54]. Early liver changes include weak lobular inflammation with scattered apoptotic bodies and minimal cell swelling. This lesion progresses within 2 to 4 weeks to a more fully developed hepatitis, consisting of portal and lobular inflammation of varying degrees with associated hepatocyte necrosis and midzonal macrovesicular steatosis. Atypical histological findings, including marked ductal injury, venulitis, profound cholestasis, bile duct proliferation and perivenular ballooning of hepatocytes are also seen in patients with recurrent HCV infection, mimicking other entities such as rejection, obstruction or ischaemia. Of practical importance, the overlap between histological features of recurrent HCV infection and rejection makes the distinction between these entities difficult. Features more suggestive of HCV infection include lymphoid aggregates and fatty changes, while those more suggestive of rejection include endotheliitis and a mixed portal inflammatory infiltrate. If doubts persist, serial biopsies should be performed. A therapeutic trial with a short course of steroids, although previously proposed as a means to differentiate the two entities, may be detrimental in the long-term, and thus is not recommended. If data exist that support the presence of both entities, treatment with corticosteroids may be attempted.

Similar to what has been described in many hepatitis B recurrences after liver transplantation [55], there is increasing evidence that HCV infection can occasionally ($\approx$6–9%) result in a severe cholestatic form of recurrent HCV infection, characterized by progressive hyperbilirubinaemia with both graft loss and patient death in fewer than 5–6 months [56]. Progressive lobular inflammation, severe cholestasis with centrilobular hepatocellular drop-out and necrosis with bridging and confluent necrosis was observed on liver biopsies. The outcome of retransplantation for patients with severe recurrent HCV disease is generally poor. Surgery is associated with high mortality, sepsis being the main cause of death, particularly in patients with concomitant renal failure. In those patients who survive, the rate of disease recurrence appears to be similar to that seen in the original allograft [56,57].

## TREATMENT OF HEPATITIS C POST-TRANSPLANTATION

Therapy for hepatitis in immunocompetent individuals is evolving, yet proven effective treatments are limited. This is even more true for immunocompromised individuals with recurrent HCV disease (Table 4).

Experience with IFN alone has been limited [58,59] and efficacy appears at best to be moderate and transient. IFN alone has failed to clear serum HCV RNA, despite normalization of alanine aminotransferase (ALT) values in 0–28% of patients depending on the series. Furthermore, relapse after discontinuing treatment is almost the rule, and post-treatment improvement in hepatic damage is uncommon. Reductions in viral RNA occur but sustained virological response to IFN is rare. The reasons for the poor antiviral effect of IFN in the transplant setting are probably due to high levels of HCV RNA during the post-transplant period and to the high rate of genotype 1b infection, both of which are associated with poor response. While there has been allograft rejection documented in transplant recipients, it appears to be a rare event in liver recipients.

IFN has also been tried in the setting of acute hepatitis post-transplantation in an attempt to decrease the progression to chronicity, as some preliminary results indicate some benefit in immunocompetent patients. Unfortunately, early use of IFN at the onset of acute hepatitis following liver transplantation was ineffective in one study, and furthermore was associated with a high rate of graft rejection (28%) [60].

In short, the data show that IFN alone is probably not going to be useful in inducing a prolonged disease remission after transplantation.

Ribavirin, a guanosine analogue, is another agent that has been recently evaluated with limited efficacy in the treatment of HCV in immunocompetent and immunocompromised individuals. In both patient groups, treatment results in biochemical but not virological responses [61,62].

Combination therapy is a recent approach with promising results. In a non-randomized pilot study [63], Bizollon *et al.* assessed the safety and efficacy of combination therapy with ribavirin and IFN for the treatment of recurrent hepatitis C. Fourteen patients with early documented recurrent HCV hepatitis were treated with IFN-$\alpha$2b (3 MU three times weekly) and ribavirin (1000 mg/day) for 6 months, and then maintained on ribavirin monotherapy until the end of the study. All patients normalized ALT, and 50% cleared HCV RNA from serum at the end of treatment. The remaining patients, although viraemic, experienced a 50% reduction in viral load. Only one patient on ribavirin monotherapy had a biochemical relapse during the 6 month period on ribavirin alone, despite reappearance of serum HCV RNA in 50% (5/10) who had initially cleared HCV RNA. Most importantly, all but one patient who tolerated the drug showed an improvement in liver histology. Safety and tolerability were satisfactory, with anaemia being the most common side-effect. No patient experienced graft rejection. This favourable outcome is noteworthy because all patients had high HCV RNA levels (mean value of 125 Meq/ml) and 92% were infected with HCV genotype 1b. One of the reasons that may explain the favourable outcome in this study is the early intervention with combined therapy at a stage when patients have developed CAH but before they progress to severe forms of liver injury. Maintenance therapy appeared critical to avoid relapse, as all three patients who stopped ribavirin because of symptomatic anaemia showed a biochemical relapse with worsening in histological score. Whether maintenance therapy could be discontinued in patients who have

responded virologically remains to be determined. This pilot study of combination therapy is encouraging and points to the need for randomized controlled trials.

A final approach is the use of prophylaxis combination therapy early after liver transplantation in an attempt to prevent HCV recurrence. In one case series [64], 21 recipients (19 of whom were infected with HCV genotype 1b) were treated with IFN-$\alpha$2b and ribavirin starting in the third week post-transplantation. After a median follow-up of 12 months, four patients (19%) had developed acute recurrent hepatitis C, but only one (5%) had evolved to CAH. Furthermore, loss of serum and liver HCV RNA occurred in nine patients (41%) after a median of 37 days of treatment. Twelve patients remained viraemic, but only one developed progressive graft damage. Common side-effects included haemolytic anaemia and astenia.

In conclusion, although 4 year patient and graft survival rates do not appear to be adversely affected by HCV, chronic hepatitis eventually develops in most patients, which in some rapidly progresses to cirrhosis and graft failure. With longer follow-up, the prevalence of graft failure is likely to increase. Strategies to prevent or reduce the effect of HCV infection after liver transplantation are therefore desirable. Unfortunately, IFN has been used with limited success and with concerns about toxicity. Ribavirin monotherapy has been ineffective in producing meaningful results. Preliminary results on combination therapy are very encouraging. However, the inability of currently available antiviral therapy to eliminate HCV in the liver transplant setting suggests that indefinite treatment designed to suppress the effects of the virus may be necessary. The feasibility of such an approach will depend on clear demonstration of a reduction of biochemical and histological activity of hepatitis, improved graft and patient survival, and the availability of an antiviral agent that has low toxicity, few side-effects and a high rate of patient compliance.

# REFERENCES

1. Anonymous. Annual report of the US Scientific Registry for Transplant Recipients and the Organ Procurement and Transplantation Network – Transplant Data: 1988–1994. Richmond, Virginia: United Network for Organ Sharing, and the Division of Organ Transplantation, Bureau of Health Resources Development.
2. Alter MJ. Epidemiology of hepatitis C in the West. *Seminars in Liver Disease* 1995; **15**:5–14.
3. Kiyosawa K, Sodeyama T, Tanaka E, Gibo Y, Yoshizawa K, Nakano Y, Furuta S, Akahane Y, Nishioka K, Purcell RH & Alter HJ. Interrelationship of blood transfusion, non-A, non-B hepatitis and

hepatocellular carcinoma: analysis by detection of antibody to hepatitis C virus. *Hepatology* 1990; **12**:671–675.

4. Fattovich G, Giustina G, Degos F, Tremolada F, Diodati G, Almasio P, Nevens F, Solinas A, Mura D, Brouwer JT, Thomas H, Njapoum C, Casarin C, Bonetti P, Fuschi P, Basho J, Tocco A, Bhalla A, Galassini R, Noventa F, Schalm SW & Realdi G. Morbidity and mortality in compensated cirrhosis type C: a retrospective follow-up study of 384 patients. *Gastroenterology* 1997; **112**:463–472.

5. Wright TL, Donegan E, Hsu HH, Ferrell L, Lake JR, Kim M, Combs C, Fennessy S, Roberts JP, Ascher NL & Greenburg H. Recurrent and acquired hepatitis C viral infection in liver transplant recipients. *Gastroenterology* 1992; **103**:317–322.

6. Feray C, Samuel D, Thiers V, Gigou M, Pichon F, Bismuth A, Reynes M, Maisonneuve P, Bismuth H & Brechot C. Reinfection of liver graft by hepatitis C virus after liver transplantation. *Journal of Clinical Investigation* 1992; **89**:1361–1365.

7. Sallie R, Cohen AT, Tibbs CJ, Portmann BC, Rayner A, O'Grady JG, Tan KC & Williams R. Recurrence of hepatitis C following orthotopic liver transplantation: a polymerase chain reaction and histological study. *Journal of Hepatology* 1994; **21**:536–542.

8. Feray C, Gigou M, Samuel D, Paradis V, Wilber J, David MF, Urdea M, Reynes M, Brechot C & Bismuth H. The course of hepatitis C virus infection after liver transplantation. *Hepatology* 1994; **20**:1137–1143.

9. Gane EJ, Portmann BC, Naoumov NV, Smith HM, Underhill JA, Donaldson PT, Maertens G & Williams R. Long-term outcome of hepatitis C infection after liver transplantation. *New England Journal of Medicine* 1996; **334**:815–820.

10. Boker KH, Dalley G, Bahr MJ, Maschek H, Tillmann HL, Trautwein C, Oldhaver K, Bode U, Pichlmayr R & Manns MP. Long-term outcome of hepatitis C virus infection after liver transplantation. *Hepatology* 1997; **25**:203–210.

11. Kim WR & Dickson ER. The role of prognostic models in the timing of liver transplantation. In *Clinics in Liver Disease*, 1997, pp. 263–279. Edited by N Gitlin & E Keefe. Philadelphia: WB Saunders.

12. UNOS. Reported deaths on the OPTN waiting list, 1988–1994. *UNOS update* 1996; **12**:25.

13. Schalm SW. Treatment of patients with cirrhosis. *Hepatology* 1997; **26** (Supplement 1):128S–132S.

14. Nishiguchi S, Kuroki T, Nakatani S, Morimoto H, Takeda T, Nakajima S, Shiomi S, Seki S, Kobayashi K & Otani S. Randomised trial of effects of interferon alpha on incidence of hepatocellular carcinoma in chronic active hepatitis with cirrhosis. *Lancet* 1995; **346**:1051–1055.

15. Roth D, Fernandez JA, Babischkin S, De Mattos A, Buck BE, Quan S, Olson L, Burke GW, Nery JR, Esquenazi V *et al.* Detection of hepatitis C virus infection among cadaver organ donors: evidence for low transmission of disease. *Annals of Internal Medicine* 1992; **117**: 470–475.

16. Pereira BJ, Wright TL, Schmid CH, Bryan CF, Cheung RC, Cooper ES, Hsu H, Heyn-Lamb R, Light JA, Norman DJ *et al.* Screening and confirmatory testing of cadaver organ donors for hepatitis C virus infection: a US national collaborative study group. *Kidney International* 1994; **46**:886–892.

17. Bouthot BA, Murthy BVR, Schmid CH, Levey AS & Pereira BJG. Long-term follow-up of hepatitis C virus infection among organ transplant recipients: implications for policies on organ transplantation. *Transplantation* 1997; **63**:849–853.

18. Laskus T, Wang LF, Rakela J, Vargas H, Pinna AD, Tsamandas AC, Demetris AJ & Fung J. Dynamic behavior of hepatitis C virus in chronically infected patients receiving liver graft from infected donors. *Virology* 1996; **220**:171–176.

19. Gretch DR, Bacchi CE, Corey L, de la Rosa C, Lesniewski RR, Kowdley K, Gown A, Frank I, Perkins JD & Carithers RL Jr. Persistent hepatitis C virus infection after liver transplantation: clinical and virological features. *Hepatology* 1995; **22**:1–9.

20. Schreiber GB, Busch MP, Kleinman SH & Korelitz JJ. The risk of transfusion-transmitted viral infections. *New England Journal of Medicine* 1996; **334**: 1685–1690.

21. Fukumoto T, Berg T, Ku Y, Bechstein WO, Knoop M, Lemmens HP, Lobeck H, Hopf U & Neuhaus P. Viral dynamics of hepatitis C early after orthotopic liver transplantation: evidence for rapid turnover of serum virions. *Hepatology* 1996; **24**:1351–1354.

22. Shiffman ML, Contos MJ, Luketic VA, Sanyal AJ, Purdum PP III, Mills AS, Fisher RA & Posner MP. Biochemical and histological evaluation of recurrent hepatitis C following orthotopic liver transplantation. *Transplantation* 1994; **57**:526–532.

23. Lok AS, Chien D, Choo QL, Chan TM, Chiu EK, Cheng IK, Houghton M & Kuo G. Antibody response to core, envelope and nonstructural hepatitis C virus antigens: comparison of immunocompetent and immunosuppressed patients. *Hepatology* 1993; **18**: 497–502.

24. Donegan E, Wright TL, Roberts J, Ascher NL, Lake JR, Neuwald P, Wilber J, Quan S, Kuramoto IK, Dinello RK *et al.* Detection of hepatitis C after liver transplantation. Four serologic tests compared. *American Journal of Clinical Pathology* 1995; **104**:673–679.

25. Chazouilleres O, Kim M, Combs C, Ferrell L, Bacchetti P, Roberts J, Ascher NL, Neuwald P, Wilber J, Urdea M *et al.* Quantitation of hepatitis C virus RNA in liver transplant recipients. *Gastroenterology* 1994; **106**: 994–999.

26. Gane EJ, Naoumov NV, Qian KP, Mondelli MU, Maertens G, Portmann BC, Lau JY & Williams R. A longitudinal analysis of hepatitis C virus replication following liver transplantation. *Gastroenterology* 1996; **110**:167–177.

27. Ohno T & Lau JYN. The 'gold standard' accuracy, and the current concepts: hepatitis C virus genotype and viraemia. *Hepatology* 1996; **24**:1312–1315.

28. Ferrell L, Wright T, Roberts J, Ascher N & Lake J. Hepatitis C viral infection in liver transplant recipients. *Hepatology* 1992; **16**:865–876.

29. Casavilla A, Mateo R, Rakela J, Starzl TE, Irish W, Demetris AJ & Fung JJ. Impact of hepatitis C virus (HCV) infection on survival following primary liver transplantation (OLTx) under FK506. *Hepatology* 1994; **20**:133A.

30. Belle SH, Beringer KC & Detre K. An update on liver transplantation in the United States: recipient characteristics and outcome. In *Clinical Transplants* 1995; pp. 19–32. Edited by PI Terasaki & JM Cecka. Los Angeles: UCLA Tissue Typing Laboratory.

31. Feray C, Gigou M, Samuel D, Paradis V, Mishiro S, Maertens G, Reynes M, Okamoto H, Bismuth H & Brechot C. Influence of genotypes of hepatitis C virus on the severity of recurrent liver disease after liver transplantation. *Gastroenterology* 1995; **108**: 1088–1096.

32. Zhou S, Terrault NA, Ferrell L, Hahn JA, Lau JY, Simmonds P, Roberts JP, Lake JR, Ascher NL & Wright TL. Severity of liver disease in liver transplantation recipients with hepatitis C virus infection: relationship to genotype and level of viremia. *Hepatology* 1996; **24**:1041–1046.

33. Vargas HE, Wang LF, Laskus T, Poutous A, Lee R, Demetris A, Dodson F, Casavilla A, Fung J, Gayowski T, Singh N, Marino I & Rakela J. Distribution of infecting hepatitis C virus genotypes in end-stage liver disease patients at a large American transplant center. *Journal of Infectious Diseases* 1997; **175**:448–450.

34. Gayowski T, Singh N, Marino IR, Vargas H, Wagener M, Wannstedt C, Morelli F, Laskus T, Fung JJ, Rakela J & Starzl TE. Hepatitis C virus genotypes in liver transplant recipients: impact on posttransplant recurrence, infections, response to interferon-alpha and outcome. *Transplantation* 1997; **64**:422–426.

35. Lau JY, Davis GL, Prescott LE, Maertens G, Lindsay KL, Qian K, Mizokami M & Simmonds P. Distribution of hepatitis C virus genotypes determined by line probe assay in patients with chronic hepatitis C seen at tertiary referral centers in the United States. *Annals of Internal Medicine* 1996; **124**:868–876.

36. Guadagnino V, Stroffolini T, Rapicetta M, Costantino A, Kondili LA, Menniti-Ippolito F, Caroleo B, Costa C, Griffo G, Loiacono L, Pisani V, Foca A & Piazza M. Prevalence, risk factors, and genotype distribution of hepatitis C virus infection in the general population: a community-based survey in southern Italy. *Hepatology* 1997; **26**:1006–1011.

37. Zein NN, Rakela J, Krawitt EL, Reddy KR, Tominaga T & Persing DH. Hepatitis C virus genotypes in the United States: epidemiology, pathogenicity, and response to interferon therapy. *Annals of Internal Medicine* 1996; **125**:634–639.

38. Nousbaum JB, Pol S, Nalpas B, Landais P, Berthelot P & Brechot C. Hepatitis C virus type 1b(II) infection in France and Italy. *Annals of Internal Medicine* 1995; **122**:161–168.

39. Prieto M, Olaso V, Verdu C, Cordoba J, Gisbert C, Rayon M, Carrasco D, Berenguer M, Higon MD & Berenguer J. Does the healthy hepatitis C virus carrier state really exist? An analysis using polymerase chain reaction. *Hepatology* 1995; **22**:413–417.

40. Terrault NA, Dailey PJ, Ferrell L, Collins ML, Wilber JC, Urdea MS, Bhandari BN & Wright TL. Hepatitis C virus: quantitation and distribution in liver. *Journal of Medical Virology* 1997; **51**:217–224.

41. Jeffers LJ, Dailey PJ, Cohelo-Little E, de Medina M, Scott C, LaRue S, Hill M, Collins MA, Chan CS, Urdea MS, Parker T, Reddy KR & Schiff ER. Correlation of HCV RNA quantitation in sera and liver tissue of patients with chronic C hepatitis. *Gastroenterology* 1993; **104**:A923.

42. Di Martino V, Saurini F, Samuel D, Gigou M, Dussaix E, Reynes M, Bismuth H & Feray C. Long-term longitudinal study of intrahepatic hepatitis C virus replication after liver transplantation. *Hepatology* 1997; **26**: 1343–1350.

43. Yun Z, Barkholt L & Sonnenberg A. Dynamic analysis of hepatitis virus polymorphism in patients with orthotopic liver transplantation. *Transplantation* 1997; **64**: 170–172.

44. Gretch DR, Polyak SJ, Wilson JJ, Carithers RL Jr, Perkins JD & Corey L. Tracking hepatitis C virus quasispecies major and minor variants in symptomatic and asymptomatic liver transplant recipients. *Journal of Virology* 1996; **70**:7622–7631.

45. Manez R, Mateo R, Tabasco J, Kusne S, Starzl TE & Duquesnoy RJ. The influence of HLA donor–recipient compatibility on the recurrence of HBV and HCV hepatitis after liver transplantation. *Transplantation* 1995; **59**:640–642.

46. Gretch D, Wile M, Gaur L, Lesniewski R, Nelson K, Strong M, Johnson R, Corey L, Perkins J & Carithers R. Donor–recipient match at the HLA-DQB locus is associated with recrudescence of chronic hepatitis following liver transplantation for end-stage hepatitis C. *Hepatology* 1993; **18** (Supplement):108A.

47. Sheiner PA, Schwartz ME, Mor E, Schluger LK, Theise N, Kishikawa K, Kolesnikov V, Bodenheimer H, Emre S & Miller CM. Severe or multiple rejection episodes are associated with early recurrence of hepatitis C after orthotopic liver transplantation. *Hepatology* 1995; **21**: 30–34.

48. Freeman R, Tran S, Lee Y, Rohrer R & Kaplan M. Serum hepatitis C RNA titers after liver transplantation are not correlated with immunosuppression or hepatitis. *Transplantation* 1996; **61**:542–546.

49. Berenguer M, Prieto M, Cordoba J, Rayon JM, Carrasco D, Olaso V, San-Juan F, Gobernado M, Mir J & Berenguer J. Early development of chronic active hepatitis in recurrent hepatitis C virus infection after liver transplantation: association with treatment of rejection. *Journal of Hepatology* 1998; **28**:756–763.

50. Rosen HR, Martin P, Shackleton CR, Farmer DA, Holt C & Busuttil RW. OKT3 use associated with diminished graft and patient survival in patients transplanted for chronic hepatitis C. *Hepatology* 1995; **22** (Supplement):132A.

51. Rosen HR, Chou S, Corless CL, Gretch DR, Flora KD, Boudousquie A, Orloff SL, Rabkin JM & Benner KG. Cytomegalovirus viremia. Risk factor for allograft cirrhosis after liver transplantation for hepatitis C. *Transplantation* 1997; **64**:721–726.

52. Huang E, Wright TL, Lake J, Combs C & Ferrell L. Hepatitis B and C coinfections and persistent hepatitis B infections: clinical outcome and liver pathology after transplantation. *Hepatology* 1996; **23**:396–404.

53. Berenguer M, Terrault NA, Piatak M, Yun A, Kim JP, Lau JY, Lake JR, Roberts JR, Ascher NL, Ferrell L & Wright TL. Hepatitis G virus infection in patients with hepatitis C virus infection undergoing liver transplantation. *Gastroenterology* 1996; **111**:1569–1575.

54. Greenson J, Svodoba-Newman S, Merion R & Frank T. Histologic progression of recurrent hepatitis C in liver transplant allografts. *American Journal of Surgical Pathology* 1996; **20**:731–738.

55. Davies SE, Portmann BC, O'Grady JG, Aldis PM, Chaggar K, Alexander GJ & Williams R. Hepatic histological findings after transplantation for chronic hepatitis B virus infection, including a unique pattern of fibrosing cholestatic hepatitis. *Hepatology* 1991; **13**:150–157.

56. Schluger LK, Sheiner PA, Thung SN, Lau JY, Min A, Wolf DC, Fiel I, Zhang D, Gerber MA, Miller CM & Bodenheimer HC Jr. Severe recurrent cholestatic hepatitis C following orthotopic liver transplantation. *Hepatology* 1996; **23**:971–976.

57. Rosen HR, O'Reilly PM, Shackleton CR, McDiarmid S, Holt C, Busuttil RW & Martin P. Graft loss following liver transplantation in patients with chronic hepatitis C. *Transplantation* 1996; **62**:1773–1776.

58. Wright TL, Combs C, Kim M, Ferrell L, Bacchetti P, Ascher N, Roberts J, Wilber J, Sheridan P & Urdea M. Interferon alpha therapy for hepatitis C virus infection

following liver transplantation. *Hepatology* 1994; **20:** 773–779.

59. Feray C, Samuel D, Gigou M, Paradis V, David MF, Lemonnier C, Reynes M & Bismuth H. An open trial of interferon alfa recombinant for hepatitis C after liver transplantation: antiviral effects and risk of rejection. *Hepatology* 1995; **22:**1084–1089.

60. Vargas V, Charco R, Castells L, Esteban R & Margarit C. Alpha-interferon for acute hepatitis C in liver transplant patients. *Transplantation Proceedings* 1995; **27:** 1222–1223.

61. Gane EJ, Tibbs CJ, Ramage JK, Portmann BC & Williams R. Ribavirin therapy for hepatitis C infection following liver transplantation. *Transplantation International* 1995; **8:**61–64.

62. Cattral MS, Krajden M, Wanless IR, Rezig M, Cameron R, Greig PD, Chung SW & Levy GA. A pilot study of ribavirin therapy for recurrent hepatitis C virus infection after liver transplantation. *Transplantation* 1996; **61:**1483–1488.

63. Bizollon T, Palazzo U, Ducerf C, Chevallier M, Elliott M, Baulieux J, Pouyet M & Trepo C. Pilot study of the combination of interferon alfa and ribavirin as therapy of recurrent hepatitis C after liver transplantation. *Hepatology* 1997; **26:**500–504.

64. Mazzaferro V, Regalia E, Pulvirenti A, Tagger A, Andreola S, Pasquali M, Baratti D, Romano F, Palazzo U, Zuin M, Bonino F, Ribero ML & Gennari L. Prophylaxis against HCV recurrence after liver transplantation. Effect of interferon and ribavirin combination. *Transplantation Proceedings* 1997; **29:** 519–521.

# 44

# Liver transplantation and hepatitis B: prophylaxis and treatment of re-infection with new antiviral agents

## Martin Krüger and Michael P Manns*

## SUMMARY

Liver transplantation in patients with end-stage liver disease secondary to chronic hepatitis B virus (HBV) infection is almost universally associated with the recurrence of infection in the transplanted liver in those patients who are hepatitis B surface antigen (HBsAg)-positive and show significant serum levels of HBV DNA prior to transplantation. The majority of recipients with HBV recurrence will develop a more aggressive course of chronic hepatitis B than is generally observed in immunocompetent patients. Thus, recent strategies have focused on decreasing HBV replication in end-stage HBV patients to prevent hepatitis B recurrence, and to treat and control HBV recurrence once viral replication occurs. During recent years, several orally active nucleoside analogues have been identified as potent inhibitors of HBV replication. Lamivudine and famciclovir have shown sustained suppression of HBV DNA levels and beneficial effects on disease activity in transplant patients. Current studies are assessing the effectiveness of these drugs as monotherapy or in combination with anti-HBs immunoprophylaxis to prevent and treat recurrent HBV infection. These new strategies profoundly change the management of HBV infection, before, during and after liver transplantation and have the potential to improve the outcome of patients undergoing liver transplantation for chronic HBV infection. Ongoing and future studies will have to define optimum combination therapies of different current and new nucleoside analogues with and without hepatitis B immunoglobulin (HBIg) to prevent and treat HBV re-infection after orthotopic liver transplantation (OLT).

## INTRODUCTION

Chronic HBV infection is a major cause of chronic liver disease, often leading to liver cirrhosis and organ failure requiring OLT [1]. In chronic viral hepatitis, recurrence of the underlying viral disease often causes graft dysfunction and diminishes long-term prognosis. The level of HBV replication before OLT is the strongest predictor of HBV recurrence [2]. Among patients with HBV-induced cirrhosis, those with detectable HBV DNA (>1 pg/ml) at the time of transplantation have a high risk (83%) of becoming or remaining HBsAg-positive 3 years after OLT [3], whereas patients who are seronegative for HBV DNA and hepatitis B envelope antigen (HBeAg) at transplantation have a lower risk of viral recurrence (58%) [3]. In addition, patients with HBV-related cirrhosis who undergo liver transplantation are at a much higher risk of recurrence (67%) than patients with fulminant hepatitis B (17%) [3]. The presence of actively replicating virus at the time of OLT not only affects the HBV recurrence rate significantly, but also causes substantial morbidity and reduces survival. If no specific prophylactic treatments are performed, the 5 year survival rate for patients undergoing liver transplantation for HBV infection is 50%, compared with survival rates of 70–85% for patients with cholestatic or alcoholic liver disease. Additional factors known to affect the outcome of transplantation include HBV DNA replication in extrahepatic sites (such as the spleen, lymph nodes, kidneys and mononuclear blood cells) [4] and immunosuppression [5]. Cyclosporin A is known to impair the cytotoxic T cell response to HBV [6,7]. A steroid-responsive enhancer region of the HBV genome and human leukocyte antigen (HLA) class I matching additionally promote HBV replication and recurrence [8,9], leading to re-infection of the graft.

During recent years, new approaches and management strategies for chronic HBV infection in the transplantation phase have been developed. As discussed below, these strategies focus on either decreasing or

*Corresponding author

**Table 1.** Pretransplantation therapeutic approaches to reduce viral replication in chronic HBV infection.

| Beneficial effect proven | Beneficial effect likely | Under evaluation | No beneficial effect/ unacceptable side-effects |
|---|---|---|---|
| IFN-α | Famciclovir | Lobucavir | Fialuridine |
| Lamivudine | | Adefovir dipivoxil | Acyclovir |
| | | Ganciclovir | Adenine arabinoside |
| | | MAb to HBsAg | Dideoxyinosine |
| | | Cytokine* | Azidothymidine |
| | | Therapeutic vaccines | Foscarnet |
| | | Adoptive immune transfer | Thymosin |
| | | | Levamisole |

*Recombinant human interleukin 12.

eliminating HBV replication in the pretransplantation phase or diminishing the frequency or intensity of HBV recurrence following liver transplantation, usually in combination with HBIg application after liver transplantation. Some of these strategies have already shown sustained beneficial effects on HBV DNA levels or disease activity (while having a favourable safety profile) and have the potential to improve substantially the outcome of HBV-infected patients undergoing liver transplantation.

## TREATMENT OF END-STAGE CHRONIC HEPATITIS B BEFORE LIVER TRANSPLANTATION

Therapeutic options to reduce viral load before transplantation are limited (Table 1). Currently, only interferon α (IFN-α) [10] and the nucleoside analogues famciclovir (diacetyl 6-deoxy-9-(4-hydroxy-3-hydroxymethyl-but-1-yl)guanine) and lamivudine [(−)-β-L 2′,3′-dideoxy-3′-thiacytidine; 3TC] have been intensively studied as potentially effective treatment options for chronic HBV infection [11–21]. Several other potential therapeutics or approaches, among them vaccination against HBV epitopes, humanized hepatitis B monoclonal antibodies and adoptive immune transfer, are currently in clinical stages of evaluation for anti-HBV activity but have not been studied in the pretransplant setting. Detailed knowledge of the HBV replication cycle has offered the potential to design specific molecular approaches to interfere with HBV replication, such as antisense oligonucleotides (synthetic nucleotide sequences that bind to mRNA and block translation of viral proteins) [22] and ribozymes (small RNA molecules with catalytic activity that inhibit HBV replication by cleaving pregenomic HBV RNA) [23,24]. However, none of these approaches is currently practical for clinical application.

Several studies suggest a role for the use of IFN-α in HBV DNA-positive patients with liver cirrhosis before liver transplantation [10,25,26]. In general, IFN-α therapy should be initiated before the onset of end-stage liver disease, although response rates in patients with decompensated HBV cirrhosis are similar to those in other chronic HBV patients, with approximately 33% achieving complete remission [25]. Unfortunately, a similar proportion do not respond to IFN-α at all [25]. Although pretransplant IFN treatment in HBsAg-positive cirrhosis does not prevent post-transplant HBV recurrence [10], a recent study demonstrated that IFN-α therapy in the peri-operative liver transplantation period improves short-term survival [26]. IFN-α therapy of HBV-related decompensated cirrhosis at the standard dose and duration is frequently associated with severe side-effects, which include acute hepatic flare-up, bacterial infections and psychiatric problems. Marcellin *et al.* [27] evaluated a prolonged (3–48 months), low-dose (3 MU) IFN-α treatment protocol in 15 patients with HBV-related decompensated cirrhosis. Ten patients (66%) had a sustained loss of serum HBV DNA associated with a decrease in alanine aminotransferase (ALT) levels into the normal range. During follow-up, seven of these 10 patients showed a marked clinical improvement. This study suggests that in patients with HBV cirrhosis, prolonged low-dose IFN-α therapy is relatively well tolerated and may induce a sustained inhibition of HBV replication with marked clinical improvement.

The nucleoside analogue acyclovir [9-(2-hydroxyethoxymethyl)guanine], despite demonstrating good preclinical properties, has no effect on human HBV replication [28].

Fialuridine [1-(2′-deoxy-2′-fluoro-β-D-arabinofuranosyl)-5-iodouracil; FIAU] has also been investigated, but is associated with an unacceptable incidence of toxicity and side-effects [29].

Recently, lobucavir, a guanosine nucleoside analogue with broad spectrum antiviral activity against HBV, human cytomegalovirus (HCMV), herpes simplex virus (HSV) and varicella-zoster virus (VZV), has been tested in adults with chronic hepatitis B and well-compensated liver disease (200 mg lobucavir either twice or four times daily) [30]. In this randomized, placebo-controlled, double-blind Phase I/II trial, both doses of lobucavir induced 2–4 log reductions in HBV DNA levels compared to placebo. However, viral load levels returned to baseline within 4 weeks after completing treatment in all but one active drug recipient [30]. So far, no data in transplant patients are available.

Adefovir dipivoxil (bis-POM PMEA), a broad-spectrum nucleoside analogue with activity against hepadnaviruses, retroviruses and herpesviruses, has been evaluated for safety and antiviral activity in a Phase I/II randomized, double-blind, placebo-controlled study [31]. Twenty patients [13 co-infected with human immunodeficiency virus (HIV)] were randomized to receive adefovir dipivoxil at 125 mg ($n$=15) or placebo ($n$=5) as a single daily oral dose for 28 days. Compared to placebo recipients, all active drug recipients experienced significant reductions in HBV DNA levels, which were sustained for the duration of treatment. However, after discontinuation of the drug, HBV DNA levels returned to baseline over 1 to 6 weeks, with a greater than fourfold rebound in one patient. The drug was well tolerated, although ALT elevation was observed during and after treatment. Neither lobucavir or adefovir has been evaluated in the transplant setting, either to prevent or to treat HBV re-infection.

Lamivudine, which has recently been approved by the US Food and Drug Administration for the treatment of HIV infection, is an effective inhibitor of duck and human HBV replication *in vitro* [32]. Lamivudine inhibits the reverse transcriptase of HBV by interfering with synthesis of the proviral DNA chain from viral RNA. Clinical trials subsequently demonstrated lamivudine to be well tolerated and effective in decreasing HBV replication in patients with chronic hepatitis B [18,21]. Unfortunately, the antiviral effects are not sustained after discontinuation of therapy [11,18,33]. Meanwhile, several studies have evaluated the effectiveness and safety of lamivudine treatment in patients with advanced and end-stage liver disease caused by hepatitis B. These studies looked at three different aspects: (i) the safety of lamivudine in end-stage liver disease patients; (ii) the effectiveness of lamivudine in decreasing HBV replication prior to liver transplantation; and (iii) the prevention of HBV reacti-

vation despite the immunosuppression associated with transplantation. In all studies, a favourable safety profile was found [12,34–36]. A substantial reduction in serum levels of HBV DNA was observed after short periods of lamivudine administration (2–12 weeks) with HBV DNA undetectable in virtually all patients receiving 100 mg daily [34,35]. Current data with lamivudine treatment in end-stage HBV liver disease strongly suggests that the drug is safe and effective in decreasing HBV replication to undetectable HBV DNA levels prior to transplantation, with a diminished risk of post-transplant HBV recurrence, especially under concomitant immunoprophylaxis with HBIg.

Famciclovir, an oral form of the purine nucleoside analogue penciclovir, has a broad spectrum antiviral activity against DNA viruses such as HSV, VZV, Epstein–Barr virus and HCMV [37,38]. Famciclovir was found to inhibit HBV DNA polymerase [39]. Clinical trials have demonstrated a favourable safety and tolerability profile [40]. A pilot study determined whether a 6 month course of famciclovir, administered before transplantation, was effective in inhibiting HBV replication in HBV DNA-positive patients ($n$=8) with end-stage liver disease [17]. Although an initial decline in HBV DNA serum levels occurred in all patients, only 25% of the patients became HBV DNA-negative and underwent liver transplantation. Both patients who became HBV DNA-negative under famciclovir post-operatively completed a 6 month course of famciclovir while continuously receiving HBIg prophylaxis. They showed a favourable post-transplant clinical and virological outcome and remained HBV DNA-negative after nearly 2 years of follow-up [17]. Ongoing multi-centre clinical trials will provide extensive data to determine the role of famciclovir for pretransplantation therapy of chronic HBV infection.

## PROPHYLAXIS OF HBV RECURRENCE

Recurrent HBV infection can be prevented to some extent with the long-term use of high-dose HBIg starting in the peri-operative period [41] (Table 2). HBV re-infection is observed in 80–90% of cases in the absence of sufficient HBIg prophylaxis, whereas under long-term HBIg treatment the risk of allograft infection is significantly reduced (to 20–40%). As demonstrated in a large European study, long-term HBIg prophylaxis not only reduces the rate of HBV recurrence, but also significantly increases the 5 year survival rate, to 80% compared to less than 50% for patients without immunoprophylaxis or those receiving only short-term immunoprophylaxis [3]. Although HBIg immunoprophylaxis has substantially

Table 2. Peri-operative prophylaxis and prevention of HBV recurrence

| Beneficial effect proven | Beneficial effect likely | Under evaluation | Candidates for clinical evaluation |
|---|---|---|---|
| HBIg | Lamivudine | Famciclovir | Lobucavir |
| | | | Adefovir dipivoxil |
| | | | Anti-HBs monoclonal antibodies |

Table 3. Therapy for reduction of HBV infection

| Beneficial effect proven | Beneficial effect likely | No beneficial effect | Candidates for clinical evaluation |
|---|---|---|---|
| Lamivudine | Ganciclovir | IFN-$\alpha$ | Lobucavir |
| Famciclovir | | | Adefovir dipivoxil |

improved the outcome for HBV-infected patients undergoing liver transplantation [42,43], a significant proportion of transplant recipients experience re-infection despite HBIg immunization, so additional treatment options are therefore required.

Nucleoside analogues have been investigated for use in the prophylaxis of HBV recurrence and as a treatment for graft infection. Nucleoside analogues investigated in the transplant setting include ganciclovir, lamivudine and famciclovir. Other new nucleoside analogues are on the verge of clinical evaluation.

Ganciclovir [9-[(1,3-dihydroxy-2-propoxy)methyl] guanine] has the advantage of being active against both herpesviruses and HCMV. Although ganciclovir failed to prevent graft re-infection after OLT for chronic hepatitis B [44], results in a small group of transplant recipients with recurrent HBV infection were promising [45], and the drug is under further investigation. However, the use of ganciclovir in patients undergoing immunosuppression is limited by a bone marrow-suppressing effect.

The effectiveness and safety of lamivudine in HBV patients with advanced and end-stage liver disease has been demonstrated in several studies. In studies where patients continued to receive lamivudine therapy post-transplantation (with or without concomitant HBsAg immunoprophylaxis), a substantial number of patients cleared HBeAg and HBsAg from serum, and post-transplant liver specimens were often negative for HBV DNA by PCR [36]. HBV reactivation was observed in only a small proportion of patients [12,46], suggesting a beneficial effect of lamivudine on HBV recurrence. Markowitz et al. [47] demonstrated that lamivudine (150 mg/day) in combination with HBIg (starting with 10000 U intravenously during the anhepatic phase) is safe and highly effective in preventing hepatitis B recurrence. Of the 13 patients who underwent transplantation, a 92% 1 year survival rate was observed, with none of the patients having serological or virological evidence of HBV recurrence. A variety of studies are currently being conducted to assess the value of lamivudine for prophylaxis of hepatitis B recurrence after liver transplantation with or without HBIg immunoprophylaxis.

Although several studies are currently investigating the prophylactic use of famciclovir against HBV re-infection after liver transplantation, no results have been published. A preliminary report has been presented as an abstract [48].

## TREATMENT OF HBV RE-INFECTION AFTER LIVER TRANSPLANTATION

A variety of studies have investigated the effectiveness and safety of lamivudine in the treatment of post-transplant HBV re-infection [14,46,49–51] (Table 3). In most studies, liver transplant patients with documented recurrence of HBV infection (elevated serum ALT levels, detectable HBsAg and HBV DNA) were treated with lamivudine at 100 mg once daily [14,46,50] or 150 mg once daily [49]. All patients tolerated the treatment well, and a majority of patients lost serum HBV DNA after approximately 8 weeks of lamivudine therapy (while most still remained HBsAg-positive). A recent study by Petit et al. [51] confirmed the efficacy of lamivudine for rapid suppression of serum HBV DNA at 1 month but also demonstrated residual HBV infection, with HBV DNA levels still higher than 100 copies/ml by quantitative PCR and a majority of cases (69%) being highly positive for pre-S1 antigen at 1 month after lamivudine treatment. In this study, complete viral suppression in response to lamivudine after 1 year of treatment was only observed in 30% of cases. Larger cohorts of patients need to be analysed for viral parameters in serum and liver specimens to substantiate further this observation. Recently, preliminary data from a large multicentre study on patients with recurrent or *de novo* HBV infection after liver transplantation were published [50]. In all 52 patients analysed after 6 months of lamivudine treatment (100 mg daily), therapy was well-tolerated with only minor adverse events reported. All patients lost serum HBV DNA by week 6 after starting lamivudine. However, breakthrough of serum HBV DNA associated with the development of mutations in the YMDD locus of the HBV polymerase gene occurred in a significant proportion of patients ($n$=14). Surprisingly, in most patients, development of lamivudine resistance was not associated with obvious disease progression during the reported follow-up period.

The development of resistance to lamivudine in patients who underwent transplantation for end-stage liver disease secondary to hepatitis B is likely to be a significant problem and has been reported by various investigators [50,52–57]. Recent studies in non-transplant chronic hepatitis B patients clearly demonstrated that prolonged treatment is associated with the development of escape mutants (in at least 16% of patients at 1 year) [58,59]. Base pair substitutions at specific sites within the YMDD locus of the HBV DNA polymerase gene seem to contribute significantly to the molecular mechanism of lamivudine resistance in HBV infection [54,58,59]. Interestingly, despite the virological relapse, HBV replication generally remained at lower levels compared to the wild-type virus, suggesting that even after development of escape mutants, continued treatment with lamivudine may be beneficial. Bartholomew *et al.* [53] assessed the susceptibility of HBV to lamivudine by analysis of viral sequences after infection of primary human hepatocytes with serum taken before the start of treatment and after HBV recurrence. A common mutation within the YMDD locus of the HBV polymerase gene was found to be responsible for the development of resistance. In addition, the authors confirmed the clinical findings of lamivudine resistance in hepatocyte cultures infected with pretreatment serum: HBV DNA concentrations were reduced to less than 6% of those in control cultures by addition of lamivudine, whereas in cultures treated with serum taken after recurrence, HBV DNA concentrations did not fall comparably, even with increased lamivudine doses.

After famciclovir was found to be effective in suppressing viral replication in HBV recurrence following OLT in one patient [60], a pilot study was initiated involving 12 individuals with HBV recurrence after OLT [20]. Patients were enrolled according to an open compassionate use protocol and received oral famci-

clovir at a dose of 500 mg three times daily for a minimum of 12 weeks following recurrent infection. Before OLT, all patients had biopsy-confirmed liver cirrhosis and were HBsAg-positive. The majority of patients were also HBeAg- and HBV DNA-positive. All patients had received HBIg prophylaxis after transplantation. This was initiated with 10000 IU in the anhepatic phase and levels of antibody to HBsAg were kept continuously above 100 IU/l thereafter. Despite HBIg immunoprophylaxis, within 2–28 months of OLT all subjects experienced recurrent HBV infection, as diagnosed by elevated ALT levels and return of HBsAg and HBV DNA in serum. HBV DNA was used as the main efficacy parameter. A remarkable reduction in serum HBV DNA was noted in 75% of patients after starting famciclovir treatment, with a mean change from baseline levels of 80% after 3 months, 90% after 6 months and more than 95% after 12 months of therapy. With continued treatment, 50% of patients became HBV DNA-negative by conventional hybridization assay and HBV DNA became undetectable by PCR in one patient. In parallel to HBV DNA reduction, ALT serum levels continuously declined in 50% of patients, with a median reduction from pretreatment ALT values of 80%. The nine patients defined as 'responders' to famciclovir therapy (sustained reduction in serum HBV DNA levels) showed a mean reduction from pretreatment ALT values of 25% after 3 months, 30% after 6 months and approximately 50% after 12 months of therapy. This continuous decrease of ALT was observed from the point at which famciclovir therapy was initiated, and was maintained thereafter. ALT levels normalized in four patients (33%).

Based on these encouraging preliminary results, a large multicentre study has been initiated. Currently, 107 liver transplant patients have been treated with 500 mg of famciclovir three times a day (dose frequency adjusted for renal function) for a period of up to 4 years [61]. A sustained response (defined as a rapid reduction in HBV DNA which is sustained during the study period) was observed in 65% of patients who were treated for at least 6 months, with a median reduction of HBV DNA levels of >90% after the initial 12 weeks of treatment. In the overall population, after 6 months a median reduction in ALT levels of 42% and a median reduction in HBV DNA of 80% was observed. In the subgroup of patients with 'sustained' responses, a 90% median reduction in HBV DNA levels was observed after the initial 12 weeks. A subgroup of patients with high baseline ALT (greater than three times the upper limit of normal) showed a median reduction in HBV DNA levels of 90% and a 72% median reduction in ALT levels after 6 months of famciclovir. In both studies, long-term famciclovir treatment was well-tolerated and no clinically significant side-effects were reported. Famciclovir treatment appears to reduce HBV replication and ALT levels effectively and safely in patients with HBV recurrence after liver transplantation. Further studies have to evaluate the molecular basis of the difference between responders and non-responders.

An additional study confirmed these encouraging observations with famciclovir for post-transplant HBV infection [62]. In this study, four out of eight patients responded to famciclovir therapy. Of the four responders, one patients showed a 50% reduction and three showed a 99% reduction in their HBV DNA levels. In addition, a reduction in ALT levels was observed in three of the four patients responding to famciclovir. Other investigators have published case reports of patients receiving oral famciclovir for the treatment of HBV recurrence [63] and the use of long-term famciclovir therapy to improve the outcome in patients who undergo retransplantation after HBV-related liver allograft failure [64].

Meanwhile, resistance to famciclovir has been further characterized by sequencing regions of the HBV DNA polymerase gene. In contrast to lamivudine resistance (which mainly involves the YMDD consensus sequence in the C region, the catalytic site of the HBV polymerase), mutations observed under famciclovir were mainly detected in region B of the HBV polymerase. Preliminary evidence suggests that these mutations might develop only after long-term therapy in immunocompromised patients and are associated with a reduced sensitivity to the drug, rather than complete resistance [65,66]. These studies are particularly important to understand further the genetic basis of sensitivity or resistance of HBV to nucleoside analogues, such as famciclovir.

At our centre, eight non-responders or breakthrough patients to famciclovir treatment (determined by HBV DNA serum levels) were subsequently treated with lamivudine and showed a reduction in HBV DNA levels (below detectable levels by hybridization) within 4 to 13 weeks after starting lamivudine [55]. In two of three patients after breakthrough on famciclovir (who subsequently developed breakthrough on lamivudine), sequence analysis of the HBV genome revealed the mutation L528M, which has been reported to be associated with famciclovir resistance [66]. Within 12 to 37 weeks of lamivudine treatment, three patients developed a breakthrough while exhibiting the known methionine to valine mutation in the YMDD motif. Lamivudine seems to be effective in the majority of patients not responding to famciclovir, and as all patients in this study responded initially to lamivudine, there is no evidence of cross resistance between famciclovir and lamivudine. However, future studies need to analyse whether the L528M mutation alone is sufficient to confer resistance or reduced sensitivity to famciclovir and is a risk factor for developing resistance to lamivudine. In addition, mutations in the polymerase gene arising under treatment with a nucleoside analogue such as famciclovir or lamivudine can also affect the overlapping open reading frame (ORF) for HBsAg and might thereby change the structure of the antigen and influence binding and recognition by anti-HBs antibodies. Valuable information will be obtained by studies currently being performed on patients who failed to respond to antiviral treatment and were subsequently treated with another antiviral approach [54,55,67,68]. Sequential treatment with nucleoside analogues may not prevent the development of resistance. Therefore, combination therapy should be systematically studied in larger trials, such as the combination of lamivudine with HBIg, or lamivudine with another nucleoside analogue (famciclovir, adefovir or lobucavir) for prophylaxis of recurrence and for treatment of HBV re-infection. In these combination approaches, the nucleoside analogues are likely to impede the replication of HBV without directly promoting its eradication, whereas combination with IFN might stimulate an immune response even in immunosuppressed transplant patients.

## CONCLUSIONS

Liver transplantation in patients with end-stage liver disease secondary to chronic HBV infection is almost universally associated with recurrence of infection in the transplanted liver in patients who are HBeAg-positive or show significant levels of HBV DNA in the serum prior to transplantation. The majority of recipients with HBV recurrence will develop a more aggressive course of chronic hepatitis than is generally observed in immunocompetent patients. The presence of actively replicating virus at the time of OLT causes significantly reduced graft and patient survival. Therefore, recent strategies have focused on (i) preventing hepatitis B recurrence; and (ii) controlling HBV replication after HBV recurrence. During recent years several orally active nucleoside analogues that are potent inhibitors of HBV replication have been developed. The initial experience with these agents in liver transplant recipients has been promising, and a number of studies are currently underway to

Figure 1. Proposed strategy for management of patients with HBV infection as candidates for OLT

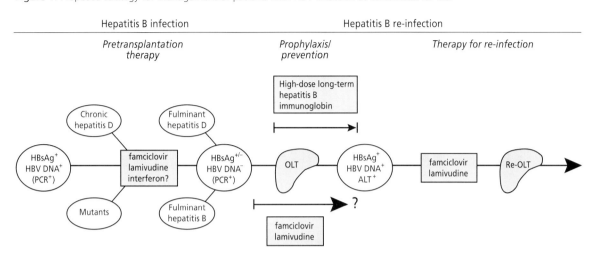

All patients receiving donor livers for HBV-related diseases should receive long-term high-dose HBIg to prevent disease recurrence. The use of famciclovir or lamivudine to supplement (or replace) this standard immunoprophylaxis is under investigation. Patients with HBV recurrence are likely to respond to famciclovir or lamivudine to stop or suppress disease progression.

determine whether these drugs, used alone or in combination with immunoprophylaxis, are effective for both the prevention and treatment of recurrent disease in those patients at highest risk of post-transplant HBV recurrence. Some of these attempts have already shown encouraging results and will profoundly change the management of HBV infection before, during and after liver transplantation. In addition, these strategies will hopefully lead to a significant better outcome for patients undergoing liver transplantation for chronic hepatitis B (Fig. 1).

Pretransplantation antiviral therapy is recommended for patients with chronic HBV infection and actively replicating virus. Multicentre clinical trials evaluating the effect of novel antiviral drugs, such as famciclovir and lamivudine, on viral replication before and after transplantation already show encouraging results. Prophylactic high-dose, long-term anti-HBIg prophylaxis should be given together with nucleoside analogues like lamivudine to reduce the rate of hepatitis B recurrence. Long-term, high-dose HBIg might be supplemented with or replaced by famciclovir, lamivudine or most probably a combination of these or other novel antiviral drugs as the standard preventive treatment for all patients receiving liver transplantation for HBV-related diseases.

Patients with recurrent HBV following transplantation are likely to respond to these new nucleoside analogues. Both agents have been extensively evaluated in animal models of HBV; they have been shown rapidly to suppress viral replication and will thereby most likely prevent disease progression.

However, nucleoside monotherapy does not seem to be sufficient to prevent HBV re-infection and the development of drug-resistant virus mutants has already been observed in transplant recipients. Further studies are needed to assess whether combination therapy may be a more effective means of avoiding development of viral resistance in patients transplanted for chronic HBV infection. Short courses with these antiviral agents generally result in rapid return of viral DNA to pretreatment levels without sustained improvement of the underlying liver disease. Therefore, in immunosuppressed transplant patients, treatment with nucleoside analogues will most likely have to be maintained indefinitely to achieve clinical benefits for HBV-infected patients. The favourable safety profile of lamivudine and famciclovir will allow long-term suppressive antiviral therapy [61,62].

Large multicentre clinical trials are required to assess all the effects of new antiviral agents as monotherapy or combination therapy on suppression of viral load and liver histology. These studies will also have to evaluate and defined endpoints of treatment, optimum compounds and combinations, dosages, schedules, duration and cost-effectiveness of combination treatment or sequential protocols. In addition, clinical and virological characteristics, frequency and clinical consequences of treatment failure will have to be elucidated. In this context, it will be particularly important to analyse mechanisms of resistance owing to the emergence of viral mutations. The molecular mechanisms involved in the activity of nucleoside analogues and HBIg need to be elucidated. It will be extremely important to analyse whether nucleoside analogues cause mutations in regions of the HBV genome where the HBV polymerase and S gene ORFs overlap, to determine whether particular nucleoside analogues when given in combination with HBIg promote resistance to anti-HBs treatment. Finally, the natural course and replication capacity of mutant HBV have to be defined and understood. Together with further molecular studies, this information will help us understand the genetic basis of sensitivity or resistance of HBV and will allow the development of more effective therapeutics to prevent and treat recurrent HBV infection.

## REFERENCES

1. Gordon R, Fung J, Tzakis AG, Todo S, Stieber A, Bronsther O, Martin M, Van Thiel DH & Starzl TE. Liver transplantation at the University of Pittsburgh, 1984 to 1990. *Clinical Transplants* 1991; 105–117.

2. Eason J, Freeman RJ, Rohrer RJ, Lewis WD, Jenkins R, Dienstag J & Cosimi AB. Should liver transplantation be performed for patients with hepatitis B? *Transplantation* 1994; **57**:1588–1593.

3. Samuel D, Müller R, Alexander G, Fassati L, Ducot B, Benhamou JP & Bismuth H. Liver transplantation in European patients with hepatitis B surface antigen. *New England Journal of Medicine* 1993; **329**: 1842–1847.

4. Yoffe B, Burns DK, Bhatt HS & Combes B. Extrahepatic hepatitis B virus DNA sequences in patients with acute hepatitis B infection. *Hepatology* 1990; **12**:187–192.

5. McMillan JS, Shaw T, Angus PW & Locarnini SA. Effect of immunosuppressive and antiviral agents on hepatitis B virus replication *in vitro*. *Hepatology* 1995; **22**:36–43.

6. Si L, Whiteside TL, Van Thiel DH & Rabin BS. Lymphocyte subpopulations at the site of 'piecemeal' necrosis in end stage chronic liver diseases and rejecting liver allografts in cyclosporin-treated patients. *Laboratory Investigation* 1984; **50**:341–347.

7. Cote PJ, Korba BE, Steinberg H, Ramirez MC, Baldwin B, Hornbuckle WE, Tennant BC & Gerin JL. Cyclosporin A modulates the course of woodchuck hepatitis virus infection and induces chronicity. *Journal of Immunology* 1991; **146**:3138–3144.

8. Lau JY, Bird GL, Naoumov NV & Williams R. Hepatic HLA antigen display in chronic hepatitis B virus infection. Relation to hepatic expression of HBV genome/gene products and liver histology. *Digestive Diseases and Sciences* 1993; **38**:888–895.

9. Calmus Y, Hannoun L, Dousset B, Wolff P, Miguet JP, Doffoel M, Gillet M, Cinqualbre J, Poupon R & Houssin D. HLA class I matching is responsible for the hepatic lesions in recurrent viral hepatitis B after liver transplantation. *Transplantation Proceedings* 1990; **22**:2311–2313.

10. Marcellin P, Samuel D, Areias J, Loriot MA, Arulnaden JL, Gigou M, David MF, Bismuth A, Reynes M, Brechot C *et al.* Pretransplantation interferon treatment and recurrence of hepatitis B virus infection after liver transplantation for hepatitis B-related end-stage liver disease. *Hepatology* 1994; **19**:6–12.

11. Lai CL, Ching CK, Tung AK, Young J, Hill A, Wong BC, Dent J & Wu PC. Lamivudine is effective in suppressing hepatitis B virus DNA in Chinese hepatitis B surface antigen carriers: a placebo-controlled trial. *Hepatology* 1997; **25**:241–244.

12. Van Thiel DH, Friedlander L, Kania RJ, Molloy PJ, Hassanein T, Wahlstrom E & Faruki H. Lamivudine treatment of advanced and decompensated liver disease due to hepatitis B. *Hepato-gastroenterology* 1997; **44**: 808–812.

13. Nevens F, Main J, Honkoop P, Tyrrell DL, Barber J, Sullivan MT, Fevery J, De Man RA & Thomas HC. Lamivudine therapy for chronic hepatitis B: a six-months randomized dose-ranging study. *Gastroenterology* 1997; **113**:1258–1263.

14. Ben-Ari Z, Shmueli D, Mor E, Shapira Z & Tur-Kaspa R. Beneficial effect of lamivudine in recurrent hepatitis B after liver transplantation. *Transplantation* 1997; **63**: 393–396.

15. Honkoop P, de Man RA, Zondervan PE & Schalm SW. Histological improvement in patients with chronic hepatitis B virus infection treated with lamivudine. *Liver* 1997; **17**:103–106.

16. Main J, Brown JL, Howells C, Galassini R, Crossey M, Karayiannis P, Georgiou P, Atkinson G & Thomas HC. A double blind, placebo-controlled study to assess the effect of famciclovir on virus replication in patients with chronic hepatitis B virus infection. *Journal of Viral Hepatitis* 1996; **3**:211–215.

17. Singh N, Gayowski T, Wannstedt CF, Wagener MM & Marino IR. Pretransplant famciclovir as prophylaxis for hepatitis B virus recurrence after liver transplantation. *Transplantation* 1997; **63**:1415–1419.

18. Dienstag JL, Perrillo RP, Bartholomew M, Vicary C & Rubin M. A preliminary trial of lamivudine for chronic hepatitis B infection. *New England Journal of Medicine* 1995; **333**:1657–1661.

19. Benhamou Y, Dohin E, Lunel FF, Poynard T, Huraux JM, Katlama C, Opolon P & Gentilini M. Efficacy of lamivudine on replication of hepatitis B virus in HIV-infected patients. *Lancet* 1995; **345**:396–397.

20. Krüger M, Tillmann HL, Trautwein C, Bode U, Oldhafer K, Maschek H, Böker KH, Broelsch CE, Pichlmayr R & Manns MP. Famciclovir treatment of hepatitis B virus recurrence after liver transplantation: a pilot study. *Liver Transplantation and Surgery* 1996; **4**:253–262.

21. Tyrrell D, Mitchell MC & De Man RA. Phase II trial of lamivudine for chronic hepatitis B. *Hepatology* 1993; **18**:112A.

22. Offensperger WB, Offensperger S, Walter E, Teubner K, Igloi G, Blum HE & Gerok W. *In vivo* inhibition of duck hepatitis B virus replication and gene expression by phosphorothioate modified antisense oligodeoxy-nucleotides. *EMBO Journal* 1993; **12**:1257–1262.

23. Welch PJ, Tritz R, Yei S, Barber J & Yu M. Intracellular application of hairpin ribozyme genes against hepatitis B virus. *Gene Therapy* 1997; **4**:736–743.

24. von Weizsäcker F, Blum HE & Wands JR. Cleavage of hepatitis B virus RNA by three ribozymes transcribed from a single DNA template. *Biochemical and Biophysical Research Communications* 1992; **189**: 743–748.

25. Hoofnagle JH, Di BA, Waggoner JG & Park Y. Interferon alfa for patients with clinically apparent cirrhosis due to chronic hepatitis B. *Gastroenterology* 1993; **104**:1116–1121.

26. Hassanein T, Colantoni A, De Maria N & Van Thiel DH. Interferon-alpha 2b improves short-term survival

in patients transplanted for chronic liver failure caused by hepatitis B. *Journal of Viral Hepatitis* 1996; **3**:333–340.

27. Marcellin P, Giuily N, Loriot MA, Durand F, Samuel D, Bettan L, Degott C, Bernuau J, Benhamou JP & Erlinger S. Prolonged interferon-alpha therapy of hepatitis B virus-related decompensated cirrhosis. *Journal of Viral Hepatitis* 1997; **4**:21–26.

28. Berk L, Schalm SW, de Mann RA, Heytink RA, Berthelot P, Brechot C, Boboc B, Degos F, Marcellin P, Benhamou JP *et al.* Failure of acyclovir to enhance the antiviral effect of alpha lyphoblastoid interferon on Hbe-seroconversion in chronic hepatitis B. A multicentre randomized controlled trial. *Journal of Hepatology* 1992; **14**:305–309.

29. McKenzie R, Fried MW, Salli R, Conjeevaram J, Di BA, Park Y, Savarese B, Kleiner D, Tsokos M, Luciano C, Pruett T, Stotka JL, Straus SE & Hoofnagle JH. Hepatic failure and lactic acidosis due to fialuridine (FIAU), an investigational nucleoside analogue for chronic hepatitis B. *New England Journal of Medicine* 1995; **333**:1099–1105.

30. Bloomer J, Chan R, Sherman M, Ingraham P & DeHertogh D. A preliminary study of lobucavir for chronic hepatitis B. *Hepatology* 1997; **26**:428A.

31. Gilson RJC, Chopra K, Murray-Lyon I, Newell A, Nelson M, Tedder RS, Toole J, Jaffe JS, Hellmann N & Weller IVD. A placebo-controlled phase I/II study of adefovir dipivoxil (bis-POM PMEA) in patients with chronic hepatitis B infection. *Hepatology* 1996; **24**:281A.

32. Doong SL, Tsai CH, Schinazi RF, Liotta DC & Cheng YC. Inhibition of the replication of hepatitis B virus *in vitro* by 2′,3′-dideoxy-3′thiacytidine and related analogues. *Proceedings of the National Academy of Sciences, USA* 1991; **88**:8495–8499.

33. Honkoop P, de Man RA, Heijtink RA & Schalm SW. Hepatitis B reactiviation after lamivudine. *Lancet* 1995; **346**:1156–1157.

34. Gutfreund K, Fischer K, Tipples G, Ma M, Bain V, Kneteman N & Tyrrell D. Lamivudine results in a complete and sustained suppression of hepatitis B virus replication in patients requiring orthotopic liver transplantation for cirrhosis secondary to hepatitis B. *Hepatology* 1995; **22**:328A.

35. Grellier L, Mutimer D, Ahmed M, Brown D, Burroughs AK, Rolles K, McMaster P, Branek P, Kennedy F, Kibbler H, McPhillips P, Elias & Dusheiko G. Lamivudine prophylaxis against reinfection in liver transplantation for hepatitis B cirrhosis. *Lancet* 1996; **348**:1212–1215.

36. Bain VG, Kneteman NM, Ma MM, Gutfreund K, Shapiro JA, Fischer K, Tipples G, Lee H, Jewell LD & Tyrrell DL. Efficacy of lamivudine in chronic hepatitis B patients with active viral replication and decompensated cirrhosis undergoing liver transplantation. *Transplantation* 1996; **62**:1456–1462.

37. Perry CM & Wagstaff AJ. Famciclovir. A review of its pharmacological properties and therapeutic efficacy in herpes virus infections. *Drugs* 1995; **50**:396–415.

38. Vere Hodge RA, Sutton D, Boyd MR, Harnden MR & Jarvest RL. Selection of an oral prodrug (BRL 42810; camciclovir) for the antiherpes virus agent BRL 39123 [9-(4-hydroxy-3-hydroxymethylbut-1-yl)guanine; penciclovir]. *Antimicrobial Agents and Chemotherapy* 1989; **33**:1765–1773.

39. Shaw T, Mok SS & Locarnini SA. Inhibition of hepatitis B virus DNA polymerase by enantiomers of penciclovir

triphosphate and metabolic basis for selective inhibition of HBV replication by penciclovir. *Hepatology* 1996; **24**:996–1002.

40. Saltzman R, Jurewicz R & Boon R. Safety of famciclovir in patients with herpes zoster and genital herpes. *Antimicrobial Agents and Chemotherapy* 1994; **38**:2454–2457.

41. Lauchart W, Müller R & Pichlmayr R. Long-term immunoprophylaxis of hepatitis B virus infection in recipients of human liver allografts. *Transplantation Proceedings* 1987; **19**:4051–4053.

42. Todo S, Demetris AJ, Van Thiel DH, Teperman L, Fung JJ & Starzl TE. Orthotopic liver transplantation for patients with hepatitis B virus-related liver disease. *Hepatology* 1991; **13**:619–626

43. Terrault NA, Holland CC, Ferrell L, Hahn JA, Jake JR, Roberts JP, Acher NL & Wright TL. Interferon alfa for recurrent hepatitis B infection after liver transplantation. *Liver Transplantation and Surgery* 1996; **2**:132–138.

44. Jurim O, Martin P, Winston D, Shaked A, Csete M, Holt C & Busuttil R. Ganciclovir fails to prevent graft rejection following orthotopic liver transplantation for chronic hepatitis B. *Hepatology* 1994; **20**:138A.

45. Gish RG, Lau JY, Brooks L, Fang JW, Steady SL, Imperial JC, Garcia-Kennedy R, Esquivel CO & Keeffe EB. Ganciclovir treatment of hepatitis B virus infection in liver transplant recipients. *Hepatology* 1996; **23**:1–7.

46. Perrillo R, Rakely J, Martin P, Wright T, Levy G, Schiff E, Dienstag J, Gish T, Dickson R, Adams P, Brown N & Self P. Lamivudine for suppression and/or prevention of hepatitis B when given pre/post liver transplantation (OLT). *Hepatology* 1997; **26**:260A.

47. Markowitz J, Martin P, Conrad AJ, Markmann JF, Seu P, Yersiz H, Goss JA, Pakrasi A, Artinian L, Holt C, Goldstein L, Stribling R & Busuttil R. Prophylaxis against hepatitis B recurrence following liver transplantation using combination lamivudine and hepatitis B immune globulin. *Hepatology* 1997; **26**:152A.

48. Manns M, Neuhaus P, Schoenborn H, Griffin KE on behalf of the FCV End-Stage Liver Disease Study Group. Famciclovir treatment of hepatitis B infection in patients with end-stage liver disease. *Journal of Hepatology* 1998; **28**:114.

49. Markowitz J, Pakrasi A, Hollis P, Martin P, Goldstein L & Busuttil R. Efficacy of lamivudine for prophylaxis and treatment of hepatitis B in liver transplant patients. *Hepatology* 1996; **24**:182A.

50. Perrillo R, Rakela J, Martin P, Levy G, Schiff E, Wright T, Dienstag J, Gish R, Villeneuve JP, Caldwell S, Brown N & Self P. Long term lamivudine therapy of patients with recurrent hepatitis B post liver transplantation. *Hepatology* 1997; **26**:177A.

51. Petit MA, Buffello D, Roche B, Dussaix E, Aulong B, Bismuth H, Samuel D & Feray C. Residual hepatitis B virus infection in liver transplant patients under treatment with lamivudine (3TC): assessment by quantification of HBV DNA by PCR and assay of preS antigens. *Hepatology* 1997; **26**:315A.

52. Ling R, Mutimer D, Ahmed M, Boxall EH, Elias E, Dusheiko GM & Harrison TJ. Selection of mutations in the hepatitis B virus polymerase during therapy of transplant recipients with lamivudine. *Hepatology* 1996; **24**:711–713.

53. Bartholomew MM, Jansen RW, Jeffers LJ, Reddy KR, Johnson LC, Bunzendahl H, Condreay LD, Tzakis AG, Schiff ER & Brown NA. Hepatitis B-virus resistance to

lamivudine given for recurrent infection after orthotopic liver transplantation. *Lancet* 1997; **349**:20–22.

54. Naoumov NV, Choksi S, Smith HM & Williams R. Emergence and characterization of lamivudine-resistant hepatitis B virus variant. *Hepatology* 1996; **24**:282A.

55. Tillmann HL, Trautwein C, Bock T, Glowenka M, Krüger M, Böker K, Jäckel E, Pichlmayr R, Condreay L, Bruns I, Deslaurias M, Gauthier J & Manns MP. Response and mutations in patients sequentially treated with lamivudine and famciclovir for recurrent hepatitis B after liver transplantation. *Hepatology* 1997; **26**:429A.

56. Gutfreund KS, Fischer KP, Tipples FG, Ma M, Kneteman N, Jewell LD, Tyrell DLJ & Bain VG. Late breakthrough of HBV viremia with lamivudine as a single agent for prevention of graft reinfection in liver transplantation for cirrhosis secondary to hepatitis B. *Hepatology* 1996; **24**:285A.

57. Tipples GA, Ma MM, Fischer KP, Bain VG, Kneteman NM & Tyrrell DL. Mutation in HBV RNA-dependent DNA polymerase confers resistance to lamivudine *in vivo*. *Hepatology* 1996; **24**:714–717.

58. Lai CL, Liaw YF, Leung NWY, Chang TT, Guan R, Tai DI & Ny KY. 12 months of lamivudine (100 mg od) therapy improves liver histology: results of a placebo controlled multicentre study in Asia. *Journal of Hepatology* 1997; **26**:79A.

59. Honkoop P, Niesters HG, de Man RA, Osterhaus AD & Schalm SW. Lamivudine resistance in immunocompetent chronic hepatitis B. Incidence and patterns. *Journal of Hepatology* 1997; **26**:1393–1395.

60. Böker KH, Ringe B, Krüger M, Pichlmayr R & Manns MP. Prostaglandin E plus famciclovir – a new concept for the treatment of severe hepatitis B after liver transplantation. *Transplantation* 1994; **57**:1706–1708.

61. Neuhaus P, Manns MP & Atkinson G. Safety and efficacy of famciclovir for the treatment of recurrent hepatitis B in liver transplant recipients. *Hepatology* 1997; **26**:260A.

62. Rabinovitz M, Dodson F & Rakela J. Famciclovir for recurrent hepatitis B infection after liver transplantation. *Hepatology* 1996; **24**:282A.

63. Klein M, Geoghegan J, Schmidt K, Bockler D, Korn K, Wittekind C & Scheele J. Conversion of recurrent delta-positive hepatitis B infection to seronegativity with famciclovir after liver transplantation. *Transplantation* 1997; **64**:162–163.

64. McCaughan G, Angus P, Bowden S, Shaw T, Breschkin A, Sheil R & Locarnini S. Retransplantation for precore mutant-related chronic hepatitis B infection: prolonged survival in a patient receiving sequential ganciclovir/famciclovir therapy. *Liver Transplantation and Surgery* 1996; **2**:472–474.

65. Locarnini S, Aye TT, Shaw T, DeMan R, Angus PW & McCaughan GW. The emergence of famciclovir resistant mutations in the hepatitis B virus polymerase during therapy in patients following liver transplantation. *Hepatology* 1997; **26**:368A.

66. Aye TT, Bartholomeusz A, Shaw T, Bowden S, Breschkin A, McMillan J, Angus P & Locarnini S. Hepatitis B virus polymerase mutations during antiviral therapy in a patient following liver transplantation. *Journal of Hepatology* 1997; **26**:1148–1153.

67. Shields PL, Ling R, Harrison T, Boxall E, Elias E & Mutimer DJ. Management and outcome of lamivudine-resistant hepatitis B virus infection after liver transplantation. *Hepatology* 1997; **26**:260A.

68. Krüger M, Böker KH, Zeidler H & Manns MP. Treatment of hepatitis B-related polyarteritis nodosa with famciclovir and interferon alfa-2b. *Journal of Hepatology* 1997; **26**:935–939.

# Section VII

## CLINICAL AND THERAPEUTIC STRATEGIES

### Part C

#### COINFECTIONS

# 45

# Effect of lamivudine on hepatitis B virus–human immunodeficiency virus coinfected patients from the CAESAR study

## David A Cooper

## BACKGROUND

It has been shown that treatment of hepatitis B virus (HBV)-infected immunosuppressed patients with 100 mg lamivudine per day, results in significant improvements in liver histology, suppresses HBV DNA replication, improves alanine aminotransferase (ALT) values and increases HBeAg seroconversion rates. However, there have only been anecdotal reports and a small series examining lamivudine efficacy among patients coinfected with HBV and human immunodeficiency virus (HIV).

The randomized trial of lamivudine in HBV–HIV coinfected patients developed out of the larger CAESAR study. This study assessed the effect of lamivudine in HIV infection to prove its clinical benefit at a time when some regarded surrogate markers as unconvincing. The objectives of the trial were to investigate the efficacy and safety of lamivudine therapy among these coinfected patients, to examine the available virological and biochemical evidence for suppression of HBV by lamivudine, and to examine HIV disease progression among the HBV–HIV coinfected population [1].

## SELECTION CRITERIA

The CAESAR study was a 52 week double-blind randomized trial conducted over a 1 year period and powered to obtain the required HIV endpoints. A total of 1895 subjects were randomly assigned drug treatment at a ratio of 1:2:1, to add double-blind lamivudine therapy (150 mg twice daily) or lamivudine therapy with loviride (100 mg three times daily) to their zidovudine-containing background antiretroviral treatment. Because loviride, a non-nucleoside reverse transcriptase inhibitor (NNRTI), does not possess *in vitro* HBV activity, the two lamivudine-containing arms were grouped for comparison with the placebo arm.

Inclusion criteria for both the study and substudy were persons aged 18 years or over with CD4 counts of 25–250 cells/µl and no prior lamivudine or non-nucleoside treatment (no protease inhibitors were available at the time). Patients were recruited at any disease stage, with previous treatment being either none or nucleoside reverse transcriptase inhibitor (NRTI), and either on monotherapy or combination therapy. Patients in the substudy had the additional criterion of being HBsAg-positive at screening.

When compared with the remainder of the CAESAR study population, the HIV–HBV coinfected study population had a similar median age of around 36 years. However, there were more males in the coinfected group compared with the HIV-infected group. As expected, the alanine aminotransferase (ALT) levels were slightly more abnormal in the coinfected group.

## BASELINE HBV SEROLOGY

Baseline HBsAg results were available for 1790 patients, of whom 122 (6.8%) tested positive (97 of these patients were on the lamivudine arms of the study and 25 were on the placebo arm). Retrospective analyses for serial HBV DNA (Roche Amplicor HBV PCR Monitor), HBsAg and HBeAg were performed on stored serum from the randomized study period. The quantification ranged from $4 \times 10^7$ down to 400 copies.

Baseline serology of the coinfected group was well matched. The baseline HBV DNA in the placebo group was $\log_{10}$ 7.3, and was 7.6 in the lamivudine group. Among those who were HBsAg-positive at baseline, HBV DNA and HBeAg were present in

83% (98/118) and 63% (74/118), respectively, with no significant difference between treatment arms.

## EFFECT OF LAMIVUDINE ON HBV ACTIVITY

At week 12, the median $\log_{10}$ HBV DNA change was −2.0 and 0.0 in the lamivudine and placebo arms, respectively. The HBV DNA suppression was maintained throughout the subsequent follow-up, with the change in $\log_{10}$ HBV DNA at week 52 being −2.7 in the lamivudine arms and 0.0 in the placebo arm.

The absence of HBV DNA defined as less than 400 copies/ml among those positive at baseline, was about 40% by week 52. Loss of HBeAg occurred in 22% (7/32) and 0% (0/7) in the lamivudine and placebo arms, respectively. A trend to a lower mean ALT level was seen in the lamivudine arms (74.7 to 54.7 U/l), whereas a stable level was seen in the placebo arm (68.2 to 74.9 U/l).

## HIV OUTCOMES

Progression of HIV disease was delayed in patients in the lamivudine arms compared with those in the placebo arm (hazard ratio 0.26; 95% confidence interval 0.08–0.80), showing a similar trend to that seen in patients enrolled in the CAESAR study who were infected with HIV alone.

## ADVERSE EVENTS

Lamivudine is known to be generally well-tolerated in the HIV-infected population. In this study there was no difference in the number or type of adverse events between the lamivudine arms and placebo arm of the HIV–HBV-coinfected subpopulation. There was also no difference in adverse events between HIV–HBV-coinfected and HIV-infected populations.

## CONCLUSIONS

In HBV–HIV-coinfected patients, lamivudine together with the standard antiretroviral therapy, in this case nucleoside analogues, was well tolerated. The study found that lamivudine significantly reduced the levels of HBV DNA and resulted in a non-significant decrease in the levels of HBeAg and HBsAg. Furthermore, lamivudine delayed HIV disease progression in HBV–HIV-coinfected patients in a trend similar to its effect on HIV-infected patients.

## ACKNOWLEDGEMENTS

The CAESAR Coordinating Committee would like to acknowledge the enormous effort involved in this study, particularly by Glaxo Wellcome in the various countries. Thanks to Catherine Barrett from the hepatitis B team, Li-Ean Goh from the HIV team, Hugh McDade, who is in charge of antiviral therapy for Glaxo Wellcome in the UK, and the statistician, Bharat Thakrar, from Glaxo Wellcome in the USA.

## REFERENCE

1. CAESAR Coordinating Committee. Randomised trial of addition of lamivudine or lamivudine plus loviride to zidovudine-containing regimens for patients with HIV-1 infection: the CAESAR trial. *Lancet* 1997; **349**: 1413–1421.

# 46 Coinfection with hepatitis B and C viruses

## Patrizia Pontisso*, Martina Gerotto, Luisa Benvegnù, Liliana Chemello and Alfredo Alberti

## INTRODUCTION

Coinfection by hepatotropic viruses, namely hepatitis B virus (HBV) and hepatitis C virus (HCV) can occur, since they share similar routes of transmission [1,2]. Increasing numbers of patients have been identified so far as having multiple hepatitis viruses [3–5] and this situation is associated with different clinical manifestations, including fulminant hepatitis, acute and chronic hepatitis, and hepatocellular carcinoma. The interplay between the two viruses and the relative contribution to the severity of liver disease among infected individuals has not yet been well defined [6,7]. Furthermore, it is not clear whether the response rate to interferon therapy in these individuals is similar to that obtained in patients infected with only HCV or HBV [8,9].

## FULMINANT HEPATITIS

The role of dual infection in the development of fulminant hepatitis is still debated and discrepant results might be related to different epidemiological settings from which clinical observations originate. In Western countries, among individuals with fulminant hepatitis, serum HCV RNA was identified in about half of HBV surface antigen (HBsAg)-positive patients, while HCV itself was not detected in acute hepatic failure without evidence of HBV infection, suggesting that HCV can concur with fulminant hepatitis, rather than being primarily responsible for this event [10]. A recent study from Japan, while confirming the low incidence of HCV infection alone as aetiologic agent of acute liver failure, does not identify mixed infection as a concurrent cause in the development of the critical clinical outcome in this geographic area [11].

## ACUTE HEPATITIS

Few data are available in the literature concerning clinical features of patients with acute hepatitis due to dual HBV/HCV aetiology. Longitudinal studies indicate that acute HCV superinfection can lead to clearance of

the pre-existing HBV [12,13]; however, clinical profiles comparing coinfected patients with those acutely infected by a single agent are lacking. In our series of 206 patients, matched for age, sex and risk factors, biochemical parameters in coinfected patients were similar to those found in acute HBV infection (Table 1). In contrast, the outcome of HCV infection was significantly different in patients with mixed infection, compared to those with HCV alone. Clearance of HCV was indeed observed in 71% of the patients with HBV coinfection but only in 14% of the cases with HCV alone ($P<0.001$). These results suggest that HBV might interfere with HCV replication, promoting viral clearance. No evidence for the opposite influence of HCV on replication of HBV has been provided in this cohort of patients. One of the responsible factors could be ascribed to the infecting genotype. The majority of the patients were indeed infected by genotype 3 and previous studies indicate that this viral type is rarely found in mixed infection [14]. One possible explanation could be a high sensitivity of this genotype to interferon endogenously induced by HBV [15], as already documented for exogenous administration of this drug [16].

## CHRONIC HEPATITIS

Clinical and pathological severity of liver disease among patients with chronic hepatitis resulting from multiple viruses is increased, as documented in several reports. Total Scheuer score, portal and lobular inflammation

Table 1. Characteristics of acute viral infection in 206 patients matched for sex, age and risk factors

| Marker | HBV/HCV | HBV alone | HCV alone |
|---|---|---|---|
| Bilirubin peak (mg/ml) | 14.7±6.7 | 10.0±7.0 | 2.0±1.3 |
| ALT peak (IU/L) | 1250±335 | 1208±374 | 659±205 |
| HBV DNA clearance | 71% | 89% | – |
| HCV RNA clearance | 71%* | – | 14%* |

*$P<0.001$

*Corresponding author:

and fibrosis have all been described to be worse in coin-fected subjects [17,18]. In agreement with these obser-vation, we have also shown that the severity of liver injury is higher when active HBV replication is detectable [19]. In HDV-negative patients, HCV replica-tion is always detectable in the liver of the patients with dual infection, while absence of HBV DNA could be due to HBsAg carriage, which does not imply active replica-tion of the virus, but only HBsAg protein synthesis by the integrated viral genome [20]. Therefore, more severe liver injury in patients with serological markers of mixed infection could be associated with replication of both viruses, while replication of HCV alone, which can occur when 'healthy HBV carriers' are superinfected with HCV, might be associated with milder histological findings. The state of replication of the infecting viruses is an important parameter that is in part modulated by the HCV genotype. Replication of HBV is more effi-ciently inhibited by HCV genotype 1 than by genotype 2 [14], while viral load of the latter is usually more sensitive to HBV interference (Fig. 1), giving rise to a composite picture in which final result depends on molecular characteristics of the infecting agents.

# HEPATOCELLULAR CARCINOMA
## Clinical data

Epidemiological studies have shown that chronic infection by hepatotropic viruses is one of the major risk factors in the development of hepatocellular carcinoma (HCC) [6,21]. The relative roles of HBV and HCV in hepatocarcinogenesis vary considerably among populations. While HBV is a primary risk factor in the People's Republic of China and in Southern Africa [22],

studies from Japan indicate that approximately 55% of patients with HCC are positive for serological markers of HCV alone [23]. However, a recent work by Koike *et al.* [24] reported a high rate of HBV DNA integration in patients with HCV-related HCC who were negative for serum HBsAg, strongly suggesting a role for HBV in tumour progression and indicating that seronegativity for HBsAg does not exclude the presence of HBV DNA sequences in the liver. In the United States, approxi-mately 30% of cases of HCC are HBV- or HCV-related and an additional 20% are coinfected by both viruses [25]. A prospective study indicates that concurrent infection predisposes cirrhotic patients to a significantly higher risk of HCC than patients with single-agent infection [26]. Indeed, over a mean follow up of $46.3 \pm 21.4$ months, tumour development was observed in 19.6% of HBsAg-positive patients, in 12.2% of anti-HCV-positive patients and in 40% of patients positive for HBsAg and anti-HCV antibodies. By multivariate analysis, mixed viral infection was found to be independ-ently related to tumour appearance ($P<0.05$), in addition to age ($P<0.01$), male sex ($P<0.05$) and alcohol abuse ($P<<0.08$). In Southern African blacks, the calculated relative risk for hepatocellular carcinoma of 23.3 for HBV and 6.6 for HCV increased to 82.5 when both viruses were present [22], confirming that coinfection by the two viruses carries a synergistic risk of HCC formation.

## Potential mechanism

The mechanism by which dual infection promotes tumour development still remains speculative. Integration of HBV DNA into cellular DNA [20], as well as HBV-associated proteins, mainly X protein [27], may act as the 'initiating factor', while the presence of HCV may behave as a 'promoting factor', possibly by direct and indirect mechanisms. Persistent cell necrosis and regeneration associated with HCV infection has been recognized as the main indirect mechanism for tumour formation. Recent findings, however, indicate that HCV proteins can also have transforming capacity *in vitro*. The N-terminal part of NS3, which encodes one of the two viral serine proteases implicated in HCV polyprotein processing, can induce transformation of NIH 3T3 cells [28]. In addition, capsid protein has been shown to modulate the expression of several cellular genes, including *c-myc*, interferon β and retinoblastoma [29,30] and interfere with apoptotic cellular processes [31,32]. Although a definite pathway has not been yet identified, these observations indicate that HCV proteins may exert a direct effect on cellular activity and may drive phenotypic expression of infected hepatocytes.

**Figure 1.** Virological findings in serum of patients with HBV and HCV coinfection in relation to HCV genotype

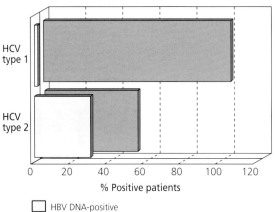

HCV type 1

HCV type 2

0   20   40   60   80   100   120
% Positive patients

☐ HBV DNA-positive
▨ HCV RNA (> 10 000 copies/ml)

# MOLECULAR BASIS OF VIRAL INTERFERENCE

Clinical evidence of reciprocal interference of virus replication has been described in patients with mixed virus infection [32–34]. This behaviour, as well as HBsAg clearance following HCV superinfection, has been repeatedly reported in the literature. Although HCV has been shown to suppress HBV replication [35], the opposite situation, namely interference of HCV replication in the presence of HBV, can occur. In patients with chronic hepatitis and mixed viral infection, a subset of patients show serological evidence of HBV replication, but at the same time-point, HCV RNA is rarely detected in serum. Analysis of the corresponding liver has revealed that HCV RNA is still present, suggesting some HBV-related interference of the replication activity of HCV (Fig. 2). Further studies have indicated that the extent of interference is not identical for different HCV genotypes, since HCV genotype 1 has a more efficient inhibitory activity on HBV than genotype 2 [14].

## Sequence analysis results

There is not only clinical but also experimental evidence that HCV can suppress HBV replication, and, in particular, HCV core protein has been identified as being responsible for this viral interference. It has been shown that an *in vitro*-engineered capsid with a C-terminal deletion is targeted to the nucleus [36]. Sequence comparison with known nuclear localization signals (NLSs) revealed that there are three NLSs located in the HCV core protein at residues 38 to 43, to 64/66 to 71 [37]. Furthermore, the fact that the core protein contains 16.8% basic amino acid residues that cluster in three regions (6–23, 39–74 and 101–121) suggested that it is a nucleic acid-binding protein [38]. In addition, a putative DNA-binding motif, SPRG, is located at residues 99 to 102. The SPXX-type DNA-binding motif is specified by several transcriptional regulators [39]; this leads to the possibility that HCV core could interact with cellular genes and would interfere with the normal function of the gene.

## *In vitro* experiments

It has been demonstrated by Shih *et al.* [40] that the HCV core protein can suppress, in the absence of host factors, the gene replication and expression of HBV. *In vitro* experiments showed that expression of HBV-specific transcripts, as well as HBsAg, e antigen and core antigen, can be reduced several fold by cotrans-

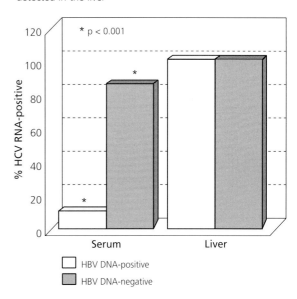

**Figure 2.** HCV RNA in serum and the liver of patients coinfected with HBV and HCV in relation to HBV replication detected in the liver

fection of HuH-7 cells with cloned HBV DNA and with the full length or a truncated version of the HCV core gene. Although the exact mechanism responsible for the suppressive effect is not clear, there is evidence that HCV core directly binds to HBV RNA, affecting HBV pregenomic encapsidation and viral particle release. This possibility concerns the specificity and ability of the N-terminal 122 amino acid residues of the HCV core protein to bind nucleic acids and to suppress HBV viral genomic RNA encapsidation [40]. More precisely, the ability to bind HBV RNA has been restricted to the segment between amino acids 101 and 122 of the HCV core protein.

## Possible interpretation

It is known that only one of several genomic HBV RNAs is selected for encapsidation, termed the pregenomic RNA (which starts at map position 3100) [41]. Within this RNA, a 137 nucleotide sequence has been identified as indispensable and sufficient for RNA encapsidation. Deletion analysis of HBV p21.5 core protein demonstrated that most of the RNA-binding and encapsidation activity of the entire protein resides in the segment down to Arg 164 [42]. Within this portion of the protein, an 8 amino acid sequence, RRRDRGRS (residues 150 to 158), has been identified as the minimal sequence required for HBV RNA-specific binding. As shown in Figure 3, this 8 amino acid sequence of HBV

Table 2. Response to interferon treatment in HBV/HCV coinfected patients

| Author | No. cases | IFN dose* | IFN response | |
|--------|-----------|-----------|--------------|---|
| | | | End of treatment | Follow up[†] |
| Genéhéot et al. [8] | 16 | 3 MU/6 months | 44% | 32% |
| Waltman et al. [7] | 8 | 3 MU/6 months | 25% | 13% |
| Liaw et al. [43] | 15 | 3 MU/6 months | 6.7% | 6.7% |
| Zignego et al. [9] | 14[‡] | 3 MU/12 months | 28% | 0% |

*IFN was given three times a week for the indicated period.
[†]6–12 months.
[‡]HBsAg-negative/HBV DNA-positive by PCR.

Table 3. Response to interferon therapy in 44 patients with HBV and HCV markers

| Group | IFN dose* | Normal ALT | HBV DNA-negative | HCV RNA-negative | Complete sustained response |
|-------|-----------|------------|------------------|------------------|------------------------------|
| HBV DNA-positive and HCV RNA-positive (16 cases) | 10 MU/6 months | 12% | 38% | 12% | 12% |
| | 3 MU/12 months | 25% | 25% | 25% | 25% |
| | 5 MU/12 months | 75% | 75% | 50% | 50% |
| HBV DNA-negative and HCV RNA-positive (20 cases) | 10 MU/6 months | 50% | – | 25% | 25% |
| | 3 MU/12 months | 40% | – | 30% | 30% |
| | 5 MU/12 months | 33% | – | 33% | 33% |
| HBV DNA-positive and HCV RNA-negative (8 cases) | 10 MU/6 months | 50% | 50% | – | 50% |
| | 5 MU/12 months | 50% | 50% | – | 50% |

*IFN was given three times a week for the indicated period.
Abbreviations: MU, mega units; ALT, alanine aminotransferase.

shares an important Arg-rich motif with the core domain 101–122 of HCV genotype 1, while at the same position HCV genotype 2 does not have the Arg-rich motif. It has been suggested that these Arg residues have a crucial role in driving the binding and hence the encapsidation of RNA. These molecular findings, while possibly explaining the observed inhibitory activity of HCV core protein on HBV replication, can also provide a potential rationale for the lack of inhibition observed clinically in patients infected with genotype 2 HCV.

## RESPONSE TO INTERFERON THERAPY

The finding of more severe histological liver disease activity in patients with mixed viral infection warrants the identification of effective therapeutic schemes. To date, not many data are available in this field and small groups of patients, treated with different interferon (IFN) schedules have been reported. Table 2 summarizes published results: in the first three studies, sustained responses were seen in 32%, 13% and 6.7% of cases, respectively. The fourth study was performed on HCV-positive/HBsAg-negative patients who were nevertheless positive for HBV DNA by PCR, and none of them showed complete response after a 12-month

Figure 3. Sequence comparison between the arginine-rich domain of the HBV core protein and core proteins from different HCV genotypes

```
          150      158
           |        |
HBV       RRRDRGRS

HCV 1a    RRRSRNLG
HCV 1b    RRRSRNLG

          113      120
           |        |
HCV 2a    RHRSRNLV
HCV 2b    RHrSRNLG
HCV 2c    RHKSRNLG

HCV 3a    RRRSRNLG
```

course of IFN. Overall, no satisfactory response to treatment was achieved in these patients and usually, low IFN doses, derived from HCV-tailored protocols, were used.

An analysis of IFN response in relation to therapeutic scheme was recently carried out in our institution. Among patients with active replication of both HBV and HCV, an increased rate of complete long-term response was achieved with higher IFN doses. In HBV DNA- or HCV RNA-negative patients, no significant differences were observed in relation to different therapeutic schemes (Table 3), and rates of persistent viral clearance were similar to those obtained in patients infected only with HCV or HBV, respectively. Although promising, these results have been obtained in a small number of patients and no analysis of the HCV genotype or viral load was carried out, which would allow us to more effectively compare the virological features of the responding patients. Prospective, controlled trials, in which the virological status of both viruses is considered as an initial parameter, are needed to better address an effective antiviral therapy.

# REFERENCES

1. Dienstag JL, Alaama M, Mosley JW, Redeker AG & Purcell RH. Etiology of sporadic hepatitis B surface antigen-negative hepatitis. *Annals of Internal Medicine* 1977; **87**:1–6.
2. Alter MJ, Hadler SC & Judson FN. Risk factors for acute non-A, non-B hepatitis in the United States and association with hepatitis C virus infection. *JAMA* 1990; **264**:2231–2235.
3. Fong TL, Di Bisceglie AM, Waggoner JG, Banks SM & Hoofnagle JH. The significance of antibody to hepatitis C virus in patients with chronic hepatitis B. *Hepatology* 1991; **14**:64–67.
4. Schiff ER. The role of hepatitis C virus in liver disease. *Journal of Gastroenterology and Hepatology* 1991; **6** (Supplement 1):29–30.
5. Sato S, Shigetoshi F, Tanaka M, Yamasaki K, Kuromoto I, Kawano S, Sato T, Mizuno K & Nonaka S. Coinfection of hepatitis C virus in patients with chronic hepatitis B infection. *Journal of Hepatology* 1994; **21**:159–166.
6. Kaklamani E, Trichopoulos D, Tzonou A, Zavitsanos X, Koumantaki Y & Hatzakis A. Hepatitis B and C viruses and their interaction in the origin of hepatocellular carcinoma. *JAMA* 1991; **265**:974–1976.
7. Sheen IS, Liaw YF, Chu CM & Pao CC. Role of hepatitis C virus infection in spontaneous hepatitis B surface antigen clearance during chronic hepatitis B virus infection. *Journal of Infectious Diseases* 1992; **165**:831–834.
8. Géhénot M, Marcellin P, Colin JF, Martinot M, Benhamou JP & Erlinger S. Alpha interferon therapy in HBsAg positive patients with chronic hepatitis C. *Hepatology* 1995; **22** (Supplement):116A.
9. Zignego AL, Fontana R, Puliti S, Barbagli S, Monti M, Careccia G, Giannelli F, Giannini C, Buzzelli G, Brunetto MR, Bonino F & Gentilini P. Impaired response to alpha interferon in patients with an inapparent hepatitis B and hepatitis C virus infection. *Archives of Virology* 1997; **142**:535–544.
10. Feray C, Gigou M, Samuel D, Reyes G, Bernuau M, Bismuth H & Brechot C. Hepatitis C virus RNA and hepatitis B virus DNA in serum and liver of patients with fulminant hepatitis. *Gastroenterology* 1993; **104**:549–555.
11. Inokuchi K, Nakata K, Hamasaki K, Daikoku M, Kato Y, Yatsuhashi H, Koga M, Yano M & Nagataki S. Prevalence of viral hepatitis B or C virus infection in patients with fulminant viral hepatitis. An analysis using polymerase chain reaction. *Journal of Hepatology* 1996; **24**:258–264.
12. Liaw YF, Lin SM, Sheen IS & Chu CM. Acute hepatitis C in virus superinfection followed by spontaneous HBeAg and HBsAg seroconversion. *Infection* 1991; **19**:250–255.
13. Tsiquaye KN, Portman B & Tovey G. Non-A, non-B hepatitis in persistent carriers of hepatitis B virus. *Journal of Medical Virology* 1983; **11**:179–189.
14. Pontisso P, Gerotto M, Ruvoletto MG, Fattovich G, Chemello L, Tisminetzky S, Baralle F & Alberti A. Hepatitis C genotypes in patients with dual hepatitis B and C virus infection. *Journal of Medical Virology* 1996; **48**:157–160.
15. Pignatelli M, Walters J, Brown D, Lever A, Iwarson S, Shaff Z, Gerety R & Thomas HC. HLA class I antigens in the hepatocyte membrane during recovery from acute hepatitis B virus infection and during interferon therapy in chronic hepatitis B virus infection. *Hepatology* 1986; **6**:249–235.
16. Chemello L, Bonetti P, Cavalletto L, Talato F, Donadon V, Casarin C, Belussi F, Pontisso P & Alberti A. Randomized trial comparing three different regimens of alpha-2a interferon in chronic hepatitis C. *Hepatology* 1995; **22**:700–706.
17. Weltman MD, Brotodihardjo A, Crewe EB, Farrell GC, Bilous M, Grierson JM & Liddle C. Coinfection with hepatitis B and C or C and delta viruses results in severe chronic liver disease and responds poorly to interferon-alpha treatment. *Journal of Viral Hepatitis* 1995; **2**:39–45.
18. Crespo J, Lozano JL, de la Cruz F, Rodrigo L, Rodriguez M, San Miguel G, Artinano E & Pons-Romero F. Prevalence and significance of hepatitis C viremia in chronic active hepatitis B. *American Journal of Gastroenterology* 1994; **89**:1147–1151.
19. Pontisso P, Ruvoletto MG, Fattovich G, Chemello L, Gallorini A, Ruol A & Alberti A. Clinical and virological profiles in patients with multiple hepatitis virus infection. *Gastroenterology* 1993; **105**:1529–1533.
20. Kam W, Rall LB & Smuckler EA. Hepatitis B viral DNA in liver and serum of asymptomatic carriers. *Proceedings of the National Academy of Science USA* 1982; **79**:7522–7526.
21. Beasley RP. Hepatitis B virus. The etiology of hepatocellular carcinoma. *Cancer* 1988; **61**:1942–1956.
22. Kiew MC, Yu MC, Kedda MA, Coppin A, Sarkin A & Hodkinson J. The relative roles of hepatitis B and C viruses in the etiology of hepatocellular carcinoma in southern African blacks. *Gastroenterology* 1997; **112**:184–187.
23. Nishioka K, Watanabe J, Furuta S, Tanaka E, Iino S, Suzuki H, Tsuji T, Yano M, Kuo G, Choo QL, Houghton M & Oda T. A high prevalence of antibody to the hepatitis C virus in patients with hepatocellular carcinoma in Japan. *Cancer* 1991; **67**:429–233.

24. Koike K, Nakamura Y, Kobayashi M, Takada S, Urashima T, Saigo K, Kobayashi S, Isono K, Hayashi I & Fujii A. Hepatitis B virus DNA integration frequently observed in the hepatocellular carcinoma DNA of hepatitis C virus-infected patients. *International Journal of Oncology* 1996; **8**:781–784.

25. Liang TJ, Jeffers LJ, Reddy KR, De Medina M, Parker IT, Cheinquer H, Idrovo V, Rabassa A & Schiff ER. Viral pathogenesis of hepatocellular carcinoma in the United States. *Hepatology* 1993; **18**:1326–1333.

26. Benvegnù L, Fattovich G, Noventa F, Diodati G, Tremolada F, Chemello L, Cecchetto A & Alberti A. Evidence that concurrent hepatitis B and C virus infection increases the risk of developing hepatocellular carcinoma in cirrhosis: a prospective study. *Cancer* 1994; **74**:2442–2448.

27. Kekulé AS, Lauer U, Weiss L, Luber B & Hofshneider PH. Hepatitis B virus transactivator HBx uses a tumor promoter signalling pathway. *Nature* 1993; **361**: 742–745.

28. Sakamuro D, Frukawa T & Takegami T. Hepatitis C virus nonstructural protein NS3 transforms NIH 3T3 cells. *Journal of Virology* 1995; **69**:3893–3896.

29. Ray RB, Lagging LM, Meyer K, Steele R & Ray R. Transcriptional regulation of cellular and viral promoters by hepatitis C virus core protein. *Virus Research* 1995; **37**:209–220.

30. Wan Kim D, Suzuki R, Harada T, Saito I & Miyamura T. Trans-suppression of gene expression by hepatitis C viral core protein. *Japanese Journal of Medical Science Biology* 1994; **47**:211–220.

31. Ray RB, Meyer K & Ray R. Suppression of apoptotic cell death by hepatitis C virus core protein. *Virology* 1996; **226**:176–182.

32. Ruggieri A, Harada T, Matsuura Y & Miyamura T. Sensitization to Fas-mediated apoptosis by hepatitis C virus core protein. *Virology* 1997; **229**:68–76.

33. Law Yun-Fan. Role of hepatitis C in dual and triple hepatitis virus infection. *Hepatology* 1995; **22**:1101–1108.

34. Ghetti S, Ballardini G, De Raffaele E, Grassi A, Lari F, Zauli D, Cavallari A & Bianchi FB. Hepatitis B (HBV) and hepatitis C (HCV) viruses can infect the same hepatocytes in vivo. *Hepatology* 1997; **26**:514A.

35. Guido M, Fattovich G, Rugge M, Alberti A, Cecchetto C & Thung SN. Effect of chronic HCV infection on intrahepatic expression of HBV antigens. *Hepatology* 1996; **24**:226A.

36. Suzuki R, Matsuura Y, Suzuki T, Ando A, Chiba J, Harada S & Saito I. Nuclear localization of the truncated hepatitis C virus core protein with its hydrophobic C-terminus deleted. *Journal of General Virology* 1995; **76**:53–61.

37. Chen PJ, Lin MH, Tai KF, Liu PC, Lin CJ & Chen CS. The Taiwanese hepatitis C virus genome: sequence determination and mapping the 5′ terminal of viral genomic and antigenomic RNA. *Virology* 1992; **188**:102–113.

38. Santolini E, Migliaccio G & La Monica N. Biosynthesis and biochemical properties of hepatitis C virus core protein. *Journal of Virology* 1994; **68**:3631–3641.

39. Suzuki R. SPXX, a frequent sequence motif in gene regulatory proteins. *Journal of Molecular Biology* 1989; **207**:61–84.

40. Shih CM, Lo SJ, Myamura T, Chen SY & Lee YH. Suppression of hepatitis B virus expression and replication by hepatitis C virus core protein in Hu-7 cells. *Journal of Virology* 1993; **67**:5823–5832.

41. Junker-Niepmann M, Bartenschlager R & Schaller H. A short cis-acting sequence is required for hepatitis B virus pregenome encapsidation and sufficient for packaging of foreign RNA. *EMBO Journal* 1990; **9**:3389–3396.

42. Birnbaum F & Nassal M. Hepatitis B virus nucleocapsid assembly: primary structure requirements in the core protein. *Journal of Virology* 1990; **64**:3310–3330.

43. Liaw YF, Chien RN, Lin SM, Yeh CT, Tsai SL, Sheen IS & Chu CM. Response of patients with dual hepatitis B virus and C virus infection to interferon therapy. *Journal of Interferon and Cytokine Research* 1997; **17**: 449–452.

# Section VII

---

# CLINICAL AND
# THERAPEUTIC STRATEGIES

## Part D
## Hepatocellular Carcinoma

# 47 Relationship between infection with hepatitis C virus and hepatocellular carcinoma in Japan

## Shiro Iino

## INTRODUCTION

Before the discovery of the hepatitis C virus (HCV), there was little awareness worldwide that non-A, non-B hepatitis was a serious, progressive liver disease [1]. Since its discovery, however, HCV has been recognized as a major cause of liver cirrhosis and hepatocellular carcinoma (HCC) [2].

In Japan, attention was focused on non-A, non B chronic hepatitis as an important cause of the continuing increase in liver cirrhosis and HCC [3]. With the discovery of HCV, it became clear that 84% of non-A, non-B hepatitis was caused by this agent [4], and basic and clinical research has seen great progress. This report will introduce the background for the unique developments in Japan in the treatment of chronic hepatitis C with interferon (IFN) [5] and will discuss the primary concern of whether IFN has reduced the incidence of HCC, as well as future therapeutic goals in chronic hepatitis C.

## STATUS OF HCV INFECTION IN JAPAN AND INCREASING INCIDENCE OF HCC

It is estimated that more than 2 million Japanese (1.7% of the population) are HCV carriers. There are almost no carriers below the age of 20, but in those older than 20, the prevalence of carriers increases with age, reaching a peak of 6% in those 60 years or older [2]. The cause of infection in about half of these carriers is exposure through blood transfusion or blood products. Past unsanitary medical practices account for most of the remaining half, while transmission through tattooing and intravenous drug use accounts for only a very small percentage of carriers in Japan.

Liver disease in HCV carriers with a history of blood transfusion is observed to progress with time from blood transfusion [1] although there is individual variation. Liver cirrhosis starts to be observed after 20 years and HCC after 25 years [6]. On the other hand, even after 20 years, chronic hepatitis C can be mild but can also then suddenly progress to liver cirrhosis.

As a result, the number of deaths due to HCC in Japan has been increasing since 1975, as shown in Figure 1, and the increase is particularly marked in males.

## TREATMENT OF CHRONIC HEPATITIS C WITH IFN UNIQUE TO JAPAN

At the time IFN was first shown to reduce serum alanine aminotransferase (ALT) levels in patients with non-A, non-B chronic hepatitis [7], Stronger Neo-

**Figure 1.** Incidence of deaths due to hepatocellular carcinoma and liver cirrhosis in Japan

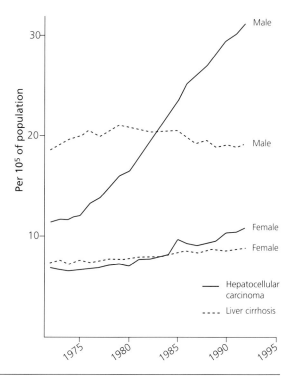

Minophagen C (SNM), an inexpensive glycyrrhizin preparation with few side effects, was already being widely used in Japan to lower ALT levels, an effect observed only during administration of the drug [8]. It was therefore considered important that IFN, an expensive drug with strong side effects, should have a beneficial effect that would be sustained even after the end of treatment, in order to justify its clinical use. With this in mind, a criterion for efficacy evaluation of IFN in non-A, non-B chronic hepatitis was established which had ALT normalization and ALT reduction after the end of treatment as indices [9]. Based on this evaluation criterion, the relationship between treatment regimen and the effect of IFN treatment was demonstrated, and high-dose IFN treatment unique to Japan was established [10]. The details of this background have been reported previously [5]. When the detection of HCV RNA became possible [11], it became clear that HCV RNA loss that is sustained for several years is observed in more than 70% of patients who achieve ALT normalization (complete response) [12].

The factors related to achieving complete response to IFN treatment are now well known, and they are: HCV genotype; serum HCV RNA levels; IFN treatment regimen; degree of severity of liver disease; and HCV genome mutation [5]. Nothing is known, however, of the factors related to sustained ALT normalization despite the persistent presence of HCV RNA (incomplete response) following IFN therapy.

Japan is characterized both by a large number of patients with HCV genotype 1b [13] that is resistant to IFN, and for the administration of high doses of IFN which was required to raise the response rate.

The standard therapy used in Japan is 9 to 10 MIU of IFN-$\alpha$ administered daily for 2 to 4 weeks, and then three times a week for 20 to 24 weeks.

## EFFECT OF IFN THERAPY IN INHIBITING THE INCIDENCE OF HCC IN JAPAN

The goal of IFN therapy in chronic hepatitis C is to inhibit progression to liver cirrhosis and HCC. Although it is difficult to determine whether the development of liver cirrhosis has been inhibited because chronic hepatitis and liver cirrhosis are sequential disease states, HCC can be identified definitively by such methods as ultrasonography, computerized tomography, angiography and measurement of alpha-fetoprotein. A survey was therefore conducted by the Non-A, Non-B Hepatitis Research Group of the Japanese Ministry of Health and Welfare at 18 affili-

ated institutes to study the incidence of HCC in patients with chronic hepatitis C who had been followed up for at least one year after IFN treatment. Patients who were diagnosed with HCC within one year were excluded from the survey.

The effect of IFN in chronic hepatitis C was evaluated as follows: complete response (CR) was defined as normalization of ALT levels within 6 months after the end of IFN therapy, sustained for at least 6 months, as well as HCV RNA not detected 6 to 12 months after the end of IFN therapy. Incomplete response (IR) was defined as normalization of ALT levels within 6 months after the end of IFN therapy, sustained for at least 6 months, but with HCV RNA detected after 6 months following the end of IFN therapy. Incomplete response was further divided into IR-1, or those having sustained ALT normalization, and IR-2, or those having normalized ALT for at least 6 months followed thereafter by re-elevation. Partial response (PR) was defined as remaining positive for HCV RNA and having ALT levels of less than two times the upper limit of normal after the end of IFN therapy. No response (NR) was when none of the above was applicable.

The results of efficacy evaluation of IFN in chronic hepatitis C based on these criteria are given in Table 1. These results are considered to be generally representative of the efficacy of IFN administered at the standard regimen for chronic hepatitis C in Japan.

The overall CR rate was 29.8%. The sustained ALT normalization rate, or the sum of the CR, IR-1 and IR-2 rates, was 41.4%. By genotype, CR was observed in 17.9% and sustained ALT normalization in 29.9% with genotype 1b. With genotype 2a, 63.7% had CR and 72.5% had sustained ALT normalization. The difference in sensitivity to IFN observed between genotypes 1b and 2a was to such a degree that they could be imagined to be different viruses. The response observed with genotype 2b was midway between that of 1b and 2a.

The cumulative incidence of HCC after IFN therapy in patients undergoing long-term follow-up, as determined by the Kaplan–Meier method, is shown in Figure 2. The number of follow-up patients is shown at the bottom of the figure.

The overall cumulative HCC rate was 2.90% and overall annual rate was 0.89%. According to response to IFN therapy, the cumulative rates and annual rates were 0.87% and 0.26% with CR, 0.74% and 0.24% with IR-1, 1.69% and 0.49% with IR-2, 3.59% and 1.04% with PR, and 4.65% and 1.49% with NR. Statistically significant differences were observed between CR and IR-1, and PR and NR. No statisti-

Table 1. Efficacy of IFN therapy in patients with chronic hepatitis C

| Genotype | Total | CR | IR1 | IR2 | PR | NR |
|---|---|---|---|---|---|---|
| 1b | 2631 | 470 (17.9%) | 179 (6.8%) | 136 (5.2%) | 595 (22.6%) | 1251 (47.5%) |
| 2a | 771 | 491 (63.7%) | 48 (6.2%) | 20 (2.6%) | 95 (12.3%) | 117 (15.2%) |
| 2b | 288 | 127 (44.1%) | 31 (10.8%) | 15 (5.2%) | 37 (12.8%) | 78 (27.1%) |
| Others | 168 | 63 (37.5%) | 12 (7.1%) | 7 (4.2%) | 26 (15.5%) | 60 (35.7%) |
| All | 3858 | 1151 (29.8%) | 270 (7.0%) | 178 (4.6%) | 753 (19.5%) | 1506 (39.0%) |

Abbreviations: see text.

cally significant difference was observed between CR and IR-1. If limited to the period within 5 years after the completion of IFN therapy, the incidence of HCC is markedly reduced as long as ALT levels are normalized, regardless of whether or not HCV has been eradicated. On the other hand, it was also noted that HCC can develop within 5 years even in patients who achieve CR.

## FUTURE APPROACHES TO CHRONIC HEPATITIS C TREATMENT

The most certain method to reduce the incidence of future HCC is to eradicate HCV, but as indicated above, the effect of IFN in inhibiting the development of HCC is dependent on ALT levels following IFN therapy, and the importance of maintaining ALT at low levels was demonstrated.

SNMC has been widely used in Japan to lower ALT levels in chronic liver diseases since 1975, when it was shown to provide a statistically significant reduction in ALT levels that was also significantly correlated to

inhibition of liver inflammation [14]. Arase *et al.* have reported that SNMC clearly inhibits the development of HCC [15]. Figure 3 shows the change in ALT levels in patients who failed to achieve ALT normalization after initial IFN therapy and received retreatment with IFN, SNMC, or no drug treatment [16]. Satisfactory control of ALT levels is obtained with SNMC. Although ALT levels are lowered with retreatment with IFN, the effect is not as pronounced as with SNMC.

The administration of ursodeoxycholic acid is also effective in reducing ALT levels [17]. Ursodeoxycholic acid can control ALT levels in patients with only mild ALT abnormality and in patients who do not respond adequately to SNMC. It is possible to maintain ALT at 50 IU/l or less in more than 70% of patients with the use of SNMC and ursodeoxycholic acid. In addition, it is also possible to maintain ALT at low levels in patients who do not respond adequately to these two drugs by the administration of low-dose (3 MIU) IFN two to three times a week. Ribavirin is also effective for this purpose.

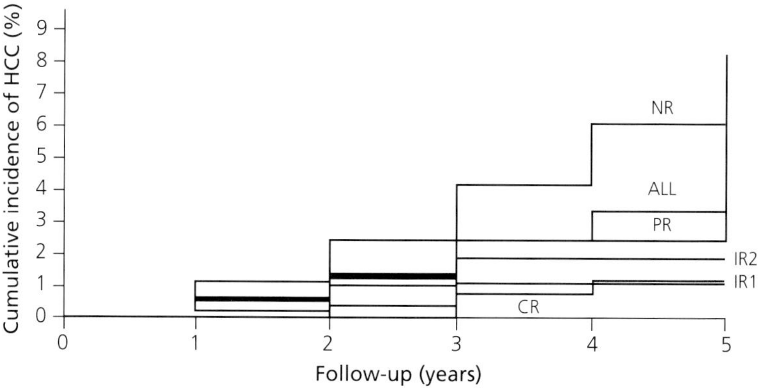

Figure 2. Cumulative incidence of HCC in patients with chronic hepatitis C after IFN therapy

| | 1Y | 2Y | 3Y | 4Y | 5Y | |
|---|---|---|---|---|---|---|
| ALL | 3858 | 3301 | 2241 | 1172 | 512 | |
| CR | 1151 | 988 | 689 | 419 | 207 | |
| IR1 | 270 | 232 | 147 | 58 | 19 | |
| IR2 | 178 | 158 | 121 | 58 | 23 | |
| PR | 753 | 673 | 490 | 253 | 137 | |
| NR | 1506 | 1250 | 794 | 384 | 126 | Number of patients |

**Figure 3.** Comparison of the effect of SNMC (Group A), no treatment (Group B) and IFN (Group C) in non-responders to IFN

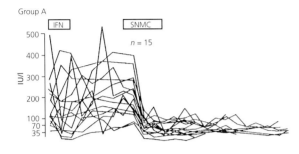

Group A

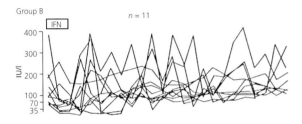

Group B

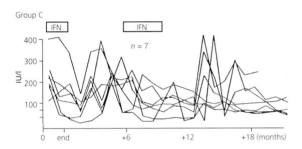

Group C

In the future, in addition to the development of therapies to eradicate HCV, treatments to lower ALT levels will also be important.

## REFERENCES

1. Kiyosawa K, Sodeyama T, Tanaka E, Gibo Y, Yoshizawa K, Nakano Y, Furuta S, Akahane Y, Nishioka K, Purcell RH, *et al.*: Interrelationship of blood transfusion, non-A, non-B hepatitis and hepato-cellular carcinoma: analysis by detection of antibody to hepatitis C virus. *Hepatology* 1990; **12**:671–675.
2. Nishioka K, Watanabe J, Furuta S, Tanaka E, Iino S, Suzuki H, Tsuji T, Yano M, Kuo G, Choo QL, *et al.* A high prevalence of antibody to the hepatitis C virus in patients with hepatocellular carcinoma in Japan. *Cancer* 1991; **67**:429–443.
3. Suzuki H. Viral hepatitis in Japan. In *Viral Hepatitis and Liver Disease* 1994; pp. 426–428. Edited by K Nishioka, H Suzuki, S Mishiro, T Oda. Tokyo: Springer.
4. Hino K. Diagnosis of hepatitis C. *Intervirology* 1994; **37**:77–86.
5. Iino S, Hino K & Yasuda K. Current state of interferon therapy for chronic hepatitis C. *Intervirology* 1994; **37**:87–100.
6. Kurai K, Iino S, Tanaka N, Nakayama T, Miyazaki J, Endo Y, Oda T, Suzuki H & Mitamura K. Clinical studies on HBsAg-negative hepatocellular carcinoma. *Acta Hepatologica Japonica* 1982; **23**:50–56.
7. Hoofnagle JH, Mullen KD, Jones DB, Rustgi V, Di Bisceglie A, Peters M, Waggoner JG, Park Y & Jones EA. Treatment of chronic non-A, non-B hepatitis with recombinant human alpha interferon. A preliminary report. *New England Journal of Medicine* 1986; **315**: 1575–1578.
8. Fujisawa K & Tandon BN. Therapeutic approach to the chronic active liver disease. In *Viral Hepatitis and Liver Disease* 1994; pp. 662–665. Edited by K Nishioka, H Suzuki, S Mishiro, T Oda. Tokyo: Springer.
9. Iino S. Interferon therapy in hepatitis C-refractory hepatitis: Report of the research subgroup of treatment of chronic hepatitis. *Gastroenterology Japan* 1993; **28** (Supplement 4): S139–S142.
10. Iino S, Hino K, Kuroki T, Suzuki H & Yamamoto S. Treatment of chronic hepatitis C with high-dose interferon α-2b. *Digestive Diseases and Sciences* 1993; **38**:612–618.
11. Okamoto H, Okada S, Sugiyama Y, Yotsumoto S, Tanaka T, Yoshizawa H, Tsuda F, Miyakawa Y & Mayumi M. The 5′-terminal sequence of the hepatitis C virus genome. *Japanese Journal of Experimental Medicine* 1990; **60**: 167–177.
12. Iino S. High dose interferon treatment in chronic hepatitis C. *Gut* 1993; **34** (Supplement): S114–S118.
13. Okamoto H, Sugiyama Y, Okada S, Kurai K, Akahane Y, Sugai Y, Tanaka T, Sato K, Tsuda F, Miyakawa Y, Magumi M. Typing hepatitis C virus by polymerase chain reaction with type-specific primers: Application to clinical surveys and tracing infection sources. *Journal of General Virology* 1992; **73**:673–679.
14. Suzuki H, Fujisawa K, Ohta Y, Suzuki H, Ohta Y, Takino T, Fujisawa K, Hirayama C, Simizu N & Asao Y. Therapeutic efficacy of Stronger Neo-Minophagen C on chronic hepatitis. *Igaku No Ayumi* 1997; **102**:562–578 (in Japanese).
15. Arase Y, Ikeda K, Murashima N, Chayama K, Tsubota A,

With these drugs which reduce ALT levels, however, extremely long-term administration is required since ALT levels re-elevate upon discontinuation.

## CONCLUSIONS

The number of deaths due to HCC is increasing in Japan. Males in particular have seen a marked increase in the past 20 years, and HCV infection accounts for this increase.

In patients treated with IFN and followed up for more than 12 months, HCV clearance was achieved in 29.8% and sustained normalization of ALT levels was achieved in 41.4% following IFN therapy.

The incidence of HCC following IFN treatment is dependent on the effect of IFN on ALT levels. The incidence of HCC was low in patients with sustained normalization of ALT levels following IFN therapy, regardless of whether or not HCV had been eradicated.

# 48 Factors influencing the course of hepatitis B virus infection

## Baruch S Blumberg

## SUMMARY

There are several possible outcomes following infection with hepatitis B virus (HBV). These include infection without disease followed by the development of antibody against the surface antigen, acute hepatitis, the asymptomatic carrier state, chronic hepatitis and hepatocellular carcinoma (HCC). Environmental and genetic factors influence the response of the host and the outcome of infection. These include susceptibility genes in the host, such as haplotypes of major histo-compatibility complex (MHC) class II, exposure to arsenic and the *Aspergillus* carcinogen aflatoxin, and interaction with other viruses including hepatitis viruses. In addition, recent studies indicate that there are host polymorphic genes at two loci that control the detoxification of aflatoxin and could influence the development of HCC

## INTRODUCTION

A large part of contemporary biological science is reductionist in nature. This implies that scientists attempt to describe natural phenomena in the simplest terms possible, such as proteins, enzymes, genes and other fundamental units. Experiments are designed to eliminate all but what are deemed to be essential variables in order to understand the essence of a problem. This has resulted in great scientific achievements and will continue to do so in the future. It is also necessary to address the complexity that is seen in nature, and to attempt to account for as many of the variables as possible. Epidemiological methods are often applied to these problems, particularly methods designed for multiple variables.

In the case of infectious diseases, the reductionist approach deals primarily with the interaction of the virus and its host. As for most natural events, however, infectious diseases do not occur in isolation. Rather, they occur in the context of their environment, any one or more components of which might have important effects on the course of the disease caused by the infectious agent. For example, interactions between the infectious agent and host gene products, between the infectious agent and other infectious agents, and between the infectious agent and exogenous substances, may all influence the course of disease. The source of an infection may also be a factor in pathogenesis, and infection from one individual may be different from infection from another, particularly in circumstances where the viral genome integrates into the genome of a host. The consideration of multiple interacting factors could lead to the identification of more effective preventative and therapeutic strategies [1].

## THE DIVERSITY OF FACTORS AFFECTING HEPATITIS B

HBV causes an infection that leads to variable outcomes. Some HBV-infected individuals remain asymptomatic carriers for long periods. Others may experience acute hepatitis but later recover and develop protective antibodies. Some develop chronic liver disease and others progress to HCC. Factors that determine which of these courses the disease can take have been identified. In this paper, several of these factors and how they interact with each other and with the host to determine the course of the infection will be discussed.

## HCC AND AFLATOXIN EXPOSURE

Aflatoxin is a carcinogenic substance produced by the fungus *Aspergillus*. When stored under poor conditions, grain, peanuts and other nuts and cereals may be colonized by *Aspergillus* and become contaminated with aflatoxin. In some parts of the world, for example Asia and Africa, the contamination of foodstuffs with aflatoxin is a major health hazard.

Aflatoxin is associated with an increased risk of progression to HCC in individuals who are infected with HBV. In a study performed in Shanghai by Qian *et al.* [2] involving 18244 men aged 45–64 years, the development of HCC was monitored in relation to urinary markers of aflatoxin. The participants were classified according to whether they were positive or

Table 1. Relative risks for the development of HCC according to HBsAg and aflatoxin status in Chinese males

| HBsAg | Risk ratio (95% confidence intervals) | |
| | Aflatoxin-negative | Aflatoxin-positive |
| --- | --- | --- |
| Negative | 1.0 | 3.4 (1.1, 10.0) |
| Positive | 7.3 (2.2, 24.4) | 59.4 (16.6, 212.0) |

Table 2. Aflatoxin $B_1$–albumin adduct distribution by EPHX and GSTM1 genotype in Ghanaian males

| Aflatoxin B1 | EPHX genotype | | | GSTM1 genotype | | |
| | 1/1 | 1/2 or 2/2 | Total | Present | Null | Total |
| --- | --- | --- | --- | --- | --- | --- |
| ≤5 pg/mg | 21 | 4 | 25 | 19 | 6 | 25 |
| >5 pg/mg | 13 | 11 | 24 | 11 | 13 | 24 |
| Total | 34* | 15* | 49 | 30† | 19† | 49 |

*$\chi^2=5.1$; $P=0.02$.
†$\chi^2=4.7$; $P=0.03$.

negative for the HBV surface antigen (HBsAg) and for high levels of urinary aflatoxin.

After approximately 70000 person-years of follow-up there were 55 cases of HCC. Individuals who were positive for either HBsAg or aflatoxin were more likely to develop HCC than those who were negative for both of these markers. However, among individuals who were positive for both HBsAg and aflatoxin, the risk of developing HCC was much greater than the risks attributable to HBV and aflatoxin independently or added together, indicating that these two factors act synergistically to cause HCC. The relative risk ratios for the development of HCC in this study are shown in Table 1.

This is an example of the interaction of an environmental agent ingested with food that affects the host and alters its interaction with the virus. There are also interactions with the genetics of the host.

Aflatoxin is metabolized in the liver by at least two human enzymes, microsomal epoxide hydrolase (EPHX) and a member of the glutathione S-transferase μ family (GSTM1). The genetic loci that encode EPHX and GSTM1 are both polymorphic. The EPHX locus has two alleles, 1 and 2, and any given individual can be either homozygous for the 1 allele, homozygous for the 2 allele or heterozygous. GSTM1 can either be *present* or *null*.

In a study performed by McGlynn *et al.* [3] in Ghanaian males, individuals were classified according to their EPHX and GSTM1 genotypes. They were also grouped according to whether their urinary aflatoxin $B_1$ concentrations were or were not elevated. Men with aflatoxin $B_1$ levels greater than 5 pg/mg were more likely to have either an EPHX 1/2 or 2/2 genotype than were men who did not have detectable amounts.

Similarly, a significantly greater proportion of individuals who were *null* at the GSTM1 locus had high aflatoxin $B_1$ levels compared with those who had the *present* allele at this locus (Table 2).

In another study, individuals were grouped according to their EPHX and GSTM1 genotypes, and whether or not they developed HCC. The frequency of the GSTM1 *null* genotype was greater among the cases than among the controls and this difference was statistically significant. Also, the frequency of EPHX allele 2 was significantly higher in the cases than in the controls.

Investigations into the mechanism of the increased risk of HCC in individuals who are exposed to aflatoxin with certain EPHX and GSTM1 genotypes suggest that it may be related to changes in the p53 tumour suppresser gene. In epidemiological studies, an association was found between an increased risk of HCC and the presence of a mutation at codon 249 of exon 7 of this gene. In one study, individuals with the EPHX and GSTM1 genotypes that cause aflatoxin to be poorly metabolized had the codon mutation more often than those with strongly metabolizing EPHX and GSTM1 genotypes, although the difference was not quite significant at the $P=0.05$ level (Table 3).

The study by McGlynn *et al.* [3] illustrates the complex interactions between the host genome, HBV, aflatoxin and mutations at the p53 locus.

## THE GENETICS OF THE HBV CARRIER STATE: MHC CLASS II AND CHRONIC HEPATITIS

Following infection, the two major host responses to HBV infection are (i) the development of antibody

Table 3. p53 codon 249 mutation status by EPHX/GSTM1 genotype in HCC carriers in China

| | Genotype | | | |
| --- | --- | --- | --- | --- |
| p53 | EPHX low risk/ GSTM1 low risk | Intermediate | EPHX high risk/ GSTM1 high risk | Total |
| Mutant | 0 | 2 | 8 | 10 |
| Wild-type | 1 | 24 | 17 | 42 |
| Total | 1 | 26* | 25* | 52 |

*$\chi^2$=5.1; *P*=0.07.

to the surface antigen, which provides protection against subsequent infection; and (ii) the development of the HBV carrier state, which increases the risk of chronic liver disease and HCC. Some of our earliest studies [4] suggested that this may be under genetic control.

There is also evidence to suggest an association between certain MHC class II haplotypes and the risk of chronic hepatitis. In a study by Thurz *et al.* [5] performed in Faraja, The Gambia, 1344 children aged up to 10 years and 260 adult male blood donors were tested for HBV serologically [anti-HBs, anti-HBc, anti-HBc (IgM) and HBsAg]. They also had their MHC antigen status determined (class I, microlymphocytotoxicity assay with 23 specificities; class II, restriction fragment length polymorphism analysis with 10 specificities).

No association was found between the clearance of HBV and MHC class I alleles. However, two of the class II haplotypes, 25-1 and 13-2, were found to be associated with elimination of the infection and the development of antibody. The presence of the 25-1 haplotype reduced the relative risk of developing the carrier state for HBV to 0.53, and the 13-2 haplotype reduced it to 0.35.

Earlier studies have shown that these two MHC class II haplotypes are also associated with a reduced risk of cerebral malaria, a more favourable response to certain interferons and a protective effect against human papillomavirus infection. The investigators therefore examined whether the individuals who cleared HBV were less likely to develop malaria than those who did not. They found that there was such an association, with individuals with severe malaria having a greater risk of becoming a HBV carrier.

The association between HBV clearance and a protective effect against malaria may be attributable to the development of a protective mechanism against malaria in individuals exposed to HBV or vice versa, or through the association with certain MHC class II haplotypes, or a combination of these three. A prospective study is planned to investigate these possibilities.

## INTERACTIONS BETWEEN THE HEPATITIS VIRUSES

Six hepatitis viruses, designated A, B, C, D, E and G, have now been identified. Hepatitis B, C, D and G viruses have similar modes of transmission. Several have overlapping geographical distributions. It is probable that coinfection with two or more types of hepatitis virus will occur frequently. This coinfection may influence the course of the disease that results from either or both of the viruses.

Since most studies of viral hepatitis involve only one type of virus, relatively little is known about the manner in which different types of hepatitis virus interact with each other. However, there are some data. Superinfection can influence the replication of other viruses. Thus, hepatitis D virus decreases the replication of HBV, and superinfection with HBV decreases the replication of hepatitis C virus. However, carriers of HBV have a higher rate of mortality when infected with hepatitis E virus and have more severe clinical consequences when infected with hepatitis C virus. These findings are reviewed in [1].

## HEPATIC CANCER AND ARSENIC

In the southwestern part of Taiwan there are areas with high arsenic levels in the drinking water. Blackfoot disease, a vascular occlusive disease, is endemic in the same area and is associated with high arsenic levels [6]. There also appears to be an association between arsenic and an increased risk of developing cancer of the liver. Mortality as a result of hepatic cancer was found to increase in relation to local levels of arsenic in the water from artesian wells.

## CONCLUSIONS

There are numerous co-factors, including genetically controlled enzymes and other proteins, environmental substances and concurrent infections, that can influence the course of chronic HBV infection and determine if the carrier of the virus will remain asymptomatic or develop chronic liver disease and/or HCC.

Many of the environmental factors can be controlled to prevent the progression of the disease. It would be useful to develop bio-mathematical models for these interactions to arrive at appropriate strategies for environmental intervention, vaccination and treatment, in order to decrease the heavy toll of disease associated with HBV and the other hepatitis viruses.

## ACKNOWLEDGEMENTS

This work was supported by USPHS grant CA-06927 from the National Institutes of Health and by an appropriation from the Commonwealth of Pennsylvania.

## REFERENCES

1. Blumberg BS. Complex interactions of hepatitis B virus with its host and environment. *Journal of the Royal College of Physicians, London* 1995; **29**:31–40.
2. Qian G-S, Ross RK, Yu MC, Yuan J-M, Gao Y-T, Henderson BE, Wogan GN & Groopman JD. A follow-up study of urinary markers of aflatoxin exposure and liver cancer risk in Shanghai, People's Republic of China. *Cancer Epidemiology, Biomarkers and Prevention* 1994; **3**:3–10.
3. McGlynn KA, Rosvold EA, Lustbader ED, Hu Y, Clapper ML, Zhou T, Wild CP, Xia X-L, Baffoe-Bonnie A, Ofori-Adjei D, Chen G-C, London WT, Shen F-M & Buetow K. Susceptibility to hepatocellular carcinoma is associated with genetic variation in the enzymatic detoxification of aflatoxin $B_1$. *Proceedings of the National Academy of Sciences, USA* 1995; **92**: 2384–2387.
4. Blumberg BS, Melartin L, Guinto RA & Werner B. Family studies of a human serum isoantigen system (Australia antigen). *American Journal of Human Genetics* 1966; **18**:594–608.
5. Thurz MR, Kwiatkowski D, Allsopp CEM, Greenwood BM, Thomas HC & Hill AVS. Association between an MHC class II allele and clearance of hepatitis B virus in the Gambia. *New England Journal of Medicine* 1995; **332**:1065–1069.
6. Chen C-J & Lin L-J. Human carcinogenicity and atherogenicity induced by chronic exposure to inorganic arsenic. In *Arsenic in the Environment, Part II: Human Health and Ecosystem Effects*, 1994; pp. 109–131. Edited by JO Nriagu. Chichester: John Wiley.

# Index

**Indexed by Laurence Errington**